Rethinking Culture in Health Communication

Rethinking Culture in Health Communication

Social Interactions as Intercultural Encounters

Elaine Hsieh and Eric M Kramer

University of Oklahoma
Norman, Oklahoma

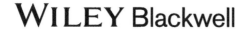

Registered Office
John Wiley & Sons, Inc., 111 River Street, Hoboken, NJ 07030, USA

Editorial Office
111 River Street, Hoboken, NJ 07030, USA

For details of our global editorial offices, customer services, and more information about Wiley products visit us at www.wiley.com.

Wiley also publishes its books in a variety of electronic formats and by print-on-demand. Some content that appears in standard print versions of this book may not be available in other formats.

Library of Congress Cataloging-in-Publication Data
Names: Hsieh, Elaine, author. | Kramer, Eric Mark, author.
Title: Rethinking culture in health communication : social interactions
    as intercultural encounters / Elaine Kramer Hsieh, University of Oklahoma,
    Norman, Oklahoma, Eric Mark Kramer, University of Oklahoma,
    Norman, Oklahoma.
Description: Hoboken : John Wiley & Sons, 2021. | Includes index.
Identifiers: LCCN 2020040724 (print) | LCCN 2020040725 (ebook) |
    ISBN 9781119496168 (paperback) | ISBN 9781119496137 (pdf) |
    ISBN 9781119496106 (epub)
Subjects: LCSH: Communication in medicine. | Communication in
    medicine--Cross-cultural studies. | Social interaction--Cross-cultural studies.
Classification: LCC R118 .H75 2021 (print) | LCC R118 (ebook) | DDC
    610--dc23
LC record available at https://lccn.loc.gov/2020040724
LC ebook record available at https://lccn.loc.gov/2020040725

Cover image: © Gabriel Perez /Getty Images
Cover design: Wiley

Set in 9.5/12.5pt STIXTwoText by Integra, Pondicherry, India

10 9 8 7 6 5 4 3 2 1

Dedication

Rudy and Tigger, thank you for your playful spirit and companionship.

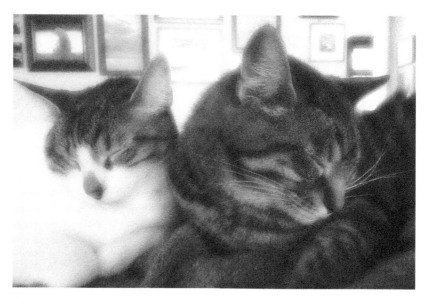

Source: Elaine Hsieh

Contents

Acknowledgment

Financial support was provided by the Research Council, the Office of the Vice President for Research and Partnerships, and the Office of the Provost, University of Oklahoma.

1

Rethinking Culture in Health Communication

The chapter provides an overview of traditional and emerging fields of health communication, highlighting its interdisciplinary and applied nature as a field of research and practice. We will then explore how culture has been incorporated in health communication and examine the failure in organizing and conceptualizing the field in general through a cultural lens. We will present theoretical backgrounds and a conceptual framework that grounds the cultural perspectives discussed in this book. We will propose some learning objectives for our readers.

I. The Expanding and Interconnected Fields of Health Communication

This book is published at a historical moment that is seared into everyone's memory and is likely to transform our everyday life and redefine who we are. On December 31, 2019, the World Health Organization (2020b) received a report of a cluster of cases of pneumonia in Wuhan, Hubei Province in China. By July 4, 2020, the COVID-19 pandemic has reached over 11 million cases and over 530,000+ deaths worldwide, including 2.8+ million cases and nearly 130,000 deaths in the United States (Johns Hopkins Coronavirus Resource Center, 2020). At this writing, the numbers are accelerating in growth (see Figure 1.1). In 15 weeks, over 48 million Americans have filed for unemployment since mid-March when President Trump declared a national emergency concerning the COVID-19 outbreak (Menton, 2020; White House, 2020). Among those who lost jobs, poor Americans were hit the hardest: 39% of former workers living in a household earning $40,000 or less lost work; in contrast, among those making more than $100,000, 13% lost jobs (Smialek, 2020; see Figure 1.2). Worse yet, it is estimated that COVID-19 may leave 27 million Americans to lose their employer-sponsored health insurance coverage after being laid off (Garfield et al., 2020) – during a time when healthcare coverage is essential to protect individual health *and* family wealth.

On May 25, 2020, George Floyd, a 46-year-old African American, repeatedly said, "I cannot breathe," and eventually died in police custody after an officer kneeled on his neck for 8 minutes and 46 seconds during an arrest (see Figure 1.3). Despite the risk of exposure to COVID-19, numerous protests were held in small towns and big cities in the United States and internationally to demand justice for George Floyd, raise awareness of

Rethinking Culture in Health Communication: Social Interactions as Intercultural Encounters, First Edition. Elaine Hsieh and Eric M Kramer.
© 2021 John Wiley & Sons, Inc. Published 2021 by John Wiley & Sons, Inc.

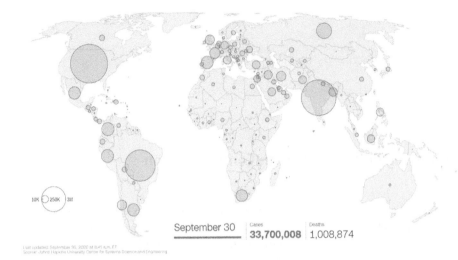

September 30   Cases **33,700,008**   Deaths 1,008,874

Last updated: September 30, 2020 at 8:45 a.m. ET
Source: Johns Hopkins University Center for Systems Science and Engineering

Figure 1.1 Global map of total cases of the COVID-19 pandemic (September 30, 2020). Adapted from the interactive map by CNN (Pettersson et al., 2020). *Source:* Adapted from Pettersson, et al. (2020, July 5).

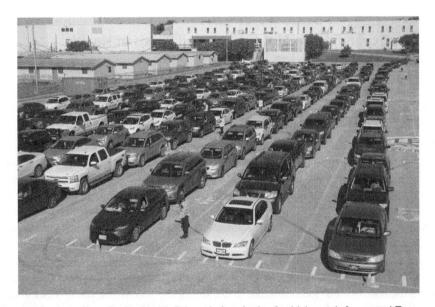

Figure 1.2 Long lines for food bank. Drivers in hundreds of vehicles wait for central Texas food bank volunteers to deliver 28-pound boxes of staples during a food giveaway in Austin, Texas. Almost 1,500 families picked up boxes in response to extensive COVID-19 pandemic job losses and general economic fallout. *Source:* Bob Daemmrich / Alamy Stock Photo

unconscious bias, and seek solutions to structural racism. During the eight days of national civil rights protests, 62,000 National Guard soldiers and airmen were deployed to protests in 24 states plus the District of Columbia (Sternlicht, 2020). Over 4,400 people have been arrested as protests occur in all 50 states (Sternlicht, 2020). Over 40 cities have instituted curfews, including Minneapolis, New York, Louisville, Philadelphia, Chicago, and San Francisco (Sternlicht, 2020).

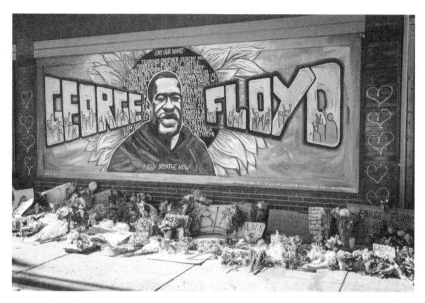

Figure 1.3 A mural dedicated to George Floyd. The mural also includes names of many other victims in honoring the Black Lives Matter movement in Minneapolis, MN, on May 29, 2020. *Souce:* Sipa USA/Alamy Stock Photo

We do not see the pandemic, the economic crash with millions losing health insurance, and the civil rights protests as three independent, random events that just happened to take place at the same time in history. Rather, these events are interconnected, highlighting the social injustice and structural barriers faced by the poor and the marginalized. Of the three, the pandemic and structural inequality along racial lines exist all over the world. However, the lack of universal health insurance in the United States is unique among wealthy industrial nations (Béland et al., 2016), which compounds the damages from the other two crises. Together, they tell a story of institutional failures to effectively protect, communicate, and listen to its most vulnerable citizens, responding to the social injustice and structural barriers that have limited their ability and potential to thrive over time, from one generation to the next.

Health and illness are pervasive in our everyday life. How we live our life, structure our social system, and respond to health disparities have consequences not only to our individual health, but also our family's financial well-being and our community's ability to thrive as a whole. How we conceptualize health and illness will define our abilities to find solutions and address injustice. To this end, we must see health and illness more than a biological phenomenon.

A. The Landscape of Health Communication

Caring for patients can be traced back thousands of years to ancient times in Greece and Roman; however, modern medicine only emerged in its current form in the 19th century (Bynum, 2008). The latest trends in medical science have become increasingly focused on advancing the institutional and scientific knowledge of the biological body (Bynum, 2008; Mukherjee, 2016). Medicine and healthcare providers also have begun to recognize that health and illness are situated in social, cultural, and economic contexts (Rosen, 1958/2015). The 19th century sanitary movement (i.e., the introduction of piped water to people's homes and sewers rinsed by water) is considered the greatest medical advance since 1840 (Ferriman, 2007). Medical sociology first emerged in the 1950s to address how the politics and of health and illness can maintain and even reinforce systemic disparities and social injustice in the post-WWII period (Brown, 1991; Bury, 1986).

Compared to these fields, health communication, first formalized in the early 1970s, is a relatively young but rapidly growing discipline (Kreps, 2014). *Health Communication* and the *Journal of Health Communication*, two leading academic journals in the field, were established in 1989 and 1996 respectively. From its beginning, health communication has been influenced by a wide range of disciplinary approaches, including communication, psychology, medical sociology, and clinical medicine (Kreps et al., 1998). A review of published articles in *Health Communication*, the first academic journal focused solely on health communication scholarship, from 1989 to 2010, found that the field has been heavily influenced by western scholarship because the nationality of first authors was mostly United States (90.5%), followed by Canada (2%) and Australia (1.5%; Kim et al., 2010). In addition, over 50% of the total publications aimed at improving the penetration of health messages (i.e., persuasion) to targeted groups (Kim et al., 2010). Notably, Kim et al. (2010) concluded that individuals have been the focal level of analysis and there is "an absence of focus on structural factors or social policies that are more conducive to improving the health conditions of social members" (p. 500).

However, the landscape of health communication has expanded significantly since 2010 (Kreps, 2014). In particular, health communication scholars have collaborated with researchers from other disciplines, including medicine, public health, social work, critical studies, cultural studies, education, history, humanities, ethics, public policy, and law, to create new understandings and new approaches to the investigation of communication in health contexts. Here are some of the major themes and trends in health communication, along with some exemplars from this book.

1. Persuasion and Behavioral Change: Public Health Campaigns

As a major theme within health communication, **health promotion** centers on the persuasive use of communication messages and media to promote public health (Kim et al., 2010; Kreps et al., 1998). Scholars of mass communication, message designs, message effects, social influence, persuasion, and even political communication scholars have long investigated the *development*, *implementation*, and *evaluation* of persuasive messages in inducing behavioral changes in the public. As a result, this is a field that includes theory-oriented research (e.g., testing and evaluating message designs and effects) as well as practice-oriented fieldwork (e.g., executing actual campaigns through mass media).

Public health campaigns represent a valuable and rewarding testing ground to examine how persuasive messages can maximize public health benefits through (a) *promoting specific health behaviors*, including one-time health behaviors (e.g., vaccination) and long-term health maintenance (e.g., safe sex practices and regular physical exercise), and (b) *targeting specific populations*, including at-risk populations (e.g., individuals with mental illness, heart disease, or substance abuse problems) and the general public (e.g., five-a-day campaign for fruits and vegetables). This is an area that is heavily influenced by the sociopsychological traditions of health communication, largely informing and informed by theories of health beliefs, risk perceptions, fear appeals, and compliance.

In Chapter 6, we will examine major theories in public health (e.g., Health Belief Model, Theory of Reasoned Action, and Theory of Planned Behavior). We will discuss how the underlying principles and presumptions in these theories reflect values grounded in the West. In Chapter 13, we will explore how tailored health communication and related theories can be informed by a cultural approach to community-based health interventions. In addition, we will examine how different cultural perspectives can bring new insights into future theories and practices of public health campaigns.

2. Interpersonal and Group Communication: Healthcare Delivery

As a field of inquiry in communication, **healthcare delivery** investigates how communication can influence the *access*, *process*, and *outcome* of care. Medical sociologists provided some of the earliest work on examining the communicative processes and power dynamics in provider-patient interactions in clinical settings (e.g., Kleinman, 1980; Parsons, 1951). By conceptualizing medicine as a cultural system, these scholars examined how communication can maintain and reinforce power hierarchy in and social control over patients' illness experiences, silencing their voices and suffering. In addition, because healthcare providers are knowledgeable professionals, their interactions with laypersons who are unfamiliar with the cultural perspectives of medicine are best understood as cross-cultural encounters (Ruben, 2016). In Chapters 3 and 4, we will compare and contrast the cultural perspectives of patients' lifeworlds and providers' culture of medicine.

Communication scholars in interpersonal communication further connected provider-patient communication to the quality of care by connecting the communicative content and processes to health outcomes, including patients' subjective experiences (e.g., satisfaction and understanding) and behavioral outcomes (e.g., treatment adherence) with clinical indicators (e.g., improved biological status; e.g., Cegala et al., 2008; Robinson & Heritage, 2016; Street, 2013). Alternatively, communication scholars also investigated how patients' characteristics (e.g., low health literacy and race) can shape their health behaviors and interactions with health professionals (e.g., Johnson et al., 2004; Miller, 2016). Expanding their analysis from clinical care, communication researchers have also explored how communication between members of social networks (e.g., family members, friends, and supportive others) can influence individuals' health behaviors and health decisions (e.g., Scott & Caughlin, 2015; Thompson & Parsloe, 2019). By conceptualizing health management as a communicative activity coordinated between multiple parties, group communication researchers also have examined how interprofessional health teams, patients, and supportive others coordinate with one another to achieve optimal care.

In Chapter 4, we examine how providers' medical training socializes them with the cultural perspective of medicine, which can create tensions with their own and patients' other cultural attitudes. In Chapter 5, we examine how healthcare providers' culture and patients' cultural perspectives can impact the quality of care. In Chapter 7, we will examine health literacy as a theoretical concept and a communicative skill in shaping individuals' health experiences. In addition, by situating health literacy in sociocultural contexts, we challenge readers to consider how health literacy may operate differently for members of the dominant versus non-dominant groups.

3. Sense-Making and Coping: Lived Experiences

Lived experiences highlight individuals' health and illness as socially situated and culturally contextualized experiences. By viewing communication as a resource and product of social constructions of meanings, both sociologists and communication researchers have relied on patients' illness narratives to gain insights into patients' lived experiences (Bury, 1982; Charmaz, 2002; Frank, 1998). These researchers recognize that the *meanings* of health and illness are coordinated between the patients as well as their supportive others and are not necessarily defined by biological symptoms. For example, a Hmong patient may believe that epileptic seizures are indicators of one's identity as a shaman, a divine gift from God, rather than misfires of abnormal electrical signals in one's brain (Fadiman, 1997). By situating individuals' health and illness in sociocultural and sociopolitical contexts, researchers have explored how patients may incorporate cultural-specific resources in their illness experiences and coping strategies.

In Chapter 2, we discuss how Native Americans' and Jehovah's Witnesses' strong identification with their cultural/religious identities are essential in shaping their health decisions. In Chapter 3, we discuss the importance of stories and storytelling in helping patients to make sense of their illness experiences *and* the larger community to uphold values and principles to which they aspire. In Chapters 9 and 13, we explore how religion can provide valuable frames in helping patients to make sense of their illness experiences and suffering. In Chapter 10, we examine how blood ties and filial piety, a Confucian cultural view that guides parent-child relationships, can empower cultural participants and motivate social support between family members in Chinese culture. In Chapter 12, we discuss how marginalized communities may adopt risky health behaviors to perform desirable identities and relationships and to engage in social resistance against dominant cultures.

4. Pan-Evolution of Medicine and Technology: Transformative Technologies

We use the term **transformative technologies** to highlight that technologies not only change the way we communicate but also create fundamental, structural changes in the surrounding environment. Advances in technologies are transforming the landscape and paradigms of medicine and health management. We use the term "pan-evolution" to highlight how the changes are not one-directional nor linear. **Pan-evolution** means that changes in one can lead to changes in all others that are connected in the system. In other words, emerging technologies create interactive, rippling effects on how people understand, communicate, and manage health and illness. In Chapter 11, we explore how advances in genetic medicine can change how an illness is conceptualized and legitimized. For example, a person who is physically healthy can become an eligible patient for a mastectomy, an aggressive surgical intervention, when they carry BRAC1 mutation, a genetic mutation that has been linked to an increased risk of cancers based on statistical models. The rippling effects of transformative technologies are not limited to advanced knowledge in medical science. For example, in Chapter 8, we examine how the early history of genetics facilitated social injustice and racial disparities as it promoted eugenics and led to the legalization of forced sterilization for marginalized and vulnerable populations.

Communication technology is vital to recent developments in risk communication. **Risk communication** refers to "the exchange of real-time information, advice and opinions between experts and people facing threats to their health, economic or social well-being" (World Health Organization, 2020a, para. 1). The availability of big data technologies and the popularity of mobile technologies and social media have made risk communication essential in disseminating information as well as detecting and responding to misinformation in emergencies and disasters. In Chapter 11, we also examine how big data technologies, mobile technologies, and social media have made it possible to identify people who may be ill *before* they know that they are sick. More importantly, we will examine how such technologies can trigger fundamental shifts in cultural perspectives, treatment paradigms, and redefine public health.

5. Social Structure and Health Disparities: Health Policies

Although investigations of structural factors and social policies were lacking in the early development of health communication (Kim et al., 2010), communication researchers recently have connected beyond disciplines in social sciences to explore how communication can maintain, reinforce, or resist social structures that legitimize disparities for marginalized and vulnerable populations. Two approaches have led the development in this trend: (a) medical humanities, and (b) social activism. **Medical humanities** is an interdisciplinary approach to conceptualize medicine through some combination of its relevant disciplines – ethics and philosophy, religious studies, history, and literature (Bleakley, 2015; Brody, 2011). By situating health and healthcare practices in sociohistorical contexts, ethics, and aesthetics, researchers are exploring how public discourse and communication about health concepts and practices can reflect and invoke sociopolitical conflicts and tensions and also serve as a resource and product of social control and of social resistance (e.g., Jensen, 2010, 2016). In Chapter 12 and Chapter 14, we will examine how medical schools are transforming their curriculum and institutional practices to (a) enhance providers' cultural competence and (b) educate students about historical and social injustice faced by marginalized populations.

Alternatively, scholars of critical studies, cultural studies, and health policy studies have collaborated with grassroots, activist organizations to engage in structural, cultural-level changes in health disparities (e.g., Dutta & Zapata, 2019; Zoller, 2006). Recognizing that individual-level prejudice and institutional-level stigma are best analyzed and addressed through structural and policy considerations, researchers are describing and analyzing how historical injustice through laws and instructional policies can create disparities in a wide range of areas in life, including social, economic, and health disparities. In Chapter 2, we will examine how the conceptualization of Black as a racial category was grounded in historical discrimination, legitimized by laws and governmental policies, and continues to shape individuals' understandings of this racial category today. In Chapter 14, we will explore the complex and nuanced working of structural barriers and consider how theories of distributive justice can provide insights into how to best address health disparities in the larger society.

B. Conceptualizing Culture in Health

In recent years, scholars have become increasingly concerned about our failure to recognize the complexity and diversity in social science research (Jones, 2010; Rad et al., 2018). A significant majority of the publications about human behaviors and psychology are based on **WEIRD** participants (i.e., relying on participants who are "overwhelming Western, Educated, and from Industrialized, Rich, and Democratic countries;" Brookshire, 2013, para. 2; see Figure 1.4). A study of publications during 2006–2010 in high impact journals in developmental psychology found that WEIRD participants account for 90.52% of the research subjects from whom claims were extrapolated and generalized (Nielsen et al., 2017). But we know that WEIRD participants differ from other populations in visual perception, spatial reasoning, reasoning styles, categorization and inferential induction, self-concepts and related motivations, as well as perceptions of fairness, cooperation, and moral reasoning (Henrich et al., 2010a, 2010b).

Communication scholars recently have utilized the platforms of the National Communication Association (NCA) and the International Communication Association (ICA), two of the largest professional organizations in the field of communication, to challenge the history, development, publication patterns of the discipline as well as the choice of NCA Distinguished Scholars and ICA Fellows (Chakravartty et al., 2018; Gardner, 2018; Mukherjee, 2020). Based on an analysis of publications and citations in communication journals between 1990–2015, Chakravartty et al. (2018) concluded that "non-White scholars continue to be underrepresented in publication rates, citation rates, and editorial positions in communication" (p. 254). #CommunicationSoWhite became the entry point of recognizing the struggles and silencing faced by some, and the point of reflection of one's privilege and responsibilities for many. Mukherjee (2020) argued, "Communication-So-White is a profoundly raced and gendered formation that polices our work methodologically, theoretically, and institutionally. ... Communication-So-White maintains the structural and ideological apparatuses of white privilege by rendering such privilege invisible in the ways we are expected to see and know" (p. 2). In short, "communication scholarship normalizes Whiteness" (Chakravartty et al., 2018, p. 262). When we fail to critically and reflexively recognize how the knowledge production perpetuates the views of a specific cultural perspective/group as the norm/standard, we inevitably maintain and reinforce a distorted reality.

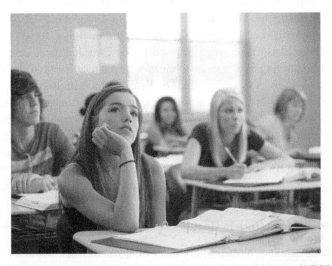

Figure 1.4 WEIRD as cultural perspectives. In what ways do you think your WEIRD status makes you different from non-WEIRD others? *Source:* Rubberball/Weston Colton/Getty Images

Because social science is a field of research that emerged from the West, we are inevitably limited by western thinking, cultural perspectives, linguistic limitations, and even imaginations (see Figure 1.5). This is not a "fault" per se as we are all limited by our cultural imaginations. We can only recognize our own cultural perspectives and limitations when we encounter "differences." Raising concerns about how citational segregation (i.e., a preference for citing authors who are members of the same group) can reinforce established patterns of disparities and professional socialization within the discipline, Chakravartty et al. (2018) argued that it is not sufficient to add more scholars of color. After all, if *all* scholars continue to be trained in and are expected to be familiar with (and cite) the literature that holds predominately western and White worldviews, such an approach will only continue to reinforce disparities and exclude other non-dominant (cultural) perspectives. Chakravartty et al. (2018) concluded that "rethinking normative theories of communication" is necessary to address the predominately White perspectives in the field (p. 261).

Culture is an essential factor in shaping individuals' understanding and behaviors in healthcare settings. Traditionally, the fields of public health and health communication have treated culture as an important caveat, noting that many of the findings may not be valid or applicable to individuals and organizations from non-western cultures. How can culture be an important contextual factor yet functions as a "caveat," an outlier that creates noise to observed patterns? More importantly, such an approach to culture in health context (or communication in general) also fails to account for the roles, functions, and impacts of culture in the West. This is reflected in the lack of systematic discussion and conceptualization about how culture, as a contextual factor, (a) serves as a resource and a product of individuals' health behaviors, (b) shapes communities' responses in offering support for some yet silencing suffering for others, and (c) shapes institutional structures and policies that reinforce disparities or minimize injustice. In other words, culture in the WEIRD-based literature becomes invisible. If western, modern, and/or industrialized societies are under the influence of culture, how can we theorize culture to explain our understanding and behaviors of

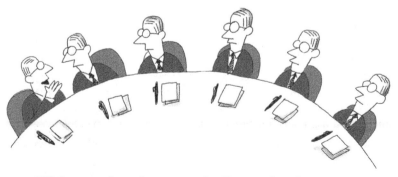

"Diversity is good. Pass it down."

Figure 1.5 Diversity is good. Until and unless we begin to see outside of our cultural perspectives, we cannot truly understand ourselves or others. *Source:* YAY Media AS / Alamy Stock Photo

health and illness – not just as a caveat or a contextual factor for non-western people but for *all* people?

In this book, we will *situate culture front and center*, examining its complex definitions and dimensions and exploring the various pathways in which culture can shape patients' illness experiences and providers' behaviors. We will examine how culture may create challenges and dilemmas in cross-cultural healthcare in which various individuals and institutions may hold diverging, if not incompatible, views of ethics and reality. More importantly, we do not view culture as something that is limited to ethnic minorities or marginalized populations. Rather, we argue that all people are cultural beings: We embody our cultures. Culture is enacted, performed, and negotiated in our everyday social interactions.

This book will begin by building a solid and comprehensive foundation on the understandings of different forms, functions, and meanings of culture and integrating health related examples. In later chapters, we will systematically examine major themes in health communication. This book adopts an interdisciplinary approach to examine culture as a resource and product of healthcare settings. In this book, we focus on three general areas: (a) culture and health behaviors (Chapter 2–5), (b) health as socially coordinated activities (Chapter 6–11), and (c) health disparities and health policies (Chapter 12–14). We are heavily influenced by the fields of cultural phenomenology, philosophy, anthropology, psychology, sociology, sociolinguistics, communication, public health, and ethics, among others.

II.   Foundational Framework: Dimensional Accrual and Dissociation

The foundational framework for this book includes the Theory of Dimensional Accrual and Dissociation (i.e., DAD; Kramer, 1997, 2013) and cultural fusion theory (i.e., CFT; Kramer, 2000, 2019). Both theories are based on prior research in the fields of comparative civilizations (Gebser, 1949–1953/1985, 1996), intercultural communication (Campbell, 1988/2011), and cultural structures (Mumford, 1934/2010). We have also extended DAD and CFT by proposing specific terms to highlight the unique aspects of the four primary cultural perspectives. We propose that cultures can be understood from three perspectives: Magic Consciousness (e.g., all lives are connected as one), Mythic Connection (e.g., stories and narratives that strengthen group norms and values), and Perspectival Thinking (e.g., science). These cultural perspectives also blend with one another, creating an Integral Fusion worldview (e.g., a scientist who is also highly religious). We then use these cultural perspectives to examine existing theories in health communication and health policies.

We chose the skeleton dressed in festive colors for the Day of the Dead as our book cover because it highlights the different perspectives of what we are trying to accomplish in this book. On *Día de los Muertos*, the Day of the Dead, people believe that the dead are just as "alive" and "real" as the living (i.e., Magic Consciousness). The day of the event is rich with stories that call for cultural beliefs and values for the living (i.e., Mythic Connection). Yet, in medicine, we often see skeletons as an impersonal object to be studied in human anatomy (i.e., Perspectival Thinking). The blending of all of our cultural frames into one is Integral Fusion (i.e., a dressed-up skeleton treated as a living person on a cultural-specific holiday to remember one's ancestors and follow community values). We will detail these cultural perspectives and explore their applications in health contexts in Chapter 2–5.

Before taking an in-depth look at each cultural perspective, we need to understand what is borrowed from Mumford (1934/2010) and Gebser (1949–1953/1985, 1996) in order to understand the DAD and CFT theories. Both Mumford and Gebser are NeoKantians. This means that they adopted many of the insights found in the works of Immanuel Kant (1798/1992, 1781/1999, 1786/2011).

A. Kant: Lifeworld as a Product of Constitutive Activity

Though we may imagine a world without human awareness, the only access we have to the universe is through our minds: our living minds render a world of sense and meaning. Our Lifeworld is constructed through our language and culture. Because there are many different languages and cultures, there are many different Lifeworlds, yielding different worldviews. We embody our Lifeworld and cannot be separated from it. This is because our experiences, perceptions, and understanding of realities are products of our human consciousness, which is shaped by our language and culture. Our consciousness structures experiences and "realities" for us – and this includes what "I" and "We" are and mean. Entire cultures tend to have collectivistic or individualistic senses of self, motives, values, and beliefs.

Kant's (1798/1992, 1781/1999, 1786/2011) great discovery was that the mind structures our perception. Kant (1781/1999) was the first to describe how awareness or consciousness is a product of the human nervous system, which includes the brain and all channels that feed into it. Kant noted that consciousness is a synthetic product: Consciousness is a result of synthesis and integration of all our memories, emotional states, sensory stimuli, and so forth. What this means is that information flows into the brain from our various senses, including complex messages (e.g., our sense of balance) and non-sensory information (e.g., memory, moods, and reasoning). **Consciousness** refers to all these different sources of information that are then combined into a coherent and consistent flowing awareness in real-time (Kramer, 1992a). In other words, consciousness forms the basic architectural structure that governs how all these different sources are combined. This process is constitutive: Out of many channels of information, one unified stream of awareness is synthesized by an active mind to create a coherent meaning (i.e., sense-making). Kant called the architectonic construct of the *human manifold* "a projection of an a priori intuition, a manufactured totality, in unconscious thought, onto the phenomenal world" (p. 46).

According to Kant's initial conceptualization, the basic dimensions of the architecture are the categorical *a priori* of space and time. The categorical *a priori* (space and time) form the structural logic that gives patterns and sense to all the information flowing into the brain. This architecture was universal and natural, grounded in *all* human minds. It was not a consequence of culture. The old nature versus nurture argument was very common during the Enlightenment when Kant was writing. He tended to see his work as discovering a universal and natural process. In other words, Kant initially believed that *all* human beings experience space and time the same way and that such experiences form the structure for the synthesis of all other experiences.

Kant (1724–1804) was writing in the seventeen and eighteen hundreds in a city in Northern Europe along the Baltic Sea. Kant initially believed he had discovered the universal structure for all human consciousness. But he began to suspect that there may be more than one architecture. His work was widely celebrated as one of the greatest accomplishments of the Enlightenment. Nevertheless, by the end of his life, he began to question the scope of his theory of consciousness, suspecting whether it was, in fact, true for all humans or limited in application. Living in a port city, Kant had the opportunity to meet with many people who had traveled to distant lands. Europe was entering its greatest period of colonial expansion and global exploration. As he met with travelers, they described to him people and distant cultures that did not share the same sense of time and space as Northern Europeans.

As he began to recognize the possibility of cultural variations, Kant started to recognize that the human brain is both a biological organ of the body and a social organ: its structure, the neuronetwork was a product of communication and culture. The human brain and the consciousness it generates are products of both biological factors such as genetics as well as being a cultural product. Even before the child is born, cultural issues (e.g., availability and form of prenatal care) can affect the brain.

The human brain is not finished at birth. The way it is formed is a result of our personal experiences, which are based on social interactions, the language we speak, and our culture (Fuchs, 2011). Compared to other modern apes, the human brain has a unique pattern of slow and prolonged development in general, only maturing into an adult brain when reaching 20 years old (Tottenham, 2014). In addition, the human brain continues to restructure itself throughout our lifetime, shaped by our lived experiences, including our lived environment, our illnesses, and our health behaviors (D'Sa & Duman, 2002; Pittenger & Duman, 2008). Culture is passed on from one generation to the next via symbol systems. Unlike our primal/animal instinct, culture can be lost.

In summary, Kant's work would lead to modern cognitivism because he argued that the brain is active and essential to the formation of a sensical, coherent, and consistent stream of consciousness. Kant's work has been widely celebrated as profoundly insightful, original, and foundational to modern studies of consciousness and neuroscience. In his later years, Kant argued that because our understandings of realities are synthesized through our brain, all our experiences are dependent on our culture and language, including our understanding of space and time. Before Kant could undertake a large-scale investigation into such variances, he died. Years later, another scholar, Jean Gebser, took up the effort.

B. Gebser: Multiple Architectures of Awareness

Jean Gebser (1905–1973) learned many languages, including non-European ones such as Hindi, Sanskrit, and some Chinese (Arneson, 2007). He also traveled and lived for extended periods of time around the globe. He was a close colleague to many scholars who traveled the world, compiling anthropological investigations. Based on his life-long studies of different languages, cultures, religions, psychologies, legal systems, arts, philosophies and so forth, Gebser proposed a modified version of Kant's theory (Kramer, 1992b). Gebser realized that there was more than one basic architectural pattern for organizing experience. It is unclear if he believed these differences were caused by cultural variation or if, in the other direction, cultural differences can be traced to different architectonic constructs. Regardless, Gebser realized that different languages and cultures perceive the world differently and experience different kinds of space and time (Kramer, 1992a). What Kant called the architectonic structure of awareness is similar to the concept of "deep structures" proposed by Noam Chomsky (1969). Gebser (1949–1953/1985) argued that there was more than one kind of structure.

One way to understand what Gebser called "**consciousness structures**" is to think of the human brain as unfinished at birth. The brain of a baby has great potential, but it cannot integrate, organize, and make sense of new information until it has a basic construct. If you think of the human brain as being like the central processing unit of a computer with a basic subroutine, then you can begin to understand what a consciousness structure and its architecture are. A subroutine is an assembly language that enables programs to operate. If a computer has no subroutine, it cannot "read" any language or program.

As a baby is socialized, its brain grows and forms a very basic (simple but profoundly important) matrix or structure that enables the organization and integration of future experiences. At the same time, those experiences also effect the structure of the brain and the way that person perceives space, time, emotion, identity, and other things: the way they see and think about the world. This rudimentary structure will form the basis for how the child will integrate and perceive all new experiences. This includes language itself. The architecture itself changes in structure as language and culture are integrated into the child's mind. Studies of "feral" children who were lost in the wilderness and never taught language by a certain age indicate that after being discovered, they are unable to acquire language (Vyshedskiy et al., 2017). It appears that the biological brain develops through stages and certain types of cognition can develop at only certain times. If these periods are missed, the child will never fully acquire those cognitive and affective abilities (Sakai, 2005; Tottenham, 2014). The basic architecture that enables the synthesis of a coherent and consistent streaming awareness is acquired very early in childhood, which then enables all future sense-making; all future "learning."

In the 20th century, Gebser (1949–1953/1985) discovered that there exists around the world at least four different architectures and consequently four different worldviews: four different ways to experience time, space, and everything that relies on duration and extension – which means everything from dreams and ideas to the perception of empirical objects. Our perception is always already influenced by past experiences, including the language we think in and the culture we grow up in. Since the basic way consciousness is organized is according to temporal and spatial requirements, and because these are dimensions, Gebser argued that the four different worldviews expressly manifest four different formations of these dimensions. They are the magic one-dimensional worldview, the mythic two-dimensional worldview, the perspectival modern three-dimensional worldview, and the postmodern aperspectival or integral worldview.

Finally, culture is not necessarily present for all humans. Gebser (1949–1953/1985) noted that archaic hominids are animal-like, living without made shelter, writing, or art. We know them mostly from skeletal remains. The lifeworld of archaic men is zero-dimensional. Zero-dimensionality means that they do not have a sense of space or time as we moderns know, and therefore no self-awareness as we understand it. Because zero-dimensional hominids did not see themselves as something other than their environment, they did not experience nature or culture, but rather, simply the world, just as other animals do. As such, the archaic cultural perspective, if it exists at all, is not covered in this book.

C. Kramer: Dimensional Accrual and Dissociation

Eric Kramer further synthesizes Gebser's work on various worldviews with Mumford's (1934/2010) notion of dissociation. Lewis Mumford (1934/2010) traced a process of increasing dissociation through history: Humans gradually separate from nature and progressively build an artificial world that enables them to control and exploit everything, including other people, animals, plants, rivers, lakes, and technology in general. A quality of dissociation is a decrease in emotional attachment to things and people as the number of dimensions to awareness increases.

Dissociation means separation from nature and an increasingly abstract way of thinking. An example of dissociation is the invention and adoption of the mechanical clock, which produces a type of time disconnected from the natural cycles of the actual seasons. Following the natural cycles of seasons, we eat when we are hungry; similarly, we work till the day turns dark or when we get tired. However, the invention of the mechanical clock dissociates us from the natural rhythm, creating a form of virtual time that has no referent to actual light or dark. After the spread and adoption of artificial clock time, we eat and work when "it's time" (as opposed to when we are hungry) and we even began to disregard our bodies and feelings (e.g., exhaustion) because we are not "off the clock" just yet. The clock becomes the new frame that orients not only our understanding of time but also regulates and defines our bodies, feelings, and everyday life.

Theory of Dimensional Accrual and Dissociation (DAD), proposed by Eric Kramer, argues that each worldview manifests through four different modes of *communication* and understanding; one-dimensional idolic communication, two-dimensional symbolic communication, three-dimensional signalic communication, and four-dimensional integral polycentricity (Kramer, 1997, 2013; Kramer & Ikeda, 1998). The integral worldview is a result of cultural fusion (Kramer, 2019). In Chapter 2–5, we will discuss each cultural perspective in detail and explore how they provide more insights into our understanding of health theories and practices. In this Chapter, our goal is to provide a brief overview of the foundational framework. As dimensions accrue, dissociation increases (e.g., identification and care decrease).

1. One-Dimensional Idolic Communication: Magic Consciousness

Scholars argued that Magic culture emerged between 40,000 to 20,000 years ago when prehistoric humans in southern African decorated their bodies and then other surfaces such as cave walls with paintings, depicting everyday life with images of humans and animals (Greenwood & Goodwyn, 2015; McNamara, 2004). Relative to archaic hominids, Magic humans began to dramatically dissociate from the rest of reality/nature and began to develop complex language, tool-making, and ceremonial rituals we call Magic (Greenwood & Goodwyn, 2015). Gebser (1949–1953/1985) called this revolution in human consciousness the dawn of the one-dimensional magic world. Paintings of beasts on cave walls were the beasts who came to life in the flickering torches of the Shaman. Anthropologists have described countless examples of "primitive art" that does not represent things but is "the thing." Naming and depicting "the thing" give Magic people control over it. In this book, we call this cultural perspective Magic Consciousness.

Magic communities are highly collectivistic. People in a magic community experience everything as a whole and all members' identities are fused as one (Kramer, 2004; Kramer & Ikeda, 1998). For people with Magic Consciousness, when a member of the tribe feels pain, everyone feels pain. They dance, cry, and laugh together. Their totem animal swimming across the river is them swimming (Neihardt, 1932/2014). Because they do not distinguish themselves from other members of the tribe or even other "beings" in their world, they share deep bonds with all beings in their magic community. There is no theater, no performers nor audience. This is because there is no fragmentation between audience and speaker.

For people with Magic Consciousness, their world is taken-for-granted – everything is finished and complete. Initially, Magic culture is still closely identified with natural rhythms and processes. But as dissociation increases, culture, like the ego, emerges as more starkly that which is *not* nature (McNamara, 2004). Bit by bit, magic humans began to attempt to cajole nature, to appease it, to appeal to its forces in order to enhance wellbeing, fertility, and prolong life. Magic systems seek to achieve balance and harmony with the universe in order to enhance health and prolong life. Magic is the first attempt by humans to step out from the rest of nature, turn toward it, and comprehend it as something different from themselves (Greenwood & Goodwyn, 2015). This is the emergence of the one-dimensional structure of Magic Consciousness (Gebser, 1949–1953/1985; Kramer & Algis, 1992).

The earliest forms of magic are attempts to control forces such as illness, fertility, and mortality. Although magic humans still have a very strong emotional attachment and a shared identity with their environment, they also exhibit a realization that the environment is fragmenting into many beings and that they can confront natural forces as things other than themselves. Tools to achieve such desires multiply. Complex magic, idolic incantation, and ritual proliferate. Magic is a tool used to alter reality to suit one's needs and desires – to increase fertility, to make it rain, to cure illness. This indicates the first nascent sense of space, of fragmentation, of directional planning, of a world to be confronted and manipulated.

Magic communication is idolic, meaning that messages and utterances are not dissociated from that which they "reference" (Kramer, 2013). Magic idolic communication has no dissociative space between the sign and what is symbolized. As words are spoken, realities are invoked. Idolic magic communication is meant to directly modify conditions. Reality is evoked and invoked as the talk/act is performed. It uses incantatory speech and acts that invoke and evoke changes that are desired. Spellcasting, ritual movements, chants, actions, and signs are not interpretable or replaceable. There is no space between the spell and its impact. The spell is uttered and either it works (transforms reality), or it does not. Spells are not arbitrary. If you pick up a magic amulet or figurine of a goddess, you are not merely picking up a dissociated symbol of the goddess but the goddess herself. Words have inherent power.

2. Two-Dimensional Symbolic Communication: Mythic Connection

As dissociation increases, it manifests as our ability to perceive a second dimension. As people increasingly dissociate from the taken-for-granted world of Magic Consciousness, two-dimensional symbolic communication manifests nascent spatial thinking such that messages become ambiguous with both literal and figural meanings simultaneously. Individualism begins to emerge with more emphasis on opinions and interpretations (McNamara, 2004). Communication becomes problematic because meanings are no longer inherent in the words. Storytelling, epic poetry emerges with the linear telling of mythic tales to reconcile differences of meanings and interpretations (Ellwood & York, 1999; McNamara, 2004). These stories define both the speakers' and the audiences' reality and *establish their shared priorities* as a community (Grant, 1998). This is the emergence of the two-dimensional structure of Mythic Connection (Gebser, 1949–1953/1985; Kramer & Algis, 1992).

Idolic communication (e.g., incantation) in the world of Magic Consciousness gives way to more spatial linear storytelling, symbolic communication in the world of Mythic Connection (McNamara, 2004). The age of the great religions commences and is based on lengthy epic poems and histories of the sacred (Eliade, 1959; Eliade, 1964/1998). Time becomes increasingly spatialized in the form of teleological cosmology. Humanity separates from nature. Individuals as historic actors begin to emerge. Concern about the self and concepts such as salvation become prominent. Nascent "progress" toward final judgment days and other terminuses become critical to judgments and spiritual life. With increased spatial thinking in the symbolic world, drama ensues with great tales of the struggle between good and evil (Eliade, 1959). Myths and stories are essential and fundamental in defining and maintaining reality and values shared by all members of the community (Campbell, 1988/2011; Ellwood & York, 1999).

3. Three-Dimensional Signalic Communication: Perspectival Thinking

With increasing dissociation, the ability to perceive the third dimension occurs, the perspectival world (Gebser, 1949–1953/1985). With the emergence of three-dimensional depth space, objects become discrete. In the world of Perspectival Thinking, the dominant mode of communication is signalic (Kramer, 2013). Things are increasingly objectified, meaning that they hold no inherent meaning. As spatial thinking further intensifies, words no longer hold inherent power but are only referential to things. Three-valued logic emerges along with the linear movement of knowledge from thesis to antithesis to synthesis. The relationships between the signifier and the signified are deemed arbitrary and hold little emotional value. Emotional attachment and care that were once rich in the world of Magic Consciousness dissipate in the world of Perspectival Thinking. Nothing is sacred or irreplaceable. People don't care. Meanings in Perspectival Thinking are dependent on the perspectives one takes (Haynes, 2000).

The "beings" that once permeated the world of Magic Consciousness are reduced to material and discrete "objects." As spirit and soul disappear from the world, the "body" becomes an object among other objects. Objects are to be observed and studied. Dissection of bodies becomes the primary path to knowledge. Biological bodies are fragmented into discrete systems. Organs are identified and expertise narrows to specialization on particular systems and diseases. Prothesis, replacement "parts" proliferate. Extraction, storage and transplantation or parts and organs become feasible.

Fragmentation and individuation characterize the three-dimensional perspectival world. Collective community dissolves and modern maladies such as alienation, isolation, and loneliness become epidemic (Kramer et al., 2014). Property and rights become personal. Individualism for humans also occurs and so formalized talk in the structure of dialectical debate becomes prominent. The emergence of this state of affairs motivates the invention of the modern social sciences as all the founding authors from Ferdinand Tönnies (1887/2017) and Max Weber (1905–1920/2002), to Karl Marx (1935) and Emile Durkheim (1953/2010) were compelled to begin analyses of modern society and the individual's "place," and "situation." Spatial conceptualization of society came to focus on roles, status, hierarchies, power distances, and other aspects of a fragmenting social world. Spatial thinking emphasizes mobility from spatial exploration to social movement within hierarchies. Systems thinking becomes dominant with sub- and super- systemic hierarchies. Identity becomes flexible, even arbitrary, and can encounter a crisis. Stark individualistic, subjective relativity is a result of three-dimensional signalic communication and its quality of being arbitrary.

4. Four-Dimensional Integral Polycentricity: Integral Fusion

Magic Consciousness, Mythic Connection, and Perspectival Thinking are three different cultural perspectives. Each represents a distinctive approach to understanding one's reality and its relationship with language and culture. These cultural perspectives can be incompatible. Either a person's body is fused with other sacred spirits and life forces in the universe (under Magic Consciousness), or it is understood to be a symbolic gift of love and life by one's ancestors (under Mythic Connection), or it is a material object that can be dissected and studied (under Perspectival Thinking). For a person with Magic Consciousness, dissecting a body can be disrespectful, dangerous, and even unthinkable. For a person with Perspectival Thinking, believing that a body is fused with spirits and needs to be in harmony with the universe to be healthy sounds silly and superstitious.

Kramer (2013) used the term "dimensional accrual" to highlight that the people with access to more dimensions continue to have the capacity to understand individuals with worldviews that have fewer dimensions, but often they do not. Or, if they do, they apply a more dissociative attitude to those forms. One result is cynicism. Although a person with Perspectival Thinking can understand, manipulate, and even exploit the thinking of people with Magic Consciousness (see also Exploitation Exists Only in Perspectival Thinking in Chapter 13), a person with Magic Consciousness may not immediately understand a Perspectival person's calculative self-interest, in part because it is foreign to them. This is the layering effect of cultural perspectives (see also Accrual of Cultural Dimensions in Chapter 5). In our modern world, in which Perspectival Thinking predominates, all cultural perspectives are co-present as potential and as essential aspects of human consciousness. However, Magic Consciousness and Mythic Connection tend to be latent. Nevertheless, each cultural perspective holds capacities and potentials we need for survival but which we may not yet understand. For now, the key point is that these three cultural perspectives have a layering effect on one's understanding and appreciation of realities.

More importantly, although the numbering of dimensions of each cultural perspective may appear to give a sense of ranking or hierarchy, it is important *not* to mistake the numbering as an indicator of developmental or linear progress of human societies or cultures. They represent different modes of understanding one's reality and the roles of culture and language. Each cultural perspective serves as one's architectural structure that governs how all other sources of information are combined to create a synthesized, coherent meaning. One is not "better" than the other. In fact, many scholars have argued that stronger identification with worldviews of Magic Consciousness and Mythic Connection is necessary to avoid the increasing deterioration and depletion of our world, which is dominated by Perspectival Thinking (Greenwood & Goodwyn, 2015; Kramer et al., 2014; McNamara, 2004). We will revisit this issue throughout the book.

An Integral Fusion worldview is a result of cultural fusion among the cultural perspectives of Magic Consciousness, Mythic Connection, and Perspectival Thinking. Essential to Integral Fusion is one's ability to view different perspectives with equal care, respect, and validity. As a cultural perspective, Integral Fusion is **polycentric** because it not only recognizes but also *appreciates* other cultural perspectives. This understanding of the ever-present functioning and ontogenesis of Magic, Myth, and Perspectivism through their differences, and their vitality in our lives, is integrality. It has profound emotional, spiritual, *and* analytical aspects. Just as two or more adjacent colors change each other, Magic emotion, Mythic story, and Perspectival measure reveal each other's qualities by contrast and complement through time.

Integral Fusion does not adopt a fixed, dominant cultural perspective that marginalizes all Others. Nor does it dislocate or eliminate others. There is no modern ideological category (e.g., the "subaltern") in an Integral Fusion worldview as all perspectives are taken into consideration, with equal weight and care. An Integral Fusion worldview is reflected in one's ability to integrate and synthesize these diverging cultural perspectives and reconcile the tensions between them. However, rather than a layering of other cultural perspectives, cultural fusion always leads to something *new*, something that is not the direct derivative of the source cultures. It creates a *new* cultural perspective that is influenced by all cultural perspectives but also unique in its blending of cultures (Kramer, 2000). An Integral Fusion worldview is a result of cultural fusion *without* the erasure of the original cultural self (Kramer, 1997, 2000, 2008). Through social interactions, new forms (of music, cuisine, art, literature, science, history, fashion, business models...) of cultural fusion proliferate.

An Integral Fusion worldview is able to see by *seeing through* the different cultural perspectives, appreciating their strengths, understanding their limitations, and developing unique and innovative blends that best accommodate everyone's needs. An Integral Fusion worldview can be a result of intentional efforts or organic, unexpected processes of intercultural encounters. It is not inherently "better" than other cultural perspectives. Cultural fusion does not guarantee a "better" result. Nevertheless, because an Integral Fusion worldview promises infinite possibilities and potentials through the blending of cultural perspectives, its flexibility and diversity are some of the greatest strengths in addressing problems faced by our society. In this book, we will explore why cultural fusion is valuable in helping our communities to meet the challenges of our times in healthcare settings and in health policies.

III. Learning Objectives

There are three primary learning objectives that guide our focus for this book. First, we will challenge our readers to see culture beyond racial and ethnic groups. We have included different conceptualizations of culture (e.g., culture as group, as speech community, as worldview, and as a living process), exploring how these distinctive approaches may allow readers to identify different problems and develop different solutions. In addition, we encourage our readers to reflect and consider how they may hold different cultural perspectives on different issues/topics, shaping their behaviors and responses accordingly.

Second, by covering a wide range of topics in cultural studies, public health, health communication, and health policies, our goal is to help the readers develop the skills to recognize and challenge the cultural perspectives inherent in theory or practice. In addition, by contextualizing cultural groups' past experiences, we hope that readers will reconsider the effectiveness and appropriateness in how we conceptualize barriers and facilitators of health and healthcare services.

Third, our goal is to help our readers develop a conceptual framework that allows them to critically and reflexively examine the issues at hand, including health theories and practices. Scheper-Hughes (1992) commented, "We cannot rid ourselves of the cultural self we bring with us into the field any more than we can disown the eyes, ears, and skin through which we take in our intuitive perceptions about the new and strange world we have entered" (p. 28). In other words, we cannot "objectively" interpret or understand the world as our subjectivity is embedded in our consciousness, nor can we truly unlearn and forget about our cultural selves (Liu & Kramer, 2019). Nevertheless, as we become more aware of cultural perspective(s), we can learn to appreciate differences and develop repertoires that allow us to identify creative, effective and appropriate strategies to achieve mutually agreeable solutions.

Finally, we also face the limits of our own cultures and languages. Although both authors have extensive background and training in different cultures, our training in social science inevitably reinforces our Perspectival Thinking, which requires analytical reasoning. There may be moments that we misappropriate analytical concepts when addressing other cultural approaches and perspectives. In addition, as citizens of democratic societies, we also recognize that some of our suggestions and recommendations are not applicable to cultures and societies where its citizens are not treated to be equal and free and do not have the agency and control over their behaviors and life destinies. We regret that we were not able to give sufficient depth and analysis to address their struggles and suffering.

As we complete our chapters during this historical time of a global pandemic, we felt a sense of purpose. We hope you enjoy this book as much as we do.

IV. Additional Resources

A. Key Terms and Theories

> health promotion
> healthcare delivery
> lived experience
> transformative technologies
> pan-evolution
> risk communication

medical humanities
WEIRD
consciousness structures
Theory of Dimensional Accrual and Dissociation (DAD)
   Magic Consciousness
   Mythic Connection
   Perspectival Thinking
   Integral Fusion
polycentricity

B. Discussion Questions

1. Many people have commented on how the September 11, 2001 attack against the United States has transformed our everyday life. Do you think the COVID-19 pandemic in 2020 transformed our everyday life? In what ways?
2. Public health campaigns represent an important area of research and practice of health communication.
   a. Can you recall the last health campaign you saw? What was it? Where did you see it?
   b. Do you think it will be effective? Why or why not?
3. In what ways do you think your interactions with your healthcare providers may influence your health behaviors?
   a. Do you ever feel discriminated or stigmatized by your physicians or nurses? How?
   b. Do you think your physicians or nurses may not have told you the whole truth? Why?
   c. Do you think your family members may influence your perceptions and interactions with your providers? How?
4. Do you think people who have the same illness may still have very different lived experiences regarding their illness? Why and how?
5. In what ways do you think your WEIRD status makes you different from non-WEIRD others?
6. Do you agree that your language and culture may influence your perception and experiences of the world?
   a. Do you think people who have different languages and cultures experience temperature (e.g., hot and cold) differently than you do? Why and how?
   b. Do you think people who have different languages and cultures experience space and time differently than you do? Why and how?
   c. Do you think people who have different languages and cultures experience quantity (e.g., numbers, hierarchies, or ranking the level of your pain/depression from 1–10) differently than you do?
   d. Do you think people who have different languages and cultures experience pain differently than you do?
7. Do you like fusion food or music? Why or why not?
8. Do you think cultural fusion is different from "cultural appropriation"? In what ways? (see also Chapter 5)

C. References

Arneson, P. (Ed.). (2007). *Perspectives on philosophy of communication*. Purdue University Press.

Béland, D., Rocco, P., & Waddan, A. (2016). Obamacare and the politics of universal health insurance coverage in the United States. *Social Policy & Administration, 50*(4), 428–451.

Bleakley, A. (2015). *Medical humanities and medical education: How the medical humanities can shape better doctors*. Routledge.

Brody, H. (2011). Defining the medical humanities: Three conceptions and three narratives. *Journal of Medical Humanities, 32*(1), 1–7.

Brookshire, B. (2013, May 8). *Psychology is WEIRD*. Slate. https://slate.com/technology/2013/05/weird-psychology-social-science-researchers-rely-too-much-on-western-college-students.html

Brown, P. (1991). Themes in medical sociology. *Journal of Health Politics, Policy and Law, 16*(3), 595–604.

Bury, M. (1982). Chronic illness as biographical disruption. *Sociology of Health & Illness, 4*(2), 167–182.

Bury, M. R. (1986). Social constructionism and the development of medical sociology. *Sociology of Health & Illness, 8*(2), 137–169.

Bynum, W. (2008). *The history of medicine: A very short introduction*. Oxford University Press.

Campbell, J. (with Moyers, B.). (2011). *The power of myth*. Knopf Doubleday. (Original work published 1988)

Cegala, D. J., Bahnson, R. R., Clinton, S. K., David, P., Gong, M. C., Monk, J., Nag, S., & Pohar, K. S. (2008). Information seeking and satisfaction with physician-patient communication among prostate cancer survivors. *Health Communication, 23*(1), 62–69.

Chakravartty, P., Kuo, R., Grubbs, V., & McIlwain, C. (2018). #CommunicationSoWhite. *Journal of Communication, 68*(2), 254–266.

Charmaz, K. (2002). Stories and silences: Disclosures and self in chronic illness. *Qualitative Inquiry, 8*(3), 302–328.

Chomsky, N. (1969). *Deep structure, surface structure, and semantic interpretation*. Indiana University Linguistics Club.

D'Sa, C., & Duman, R. S. (2002). Antidepressants and neuroplasticity. *Bipolar Disorders, 4*(3), 183–194.

Durkheim, E. (2010). *Sociology and philosophy*. Routledge. (Original work published 1953)

Dutta, M. J., & Zapata, D. B. (Eds.). (2019). *Communicating for social change: Meaning, power, and resistance*. Palgrave Macmillan.

Eliade, M. (1959). *The sacred and the profane: The nature of religion* (W. R. Trask, Trans.). Harcourt.

Eliade, M. (1998). *Myth and reality*. Waveland Press. (Original work published 1964)

Ellwood, R., & York, S. U. N. (1999). *The politics of myth: A study of C. G. Jung, Mircea Eliade, and Joseph Campbell*. State University of New York Press.

Fadiman, A. (1997). *The spirit catches you and you fall down: A Hmong child, her American doctors, and the collision of two cultures*. Farrar, Straus and Giroux.

Ferriman, A. (2007). *BMJ* readers choose the "sanitary revolution" as greatest medical advance since 1840. *BMJ, 334*(7585), 111.

Frank, A. W. (1998). Just listening: Narrative and deep illness. *Families, Systems, & Health, 16*(3), 197–212.

Fuchs, T. (2011). The brain – A mediating organ. *Journal of Consciousness Studies, 18*(7–8), 196–221.

Gardner, P. M. (2018). Diversifying ICA: Identity, difference, and the politics of transformation. *Journal of Communication, 68*(5), 831–841.

Garfield, R., Claxton, G., Damico, A., & Levitt, L. (2020, May 13). *Eligibility for ACA health coverage following job loss*. Kaiser Family Foundation. https://www.kff.org/coronavirus-covid-19/issue-brief/eligibility-for-aca-health-coverage-following-job-loss

Gebser, J. (1985). *The ever-present origin* (N. Barstad & A. Mickunas, Trans.). Ohio University Press. (Original work published 1949–1953)

Gebser, J. (1996). Cultural philosophy as method and venture (G. Feuerstein, Trans.). *Integrative Explorations: Journal of Culture and Consciousness, 3*(1), 78–83.

Grant, C. (1998). *Myths we live by*. University of Ottawa Press.

Greenwood, S., & Goodwyn, E. D. (2015). *Magical consciousness: An anthropological and neurobiological approach*. Routledge.

Haynes, J. D. (2000). *Perspectival thinking: For inquiring organisations*. Informing Science Press.

Henrich, J., Heine, S. J., & Norenzayan, A. (2010a). Most people are not WEIRD. *Nature, 466*(7302), 29.

Henrich, J., Heine, S. J., & Norenzayan, A. (2010b). The weirdest people in the world? *Behavioral and Brain Sciences, 33*(2–3), 61–83.

Jensen, R. E. (2010). *Dirty words: The rhetoric of public sex education, 1870–1924*. University of Illinois Press.

Jensen, R. E. (2016). *Infertility: Tracing the history of a transformative term*. Penn State University Press.

Johns Hopkins Coronavirus Resource Center. (2020). *Coronavirus COVID-19 global cases by the Center for Systems Science and Engineering (CSSE) at Johns Hopkins University (JHU)*. Retrieved July 4, 2020, from https://coronavirus.jhu.edu/map.html

Johnson, R. L., Roter, D., Powe, N. R., & Cooper, L. A. (2004). Patient race/ethnicity and quality of patient–physician communication during medical visits. *American Journal of Public Health, 94*(12), 2084–2090.

Jones, D. (2010). A WEIRD view of human nature skews psychologists' studies. *Science, 328*(5986), 1627.

Kant, I. (1992). *The conflict of the faculties [Der streit der fakultäten]* (M. J. Gregor, Trans.). University of Nebraska Press. (Original work published 1798)

Kant, I. (1999). *Critique of pure reason* (P. Guyer & A. W. Wood, Eds. & Trans.). Cambridge University Press. (Original work published 1781)

Kant, I. (2011). *Groundwork of the metaphysics of morals* (M. Gregor, J. Timmermann, & J. Timmermann, Eds.; German–English ed.). Cambridge University Press. (Original work published 1786)

Kim, J.-N., Park, S.-C., Yoo, S.-W., & Shen, H. (2010). Mapping health communication scholarship: Breadth, depth, and agenda of published research in *Health Communication*. *Health Communication, 25*(6–7), 487–503.

Kleinman, A. (1980). *Patients and healers in the context of culture: An exploration of the borderland between anthropology, medicine, and psychiatry*. University of California Press.

Kramer, E. M. (1992a). Consciousness and culture. In E. M. Kramer (Ed.), *Consciousness and culture: An introduction to the thought of Jean Gebser* (pp. 1–60). Greenwood.

Kramer, E. M. (Ed). (1992b). *Consciousness and culture: An introduction to the thought of Jean Gebser*. Greenwood.

Kramer, E. M. (1997). *Modern/postmodern: Off the beaten path of antimodernism*. Praeger.

Kramer, E. M. (2000). Cultural fusion and the defense of difference. In M. K. Asante & J. E. Min (Eds.), *Socio-cultural conflict between African and Korean Americans* (pp. 182–223). University Press of America.

Kramer, E. M. (2004). The body in communication. In V. Berdayes, L. Esposito, & J. Murphy (Eds.), *The body in human inquiry: Interdisciplinary explorations of embodiment* (pp. 51–86). Hampton.

Kramer, E. M. (2008). Theoretical reflections on intercultural studies: Preface. In S. M. Croucher, *Looking beyond the hijab* (pp. ix–xxxix). Hampton.

Kramer, E. M. (2013). Dimensional accrual and dissociation: An introduction. In J. Grace & E. M. Kramer (Eds.), *Communication, comparative cultures, and civilizations* (Vol. 3, pp. 123–184). Hampton.

Kramer, E. M. (2019). Cultural fusion theory. In J. F. Nussbaum (Ed.), *Oxford research encyclopedia of communication*. Oxford University Press. https://doi.org/10.1093/acrefore/9780190228613.013.679

Kramer, E. M., Adkins, G., Kim, S. H., & Miller, G. (2014). *Environmental communication and the extinction vortex: Technology as denial of death*. Hampton.

Kramer, E. M., & Algis, M. (1992). Introduction: Gebser's new understanding. In E. M. Kramer (Ed.), *Consciousness and culture: An introduction to the thought of Jean Gebser* (pp. xi–xxxi). Greenwood.

Kramer, E. M., & Ikeda, R. (1998). Understanding different worlds: The theory of dimensional accrual/dissociation. *Journal of Intercultural Communication, 1*(2), 37–51.

Kreps, G. L. (2014). Health communication, history of. In T. L. Thompson (Ed.), *Encyclopedia of health communication* (Vol. 2, pp. 567–572). Sage.

Kreps, G. L., Bonaguro, E. W., & Query, J. L. Jr. (1998). The history and development of the field of health communication. In L. D. Jackson & B. K. Duffy (Eds.), *Health communication research: A guide to developments and directions* (pp. 1–15). Greenwood.

Liu, Y., & Kramer, E. (2019). Conceptualizing the other in intercultural encounters: Review, formulation, and typology of the other-identity. *Howard Journal of Communications, 30*(5), 446–463.

Marx, K. (1935). *Wage-labour and capital: Value, price, and profit*. International Publishers.

McNamara, T. E. (2004). *Evolution, culture, and consciousness: The discovery of the preconscious mind*. University Press of America.

Menton, J. (2020, July 2). *48M Americans filed jobless claims in 15 weeks*. USA Today. https://www.usatoday.com/story/money/2020/07/02/layoffs-1-4-m-workers-file-unemployment-covid-19-signals-slow-recovery/5357970002

Miller, T. A. (2016). Health literacy and adherence to medical treatment in chronic and acute illness: A meta-analysis. *Patient Education and Counseling, 99*(7), 1079–1086.

Mukherjee, R. (2020). Of experts and tokens: Mapping a critical race archaeology of communication. *Communication, Culture and Critique, 13*(2), 152–167.

Mukherjee, S. (2016). *The gene: An intimate history*. Scribner.

Mumford, L. (2010). *Technics and civilization*. University of Chicago Press. (Original work published 1934)

Neihardt, J. G. (2014). *Black Elk speaks: The complete edition*. University of Nebraska Press. (Original work published 1932)

Nielsen, M., Haun, D., Kärtner, J., & Legare, C. H. (2017). The persistent sampling bias in developmental psychology: A call to action. *Journal of Experimental Child Psychology, 162*, 31–38.

Parsons, T. (1951). Illness and the role of the physician: A sociological perspective. *American Journal of Orthopsychiatry, 21*(3), 452–460.

Pettersson, H., Manley, B., & Hernandez, S. (2020). *Tracking coronavirus' global spread*. CNN. Retrieved September 30, 2020, from https://www.cnn.com/interactive/2020/health/coronavirus-maps-and-cases/

Pittenger, C., & Duman, R. S. (2008). Stress, depression, and neuroplasticity: A convergence of mechanisms. *Neuropsychopharmacology, 33*(1), 88–109.

Rad, M. S., Martingano, A. J., & Ginges, J. (2018). Toward a psychology of *Homo sapiens*: Making psychological science more representative of the human population. *Proceedings of the National Academy of Sciences, 115*(45), 11401–11405.

Robinson, J. D., & Heritage, J. (2016). How patients understand physicians' solicitations of additional concerns: Implications for up-front agenda setting in primary care. *Health Communication, 31*(4), 434–444.

Rosen, G. (2015). *A history of public health*. Johns Hopkins University Press. (Original work published 1958)

Ruben, B. D. (2016). Communication theory and health communication practice: The more things change, the more they stay the same. *Health Communication, 31*(1), 1–11.

Sakai, K. L. (2005). Language acquisition and brain development. *Science, 310*(5749), 815.

Scheper-Hughes, N. (1992). *Death without weeping: The violence of everyday life in Brazil*. University of California Press.

Scott, A. M., & Caughlin, J. P. (2015). Communication nonaccommodation in family conversations about end-of-life health decisions. *Health Communication, 30*(2), 144–153.

Smialek, J. (2020, May 14). *Poor Americans hit hardest by job losses amid lockdowns, fed says*. The New York Times. https://nyti.ms/2X32fq2

Sternlicht, A. (2020, June 2). *Over 4,400 arrests, 62,000 National Guard troops deployed: George Floyd protests by the numbers*. Forbes. https://www.forbes.com/sites/alexandrasternlicht/2020/06/02/over-4400-arrests-62000-national-guard-troops-deployed-george-floyd-protests-by-the-numbers/#6b2ea427d4fe

Street, R. L., Jr. (2013). How clinician–patient communication contributes to health improvement: Modeling pathways from talk to outcome. *Patient Education and Counseling, 92*(3), 286–291.

Thompson, C. M., & Parsloe, S. (2019). "I don't claim to be the world's foremost expert, but ...": How individuals "know" family members are not experiencing health issues as severely as they claim. *Qualitative Health Research, 29*(10), 1433–1446.

Tönnies, F. (2017). *Community and society*. Routledge. (Original work published 1887)

Tottenham, N. (2014). The importance of early experiences for neuro-affective development. *Current Topics in Behavioral Neurosciences, 16*, 109–129.

Vyshedskiy, A., Mahapatra, S., & Dunn, R. (2017). Linguistically deprived children: Meta-analysis of published research underlines the importance of early syntactic language use for normal brain development. *Research Ideas and Outcomes, 3,* Article e20696. https://doi.org/10.3897/rio.3.e20696

Weber, M. (2002). *The Protestant ethic and the "spirit" of capitalism and other writings* (P. Baehr & G. C. Wells, Eds. & Trans.). Penguin. (Original work published 1905–1920)

White House. (2020, March 13). *Proclamation on declaring a national emergency concerning the novel coronavirus disease (COVID-19) outbreak.* https://www.whitehouse.gov/presidential-actions/proclamation-declaring-national-emergency-concerning-novel-coronavirus-disease-covid-19-outbreak/

World Health Organization. (2020a). *General information on risk communication.* https://www.who.int/risk-communication/background/en

World Health Organization. (2020b, September 9). *Timeline of WHO's response to COVID-19.* https://www.who.int/news-room/detail/29-06-2020-covidtimeline

Zoller, H. M. (2006). Health activism: Communication theory and action for social change. *Communication Theory, 15*(4), 341–364.

2

Cultural Consciousness I

Magic Consciousness and Emotions in Health

Chapter 2 begins with a brief review of how culture has been conceptualized in different fields, providing a structure for Chapters 2 to 5. By examining and reflecting on the primordial and existential elements of culture, we will examine how Magic Consciousness as a cultural consciousness shape individuals' instinctual understanding and interpretation of health behaviors. By noting that emotion is inseparable to Magic Consciousness, we will explore how such emotions can become motivating factors in influencing individuals' health practices.

I.   What is Culture?

Scholars from different disciplines have different ways to think and talk about culture. Some see culture as a relatively fixed or stable set of beliefs, values, and behavior patterns, often demarcated by national or ethnic boundaries (Hofstede 2001; Ting-Toomey 2012). Others see culture as a continual process of renewal and of integrating new information from outside forces (e.g., climate change, overexploitation of natural resources, and invading cultures) and also from indigenous experiences (Kramer 2019; Kramer & Liu 2015; Streeck 2002). In this Chapter, we will review four of the primary ways scholars have conceptualized culture: (a) culture as ethnicity and race, (b) culture as speech communities, (c) culture as worldviews, and (d) culture as a living process.

A.   Culture as Ethnic and Racial Group

Ethnic group, race, and nation are three distinct concepts that often share a single core that implicates a shared culture. According to Fenton (2013), **race** is defined by a group of persons connected by common descent or origin; in contrast, a **nation** involves an aggregate of people closely associated with each other by common descent, language, or history as to form a distinct race of people usually organized as a separate political state, occupying a definite territory. **Ethnic group** pertains to a race or nation, having common racial, cultural, religious, or linguistic characteristics shared by a specific group within a larger system. Although laypeople may think of race or ethnic categories as biological categories that involve distinctive phenotype or unique traits (e.g., Caucasians are white; Hispanic people have dark hair; Asians have brown eyes;

Rethinking Culture in Health Communication: Social Interactions as Intercultural Encounters,
First Edition. Elaine Hsieh and Eric M Kramer.
© 2021 John Wiley & Sons, Inc. Published 2021 by John Wiley & Sons, Inc.

or indigenous people are vulnerable to diabetes), researchers are increasingly wary of imposing racial or ethnic categories, a *social construct*, to examine genetic variations because such an approach overemphasizes the influences of genetic components and can overexaggerate the salience of race (Paradies et al. 2007). Some researchers cautioned that genetic variations between populations are issues framed through political and commercial motivations, which can lead to the conflation of race, ethnicity, and nationality with biological differences as well as discrimination of certain groups (Kahn 2014; Lee 2015). Nevertheless, in this book, we recognize that they tend to overlap so much that they are almost interchangeable designations in much of the literature prior to the 1980s.

The word ethnic derives from the Greek *ethnikos*, meaning heathen. Later in Middle English (i.e., the form of English spoken after the Norman conquest until the late 15th century), "ethnic" came to mean a person who was not a Christian ("Ethnic," 2016). Today these connotations remain, but more commonly, **ethnic identity** is related to one's origin by birth or descent and/or membership in a subgroup as contrasted with a person of the so-called "mainstream" majority of present nationality. For instance, in the United States, "ethnic" cuisine often means non-Western food. In terms of music, it tends to mean non-English lyrics.

Ethnic tends to mean someone *other* – someone not descendent from the majority cultural tradition within designated boundaries (Fenton, 2013). The word ethnic has become increasingly problematic as it fragments populations into groups. Such fragmentations typically involve notions of mainstream power and privilege: what is "normal" as opposed to foreign or exotic. Hence, identification of mainstream versus subgroups often involves inequality of opportunity. Such categorical designations constitute structural distinctions often related to race, language, and religion.

In more enlightened societies, ethnic diversity may not have the negative connotations of "heathen" Other, but instead may be celebrated. Under such sociocultural tolerance, each tradition may be recognized as providing unique and valuable cultural knowledge, fashions, beliefs, practices, styles, and solutions that enrich society. All cultures face a relatively common set of challenges such as child-rearing, building shelter, procuring sustenance, organizing work, passing on knowledge to the next generation, coping with aging, and so forth. The more essential a need (e.g., shelters, food, or healthcare), the more likely people are willing to tolerate differences. A starving man will not pass up an American hamburger just because he prefers sushi.

Diversity in any ecosystem enables that system to cope with stresses. Monocultural systems are very vulnerable to failure because they have only one solution to a problem (Kramer, 2003). The Irish starved because they had been forced to replace their traditional agriculture made up of a variety of plants with just the potato. Consequently, when that one food source failed, they were in trouble (Brown, 2019). Similarly, ethnic diversity provides an expanded repertoire of solutions to problems people face in daily life. It also presents a multiplicity of cuisines, clothing fashions, philosophies, spiritual systems, sports, and entertainments, pedagogical practices, and so forth that people can select from, combine in various ways, and enjoy.

Streeck (2002) critiqued the conceptualization of cultures as distinctive entities or categories of people is "a product of late 19th-century anthropology and its contexts, colonialism" (p. 301). Additionally, Streeck (2002) notes that we tend to "assume discreteness and distinctions where in reality there are only fuzzy boundaries, [and] we inadvertently homogenize the entities that we call *cultures*; we abstract from history, notably histories of migration, as well as its effects, such as cultural borrowing and hybridization" (p. 301). Ethnic ways offer various lifestyles, including dietary regimes that modern science is studying for solutions to illness and infirmity. Being open to diversity is a strategy that enables us to expand our repertoire of solutions. Rather than ethnocentrically rejecting solutions from other cultures, increasingly in our global world of information exchange, people are seeking out and testing solutions no matter their geographical or ethnic origins. Because we all face illness, accidents, aging, and death, such aspects of the human condition transcend ethnic, racial, and even national boundaries. But cultural and linguistic barriers exist. When conflicting values become salient, simple adoption of foreign ways is difficult.

Cultural distance (i.e., how similar one culture is to another) influences how much a specific practice is adopted unchanged. The closer two cultures are, the more likely the solutions will be transferred with little alteration. The more distant cultures are, the more likely solutions (e.g., yoga or cancer treatment) will take on an accent so to speak, meaning a modality or way of doing it that is more acceptable and functional for local populations and their norms, beliefs, values, motives, and expectations. Although people may strive to preserve "authentic" styles and practices, the ways health maintenance and healthcare are practiced still varies from place to place. As modern medical practices spread and fuse with local practices, healthcare, and health maintenance mix global with local tendencies. Such differences include what people prefer in terms of food and what foods are available. Such differences include gender norms so that exercise classes in one culture may include both sexes but in other cultures are strictly unisex. Such differences include the level of participation and access of spiritual leaders with medical practitioners. Such differences include the participation of family members in medical interventions, including information sharing. These and many other differences are rooted in cultural traditions that are shaped by sociocultural histories and geopolitical environments. The fusional product is a **glocal** (i.e., global + local) set of normative practices, motives, and expectations guided by local values, beliefs, and access. Even within a country, there are differences between rural and urban healthcare cultures. Thus, all healthcare has an accent. Rural American health practices are limited by economic and other factors that make them different from urban American healthcare.

Rather than seeing culture as the "natural order of things," cultural scholars increasingly recognize that cultural difference is "a product of human agency" that involves "the contested and shifting nature of cultural identities and cultural borders" (Streeck, 2002, pp. 301–302). This emerging approach allows scholars to move away from a static, passive understanding of culture and cultural groups imposed by dominant groups and instead examine culture as dynamic activities to be performed and negotiated between cultural participants.

B. Culture as Speech Community

The fields of linguistics, anthropology, neuroscience, and communication agree that the language you speak structures how you perceive and understand the world (O'Neill, 2015; Zlatev & Blomberg, 2015). Sociolinguist John J. Gumperz (1968/2009) argued that a **speech community** is defined by "the speech varieties employed within [the community] because they are related to a set of social norms" (p. 67). In other words, conceptualizing culture as speech communities means that a cultural group can be classified according to their communicative practices: "their usage, their origins, and the relationship between speech and social action that they reflect" (Gumperz, 1968/2009, p. 67).

The language you speak enables (and limits) how you can express everything from the sense you have of your body, to your identity, your feelings, your desires, fears, ambitions, and so forth. Language and culture combine and integrate to form the human lifeworld of sense and meaning that is conveyed and shared by communication. Some, such as cultural anthropologist Edward T. Hall (1976) even argued that culture is communication. Cultural anthropologist Clifford Geertz (1973) argued, "The concept of culture I espouse... is essentially a semiotic one" (p. 5). **Semiotics** is the study of signs, including the meanings, productions, and impacts of signs. He believed that the best way to study culture is to do so using phenomenological semiotics because culture is a thick web of meanings articulated through signs and symbols. Semiotics is the study of "the life of signs in society" (de Saussure, 2011, p. 16).

Talk structures reality. Language is the ultimate system with structures that evolve. As cultures meet, they borrow from each other. And with modern globalization, languages, and cultures are evolving faster than ever before. People are more connected and less isolated by geographical distance or barriers. More than ever, many languages and their worldviews are being displaced by others and going extinct (Trudgill, 1991).

The approach Geertz takes is to recognize both the attempt to draw broad generalizations about culture as a distinctly human phenomenon across time and place and to also demand that we focus on the differences that make the study of culture valuable. Similarly, we can speak of language as a quintessential human product and activity, but it is the difference between languages that present different ways of being in the world. This is the source of and motivation for our social scientific investigations into comparative healthcare systems and how glocalization (i.e., globalization and localization) is resulting in a mixing of ideas, solutions, and techniques. These differences are both interesting in and of themselves, and also present opportunities for exchange and sharing along with the difficulties of translating meanings that motivate our study. Not everyone is the same. It is the differences that are most intriguing and challenging.

Geertz (1973) defined culture as "a system of inherited conceptions expressed in symbolic forms by means of which men [sic] communicate, perpetuate, and develop their knowledge about and attitudes toward life" (p. 89). What emerges then is the confluence of community and culture as *shared symbol systems* rooted in linguistic diversity. Geertz (1973) explained:

> One of the most significant facts about us may finally be that we all begin with the natural equipment to live a thousand kinds of life but end in the end having lived only one.
>
> The "control mechanism" view of culture begins with the assumption that human thought is basically both social and public – that its natural habitat is the house yard, the marketplace, and the town square. Thinking consists not of "happenings in the head" (though happenings there and elsewhere are necessary for it to occur) but of a traffic in what have been called, by G. H. Mead and others, significant symbols – words for the most part but also gestures, drawings, musical

> sounds, mechanical devices like clocks, or natural objects like jewels – anything, in fact, that is disengaged from its mere actuality and used to impose meaning upon experience. From the point of view of any particular individual, such symbols are largely given. He finds them already current in the community when he is born, and they remain, with some additions, subtractions, and partial alterations he may or may not have had a hand in, in circulation after he dies. (p. 45)

Unlike instinct, culture is learned behavior and learning does not take place "in our heads" but through interactions with the world, including others, *outside* our heads. We are cultural beings but that also means we are social beings. Culture is passed on from one generation to the next via symbolic interaction. The world is sustained by conversation.

C. Culture as Worldview

By noting that social worlds are constructed through social actions, Geertz (1973) emphasized the importance of not viewing culture as a general catch-all concept, which provides little insights into the actual lived-world of real human beings. Instead, he noted that situating cultures in the context of other cultures (for identity relies on difference), recognizing the complexity of social norms and practices, can help uncover rich information and in-depth understanding of cultural nuances and diversities to enrich our worlds. As languages and communicative practices structure and sustain our reality, cultural **worldviews** embedded in these social actions are implied, often taken-for-granted as essential pillars of such realities. The concept of worldviews has different roots, including in the fields of philosophy, history, and anthropology (Hiebert, 2008). Worldviews are more than speech practices or social actions. They also consist of social norms. Worldviews are the "fundamental cognitive, affective, and evaluative presuppositions a group of people make about the nature of things, and which they use to order their lives;" in other words, worldviews are "what people in a community take as given realities, the maps they have of reality that they use for living" (Hiebert, 2008, p. 15). People do not "make" their worldview but presume their worldview, which enables them to live a life of meaning and purpose.

Worldviews allow cultural participants to *orient* to their social worlds and to *comprehend* events taking place in their realities (Note et al., 2008). By orientation, we mean that worldviews function as a compass, creating boundaries of what is "right," "true," "real," "ethical," and "moral." These guiding posts allow cultural participants to make sense of their experiences, creates meanings in their everyday life. Note and colleagues (2008) argued that cultural participants "semi-consciously or consciously" interpret their experiences as insights – which "functions as beacons, guiding people through their lives in two basic matters: ethical matters and matters regarding the 'being'/ becoming of the world" (p. 2). We are lost without these beacons. Without a worldview, we are no more than zombies moving through the world because whatever happens or does not happen – has no meaning. From this perspective, worldviews are not just implied in our social realities, they are the fundamentals of our realities – they are the basis of all meanings and values within a culture. As such, people rarely question their worldviews in part because that involves questioning their own identity and perceived reality.

In this book, we will introduce the readers to three major cultural perspectives: Magic Consciousness, Mythic Connection, and Perspectival Thinking. Each world-view relies on a specific approach to reality and mode of communication. We will continue to revisit these cultural approaches throughout the book.

D. Culture as a Living Process

The world is constituted of an infinite number of channels of information. And the flowing of information is combined by us. This process of combination is fusional. One way to think about culture and identity is not as things but as *processes*. By conceptualizing culture as processes of communication within "systems of distributed cognition," which include human actors, material representation systems (e.g., machines and artificial intelligence), built space (e.g., farms and urban cities), sociocultural environments (e.g., temporal dimensions and geopolitical tensions), and other actors (e.g., family members), researchers have begun to recognize the dynamic and interactive nature of culture (Streeck, 2002). Hence, we can say that the word culture is not a noun but a verb: **culturing**. Rodriguez (2002) proposed that by verbing our understanding of culture, we recognize that "human beings are fundamentally relational beings with a striving and potentiality for communion with the world and each other" (p. 9). We never stop learning and changing. Past experiences effect how we learn in the future. Culturing conceptualizes cultures as a process of constant integration of past experience with new experience.

Out of this process emerges consciousness. Human consciousness is always linguistic and cultural. Consciousness is constantly transforming (Husserl, 1962; Kramer, 1992, 2019). This means that we always think in words and have a perspective but also that awareness itself is always an awareness of difference, of things changing. It also means that our perspectives are always changing. And the words we use both enable and limit our ability to conceive and to express. Language does not belong to us. Rather it is a social phenomenon and as Michel Foucault (1966/2005) put it, we belong to the language that enables us to communicate. Language is transcendental, which means it transcends us and gives us access to others. We must conform to its conventions or else we cannot participate as a member of our community. Without language, the world has no sense and events and objects have no meaning. Since our language is limited and changes slowly, our reality is fairly stable. The sense and meaning of things endure making possible culture and identity as reliable referents. Though language is conventional, it is so fundamental to our worldview that it anchors our reality. As we change (e.g., become more educated), our vocabulary also changes and so does our way of seeing and talking about the world, including ourselves.

When different linguistic communities meet, they almost always borrow words from each other to expand their worldview, to be able to reference phenomena that are new to their experience. Examples we find in Japan today are enjin (engine), kamera (camera), karendaa (calendar), arubaito (from the German arbeit meaning a part-time job), kiss suru (to kiss), taipu suru (to type), konputa (computer), jetto (jet), biiru (from Dutch bier), kohi (coffee), gamu (chewing gum), and so forth. But is this even "Japanese?"

Language, like the rest of reality and our consciousness, is always evolving and as languages mix, the notion of a "pure" language or culture proves to be an obsolete belief. As Japan was exposed to these foreign things and adopted them, they also adopted the words to talk about them. And with the transfer of foreign things such as food and technology comes new expectations, beliefs, and values. Examples of Japanese words adopted by English speakers include honcho (boss), skosh (a small amount of something), origami, bokeh (the aesthetic quality of out-of-focus areas in an image), bonsai, karaoke, tycoon (businessperson with exceptional wealth and power), kimono, hibachi, emoji, ramen, soy, futon, koi, tsunami, and so forth. And many "Japanese" words are borrowed from Chinese, just as many English words are derived from Greek and Latin.

Similarly, when investigating the clinical impacts of acupuncture, an important medical skill in East Asian medicine, scientists do not simply follow the prescriptive boundaries and norms of a homogenous, scientific community of biomedicine. Rather than seeking a direct theoretical correspondence between acupuncture and science, biomedical scientists have actively negotiated and constructed different "practices" (Pickering, 2010) – resulting in an "active and emergent 'production' in the exchange of two cultures, not a 'reproduction' from one culture to another" (Kim, 2006, p. 2971). *When cultures collide, the corresponding worldviews do not stay intact; rather, the resulting discourse often reflects a fused world.* Dissemination of meaning and innovation is a continuous process (Derrida, 1973).

In conservative societies, change is slow; in contrast, change is accelerated in progressive societies. One might believe, for instance, that Japan is a conservative society. But in the last century, few societies have embraced so many foreign ideas, technologies, customs, beliefs, and values as have the Japanese. And this includes not merely borrowing the practice of wearing blue jeans, attending university, giving a girl an engagement ring or celebrating Christmas, but also in healthcare and medicine. A technology such as air conditioning brings with it a whole host of innovations and potentialities that change how people behave as well as their expectations and motivations. This is a process of **cultural fusion**, which is the adoption and modification of foreign ways into an already functional cultural system.

As you may have noticed, some scholars have conceptualized culture as a fixed set of shared beliefs, values, and behavior patterns. We propose that expectations and motivations are vital to understanding the meanings and practices of culture. In addition, our values, beliefs, motives, and expectations do not remain eternally stable especially in a modern society. The convenience of international travel and advanced technology can create fundamental shifts in our worldviews. Because of smartphones and the Internet, I expect to be able to communicate all the time no matter where I am or what I am doing. Such an expectation did not exist before the invention of cellular communications. In the medical field, technologies, and techniques are changing rapidly and so too are our expectations and even our values. Today, we are confronted with previously unimagined choices that impact our culture, our selves, and force us to reassess our motives and values.

II. Learning and Experiencing Magic Consciousness in Health Contexts

Our goal in this book is to help you recognize culture and cultural perspectives in your everyday life. This approach will enable you to build practical skills to collaborate with one another and achieve mutually shared objectives. Now that you know about how cultures have been conceptualized and studied, we want to introduce you to three primary ways we will be talking about cultures when thinking about health-related topics from cultural perspectives: Magic Consciousness (i.e., Idolic Communication; Chapter 2), Mythic Connection (i.e., Symbolic Communication; Chapter 3), and Perspectival Thinking (i.e., Signalic Communication; Chapter 4). These three perspectives and forms of communication are conceptually distinct from one another, yet they are also interrelated. You may find yourself more inclined to a particular type of cultural perspective than others depending on the contexts or the issues that arise. In the next few chapters, we will discuss these cultural perspectives in detail. For now, let's start with the most fundamental and primal of the three cultural perspectives: **Magic Consciousness**.

The ways we "learn" about Magic Consciousness is very different from the ways we learn literature or science. We do not learn Magic Consciousness in a school-like setting. Magic Consciousness is learned through socialization.

The main difference between Magic Consciousness, Mythic Connection, and Perspectival Thinking is how much messages matter to you, how much reality changes, including identities, when something is communicated. Reality under Magic Consciousness is created as the speech is uttered. There is no distinction between speech and reality. What is said is what it is. As the social action is performed, realities come to existence. Identities and boundaries are formed accordingly.

For example, when a king is coronated, a judge is installed, a priest is ordained, a president is inaugurated, a doctor takes the Hippocratic Oath, they must publicly pronounce their allegiance to a set of principles and duties and repeat an oath out loud. It is a formal and solemn promise. Once the ritual is performed, their identities, including their power, duty, authority, and obligation, are transformed (see Figure 2.1). What they cannot do also changes. A judge cannot remain a judge if she is found publicly to have violated the law. A physician can also lose their right to practice medicine if they are found to have violated law and oath.

When President John F. Kennedy was assassinated, just a little over one hour after he died, Lyndon Johnson took the "oath of office" on an airplane from Texas to

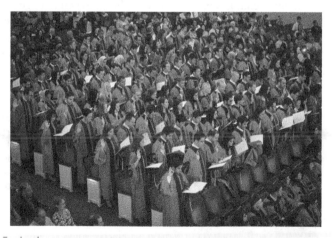

Figure 2.1 Graduation ceremony at Weill Cornell Medical College. Rituals and ceremonies are central to Magic Consciousness as they mark "rite of passage" when one becomes an official member of a group. *Source:* Taken by Author during Graduation ceremony at Weill Cornell Medicine

Washington D.C. Onboard the plane, there was a scramble to find a Bible so that Federal Judge Sarah T. Hughs could "swear in" the new President. Kennedy's widow and other authorities packed into the airplane to witness and authenticate the transition of power. Such authentication confirms that something has changed. Judges too are confirmed, and "confirmation" is the label used to describe the process of a person becoming a member of a religion. Confirmation means agreement among people. It is a community event that recognizes a change in a person's identity and their relationship to the rest of us. As Johnson became President of the United States, all duties and obligations were transferred to him (see Figure 2.2). At the moment of "swearing-in," power literally shifted from one person to the next. One minute a person has little power, the next he or she literally commands armies. They become the "head of state," and they are called a new name, "Mr. President." How that person behaves, what they are able to do, and the behavior of all around that person changes dramatically. Reality changes and history is made. It was very serious and emotional, with profound and real consequences.

Under Magic Consciousness, we engage in idolic communication. **Idolic communication** refers to communication that the talk itself "embodies the power to change reality" (Kramer, 2013, p. 148). Under Magic Consciousness, when someone says, "I love you," the talk itself evokes the reality of love. The statement is not to explain or indicate that one has love for another; rather, as the words are uttered, something profound has changed in reality. A study of 1459 multilingual adults (of 77 different languages) found that 45% of the participants reported to the greatest emotional weight of the phrase *I love you* when it is spoken in their first language, which is often the language closest to our heart (Dewaele, 2008). Several studies also suggest that we feel the strongest *emotional forces* of our language in emotion-related expressions (e.g., cursing, taboo words, and reading fictions) in our native language, which is the first language we use to develop identities and build relationships (Dewaele, 2004; Harris et al., 2003; Hsu et al., 2015). Because identities and reality are literally changed by idolic invocation and evocation, they are very emotional. Being pronounced a "winner" may evoke joy. Being pronounced a loser, heartbreak. We tend to remember idolic moments the most. Such changes may often be for life as when a judge is appointed, confirmed, and takes the oath of office to become a Supreme Court Justice. As words are said, a new reality takes place (see Figure 2.3). The new reality is as real and concrete as any "real" and "concrete" things. It is not make-believe. It is what it is, defining who we are and what we do. Magic Consciousness is powerful.

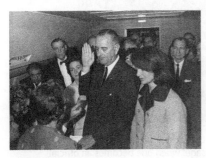

Figure 2.2 Oath of office by Lyndon Johnson. Sarah T. Hughes, U.S. District Judge, Northern District of Texas, administering the oath of office to Lyndon B. Johnson in the conference room aboard Air Force One at Love Field, Dallas, Texas. *Source:* Library of Congress, Prints & Photographs Division, NYWT&S Collection, [LC-USZ62-126329]

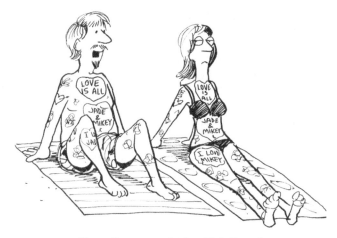

"I mostly communicate with tattoos."

Figure 2.3 When and how to best say, "I love you." For many, tattoos involve Magic Consciousness: What is tattooed is literally who we are.

Magic requires little interpretation. Either it happens, or it does not. Mythic Connection relies on symbolism. Such connections are subject to interpretation and are therefore vulnerable to confusion and conflicts among rival interpretations. Meaning fragments into sections and thus sectarian contention emerges even as efforts at clarification increase. Sometimes, the more an expert such as a medical doctor attempts to clarify what an ailment is and means to a patient, the effort to be more precise can become confusing. Specialized language is necessary for greater precision, but this also challenges the patient's health literacy and ability to understand what is being said. Such confusion can increase anxiety for the patient trying to comprehend what is being said. In contrast, Magic Consciousness involves little interpretation or competition of meanings. The reality is what it is and cannot be subject to individuals' subjective understanding or interpretation. As long as the rituals to coronate a king, confirm a judge, ordain a priest, or inaugurate a president are performed properly, their new identities and authorities cannot be denied.

One cannot not communicate. We try to make sense of everything we see and hear. Storm clouds mean something to us just as a single letter on a report card can mean so much. Sometimes we take things personally, sometimes we don't care. Depending on the context, we can understand things in an idolic sense through Magic Consciousness, in a symbolic way through Mythic Connection, or in a signalic style through Perspectival Thinking. A tumor you have may frighten you very much, prompting you to change your life plans. Or a tumor may be used to describe the source of negative energy in an office environment so that we figuratively say that this attitude is a "cancer" on the organization. As a biology student, a tumor is a group of cells and there are many different kinds that you have to memorize for a test. The first may keep you awake at nights worrying. The second type allows you to express emotion but does not literally mean everyone in the office has cancer. The third is an abstract set of labels you have to remember for a test.

A. Magic Consciousness in Everyday Life

In *Harry Potter*, Lord Voldemort was often not named by most characters but instead they referred to him with expressions such as "You-Know-Who" or "He-Who-Must-Not-Be-Named." But why? It is as if uttering the name itself would call him into being, and that everyone wanted to avoid. Magic communication is incantatory. It invokes and evokes things as it names them. They are identical. If you say the words, the thing appears. The verdict in a courtroom is read, the gavel comes down, and you are guilty. The court may be wrong, and we know sometimes they are. But for you, the person charged with a crime, and everyone who knows you, that concluding statement will change your life; all your relationships are altered and your identity may be forever changed. Another common example is when an authority (or author of reality) "pronounces" a fundamental change in someone's identity such as "I pronounce you husband and wife" or "We see no cancer. I give you a clean bill of health." We put great emotional investment in incantatory and evocative communication. It is a great relief when our doctor tells us we are okay, just as it can create powerful anxiety if she tells us the prognosis is "not good." What they are saying is your identity. You *are* literally healthy, or not. Just as I may tell you, "I am Eric," so too, I might say, "I am healthy."

Another example of Magic Consciousness is oath-taking: when a person publicly swears allegiance to transition from civilian life to become a member of the military or to become a naturalized citizen of a host country. Magic Consciousness is often performed through rituals (i.e., idolic communication). The "proper" ways to do things can make or break a reality under Magic Consciousness. Rule 603 of the Federal Rule of Evidence states, "Before testifying, a witness must give an oath or affirmation to testify truthfully." To be a credible, acceptable witness in a courtroom, one must be willing to swear to tell the truth. You must stand, be recognized by name, and say, "I swear to tell the truth..." out loud. If one refuses to take the oath, she cannot testify in court (see Figure 2.4). Magic communication is often ritualistic. Failure to assume the proper form breaks the Magic.

Magic Consciousness is intensely personal but also extremely public. Performance of the rituals to invoke Magic Consciousness often are both public and personal in nature (Jonassen, 2012). For example, when examining the Founding Fathers' visions of the Presidential Oath of office, Sheppard (2009) noted,

> The oath, by definition, is created by a public institution, indeed drafted by officials of those institutions, but it must be taken personally by the individual, who is required to perform the office with particular care and (sometimes impliedly and sometimes explicitly) for the benefit of the public. This duality [is] inherent in the "subscription" by which a person takes an oath, and the "office" that requires the oath itself. (p. 276)

Witnessing such incantatory communication is an essential part. Speaking out loud is a public act that changes the socially shared and constructed reality. The transformation is not limited to the person who performed the oath but also the public that witnessed the performance.

Magic Consciousness identifies us with others – as we talk, the participants are unified as one. Talking with others is an end in itself. We seek friends out just to talk and be social. It is the foundation of a community. When members of the northern Natal

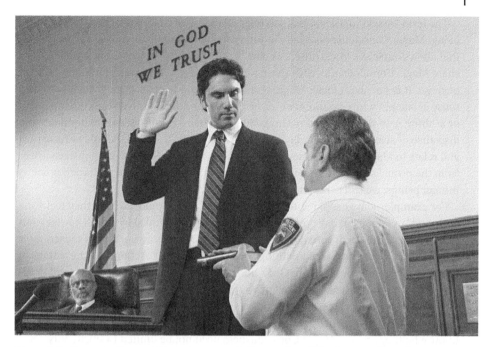

Figure 2.4 Sworn testimony. Although some variations and modifications are allowed to accommodate people who feel uncomfortable swearing religious oath in courts, a common oath in the U.S. courts is: "Do you solemnly swear that the testimony you may give in the case now pending before this court shall be the truth, the whole truth, and nothing but the truth, so help you God?" *Source:* Image Source/Getty Images

tribes of South Africa greets one another every day, they say, "Sawabona," which literally means "I see you." The proper response is "Sikhona," which means "I am here." The order of the greeting is important because *one come into existence as s/he is seen by others.* It is their belief that "a person is a person only through human connection, through recognition of one another" (Nelson & Lundin, 2010, p. 2). To see is not just about the physical vision. It is to understand one another, to open our mind and heart to experience one another and to share the present. At that moment, we come to being because we are connected to one another, unified as a single unit of *one.*

In contrast, symbolic communication through Mythic Connection (in Chapter 3) also supports communities but with less commitment and relational intensity. Since stories involve interpretation, symbolic mythic communication also tends to promote diverging meanings due to competing interpretations. Signalic communication through Perspectival Thinking (in Chapter 4) tends to be very abstract and functional. Signalic communication is instrumental, meaning that I talk with someone as a means to do something else, like pay for my groceries, and nothing more.

Pronouncing aloud to others expresses a manifest change in identity. Under Magic Consciousness, to say something out loud or to personally sign a document in "your own hand" – makes it so. In *Armance*, the hero's mother refuses to say "tuberculosis," for fear that pronouncing the word will hasten the progress of her son's illness (Stendhal, 1827/2016). Somehow, by uttering these taboo words, a corresponding "magic" reality will be invoked and materialized. Best to not speak them.

The term "magic" does not mean to refer to a sense of superpower or a supernatural being. Magic Consciousness exists in interpersonal relationships: it is a primal bond that allows ourselves to see others as part of ourselves – an extension of our being. We share Magic Consciousness with those we love and hate. It is the emotional source of purpose. It is not about logic. Magic relationships and feelings grow from a profound sense of *oneness* with one another (i.e., become one with the universe, another person, or a "thing"). In the modern-day United States, when logic and statistics dominate the discourse of science and everyday life, it may be difficult for individuals to recognize and relate to Magic Consciousness. Nevertheless, because Magic Consciousness arises from the primal sentiment that we share with the larger world and with each other as human beings, we still experience it in our everyday lives.

For example, some people with strong religious faith would say that they feel "one with God" in their everyday life. They are connected and guided by God. They feel that God is doing good deeds *through* them. They are his hands at work. God's teaching is felt and experienced as real as anything in the earthly world. Actions are the actions of God. "My" accomplishments are God's accomplishments. Empirical events and products are manifestations of God's will. If you ask them who they would be without God, they would be at a loss for words. If God is not in their life, not part of who they are and how they live their life, their loss of identity would be so profound that they would not know who they are. But Magic Consciousness need not be limited to spirituality.

When we experience Magic Consciousness, we do not rely on knowledge, logic, or analytical reasoning to navigate our world. Instead, it is experienced "as is" – it is real. No additional justification or reasoning is required. One of the most common magic bonds in individuals' interpersonal relationship is the parent-child relationship. Parents and children hold such a Magic Consciousness that renders the two entities inseparable and indistinguishable. When you are hurt, your parents feel hurt. The hurt and pain are not because of a sense of empathy or that they "share" your pain. Your parents are hurt, literally, because you are hurt. There are no differences between you and your parents. The feelings are shared as one. When someone punches you in your stomach, your parents do not think that "their child" was attacked – they feel that *they* were the one that was punched in the stomach. They felt *we* were victims of an attack. The shared bond between your parents and you motivate them to do anything for you. They cannot separate their life meanings without you. Losing you would render their lives meaningless and their future hopeless. This is because you are not separate from them, *you are them*, a fundamental, essential part of who they are, how they see themselves. Magic Consciousness is extremely powerful because there is no limit to their belief or love in you. They can always find more strength and love regardless how difficult the situation. It is self-(re)energizing. There is no giving up until the "magic" is broken.

B. Emotions and Magic Consciousness

Magic Consciousness is intensely personal because holding Magic Consciousness intact and protecting its survival is essential to the existence of the person. Losing a child is a destabilizing experience of identities and life meanings for any parent. For many, such an experience is unthinkable and unacceptable. Because Magic Consciousness calls out the profound, fundamental bonds we hold dear to our social world and worldviews, it is also deeply emotional. Magic Consciousness is pre-cognition. When operating under Magic Consciousness, we do not calculate the cost-benefit analysis, weighing one option against another. We are not disinterested observers. It would be silly to ask a mother how much she is willing to sacrifice for her child. No price is too high. The sky is the limit. In other words, when Magic Consciousness guides our decision-making and sense-making, we stick to our gut instinct, which cannot be questioned or challenged through logic or reason.

For example, if you are diagnosed with end-stage cancer, the last thought on your parents' mind would be about how much your treatment is going to cost them. They will not be thinking about whether it is "worth it" to remortgage the house so that you can have the new experimental treatment that may give you a 20% chance of living for another five years. Your siblings will not be angry at you that they have to take up part-time jobs to pay for their education because you are "using up" their resources. When a family member faces a serious illness, the whole family bonds together and face the challenge as a whole. In fact, it would break your heart if your parents never told you that one of them has been struggling with terminal cancer for months and they did not want to "bother" you with the bad news. You'd probably feel extreme anger and complete desertion if you then learned that all your other siblings knew about this but you. Experiencing calamity *together* as one is Magic Consciousness. To not to be included in the process is like being told that you are not one of "us."

C. Magic Consciousness: Non-White by Laws

Different cultures may hold different forms of Magic Consciousness that shape their worldviews and guide their everyday thinking and practices. Magic Consciousness is a deeply felt experience. Individuals who hold such a Magic Consciousness have an intense emotional investment towards its meanings and implications. As such, it is not uncommon to see cultures creating a discourse that impute morality through Magic Consciousness and even codify such moral values through laws.

For example, in many cultures, blood represents a form of Magic Consciousness. The concept and sentiment of blood purity was prominent in Nazi Germany when the government instituted laws that required people who wished to join the Nazi Party to obtain a German Blood Certificate (German: Deutschblütigkeitserklärung), a document provided by Hitler to Mischlinge (those with partial Jewish heritage), declaring them deutschblütig (of German blood). The efforts to maintain the purity of the Aryan race was so strong that those who had three or four generations of Jewish grandparents were considered Jews. Aryan and Jewish families already married were encouraged to divorce because such relationships were deemed "blood treason," an extremely emotional rhetoric. These legal efforts and social pressures to maintain blood purity paved the path toward the Holocaust.

In the United States, the **one-drop rule** is a social and legal principle of racial classification, asserting that any person with even one ancestor of sub-Saharan-African ancestry is considered Black (i.e., "one-drop" of Black blood makes a person Black). The one drop rule has shaped countless lives and shaped the history of the United States for centuries (Green, 2006). One of the earliest judicial rulings is a Virginia case, *In Re Mulatto*, issued in 1656 in which the court held that although the litigant had both European and African ancestries, it was the African ancestry that both defined his status and determined his fate as a slave (i.e., his European ancestry made no legally significant difference at all in defining his multi-racial status; Hickman, 1997).

Because Magic Consciousness is often about preserving and protecting something so valuable to the very being (not just an identity, but the "essence") of an entity, whether it is an individual or a nation, people are highly motivated to protect it without concerns about the ensuing implications, consequences, or costs. For example, a 1691 Virginia statute not only banished Whites who intermarried with a Black or a biracial person but also fined a White woman who had a "bastard child by a Negro," added five years to her term if she was an indentured servant (Hickman, 1997). Such "bastard" biracial children then were committed to slavery until the age of thirty, regardless of the status of the White mother (Hickman, 1997). For a time, Maryland took an even a stronger stand, *enslaving* White women who, "to the disgrace of our nation," married Blacks, as well as enslaving their children (Williamson, 1995). For White supremacists, because the purity of blood is so sacred that anyone, including White women, who pose risks to tainting the blood deserves to be punished. The White-nonwhite color line continued to impact U.S. history well into the 20th century. For example, Virginia passed a Racial Integrity Law in 1924, creating two racial categories: "pure" White and all others. The statute defined a "White" person as one with "no trace whatsoever of blood other than Caucasian" and legally ban interracial marriages (Sherman, 1988, p. 75).

The power of Magic Consciousness in a culture is pervasive and long-lasting. The racial classification through the one-drop rule is so profound that despite the changes made through the Civil Rights Movement in the 1960s, the legalization of interracial marriages (anti-miscegenation laws were deemed unconstitutional in the 1967 Supreme Court case, *Loving v. Virginia*), and the following movements on racial equality, many Black-White Americans' appraisals about their identities are still fundamentally shaped by the one-drop rule today (Khanna, 2010), viewing themselves and their peers as Black despite their biracial status. The 44th President of the United States, Barak Obama, is often referenced as the first African American to be elected to that Office – even though he is biracial, born to a White mother and a Black father.

In the U.S. Census, between 1790 and 1950, "White" was a racial category to be determined by census takers sometimes "taking into account how individuals were perceived in their community or using rules based on their share of 'black blood'" (Williams, 2019, p. 12). It was not until 1960, almost two hundred years later, that U.S. residents were allowed to choose their own race. Until 2000, U.S. residents do not have the option to identify with more than one racial category in the census (Parker et al., 2015). Due to the historical and cultural contexts in the United States, researchers concluded, "Blackness continues to constitute a fundamental racial construction in American society" (Lee & Bean, 2007). Black multiracial individuals face persistent and rigid constraints in defining their racial identities that reinforce and limit their identities as "Black." The Magic Consciousness of blood remains influential in the United States.

Recognizing how Magic Consciousness can shape a cultural response and understanding of values, identities, and practices allows practitioners to understand the issues that motivate a person's decision-making in health contexts.

III. Magic Consciousness a Motivating Factor in Health Practices

One of the most common mistakes when it comes to Magic Consciousness is that we instantly recognize the "illogical" and "unreasonable" nature of others' thinking without recognizing the Magic Consciousness held by ourselves. Thinking through the following two scenarios will allow us to reflect on the Magic Consciousness we hold in shaping our thinking and responses when managing health-related issues.

If you are a physician or a nurse, what would you do in the following situations:

1. Ms. Dyani Hunt, a 61-year-old woman with diabetes mellitus (DM) type II and peripheral vascular disease (PVD), presented with several purulent, nonhealing ulcers of the right medial malleolus, sepsis, and wet gangrene of the right leg. She arrived at the hospital because she could no longer walk. After a careful study of her lab work, a surgical consultant recommended a right-sided below-the-knee amputation. However, Ms. Hunt is from a Native American tribe that believes that the body should be kept intact and buried as a whole. When she learned about the recommendation, she said, "I have lived a good life. Being a Native American, I know having diabetes is part of my destiny. I'd rather die now than risk going to hell because I amputated my limb."

2. Mr. John Prince just learned that he has a heart condition that requires an open-heart surgery. However, as a Jehovah's Witness, he cannot accept a blood transfusion. When asked why he cannot accept blood, Mr. Prince explained, "It's my religious belief. Both the Old and New Testaments clearly command us to abstain from blood. Also, God views blood as representing life. So we avoid taking blood not only in obedience to God but also out of respect for Him as the Giver of life." You informed Mr. Prince that an open-heart surgery would be extremely challenging. Mr. Prince responded, "I'd only accept surgery without a blood transfusion."

Can you identify any Magic Consciousness held by Ms. Hunt and Mr. Prince? What are they? How would you respond to their requests? Do you find yourself feeling conflicted or frustrated? Why? Do you think your feelings are shaped by your Magic Consciousness? What are they?

A. Native American Women with Diabetes

1. Bodily Integrity

Many of you will immediately recognize that Ms. Hunt holds a Magic Consciousness about bodily integrity. Here, **bodily integrity** is not just about keeping the body intact or maintaining autonomy over one's body. Rather, bodily integrity is "the point of integration" between a person's subjectivity and the external world (Herring & Wall, 2017, p. 576). In other words, bodily integrity represents an embodied experience through which a person connects to the world and the corresponding worldviews and realities. Even though DM and PVD are chronic conditions that account for the majority of nontraumatic lower extremity amputations, most patients are unprepared for such treatment recommendations and experience a grieving process (Bhuvaneswar et al., 2007), including experiences of anxiety and depression (Coffey et al., 2009).

However, Hunt's refusal to accept amputation as a treatment is not just about being unprepared for or grieving of the loss of a limb. The sorrow is more fundamental – a person needs to be buried "whole" at death in order to have a "good" afterlife. Many Native American tribes believe that the integrity of the body is sacred, and surgery is taboo (Alvord & Van Pelt, 2000). Similar beliefs are shared by some Asian and Arabic patients, whose cultures emphasize the integrity of the whole body for future life (Tseng & Streltzer, 2008). For Chinese people, returning one's body in its original state is essential in demonstrating respect for one's parents and ancestors (Lam & McCullough, 2000). In fact, individuals who hold a strong desire to have the body remain whole, postmortem (e.g., believing bodily integrity is necessary for the next life), is one of the strongest factors in predicting whether a person will volunteer for organ donations (Stephenson et al., 2008). The Magic Consciousness a culture holds toward the integrity of the body postmortem can shape not only a person's decision about whether to accept a life-saving surgery but also whether to donate their organs after death.

2   Diabetes as Fate

Sometimes Magic Consciousness can appear fatalistic because individuals' experiences are perceived to be a part of a larger destiny (Cavanaugh et al., 2008). A study of Prima Indians of southern Arizona found that due to the prevalence of type II diabetes in local communities (i.e., approximately 50% of Prima population over 35 years old have diabetes), many Primas have come to view diabetes as part of their life history (Kozak, 1997). They expect to be sickened by, and to die from, diabetes: Diabetes is inevitable and uncontrollable as an inherited condition that foretells their destiny and even their death (Kozak, 1997). However, such a "surrender" to living with diabetes should not be viewed simply as a passive experience. These Primas have not "given up on life" in a fatalistic sense (Kozak, 1997). Instead, individuals and communities with limited resources often actively interpret and construct their experiences with diabetes to create meanings to their existence and identities in everyday life (e.g., a show of grace and faith in the face of adversity; Pitaloka & Hsieh, 2015). The debilitating illness becomes an essential part of their identities and everyday life, providing resources for them to claim virtues, validate faith, and find peace in everyday suffering (Pitaloka & Hsieh, 2015). From this perspective, Magic Consciousness is not passively accepted by its cultural participants but is actively incorporated, utilized, and performed. In other words, as Ms. Hunt asserts her desire to die from complications of diabetes and to be buried intact, she performs and reinforces her identity as a faithful Native American who is destined to go to heaven after death.

B.   Jehovah's Witnesses Needing an Open-Heart Surgery

1.   Purity through Blood

In 1945, Jehovah's Witnesses promulgated the rule of blood transfusion prohibition in the *Watchtower and Bible and Tract Society* (based on Genesis 9:4; Leviticus 17:10; Deuteronomy 12:23; and the Pauline New Testamentary reiteration in Acts 15:28, 29; Singelenberg, 1990). The issue of refusing blood transfusion did not become a salient issue until the early 1970s (Singelenberg, 1990). Although the emergence of such a belief is more mythologically-oriented (i.e., a desire to define Jehovah's Witnesses as a unique group separated from the outside, "the World"), Jehovah's Witnesses eventually elevated the Biblical scripture (a form of Mythic Connection, which will be explored in greater details in Chapter 3) to the concepts of in-group purity: Blood transfusion becomes an "act of pollution" (Singelenberg, 1990, p. 521). Blood is not simply a bodily fluid or a protein compound. Rather, it defines the very being of a Jehovah's Witnesses. Following the rule "demarcates the believers from the non-believers, thus being one of the most salient identity markers" (Singelenberg, 1990, p. 521). From this perspective, a Jehovah's Witnesses' experiences of blood transfusion are not only emotionally distressing but can be identity-shattering.

2   Claim for a Collective Identity

"For the Faithful, the relinquishing of this possibly life-saving medical therapy can be considered sacrifice as a part of membership" (Singelenberg, 1990, p. 521). Accepting the sacrifice that is prescribed as a moral and valued choice also is "a gesture of trust in the group" that "symbolizes to the group the lengths to which members are willing to go in order to belong – how positively cognized membership is" (Kanter, 1968, p. 505). It is not that the patients who refused blood transfusions do not recognize the significance of their decision and naively believe that God will guarantee positive outcomes. Rather, Magic Consciousness allows Jehovah's Witnesses to find strength in the collective faith and identity to face adversities. Similar to the earlier discussion of "surrender" of patients with diabetes, Jehovah's Witnesses do not see or feel their commitment to refuse all blood products and blood transfusions as a "sacrifice" in the sense that requires them to "lose" something. In contrast, this is an act that empowers them and validates their identities as they live the faithful life of Jehovah's Witnesses. On the other hand, failure to embrace such a practice (e.g., accepting blood donation) would be followed by excommunication (Singelenberg, 1990). In other words, for someone who refuses to accept the Magic Consciousness (i.e., a non-believer to the truth about blood, identity, and salvation as defined by the church), the person loses his or her standing and existence in the group, the one and only group that matters. Individuals may face a significant loss of resources and interpersonal networks when disavowing or ignoring a Magic Consciousness shared by a cultural group. More importantly, they lose themselves.

C.   Reflecting on Our Own Normative Beliefs

These scenarios have presented real-life dilemmas that have serious consequences. The differences in cultural perspectives can be so great that deviations from one's social norm may feel like their "moral compass" is being destroyed (Solomon, 1997). If you feel that some of the arguments presented are problematic, it may be time to consider if your social norms are being tested. Some of these normative beliefs may serve as Magic Consciousness for some people, but as Mythic Connection or Perspectival Thinking for others. Nevertheless, the differences in cultural perspectives underline potential conflicts that a patient may need to navigate and negotiate with others. In addition to the normative beliefs listed below, there are many others that we hold that may conflict with the treatment preferences held by Ms. Hunt and Mr. Prince. We will explore more about these topics and the differences between these three cultural perspectives in later chapters.

In the final section of the Chapter, we will focus on some of the core beliefs that may heighten the tensions between cultural perspectives.

1 *Above All, Do No Harm! (Primum Non Nocere)*

For many physicians, a patient's refusal for a simple life-saving procedure, whether it is a lower-extremity amputation or a blood transfusion, is deeply disturbing. After all, "do no harm" is part of the Hippocratic Oath in *Epidemics* (Book I, Chapter XI): "As to diseases, make a habit of two things – to help, or at least to do no harm" (Markel, 2004). "Do no harm" does not officially appear in the Hippocratic Oath; however, the expression *primum non nocere* (do no harm) has had and continues to have a strong oral tradition in guiding medical practice since the 1800s (Smith, 2005). However, the concept is deficient and problematic when the definitions of benefit and harm are contested (Smith, 2005). Is it harmful to ensure a patient's immediate survival even when the act damages the patient's Magic Consciousness? Is it harmful to prolong a patient's life at the expense of quality or dignity of life? Who gets to decide whether a harm exists and whether and how to best avoid it? What happens if a physician does not share the same Magic Consciousness with his or her patient (e.g., believing that a person does not have an afterlife and thus, does not need to be concerned about the integrity of a body in life or after death or alternatively, believing that committing/ assisting suicide is a mortal sin)? Asking a physician to forgo a life-saving procedure or to perform assisted suicide may pose fundamental ethical questions that challenge the oath and ethical guidelines one is compelled to follow.

2 Freedom of Religion

One of the most difficult medical-legal problems faced by healthcare facilities is the treatment of Jehovah's Witnesses who need a blood transfusion but refuse it based on religious grounds (Bamberger, 1987). Religious freedom is of such importance to the identity and culture of the United States that it is ascribed to its Constitution. The First Amendment, adopted in 1791, states, "Congress shall make no law respecting an establishment of religion, or prohibiting the free exercise thereof[.]" It forbids Congress from both promoting one religion over another or restricting an individual's religious practices.

The desire to protect individuals' religious freedom is so intense that 45 states and Washington D.C. (with the exception of California, Maine, Mississippi, New York, and West Virginia) also instituted **religious exemptions** to the mandatory vaccination requirements for children despite the increased risk of jeopardizing the health of local communities (National Conference of State Legislatures, 2020). As religious and phil-osophical (i.e., non-medical) exemptions have drastically increased since the early 2000s, researchers have found an increase in outbreaks of preventable disease rates in areas with high exemption rates (Bradford & Mandich, 2015; Gostin, 2015). More recently, employers have relied on religious exemptions to deny employees certain health insurance coverage (e.g., birth control; de Vogue, 2020; Gasper, 2015). Patients may not realize they received limited care because some hospitals not only deny patients certain healthcare services (e.g., emergency contraception for rape victims) but also prohibit healthcare providers from discussing the availability of such health options elsewhere due to the hospitals' religious affiliation (Smugar & Spina, 2000; Takahashi et al., 2019). In July 2020, the Trump Administration proposed to allow homeless shelters to turn away transgender people from single-sex facilities to better accommodate the "religious beliefs of shelter providers" (Cameron, 2020, para. 2).

Although the Founding Fathers may have started with Perspectival Thinking when they incorporated religious freedom in the Constitution to ensure the separation of Church and State, for some, freedom of religion is so fundamental to the identity, existence, and meanings of the United States that it represents a Magic Consciousness of the United States. As such, it is not to be questioned or challenged. From this perspective, the United States without religious freedom will no longer be "the United States." As a result, though other countries may be less willing to accommodate a person's religious belief, the United States (and its healthcare environment) is willing to go to great length to protect a person's right to exercise religion, including imposing increased risk, compromising the quality of care, and incurring unequal treatments to many others.

3 Right to Bodily Integrity

In the United States, individuals' right to refuse medical treatment, including life-saving procedures, is grounded in the common-law right of self-determination (i.e., a person has right to control one's own body and to free from nonconsensual bodily invasion) and the constitutional right of privacy (Kanaboshi, 2006). As such, a physician or a government may feel that they do not have the right to force a person to accept a life-saving medical procedure, even if the procedure is minor (e.g., blood transfusion) or important to public health (e.g., vaccination). During the COVID-19 pandemic in 2020, many resisted wearing facemasks, arguing that they have the right to decide for themselves (Wong, 2020). On the other hand, in healthcare settings, the normative belief for bodily integrity can be challenged when an adult parent refuses medical treatment on behalf of their minor children. To what extent should we protect a parent's right to care for his/her children? To what extent should we protect a person's right to bodily integrity even if it imposes risks to the general public (e.g., not wearing a facemask during the COVID-19 pandemic)?

IV. Additional Resources

A. Key Terms and Theories

race
nation
ethnic group
ethnic identity
cultural distance
glocal (or glocalization)
speech community
semiotics
worldviews
culturing
cultural fusion
Magic Consciousness

idolic communication
one-drop rule
bodily integrity
religious exemption

B. Discussion Questions

1. What are your race, ethnicity, and nation? Why do you describe it that way?
   a. Do you agree that race and ethnicity is a social construct?
   b. In what ways are race and ethnicity as labels of people beneficial?
   c. In what ways are race and ethnicity as labels of people harmful?
2. Can you identify the speech community or communities you to which you belong? How do you know? What are the noticeable communicative practices or speech patterns of the community?
3. Can you identify your worldviews? If you were to describe the pillars that form your understanding of your "being/becoming of the world" or your ethical principles, what would they be? Are there certain things or values that without which you would not know your place in the world?
4. If we think of culturing as a verb, a living process that we experience as we travel between and across cultures, what kinds of culturing have you experienced? Does it change who you are? In what ways?
5. Do you have rituals in your life? What are they? Remember, rituals are not habits. Habits are things you do without thinking or planning. On the other hand, rituals have meanings and are important to your identity and relationships – your reality.
6. Looking at your interpersonal relationships? Who do you share an interpersonal bond reach the level of Magic Consciousness? Provide examples to explain what this is an example of Magic Consciousness?
7. Do you think that people should be able to assert their right to free exercise of religion as a legitimate reason to refuse health services in the following scenarios? Why or why not? Can you identify any answers that invoke Magic Consciousness? What are they?
   a. To refuse vaccination?
   b. For healthcare providers to refuse the provision of contraception to patients?
   c. For healthcare providers to refuse medical services to certain groups of people?

C. References

Alvord, L. A., & Van Pelt, E. C. (2000). *The scalpel and the silver bear: The first Navajo Woman surgeon combines Western medicine and traditional healing.* Bantam.

Bamberger, D. H. (1987). Mercy Hospital, Inc. v. Jackson: A recurring dilemma for health care providers in the treatment of Jehovah's Witnesses. *Maryland Law Review, 46*(3), 514–532.

Bhuvaneswar, C. G., Epstein, L. A., & Stern, T. A. (2007). Reactions to amputation: Recognition and treatment. *Primary Care Companion To The Journal Of Clinical Psychiatry, 9*(4), 303–308.

Bradford, W. D., & Mandich, A. (2015). Some state vaccination laws contribute to greater exemption rates and disease outbreaks in the United States. *Health Affairs, 34*(8), 1383–1390.

Brown, D. (2019). Palmerston's conquest of Sligo. In M. Kelly (Ed.), *Nature and the environment in nineteenth-century Ireland* (pp. 35–54). Liverpool University Press.

Cameron, C. (2020, July 24). *HUD rule would dismantle protections for homeless transgender people.* The New York Times. https://nyti.ms/3iob9YH

Cavanaugh, C. L., Taylor, C. A., Keim, K. S., Clutter, J. E., & Geraghty, M. E. (2008). Cultural perceptions of health and diabetes among Native American men. *Journal of Health Care for the Poor and Underserved, 19*(4), 1029–1043.

Coffey, L., Gallagher, P., Horgan, O., Desmond, D., & MacLachlan, M. (2009). Psychosocial adjustment to diabetes-related lower limb amputation. *Diabetic Medicine, 26*(10), 1063–1067.

de Saussure, F. (2011). *Course in general linguistics* (W. Baskin, P. Meisel, & H. Sussy, Eds.). Columbia University Press.

de Vogue, A. (2020, July 8). *Supreme Court says Trump can weaken Obamacare contraceptive mandate.* CNN. https://www.cnn.com/2020/07/08/politics/supreme-court-obamacare-contraceptive-mandate

Derrida, J. (1973). *Speech and phenomena, and other essays on Husserl's Theory of Signs.* Northwestern University Press.

Dewaele, J.-M. (2004). The emotional force of swearwords and taboo words in the speech of multilinguals. *Journal of Multilingual and Multicultural Development, 25*(2-3), 204–222.

Dewaele, J.-M. (2008). The emotional weight of I love you in multilinguals' languages. *Journal of Pragmatics, 40*(10), 1753–1780.

Ethnic (2016). In Editors of the American Heritage Dictionaries (Ed.), *The American Heritage Dictionary of the English Language* (6th ed.). Houghton Mifflin.

Fenton, S. (2013). *Ethnicity* (2nd ed.). Polity.

Foucault, M. (2005). *The order of things: An archaeology of the human sciences.* Routledge. (Original work published 1966)

Gasper, T. (2015). A religious right to discriminate: *Hobby Lobby* and "religious freedom" as a threat to the LGBT community. *Texas A&M Law Review, 3*(2), 395–416.

Geertz, C. (1973). *The interpretation of cultures.* Basic Books.

Gostin, L. O. (2015). Law, ethics, and public health in the vaccination debates: Politics of the measles outbreak. *JAMA, 313*(11), 1099–1100.

Green, K. M. (2006). Who's who: Exploring the discrepancy between the methods of defining African Americans and Native Americans. *American Indian Law Review, 31*(1), 93–110.

Gumperz, J. J. (2009). The speech community. In A. Duranti (Ed.), *Linguistic anthropology: A reader* (2nd ed., pp. 66–73). Blackwell. (Original work published 1968)

Hall, E. T. (1976). *Beyond culture.* Anchor Books.

Harris, C. L., Aycicegi, A., & Gleason, J. B. (2003). Taboo words and reprimands elicit greater autonomic reactivity in a first language than in a second language. *Applied Psycholinguistics, 24*(4), 561.

Herring, J., & Wall, J. (2017). The nature and significance of the right to bodily integrity. *The Cambridge Law Journal, 76*(3), 566–588.

Hickman, C. B. (1997). The devil and the one drop rule: Racial categories, African Americans, and the U.S. Census. *Michigan Law Review, 95*(5), 1161–1265.

Hiebert, P. G. (2008). *Transforming worldviews: An anthropological understanding of how people change*. Baker Academic.

Hofstede, G. (2001). *Culture's consequences: Comparing values, behaviors, institutions and organizations across nations*. Sage.

Hsu, C.-T., Jacobs, A. M., & Conrad, M. (2015). Can Harry Potter still put a spell on us in a second language? An fMRI study on reading emotion-laden literature in late bilinguals. *Cortex*, *63*, 282–295.

Husserl, E. (1962). *Ideas: General introduction to pure phenomenology* (W. R. B. Gibson, Trans.). Collier Books.

Jonassen, F. B. (2012). Kiss the book... You're President...: "So help me God"and kissing the book in the Presidential Oath of office. *William & Mary Bill of Rights Journal*, *20*(3), 853–953.

Kahn, J. (2014). *Race in a bottle: The story of BiDil and racialized medicine in a post-genomic age*. Columbia University Press.

Kanaboshi, N. (2006). Competent persons' constitutional right to refuse medical treatment in the U.S. and Japan: Application to Japanese law. *Penn State International Law Review*, *25*, 5–72.

Kanter, R. M. (1968). Commitment and social organization: A study of commitment mechanisms in utopian communities. *American Sociological Review*, *33*(4), 499–517.

Khanna, N. (2010). "If you're half Black, you are just Black": Reflected appraisals and the persistence of the one-drop rule. *Sociological Quarterly*, *51*(1), 96–121.

Kim, J. (2006). Beyond paradigm: Making transcultural connections in a scientific translation of acupuncture. *Social Science & Medicine*, *62*(12), 2960–2972.

Kozak, D. L. (1997). Surrendering to diabetes: An embodied response to perceptions of diabetes and death in the Gila River Indian Community. *Omega: Journal of Death and Dying*, *35*(4), 347–359.

Kramer, E. M. (1992). Consciousness and culture. In E. M. Kramer (Ed.), *Consciousness and culture: An introduction to the thought of Jean Gebser* (pp. 1–60). Greenwood.

Kramer, E. M. (Ed.). (2003). *The emerging monoculture: Assimilation and the "model minority."* Praeger.

Kramer, E. M. (2013). Dimensional accrual and dissociation: An introduction. In J. Grace & E. M. Kramer (Eds.), *Communication, comparative cultures, and civilizations* (Vol. 3, pp. 123–184). Hampton.

Kramer, E. M. (2019). Cultural fusion theory. In J. F. Nussbaum (Ed.), *Oxford research encyclopedia of communication*. Oxford University Press. https://doi.org/10.1093/acrefore/9780190228613.013.679

Kramer, E. M., & Liu, Y. (2015). 全球化语境下的跨文化传播 [Intercultural communication in the context of globalization]. Tsinghua University Press.

Lam, W. A., & McCullough, L. B. (2000). Influence of religious and spiritual values on the willingness of Chinese–Americans to donate organs for transplantation. *Clinical Transplantation*, *14*(5), 449–456.

Lee, J., & Bean, F. D. (2007). Reinventing the color line immigration and America's new racial/ethnic divide. *Social Forces*, *86*(2), 561–586.

Lee, S. S.-J. (2015). The biobank as political artifact: The struggle over race in categorizing genetic difference. *The ANNALS of the American Academy of Political and Social Science*, *661*(1), 143–159.

Markel, H. (2004). "I swear by Apollo" – On taking the Hippocratic Oath. *New England Journal of Medicine, 350*(20), 2026–2029.

National Conference of State Legislatures. (2020, June 26). *State with religious and philosophical exemptions from school immunization requirements.* https://www.ncsl. org/research/health/school-immunization-exemption-state-laws.aspx

Nelson, B., & Lundin, S. (2010). *Ubuntu!: An inspiring story about an African tradition of teamwork and collaboration.* Crown.

Note, N., Fornet-Betancourt, R., Estermann, J., & Aerts, D. (2008). Worldviews and cultures: Philosophical reflections from an intercultural perspective. An introduction. In N. Note, R. Fornet-Betancourt, J. Estermann, & D. Aerts (Eds.), *Worldviews and cultures: Philosophical reflections from an intercultural perspective* (pp. 1–9). Springer.

O'Neill, S. P. (2015). Sapir–Whorf hypothesis. In K. Tracy , T. L. Sandel, & C. Ilie (Eds.), *The international encyclopedia of language and social interaction* (pp. 1325–1334). Wiley.

Paradies, Y. C., Montoya, M. J., & Fullerton, S. M. (2007). Racialized genetics and the study of complex diseases – the thrifty genotype revisited. *Perspectives in Biology and Medicine, 50*(2), 203–227.

Parker, K., Horowitz, J. M., Morin, R., & Lopez, M. H. (2015). *Chapter 1: Race and multiracial Americans in the U.S. Census.* Pew Research Center. https://www. pewsocialtrends.org/2015/06/11/chapter-1-race-and-multiracial-americans-in-the-u-s-census/

Pickering, A. (2010). *The mangle of practice: Time, agency, and science.* University of Chicago Press.

Pitaloka, D., & Hsieh, E. (2015). Health as submission and social responsibilities: Embodied experiences of Javanese women with type II diabetes. *Qualitative Health Research, 25*(8), 1155–1165.

Rodriguez, A. (2002). Culture to culturing: Re-imagining our understanding of intercultural relations. *Journal of Intercultural Communication,* (5), 1–10. https://www. immi.se/intercultural/nr5/rodriguez.pdf

Sheppard, S. (2009). What oaths meant to the Framers' generation: A preliminary sketch. *Cardozo Law Review De Novo,* 273–283. http://cardozolawreview.com/what-oaths-meant-to-the-framers-generation-a-preliminary-sketch/

Sherman, R. B. (1988). "The last stand": The fight for racial integrity in Virginia in the 1920s. *The Journal of Southern History, 54*(1), 69–92.

Singelenberg, R. (1990). The blood transfusion taboo of Jehovah's Witnesses: Origin, development and function of a controversial doctrine. *Social Science & Medicine, 31*(4), 515–523.

Smith, C. M. (2005). Origin and uses of primum non nocere – Above all, do no harm! *The Journal of Clinical Pharmacology, 45*(4), 371–377.

Smugar, S., & Spina, B. J. (2000). Informed consent for emergency contraception: Variability in hospital care of rape victims. *American Journal of Public Health, 90*(9), 1372–1376.

Solomon, M. Z. (1997). From what's neutral to what's meaningful: Reflections on a study of medical interpreters. *Journal of Clinical Ethics, 8*(1), 88–93.

Stendhal (2016). *Armance – Some scenes from a salon in Paris in 1827.* Read Books. (Original work published 1827)

Stephenson, M. T., Morgan, S. E., Roberts-Perez, S. D., Harrison, T., Afifi, W., & Long, S. D. (2008). The role of religiosity, religious norms, subjective norms, and bodily integrity in signing an organ donor card. *Health Communication, 23*(5), 436–447.

Streeck, J. (2002). Culture, meaning, and interpersonal communication. In M. L. Knapp & J. A. Daly (Eds.), *Handbook of interpersonal communication* (2nd ed., pp. 300–335). Sage.

Takahashi, J., Cher, A., Sheeder, J., Teal, S., & Guiahi, M. (2019). Disclosure of religious identity and health care practices on Catholic hospital websites. *JAMA, 321*(11), 1103–1104.

Ting-Toomey, S. (2012). *Communicating across cultures.* Guilford Press.

Trudgill, P. (1991). Language maintenance and language shift: Preservation versus extinction. *International Journal of Applied Linguistics, 1*(1), 61–69.

Tseng, W.-S., & Streltzer, J. (2008). *Cultural competence in health care.* Springer.

Williams, T. C. (2019). *Self-portrait in Black and White: Unlearning race.* W. W. Norton.

Williamson, J. (1995). *New people: Miscegenation and mulattoes in the United States.* LSU Press.

Wong, B. (2020, July 2). *The psychology behind why some people refuse to wear face masks.* HuffPost. https://www.huffpost.com/entry/psychology-why-people-refuse-wear-face-masks_l_5efb723cc5b6ca970915bc53

Zlatev, J., & Blomberg, J. (2015). Language may indeed influence thought. *Frontiers in Psychology, 6*, Article 1631. https://doi.org/10.3389/fpsyg.2015.01631

3

Cultural Consciousness II

Mythic Connection and the Social Meanings of Health and Illness

Chapter 3 examines Mythic Connection as cultural consciousness in influencing individuals' health-related worldviews. By contrasting Magic Consciousness with Mythic Connection, we will demonstrate how myths assume its powerful function in culture, allowing people to derive meanings through symbolic communication. In this book, we use stories and myths interchangeably. We view story and storytelling not as simple descriptions of factual or fictional events but as a process of sense-making in a social world. By exploring the reasons, processes, functions, and impacts of creating social meanings of health and illness, we will examine theories on illness identities and the transformational power of illness stories. We will also examine how illness narratives allow the cultural system to enforce certain values and celebrate specific illness performance yet silence other forms of suffering.

I.   Magic Consciousness v. Mythic Connection

A. Magic Consciousness is Holistic – Meaning is Inherent

Magic Consciousness and Mythic Connection represent two distinctive approaches to health and illness. The Magic Consciousness view of health and illness is pre-spatial. Therefore, it does not fragment different aspects of health and illness. Magic Consciousness sees health and illness as a seamless continuum of material and spiritual issues. Likewise, the worldview of Magic Consciousness does not separate the supernatural from the natural. There is simply the world (i.e., a *single* world). The shaman who treats a sick person may well see the illness as a spiritual phenomenon as much as a physical fact. Even a seemingly simple physical condition such as a broken leg, for the shaman, may involve a curse, or the act of malicious spirits, or just punishment for disrespecting powers and forces within the world. In the idolic world, everything is alive and aware. The Magic Consciousness worldview is animistic and primal – it does not see accidents so much as active forces that moderns might call "supernatural." Because Magic Consciousness does not separate cause from effect, disease and misfortune are "natural" extensions of disharmonic conditions. The only way to heal is to attempt to reharmonize with the world. Hence, moderns tend to see the Magic Consciousness approach to healthcare as "holistic." Everything is part of health and illness. **Holistic medicine** requires physicians to attend to individuals'

Rethinking Culture in Health Communication: Social Interactions as Intercultural Encounters,
First Edition. Elaine Hsieh and Eric M Kramer.
© 2021 John Wiley & Sons, Inc. Published 2021 by John Wiley & Sons, Inc.

whole person well-being by situating individuals' health and illness in the wider contexts of patients' everyday life (Hastings et al., 1980/2018). **Holism** recognizes that the whole is greater than the sum of its parts – being healthy is more than just not feeling physical or even psychological ailments.

This holism includes the right attitude or heart. For instance, a correct diet includes the proper way to sow and harvest, to hunt and fish, and to prepare and share food. Idolic agriculture and hunting are infused with magic rituals stressing respect for the world. One of the best examples is the Na'vi, who lives on the moon Pandora in the movie *Avatar*. Whereas humans view Pandora as a planet with rich resources to be exploited (and thus, adopting the cultural view of Perspectival Thinking; see Chapter 4), Na'vi, a highly spiritual clan, believe that all living things on Pandora are connected through the Tree of Souls, which has the ability to allow the Na'vi to connect to the energy/life of the entire planet – a Magic Consciousness worldview (Istoft, 2010). Na'vi believes that their lives are interconnected with other animals, which is reflected (quite literally) in the bonding rituals they have when choosing their animal companions. As the two bonds, their nerves are connected – a symbiosis is formed: the rider feels what the animal feels and vice versa. For Na'vi, killing of animals is ritualistic and requires reverence, which involves "reciting a prayer of thanks and a quick kill with a sharp and carefully aimed knife" (Sideris, 2010, p. 470). The world of Magic Consciousness is saturated with care. The Magic Consciousness world is infused with passion. The separation of reason from emotion is not part of the Magic Consciousness worldview. It is utterly reasonable for the person with Magic Consciousness to be concerned about spirits. Pain and suffering, joy and celebration are shared by all in what is called sympathetic social ecology.

When a fanatical follower of a sports team speaks about the team's efforts they often say "we." "We" won or lost this weekend. This unity indicates a Magic Consciousness identification with the group. When their team suffers a terrible blunder or spectacular success during play, the fanatical follower will literally suffer or celebrate with the team. This is a form of Magic Consciousness that you might recognize in the modern world. Another example is the giving over of oneself, or a total surrender to a highly emotional and shared experience in church or a political rally. Under such conditions the self is lost to the crowd, and with it, the modern sense of ego and embarrassment. Emotional tides sweep through the throng as one. Crying during a sad movie defies rational control. It is a mild expression of Magic Consciousness identification with the plight of the characters on the screen.

Everything in the idolic world of Magic Consciousness is not merely "meaningful" but infused with life and passion. The Magic Consciousness worldview is not a worldview per se because there is no view: as all are unified as one. It is one without distance, detachment, disinterest, or neutrality. There are no perspectives to be taken because everything is unified as one.

B. Mythic Connection is Symbolic – Meanings to be Found

1. Language, Myths, and Time

Through idolic communication under Magic Consciousness, reality is invoked as the words are uttered (e.g., when I call for God, God is invoked and become "real" in my presence). Reality is not dissociated from our talk. In the Mythic Connection world, one experiences dissociation from the oneness of the Magic Consciousness world (Munn, 1992). The Mythic Connection world exhibits nascent dissociation and distancing in all aspects, including physical, psychological, and spiritual domains. Rather than seeing the world "as is," a Mythic Connection worldview finds meanings through "things" – symbols to carry meanings and lessons of life. In other words, under Mythic Connection, individuals engage in **symbolic communication**. Symbolic communication means that as we talk, the "things" referenced in our talk is more than just things; they have meanings beyond the "things" itself. For example, when I say God or wear a cross as my necklace, I know that I cannot invoke the presence of God (like people under Magic Consciousness would have believed) but I also believe that when I call out for God and hold the cross in my hand, I feel more connected to the spiritual and physical world in a way that makes the world meaningful and *moral*. Symbolic communication implies a pursuit of cultural and ideological virtues as human connects the "objective" reality with meanings in their Lifeworlds through imagination and creativity. As we continue to dissociate from the world, Perspectival Thinking emerges (see more in Chapter 4). Under Perspectival Thinking, communication is instrumental (i.e., signalic communication) – we use language to *reference* "things" without a deeper connection for meaning. For example, when I say the word God, I am referring to a spiritual presence but I do not feel that God is in my presence nor a sense of connection or humility with God. A cross neckless is just a decoration and does not hold symbolic meanings or moral claims about who I am.

As dissociation increases, two concurrent things occur. First, the individual ego begins to emerge from the whole of reality and continues to solidify and concretize until individualism becomes intolerant and universal. All people, things, and events become objectified, meaning they stand alone in space as objects. We experience increasing isolation and alienation from the rest of the world.

Second, (the concept of) time emerges – the "timeless" eternal in Magic Consciousness dissipates (Munn, 1992). At first, it appears as cyclical recurrence (i.e., circular time). However, as dissociation increases, time becomes increasingly spatialized as a form, a line (i.e., linear time). Magic Consciousness is "timeless." Time has no beginning or ending. In fact, it does not exist – as the cultural participants have no sense of time. They live in the now. There's no past or future because we are all in the flow of life. We all live in the moment. Things come into existence and things die. Everything is alive, finished, and complete. A world of Magic Consciousness does not worry about purpose or progress. Everything is complete – in harmony and perfect "as is."

In contrast, in the world of Mythic Connection world, as people dissociate from the holistic, oneness world, time is dissociated as well. In Mythic Connection world, time is circular or cyclic (i.e., **circular time**), rather than linear. For example, in many ancient societies, time is understood though repetitions of natural and social events (e.g., birth, reproduction, and death). The recurring rhythm is illustrated by the lyrics of Elton John's Circle of Life for the Disney movie *Lion King*:

> Some say, "Eat or be eaten."
> Some say, "Live and let live."
> But all are agreed as they join the stampede
> You should never take more than you give

> In the circle of life
> It's the wheel of fortune
> It's the leap of faith
> It's the band of hope
> 'Til we find our place
> On the path unwinding
> In the circle, the circle of life

In contrast, **linear time** conceptualizes time as a unilinear structure – "we will never pass this way again." In the modern world of Perspectival Thinking, time is linear. Our understanding and perception of time are often embedded in languages (Klein, 1994/2013). For example, one cannot speak proper English if one is unable to properly distinguishes past, present, and future times, let alone using the right tense structure for past/present/future perfect (e.g., "I have eaten/had eaten/will have eaten the steak") or past/present/future perfect continuous (e.g., "I have been working/had been working/will have been working for 30 hours"). Without adopting an English speaker's understanding of time, a second language learner's English may appear incoherent or incomprehensible. In linear time, each event is unique, individuated, and finite. Time becomes fragmented into individual events and they are each fleeting. Although you can always have a family Christmas dinner every year, if you missed the dinner one year, the opportunity is forever lost. Future gatherings, even with the same people at the same location, are considered separate (rather than the "same") family activities.

When examining the conceptualization of time in pre-Christian spirituality and religions (especially in archaic life), the philosopher and historian Mircea Eliade (1959) explained that circular time was "reversible and recoverable, a sort of eternal mythical present that is periodically integrated by means of rites" (p. 70). Because time is circular and the present can be integrated into eternity through rituals, time in the Mythic Connection world begins to have beginnings and endings to "mark" the movement of time. Unlike the timelessness of Magic Consciousness, time in Mythic Connection world begins to emerge by dating, to be "marked," and recurrently "observed." Eliade (1959) explained:

> [F]or religious man of the archaic cultures, every creation, every existence begins in time: *before a thing exists, its particular time could not exist.* Before the cosmos came into existence, there was no cosmic time. ... every creation is imagined as having taken place *at the beginning of time, in pricipio.* Time gushes forth with the first appearance of a new category of existents. This is why myth plays such an important role... the way in which a reality came into existence is revealed by its myths. (p. 76)

Origin myths mark the beginning of time as a recurring cycle. Origin myths are stories that explain how we come into being. Origin myths are common in all cultures (Leeming, 2010; Niesiolowski-Spano & Laskowski, 2016). Thinking about time, thus, marks the beginning of mythic consciousness. Myths provide the first sense of dissociation between individuals and their lived environments. We are no longer part of the oneness with the rest of the world. As we create stories about how "we" come into being, we are no longer the same as others that are "not us." We are unique and special.

This dissociation manifests as the emergence of cyclical and mystical storytelling that, with further dissociation and abstraction, will become linear secular history (Munn, 1992). Mythic time begins to take the form of history. As the human emerges from the rest of reality, time increasingly becomes a linear human story. Through storytelling, we aim to "explain events in terms of *human actors striving to do things over time*" [emphasis added] (McAdams, 1993, p. 30). Time in Mythic Connection world becomes the essence of drama. It is *not* disinterested record keeping. It is paramount to identity. This is the story of my people.

When end times seem eminent, people reaffirm the mythic systems that give them identity and a sense of purpose. Approaching apocalyptic ends is an example. Many cultures have apocalyptic stories, a judgment day in a supernatural world that entails not only the end of the world but also the fate of the dead (Collins, 2014). Apocalyptic stories intend "to interpret present, earthly circumstances in light of the supernatural world and of the future, and to influence both the understanding and the behavior of the audience by means of divine authority" (Collins, 1986, p. 7). All the greatest mythological systems are teleological in form. Myth and music share the same etymological root *mu*. Chanting liturgy and binding songs are prominent in religious rituals. Beat binds the people. Myths bind the community: The cosmos and human history emerge as one grand story with a beginning and a destiny (Eliade, 1959). Anthropologist Claude Lévi-Strauss (1978) argued that myth, like music, can only be understood in the *totality* of contexts (e.g., cannot be separated from its historical, sociocultural, and interpersonal environments) and its meaning is always *continuously and interactively constructed* by the performer and the audiences. They are continuously constructed by the myths they live by and embody in their practices such as agriculture, child rearing, funerary practices, and so forth. In other words, the meaning of myth is alive and responds to the call of its cultural participants, and they to it.

It is important to note that in this book, myths should *not* be understood as falsehood. Myths are not "fairytales" or lies. Rather, we view myth as a particular type of speech or story that aims to create, connect, and maintain meanings in our everyday life. Mircea Eliade (1959) said that the modern people ask the wrong question of myths: Rather than asking whether a myth is true or false, the question to ask is whether the myth is alive or dead. If it is dead, it has become merely an arbitrary tale among countless others. It has no emotional impact on a person's life or behavior. It is reduced to a form of literature. *If a myth is alive, it is essential to one's identity as a member of a culture and society.*

When iconic, symbolic buildings and institutions were attacked in the United States on 9/11, churches and synagogues were overflowing with people, many of whom rarely attended regular services. Flags and Bibles sold out across the country. Emotions rose and people wept and raged in anger though they were not physically affected. However, they were magically and mythically bound to the symbols. President George W. Bush stood in the ruins of the World Trade Center Towers in New York City and announced to the world that "we" would have "our" revenge against those who attacked "our way of life." Desmond Morris (1969/1994) notes that perceived attack binds people collectively more efficiently than any other set of messages or conditions. During such convergences, people rally around sacred and semi-sacred symbols in ritual fashion in order to reaffirm the mythic power to confer identity and purpose.

2. The Emergence of the Duality of "Reality"

As dissociation intensifies, a more disinterested universe emerges. The animistic spirits that filled the idolic world of Magic Consciousness recede as space emerges. They coalesce into multiple identifiable and discrete gods that move away spatially and emotionally. They reside far away on mountain tops and may not care about our lives. In addition, the spirits become increasingly **anthropomorphic** (i.e., having human characteristics), indicating the emergent importance of human egoism via projection. An example is Ovid's epic tale Metamorphoses wherein Daphne, a Naiad-nymph of the Ladon River calls out to Gaia, the Earth goddess to turn her into a laurel tree to avoid being raped by Apollo. Many are tales of **therianthropy** which is the ability of humans to shapeshift or metamorphose into other animals, plants, rocks, and things. Perhaps the most famous one in the West is the werewolf story and in the East the story of humans turning into foxes. With this anthropomorphism comes psychological complexity, deceit, seduction, wonton cruelty, judgment, appetites, ambition, and other aspects of the modern psyche. Psychic depth emerges with the polarization of the subconscious and conscious worlds. Dreams in Magic Consciousness world are seamless with wakefulness – dream world is one with the lived world. Zhuangzi (2013), a Chinese philosopher, told a story to illustrate the point:

> Once Zhuang Zhou dreamed he was a butterfly, a butterfly flitting and fluttering around, happy with himself and doing as he pleased. He did not know he was Zhuang Zhou. Suddenly he woke up, and there he was, solid and unmistakable Zhuang Zhou. But he didn't know if he were Zhuang Zhou who had dreamed he was a butterfly or a butterfly dreaming he was Zhuang Zhou. (p. 18)

The duality of what is real and what is not real does not exist in Magic Consciousness. All are experienced "as is" and are taken-for-granted. Because one cannot decide which phenomenon is "only" a dream and which is the "reality," both realms are equally "authentic" (Möller, 1999).

In contrast, dreams in the Mythic Connection world represent symbolic clues to be interpreted for the present. The ambiguity of metaphor calls forth a need for interpretation which is the beginning of the reflective method. The Mythic Connection world is filled with dream interpretations and polarization gives rise to the potential to have conflicting interpretations via emerging points-of-view.

The Mythic Connection person begins to feel the first hints of isolation characteristic of the "internal" world of the modern psyche. Sacred stories are developed to describe in-group and out-group identities. To confront the crippling sense of meaninglessness, grand stories are written to describe a universe that has a *purpose* and, as such, is dramatic (i.e., the universe has a sense of virtue, morality, and ethics). In the story, the person becomes increasingly individuated as an actor with responsibilities. The more spatial the story, the more terminal beginnings and endings generate drama.

Mythological stories and characters epitomize the first reflections on psychological states (Eliade, 1959). Truth and falsehood remain entwined, but their outlines begin to form. With the eruption of the third-dimension formalism and structure occurs. Logical forms govern rational thinking and discourse. **Two-valued logic**, dualistic thinking, the law of the excluded middle, with strict separation of positions emerge in the form of the law of noncontradiction. In other words, two-valued logic classified almost everything and everyone into one of two competing groups (e.g., good-evil; male-female; animate-inanimate; White-nonwhite). The idolic world of Magic Consciousness has no good or evil. Things are just the way they are. The symbolic world of Mythic Connection is ambivalent, but dramatic. Folk stories and ancient myths begin to exhibit a polarization of right and wrong in the Mythic Connection world. An example of the dissociation from Magic Consciousness can be found in the story of *Hundun* (混沌) in Zhuangzi (Zhuangzi, 2013).

Hundun is a "legendary faceless being" and a primordial God of chaos in Chinese mythology. Because of Hundun's hospitality, other Gods decided to return his generosity by chipping him a face, giving him human-like senses through drilling seven openings to allow Hundun to "see, hear, eat, and breathe" like all men. However, as soon as *Hundun* has a real face, he died. Magic Consciousness does not have perspectives. The "chaos" is not chaotic: all exist in harmony. There is no need to reconcile meanings or senses. Things are just the way they are – meanings are inherent and thus, cannot be questioned. However, as one dissociates from the oneness of the Magic Consciousness and develops perspectives through our senses, we become increasingly distant from the idolic world of Magic Consciousness.

What does it mean when you see a beautiful flower that has a foul order? What does it mean when you feel happy when you saw a $100 bill left on the road, knowing that someone may feel sad about losing the money? Our senses and experiences can create competing (and conflicting) feelings and meanings. Such contradictions and tensions require reconciliations; otherwise, confusion ensues. Sense-making is essential in Mythic Connection because we try to find coherent meanings to our worlds – failure to do so can be confusing and even traumatizing. In the case of *Hundun*, he died. Hundun could no longer exist in the Magic Consciousness world as his holistic existence was narrowed into five senses. Hundun's increasing dissociation from the magic world and failure to generate coherent meanings through the independent and separate meanings of smell, hearing, sight, and taste rendered him lifeless.

II. Mythic Connection and the Creation of Meanings

A. Emergence of Myth: Mythic Connection as Dissociation from Magic Consciousness

With dissociations, the idolic communication of the Magic Consciousness world gives way to the symbolic communication of the Mythic Connection world. Because the same texts may carry different meanings and voices, they are **polyvocal** (Bakhtin, 1981). For example, a physician may say to a grieving wife, "It'd take a miracle for your husband to survive the massive bleeding caused by the stroke." The comment can mean that the patient has little chance to survive, or it might mean the wife should seek others' prayers to help the husband to pull through the illness, or that there is little that the biomedical physician can do. All these meanings co-exist within a single statement, but also manifest tensions in their corresponding worldviews, illness models, and social identities.

Polyvocal versions of texts lead to conflicts of interpretation. Understanding and conveying intent becomes an issue to be contested, negotiated, and coordinated.

Prophets may be "false." Although magicians, shaman, and sorcerers in the Magic Consciousness world used incantatory speech to directly transform reality, prophets in Mythic Connection world see reality as something other, something that will unfold without human intervention, but which can be predicted. Reflection on communication itself commences and takes the form of sectarian disputes over the meaning of sacred texts, of the proper understanding ("reading") of divine signs such as a cross appearing in the clouds. Authority and power distance increase. Oracles gain prominence as those who can interpret signs and see the fatalistic future.

The first reflection on the "problem" of interpretation takes the form of **hermeneutics** (i.e., the study of the principles of interpretation). Hermes, the messenger god in Greek mythology, does not simply relay the intent of the gods to humans. Rather he must interpret divine intent for them (Moules, 2002). Mythic language begins to separate form from content, intent from utterance.

Under Magic Consciousness, idolic communication is manifest (Kramer, 2013). People in Magic Consciousness do not need symbols. Nothing is arbitrary or in need of interpretation. There is no symbol because there is no distance between "things" and the power they hold. Magic Consciousness resists interpretation as incantation and amulets tend to be devoid of narrative. Magic emblems do not refer to anything. They act, function, and work by mere presence. The sacred tree is God. It's not a representation or a symbol of God. Incantation and other forms of communication under Magic Consciousness do not tell stories. Rather they manifestly invoke and evoke a state of reality. Incantations, tattoos, hex signs, and other "symbols" do their magic of protecting the bearer and binding the person to the whole, including the totem animal/spirit. There is nothing to discuss. People do not choose their tattoos or scarification based on personal preference or symbolic expression. The tattoos that identify an individual as a member of a tribe and protect him or her from maladies (e.g., an illness or a curse) are not arbitrary. As a result, people in Magic Consciousness world do not rally around symbols at times of crisis because the power, meaning, and strength of the culture do not reside somewhere out there to be found: They, the people, embody the Magic Consciousness (see Figures 3.1–3.3). The power (and the inherent meaning) of the magic, idolic world is literally inscribed into their flesh, the surfaces of their homes, their boats, their weapons; everything.

Mythic Connection demands interpretation because symbolic communication is more arbitrary and thus, ambiguous. The telling of the story is itself an interpretation. A **symbol** stands in for something that is semi-absent (i.e., something that is not quite there). An important distinction here is that symbols in Mythic Connection are not the same as "signs" in signalic communication. In Mythic Connection, symbols are not *abstract, arbitrary* signs; rather, a symbol is "a concrete phenomenon – religious, psychological, and poetic" (Rasmussen, 2012, p. 1). Language can be an important medium of symbols; nevertheless, symbols need not be limited to linguistic forms. All things (e.g., a tree, a relic, a wall, a wink, a scream) can serve as symbols. Symbols require interpretation. Symbols are not identical to the thing they represent. Thus, communication becomes abstract and problematized. Symbols allow people to connect meanings to things. The idea of "connection" begins to emerge as something that can fail. Words and images can misrepresent. Interpretations can be wrong. Mythic Connection presumes the possibility of disconnection. Under Mythic Connection, the possibility of poor or invalid representation cannot be avoided. Misunderstanding becomes a central concern.

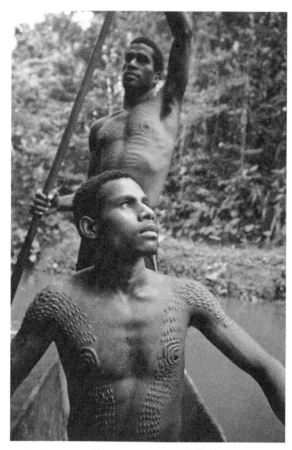

Figure 3.1 Crocodile scarification. Initiates from the crocodile scarification ceremony at Papua New Guinea. His scarification makes him a crocodile. *Source:* Design Pics Inc / Alamy Stock Photo

A symbol has an am-bi-valent relationship with reality. By *am-bi-valent*, we mean that a symbol always carries at least two meanings (or voices): a literal meaning and a figural meaning. A crucifix (i.e., an image of Jesus on the cross) is "just a symbol" yet it also evokes strong emotional responses and may change behaviors from believers. With further dissociation, signalic communication in the Perspectival Thinking world becomes totally abstract and separate from reality. It has no relationship with reality. "Words are just words," and they can be replaced at will because they are utterly arbitrary inventions with no attachment to reality. They are at best a tool for the convenience of convention, a momentary agreement among interlocutors to share some signs for enhancing social interactions.

B. Meaning-Creation in Mythic Connection

Mythic Connection as a cultural perspective provides the narrative frame for an individual (or a cultural group) to construct social meanings of health and illness. By creating and shaping narratives of illness events, one can create meanings that support cultural values and moral claims that are important to the cultural group. Under Magic Consciousness, cultural participants accept their world "as is." Issues of health

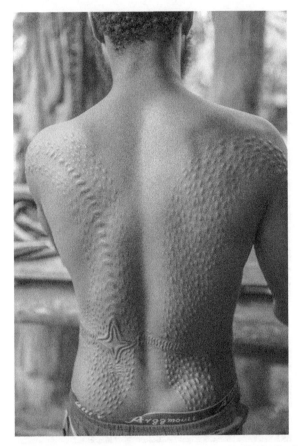

Figure 3.2 Tribal crocodile scarification. The intricate patterns on the back of a Chambri man resemble crocodile skin. *Source:* Roberto Cornacchia / Alamy Stock Photo

and illness are taken-for-granted in the culturally ordered magic world which dictates the meanings and implications of individuals' activities. In contrast, Mythic Connection strives to generate meanings, values, and morality claims in order to support the cultural system. Within Mythic Connection, cultural participants assume active roles in constructing and maintaining the values and meanings of the social world.

The language we use in everyday life provides rich resources in how we understand the world and construct our social experiences. In his book, *The Wounded Storyteller*, Arthur Frank (2013) examined how patients develop elaborate stories and rely on metaphors to help them generate and process the meanings and implications of their illness events. Stories provide an alternative reality that allows storytellers to establish coherence and meaning in their experiences (Miller et al., 2000). Patients often rely on stories to create a coherent self, making sense of their experiences and empowering their existence (Charmaz, 1999; Frank, 2013). Frank (2013) introduced the concept of **automythology**, through which patients create storylines and narratives that illustrate how they not only survived but also were transformed (and reborn, like the Phoenix,) as a result of the illness experience. Patients talk about how their illness experiences create a transformative process that allows them to create and identify new values and perspectives that their old selves would not have otherwise recognized or appreciated.

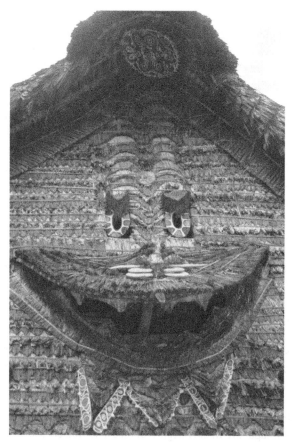

Figure 3.3 House with spirit faces. The homes of the Sepik River people of Papua New Guinea have spirits in them, literally. *Source:* blickwinkel / Alamy Stock Photo

Frank (2013) called such narratives **quest stories**. He explained:

> Quest stories meet suffering head on; they accept illness and seek to use it. Illness is the occasion of a journey that becomes a quest. What is quested for may never be wholly clear, but the quest is defined by the ill person's belief that something is to be gained through the experience. ... The quest narrative affords the ill person a voice as teller of her own story, because only in quest stories does the *teller* have a story to tell. (p. 115)

When summarizing her experiences with breast cancer, a patient explained, "And, as a result, I've done some things I never would have done. I took my first hot air balloon ride last Sunday. It was just simply beautiful ... And I've learned to swim" (Thomas-MacLean, 2004, p. 1654). While the patient's discussion of her lived experiences may appear "matter-of-fact," what is implied, however, is the expansion of her life horizon. The corresponding moral claims of her triumph are situated in the context of a devastating diagnosis. The meanings of the hot air balloon ride or learning to swim are different because of the illness.

Inherent in Mythic Connection is its moral dimension and value orientation. The stories are meaningful and powerful because they echo with the larger sociocultural system that embraces specific values (Bakhtin, 1981). Specific stories are embraced and celebrated yet others are silenced or reframed as moral lessons to be avoided. Frank (2013) noted, "Both institutions and individual listeners steer ill people toward certain narratives, and other narratives are simply not heard" (p. 77). Charmaz (2002) explained, "Stories and silences simultaneously frame and constitute meanings among people who experience disrupted lives ... [They] are emergent but seldom wholly idiosyncratic; they emerge within social contexts and thus are historically, socially, and culturally specific" (pp. 302–303). For example, audiences of a story shared in a support group may show their support or objection to the stories told as a way to socialize valued identities, prompting the storyteller to modify their stories accordingly (Hsieh, 2004). In this way, storytellers learn to develop meaningful stories that appeal to the values of their communities, allowing them to obtain the most support and resources to support their illness journeys.

Even though the stories may be told or experienced by individuals, they are situated in and evaluated by larger cultural systems (i.e., What is good or bad? What counts as a success or a failure? What is to be honored or disdained?). Swidler (2003) explained, "Becoming a certain kind of person is learned, practiced, and sustained through culture" (p. 73). For example, the larger cultural discourse has relied on the metaphor and the concept of "survivorship" to reconstruct women with breast cancer given that the illness experiences often require them to cope with disfigurement, disruption, and identity/relational insecurities. However, what if a person refuses to embrace the moral stories that emerge within and are sustained through a Mythic Connection? What happens to women who question or reject the concept of cancer survivorship when alternative images are mostly negative? (see also Kaiser, 2008).

It is important to remember that just as much as Mythic Connection has the power to create cultural heroes and heroines, it also has the power to create villains, the ones who failed to honor the cultural codes. By encouraging an optimistic, "cheerful," and "concealed disfigurement" image of breast cancer "survivors" (see Figure 3.4), the

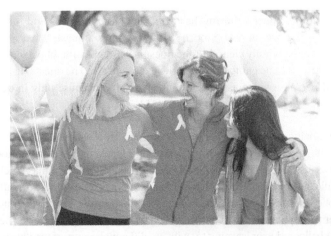

Figure 3.4 Breast cancer awareness activities. The expected performance of "cheerful survivors." *Source:* SDI Productions/Getty Images

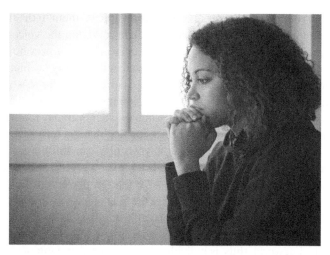

Figure 3.5   The unheard stories. The silenced stories of alienation, grief, and anger.
Source: Shutterstock / tommaso79

cultural system also successfully silences the stories of anger and grief and overlooked the permanence of physical and emotional marks on one's illness experience (see Figure 3.5). A patient who decided to forgo cure-oriented treatment may face significant social pressure for "giving up" (Makoul, 2004). On the other hand, women who worked to portray an image of perfect health after cancer treatment often paid an emotional (and monetary) price pertaining to being well and whole (Batt, 2003). In the end, both the "survivors" and "victims" pay the price under the cultural system. The cultural values and moral claims (as opposed to individual struggles or realities) are the ones to be protected and sustained in the Mythic Connection world.

III. The Social Meanings of Health and Illness

A. The Voice of the Lifeworld

We understand and interpret our world and social experiences through our languages. In the **Theory of Communicative Action**, Habermas (1981/1985) proposed that individuals' understandings of the world are not grounded in instrumental or objectivistic terms but are structured through communicative acts. By highlighting the tension between human communications in the *Lifeworld* and the *System*, Habermas noted that the two communication modalities are motivated by different types of "rationality." Communication in the Lifeworld echoes with Mythic Connection that serves the core theme of the current chapter. We will explore Habermas's understanding of the System in Chapter 4 when we examine Perspectival Thinking. For Habermas, communication in the Lifeworld is communicative actions that are sensitive to contexts, orient to mutual understanding, and result in coordinated actions through consensus (Lo & Bahar, 2013). A patient's understanding of his or her Lifeworld is situated within *value rationality* and is contextually grounded by the experiences of everyday events. By value rationality, Habermas emphasized the moral, ethical, and value-oriented structures that promote the prosperity and survival of social systems.

Mishler (1984) drew on Habermas's concepts and applied them to the field of medicine, proposing the concepts of the Voice of the Lifeworld and the Voice of Medicine (to be discussed in Chapter 4). The Voice of the Lifeworld recognizes how a patient's experiences of health and illness are always situated in their everyday life, encompassing their unique perspectives and understandings. For example, for most people, having a torn anterior cruciate ligament (ACL) is a common knee injury. For a software programmer, a torn ACL may pose little intrusion into her everyday routines, let alone perceived identity. However, For many professional athletes, a torn ACL, though not necessarily a career-ending diagnosis like 30 years ago, can still have a tremendous impact on their career (McMahan, 2017). An examination of NFL players suffering an ACL injury from 2010 to 2013 found that ACL injured players in the NFL earned $2,070,521 less than their uninjured peers over the four years after injury (Secrist et al., 2016). For NFL players, a torn ACL entails significant crises to his financial outlook, professional trajectory, and even identity management and interpersonal network. The Voice of the Lifeworld, thus, is individually experienced and interactionally negotiated with a patient's social network.

Because a patient relies on his everyday life and language to understand and interpret his illness experience, a patient may have miscommunications with his physician when they do not share the same understanding of the Lifeworld. In *Doctors' Diary* (Barnes, 2009), a documentary by PBS, a young physician, Jay Bonnar, had the following conversation at the initial appointment with an elderly, male patient who experienced numbness in his leg (PBS, 2001):

PATIENT: It started out in the back of my leg; this was in September. I had the operation. Now the front of my leg, from here down, is numb, and every time I take a shower, my whole leg gets numb.

BONNAR: So, when you shower, you take your clothes off?

PATIENT: Well, I don't take a shower with my clothes on. Of course, I do.

BONNAR: I'd like to ask you what exactly it is that you feel and then come to a...

PATIENT: My leg is numb. What else can I say to you?

BONNAR: That's fine. It may interest you to know that different people mean different things by that phrase.

PATIENT: My leg, from here to the tip of my toe, is numb.

BONNAR: I appreciate that this is something that has you very concerned, and you appear to be a little irritated at some of my questions.

PATIENT: I'm not irritated. I'm just tired of not getting any answers. That's what I'm irritated about.

BONNAR: I still don't understand exactly what's happening.

PATIENT: Well, if you've got my file. All right. You're supposed to have all of this stuff when I get down here, so you'll know what the hell you're talking about. Do I have to explain the operation to you?

BONNAR: No. I'd like to ask you what exactly it is that you feel and then come to an understanding.

PATIENT: My leg is numb. What else can I say to you? I want to know what the hell is going on with my foot.

BONNAR: We'll do everything within our power to come to that decision today.

PATIENT: I certainly hope so. I certainly hope so.

What happened here? Patients' understanding of their illnesses and illness symptoms are situated in their Lifeworld (Lo & Bahar, 2013; Todres et al., 2007). Their Lifeworld is infused with their cultural beliefs, social experiences, and folk ideologies. Although Dr. Bonnar tried to control the patient's illness narratives through a medical understanding (i.e., the Voice of Medicine), the patient resisted Dr. Bonnar's imposition to restrict his experiences in technical, mechanical, and medical terms and frames. The patient demanded the doctor recognize his uncertainty ("I want to know what the hell is going on with my foot.") of the "numbness" after the "operation" from his Lifeworld perspective. In a follow-up interview 20 years later (PBS, 2009), Dr. Bonnar reflected,

> When I see the scene [again], I kind of winced because I was doing a pretty bad job of making the patient comfortable and helping him tell me his story. I had a very locked mind of what are needed to know. I think that was facilitated in part because I felt that I was going to be quizzed immediately after by somebody else. I knew he wanted to know a particular thing and I was determined to get that information. The fact that I was being judged and evaluated then made me sort of stuck in a particular mindset. I failed to connect to the patient entirely.

B. Functions of Stories: Cultural Construction of Health and Illness

Culture has a pervasive influence on health-related behaviors. When examining the influences of culture in individuals' emotional management and experiences of social anxiety, Kirmayer (2001) explained,

> Culture provides categories and a lexicon for emotional experience, making some feelings salient and others more difficult to articulate. Culture sets limits of tolerance for specific emotions and strong affect; it also provides lay theories and strategies for managing dysphoria. Culture influences the sources of distress, the form of illness experience, symptomatology, the interpretation of symptoms, modes of coping with distress, help-seeking, and the social response to distress and disability. (p. 23)

Culture is not limited to abstract values or group preferences. Human experience, understanding, and sense are cultural. There is no such thing as a human without language or culture. Culture is embodied. The way we live literally changes the neuronal structures in our physical brain and the form of our bodies. Education and life experience change a person's brain. The kind of labor and leisure one does changes one's body. A person who spends time toiling in fields or doing rigorous athletics has a different body from a person who does not. This means that individuals' experiences and perceptions, even their physical bodies and minds, are always already cultural products (Gadamer, 1960/2005). Culture defines not only individuals' psyche but also their biology.

The cultural construction of health and illness can entail different aspects of health behaviors. Many have examined cultural similarities and differences of illness ideology and preferred treatment. For example, different cultures may attribute different causes to (and, thus, expect different treatment for) similar symptoms. In Caribbean voodoo, Chinese neurasthenia, and French crise-de-foie all describe general exhaustion that is attributed to liver problems (Rohlof et al., 2014). Fadiman (1997) investigated the cultural conflicts between the parents of a Hmong child with severe epilepsy and American doctors in California (for films on a Hmong shaman's experiences of living in American, please see Siegel, 1984, 2001). To the American doctors, the Hmong parents were incompetent and noncompliant because they did not administer the strict treatment regimens required for the seriously ill child. For the Hmong parents, American physicians were controlling and indifferent because they focused on eliminating all epileptic episodes and were not interested in the family's cultural beliefs about epilepsy (i.e., epilepsy is a gift from God and their child has the potential to be a noble shaman).

The cultural construction of health and illness is also about **embodied experiences**. In other words, individuals' biological body is a medium through which the "lived experience" of culture manifests. People who have similar clinical diagnosis may experience very different biological symptoms as a result of their culture (Kirmayer & Young, 1998). Waitzkin and Magana (1997) found that culture shapes individuals' somatic symptoms of stress: In Southeast Asian cultures, which place importance on the head, the somatic symptoms of war victims often manifest themselves as a headache; in contrast, in Latino culture, where the conceptions of "nerves" are commonplace, complaints referable to the nervous system appear more frequently. Arthur Kleinman (2004), a renowned professor of medical anthropology and cross-cultural psychiatry, explained:

> The term "culture" is often misused. In its early anthropologic usage, culture referred to the shared patterns of life that define social groups. This usage tended to portray cultures as bounded, fixed entities, neglecting crucial differences among and within groups, and it risked reducing culture to an autonomous variable among others. But culture is not a thing; it is a *process* by which ordinary activities acquire *emotional* and *moral* meaning for participants. Cultural processes include the *embodiment of meaning* in habitus and physiological reactions, the understanding of what is at stake in particular situations, the development of interpersonal connections, religious practices, and the cultivation of collective and individual identity. Culture is inextricably caught up with economic, political, psychological, and biologic conditions. Treating culture as a fixed variable seriously impedes our ability to understand and respond to disease states such as depression. [emphasis added] (p. 952)

Mythic Connection provides valuable insights to view culture as a "process by which ordinary activities acquire emotional and moral meaning for participants" (Kleinman, 2004, p. 952). Joseph Campbell (2004), a leading scholar of myth, proposed that myth serves four vital functions: metaphysical, cosmological, sociological, and pedagogical functions. These functions are not mutually exclusive. We believe that symbols in Mythic Connection serve similar functions as well.

The **metaphysical function** questions and redefines the nature of being (e.g., existence or identity). For example, personal myths are stories that define who I am and are stories that "I continue to revise, and tell to myself (and sometimes others) as I continue to go on living" (McAdams, 1993, p. 11). Illness imposes intrusion to individuals' identity, often disrupting their taken-for-granted understanding of Self and sense of time. As a result, patients often rely on illness narratives to reconstruct and (re)integrate the new self that emerged from their illness experiences to create continuity of and coherence to their life stories (Rimmon-Kenan, 2002). For example, in their investigation of patients with schizophrenia, Roe and Davidson (2005) found that patients do not focus on the permanent loss of self, but actively worked to "regain and strengthen an effective sense of self and coherent life narrative" (p. 93).

The **cosmological function** explains the form and formation of the cosmos and one's place in it. Origin myths and religious myths often involve cosmological functions. Although both Islam and Christianity are monotheistic religions, the differences in their cosmology may have contributed to the differences in their attitudes toward illness. Christian faith promotes **self-determinism**, which argues that individuals are responsible for the consequences of their free will (Atkinson & Field, 2013); in contrast, Muslim faith emphasizes "divine predestination" (i.e., God's direct intervention in the creation of existents) and humans are encouraged to orient themselves to God's will (De Cillis, 2013). The performance of Salat, the obligatory Muslim prayers to be performed five times a day, is a true embodiment of total submission to Allah (Bridgeman, 2017). Submission, thus, is often reported as a coping strategy for Muslims at times of stress, in addition to seeking support from their families and communities (Fischer et al., 2010; Pitaloka & Hsieh, 2015). In contrast, Christians are less likely to report submission but prefer individualistic, intrapersonal coping strategies such as looking for personal spiritual support, self-reliance, and problem solving (Fischer et al., 2010). A study found that 94% of Arabic patients (all Muslim) believe that illness has "no influence on life as it is fixed by fate" and 94% reported to "accept illness and bear it calmly;" in contrast only 54% and 36% of German patients (86% Christian, 10% atheist, and 5% other) hold the same attitudes (Bussing et al., 2007).

Through religious beliefs, patients of chronic illness (e.g., cancer and diabetes) have been found to transform a seemingly fatalistic attitude into an empowering motivation as a coping strategy (Bussing et al., 2007; Büssing et al., 2009; Pitaloka & Hsieh, 2015). By viewing illness as "God's will" and a "test of spiritual strength," Indonesian women with diabetes were able to perform a valued cultural virtue, submission – accepting everything in life as fate. "Submission, as a coping strategy, is the embodiment of the Javanese teaching by achieving a peaceful mind (*tentreming ati*) through patience, grace, and gratitude under stress" (Pitaloka & Hsieh, 2015, p. 1162). Similarly, when patients with cancer seek help from God through prayers, their fatalistic attitudes transform into a positive coping strategy by strengthening their sense of hope and empowerment (Sadati et al., 2015).

The **sociological function** validates and supports the social order and social norms for self and others. The **pedagogical function** teaches us how to behave through the stages of our lives. By identifying these two functions, Campbell (2004) aimed to highlight that myths not only maintain social structures of the System but they also function to teach its cultural participants about proper norms, "manners." In reality, although theoretically distinctive, these two functions generally co-exist with one another in reinforcing individual behaviors within the System. For example, parents may actively share stories about inheritable illnesses of individual family members (e.g., diabetes, dementia, and mental illness) to educate their children about family medical histories, socialize them with lessons and expectations of illness management, and develop a new framework of the illness to facilitate positive coping behaviors (Flood-Grady & Koenig Kellas, 2019; Manoogian et al., 2010).

Researchers have found that the telling and retelling of stories are essential in the formation and maintenance of values and identities of not just individuals, but also organizations (Brown, 1985; Putnam, 1982). For example, in one study, we found that physicians and nurses of a hospital repeatedly shared a story about an interpreter. Different versions of the story emerged though the actual identity of the interpreter and the actual misconduct remained uncertain. When stories are shared for the purpose of Mythic Connection, it is irrelevant whether the stories are "factual." Stories are not meant to be "facts;" rather, the purpose of storytelling is to connect the individuals to the values and principles of the community. Allegories may have no factual basis but they can be very good vehicles for imparting moral stories and socializing members of a moral community. In other words, the key to the providers' stories – the function of the institutional myth – is about institutional hierarchy, organizational standards, and the danger posed by problematic interpreters. This institutional cautionary tale aims to warn providers about the power and danger of an interpreter and the necessity of maintaining vigilance against interpreters' performance (Hsieh, Ju, & Kong, 2010).

Finally, it should be understood that to a person of the Mythic Connection world, myth does not have a "purpose" or "function" as such. Worldviews (i.e., consciousness structures) do not function in a means-ends process. This is a perspectival way of reducing myth to its own terms and way of understanding. This way of understanding myth manifests a dissociation between explanation and thing explained that is most apparent in the three-dimensional world of Perspectival Thinking.

IV. Sense-Making in an Illness Event

An essential characteristic of Mythic Connection is its transformative nature. Mythic Connection allows cultural participants to create, attach, and integrate new meanings to existing "things," generating symbols of moral claims.

A. Illness as Storied Self

Illness events can pose significant disruptions to one's life trajectory. At times, an illness disruption can be so profound that it creates **biographical disruption**, a biographical crisis that forces a person to reconsider their anticipated biography and self-concepts (Bury, 1982). Individuals' expectation of life progression in a linear timeline can no longer be taken-for-granted. For example, Mothers of kids with Down syndrome talk about mourning for the loss of the taken-for-granted future that they had anticipated for their kids' future prior to the diagnosis (Kong, 2016). When reflecting on her own experience when she learned of her child's Down syndrome diagnosis, Kong (2016) explained, "As a mother of a child with Down syndrome, I have experienced the devastation and traumatic loss of my dreamed baby. Along with the identity loss of being a typical mother, I have also lost all my dreams, hopes, and become disconnected with my life" (p. iv). Kong concluded, "The person who I was died on the day Daniel was born" (p. 4). For Dr. Kong, her life trajectory was completely transformed. Similarly, after a stroke, Swedish patients reported "a biographical disruption and anxiety of what the future had to bring" and focused on the day-to-day or week-to-week activities (i.e., life as cycles with repeated routines) to manage their uncertainty (Hjelmblink & Holmstrom, 2006, p. 371). On the other hand, researchers have observed that at times, illness diagnosis also can serve as **biographical reinforcement**, reinforcing identities that have been built prior to the diagnosis. For example, for gay men, the diagnosis of HIV reaffirmed lifelong social struggles; in contrast, for men who were hemophiliacs, an HIV diagnosis confirmed a lifetime of illness (Carricaburu & Pierret, 1995). A low-income woman may normalize her diagnosis of diabetes, constructing the diagnosis as part of their lifelong struggles with poverty and violence in everyday life (Pitaloka & Hsieh, 2015).

More recently, Tan (2018) has proposed the concept of **biographical illumination**, a transformative process of self and identity that is facilitated by, but also extends beyond, medical meaning and context, enriching personal biography and social relationships. Biographical illumination allows individuals to develop new insights and knowledge about themselves. For example, adults who learned of their Autism Spectrum Disorder later in life often reviewed their past experiences through the new diagnosis, allowing them to make sense of their behaviors and perspectives in a way that integrates the new understandings that acknowledge their atypicality and develop a more valued identity. The medical diagnosis allowed the patient to transform, enrich, and cultivate new self-concepts.

Biographic disruption, biographic reinforcement, and biographical illumination are not necessarily mutually exclusive. Kong (2016) reflected on her journey of motherhood and explained, "I didn't become a mother on [the day when my boy was born], but I really became a mother when I managed to survive in caring and raising a son with Down syndrome" (p. 4). Whether an illness event serves as biographical disruption or biographical reinforcement is not dependent on the actual details of the event. Rather, it is about perspective-taking and sense-making: How individuals choose to frame their illness experiences (through their storytelling and narratives) has a profound impact on their understanding of their social world and identities.

Kathy Charmaz identified different identities that a patient with chronic illness may generate at different stages of coping (Charmaz, 1987, 1991). At an initial stage of diagnosis, a patient may claim a **supernormal identity**, emphasizing that their illness would not interfere with their existing identity. In fact, at this stage, a patient often actively and aggressively participated in everyday activities that are more intensive than their non-ill peers. When claiming a supernormal identity, a patient not only refuses others' assistance but also tries to do "more" than what others would consider appropriate. For example, friends and family may tell a patient with a spinal injury that he is "crazy" to go hunting with the dog (Yoshida, 1993). Nevertheless, participating in these activities are essential to the patient to feel and claim that they are not defined by their illness.

Because the performance of a supernormal identity requires added energy and effort, patients often later settle into a **restored self**, in which the patient typically denies that the illness has changed them and claims that they are back to their previous "true" identity. However, if the chronic illness continues to intrude into their everyday life (e.g., feeling debilitating fatigue or pain that disrupts their taken-for-granted life), a patient may create a **contingent personal identity**, recognizing that their illness has presented constraints to their lives forcing them to reconcile the consequences of a changed identity. At the final stage, a patient develops a sense of **salvaged self**, embracing the emerged identity despite its new limitations imposed by the illness.

Although there is a sense of linear progression, researchers have found that the process of identity management can be cyclical. Individuals also do not necessarily exhibit all stage-specific identities. For example, progressive, chronic illnesses often require patients to renegotiate their identities, recreating narratives to find a sense of coherence or control over their illness events (Frank, 2013). A new diagnosis of peripheral vascular disease and a treatment recommendation of lower-extremity amputation may prompt a patient with diabetes who has developed a stabilized, restored or salvaged self into a new search of meanings and stories as a potential amputee. A patient whose cancer is in remission may need to renegotiate the boundaries of health and illness (Charmaz, 1994). From this perspective, stories and storytelling are never-ending communicative activities that demand storytellers and their audiences to identify and perform the embedded moral claims (Hsieh, 2004).

B. Illness Narratives as a Resource for Transformation

Through Mythic Connection, individuals (and cultural groups) generate stories that create, sustain, and reinforce values and moral claims within the cultural system. As such, the same behaviors or activities may result in different interpretations and entail diverging meanings due to different cultural groups. For example, an ethnographic study of heroin addicts who were homeless found that they frequently engaged in needle-sharing practices, which allowed them to maintain their "dope fiend" identities, communicate mutual bonding, and demonstrate trust in their fragile social network (Bourgois, 1998). Needle-sharing, as a health practice, communicates diverging meanings and values on the street (i.e., trust and bonding) and in the larger society (i.e., risky, reckless health behaviors). For homeless, heroin addicts, needle-sharing is the embodiment of positive meanings (e.g., bonding, trust, and stability) that are essential to build and maintain supportive relationships that are fundamental to their survival on the street. Without recognizing the symbolic meanings and the real-life implications of these actions, it is easy for one to attribute "problematic" behaviors to negative traits and implications (e.g., lack of knowledge, poor self-discipline, or recklessness).

In an illness event, individuals can rely on illness conditions or symptoms for Mythic Connection, creating stories that honor their struggles and moral claims in the face of adversity. An Indonesian woman explained her struggles with diabetes, "This disease is like a demon, haunted [sic] my life. But, we don't have to be afraid, we can become a doctor for ourselves, we are free, we can fly high and determine our life, be independent and not depend on others" (Pitaloka & Hsieh, 2015, p. 1059). The temporal dimension of an illness event provides opportunities for a person to revise their storyline and identify with new virtues and moral claims. In a study of women's coping experiences with infertility, Bute and Vik (2010) found that some patients viewed infertility as a "change agent" in promoting them to gain new perspectives on the issues of infertility. Nancy, a woman who had a successful pregnancy after a miscarriage, talked about her desire to educate others, "In the future if I know someone who has a miscarriage, I would probably let them know [my struggles with infertility]" (Bute & Vik, 2010, p. 12). For these patients, illnesses (e.g., diabetes and infertility), despite their compromised and weakened biological implications, are transformed into resources that allow them to assert moral claims (e.g., resilience and empathy).

The process of Mythic Connection is not limited to the patient but can be a joint, collaborative activity between multiple participants. When discussing the role of a physician in a patient's illness experiences, Brody (1994) noted, "Suffering cannot be relieved, however elegant a cure [a physician] performs, unless the patient's subjective sense of split and isolation [caused by illness] has been assuaged" (p. 84). Physicians assume an essential role in co-constructing a patient's illness narratives, helping them to navigate the biomedical terrain, identify meaningful healing actions, and develop a sense of coherence in the patient's life story (Brody, 1994). When a family member faces a difficult illness, the whole family engages in **joint storytelling**, as they collaborate to define the shared problem, engage in sense-making and perspective-taking, generate a shared understanding of what the experience means for the family (Koenig Kellas & Trees, 2006). An individual's illness story is transformed into a shared narrative among family members, creating "a shared system of belief for understanding their environment" (Koenig Kellas & Trees, 2006, p. 53). This serves as a Mythic Connection between members within a family unit. In essence, joint storytelling is a form of **symbolic convergence**, in which different individuals and groups collaborate together to define and shape a co-constructed reality (Bormann, 1985).

The shared storytelling does not necessarily become a consolidated, single story. For example, support group participants have been found to use stories dialogically to formulate a *collective* as well as an *individual* understanding of their experiences and identities (Hsieh, 2004). Similarly, in family joint storytelling, individual members also engage in collaborative, collective understanding and, at the same time, develop their individual interpretation (Koenig Kellas & Trees, 2006). The layering and consequent potential tensions between stories reflect possible challenges an individual faces when different cultural systems may present conflicting Mythic Connection (e.g., how can a patient assert his own agency and opinion and act as a "good" patient who follows the physicians' guidance at the same time?).

C. Creating and Maintaining Symbols

Mythic Connection centers on creating symbols, through which cultural values are attached, maintained, and sustained. The symbols can be almost anything that cultural participants attach meanings to, and by which Mythic Connection can be supported and sustained. For example, for many people, prayer "is an activity of the human spirit reflecting connectedness with God – a defining attribute of spirituality" (Meraviglia, 1999, p. 26). As such, prayers become the symbol for Mythic Connection, allowing a patient to perform valued identity (e.g., devout believer) and find strength and resources by tapping into a cultural system.

It is important to recognize it is not the prayer (i.e., the "thing") itself that creates Mythic Connection. Rather, it is how the cultural participants understand prayers that define the functions and meanings of a prayer. Under Magic Consciousness, a cultural participant views a ritualized chant (e.g., a curse, a spell, or "abracadabra") or "magic" object (e.g., an amulet or a relic) to hold actual (healing) power. For example, in Arbëreshë and Italian villages in Southern Italy, a healer would use a blessing ceremony followed by an illness-specific prayer that is repeated either three or nine times to treat malocchio (i.e., a complex illness which is also known as "evil eye;" Quave & Pieroni, 2005). Saying the chant or using the object wields real changes to the real world. The power is inherent in these acts and objects. If these acts/object fail, it's because the magic is broken. There is no one to blame. It simply failed.

In contrast, when a person uses prayers as the symbol for Mythic Connection, the cultural participant hopes that the prayer would have some effect (i.e., prayers offer the hope of divine intervention in a life crisis). However, there is no inherent power within the prayer that guarantees its effect (Smilansky, 2012). Nevertheless, prayer serves as a transformative agent that connects individuals to a collective identity (e.g., a faith group) and a value system that transforms the meanings of individual suffering. For example, Mother Theresa once said, "There is something beautiful in seeing the poor accept their lot, to suffer it like Christ's Passion. The world gains much from their suffering" (Varagur, 2017, para. 5). When asked about their experiences coping with diabetes, Indonesian women emphasized the importance of "submission" as a virtue (Pitaloka & Hsieh, 2015):

> Fitri argued, "The key is 3Bs: pray (*berdoa*), be grateful (*bersyukur*), and surrender (*berserah*)." Ningsih concluded, "You have to give thanks for every blessing, sickness, sadness, and happiness. Not just the happiness. If you enjoy yourself and are grateful for what you've got, you will feel so much better!" ... Marni echoed, "I totally surrender to God. If I must die, then so be it. I have a satisfied life!" (p. 1160)

Embracing suffering and poverty are essential as they transform cultural participants into valued identities even when God does not necessarily answer prayers in the ways that the cultural participants desire.

Symbols in Mythic Connection need not be for religious or spiritual purposes. For example, researchers have found that elderly Chinese immigrants in the United States cook dishes using food therapy in Chinese medicine as a way to pass on their cultural knowledge, "allowing their children to connect with the cultural roots" (Kong & Hsieh, 2012, p. 874). In this way, these Chinese dishes serve as the symbol to connect the cultural participants to their culture, transforming the immigrant children who were not interested in or familiar with Chinese culture into a member of the Chinese community. By relying on "pink ribbons" and breast cancer "survivors" as the movement of breast cancer awareness, Komen Foundation and the Race for the Cure created "an ideal citizenship that gains virtue and elicits identification and support because of its innocence and apparent distance from the corruption and conflict of all things political" (King, 2004, p. 488) – despite the fact that the image of these "cheerful survivors" silences the experiences of alienation, grief, and anger of many patients with breast cancer (Kaiser, 2008; see Figures 3.6 and 3.7).

In summary, stories and sense-making are essential in maintaining the symbolic world of Mythic Connection. Patients' stories are fused with the Voice of the Lifeworld, allowing them to assert moral claims through their illness experiences. Because the stories are not meant to be an authentic representation of the facts but are symbols of the values asserted, the storytellers and audiences evaluate and negotiate the appropriateness and significance of the stories based on their ability to

Figure 3.6 Breast cancer survivor I. Is there a place for a survivor who chooses not to have an implant? What defines one's femininity? Are survivors still expected to be "pretty"? *Source:* Justin Paget/Getty Images

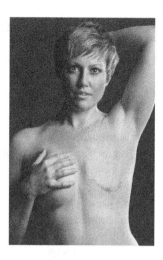

Figure 3.7 Breast cancer survivor II. What if you do not have any pretty or happy stories to tell? What is in this image of a breast cancer "survivor" that makes us uncomfortable? *Source:* Aaron Goldman / EyeEm/Getty Images

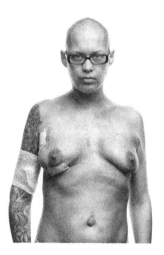

uphold the cultural System of the Mythic Connection (as opposed to the degree to which they represent independent objective realities). A good illness narrative, one that is embraced and honored by the society, is not the one that is "objectively true" but the one that is alive and supports proper identity performance and the values of the cultural world (e.g., "never give up on life;" "God has a plan for all of us;" and "suffering allows us to appreciate little things in life").

An illness story can be challenged and even disdained when it fails to honor the ethics of the System (e.g., a patient with terminal cancer embracing assisted suicide; a cancer patient who enjoys the exploitation of others' empathy and support). In other words, illness narratives are not taken-for-granted. They are performed by the patient and judged by the audience. Some stories are better and more celebrated than others. In this sense, both the storytellers and audiences of stories are active participants in the construction and maintenance of the social world of Mythic Connection. Through stories, storytelling, and story listening, we gain insights into the symbolic world of Mythic Connection.

V. Additional Resources

A. Key Terms and Theories

Magic Consciousness
holistic medicine
holism
Mythic Connection
symbolic communication
circular time
linear time
origin myths
anthropomorphic
therianthropy
two-valued logic
polyvocal
hermeneutics
symbol
automythology
quest stories
Theory of Communication Action
Lifeworld
System (see also Chapter 4)
Voice of Medicine (see also Chapter 4)
Voice of the Lifeworld
embodied experiences (or embodiment)
functions of stories by Campbell
    metaphysical function
    cosmological function
    sociological function
    pedagogical function
self-determinism
biographical disruption
biographical reinforcement
biographical illumination
illness identities (for patients with chronic illness) by Charmaz
    supernormal identity
    restored self
    contingent personal identity
    salvaged self
joint storytelling
symbolic convergence

B. Discussion Questions

1. In the film *Avatar* (Cameron, 2009), the Na'vi holds predominately Magic Consciousness and Mythic Connection worldviews; in contrast, Humans hold predominately Perspectival Thinking worldviews. What type of worldviews best

describe Na'vi's understanding and experiences of the following events? Explain why these reflect Magic Consciousness, Mythic Connection, or Perspectival Thinking worldviews held by the Na'vi and/or Humans.

    a. The Na'vi make "tsaheylu" – bonding with an animal by connecting physically with other animals via an entangling membrane or "queue" (neural connector) on the backs of animals' heads.

    b. *Eywa*. The Na'vi believes that Eywa helps all living things on Pandora to maintain perfect equilibrium. Norm, an anthropologist, explained to Jake, "Who's Eywa? Only their deity! Their goddess – made up of all living things. Everything they know! You'd know this if you had any training whatsoever."

    c. The clan was instantly reverent of Jake when he returned to the Omaticaya clan, bonded to a great leonopetryx. (The elaborate Na'vi folklore of *Toruk Makto*, a mythical hero who rides the great leonopteryx and leads the people to victory during times of great sorrow.)

    d. RDA's security forces destroyed the "one big damn tree," *Kelutral*, forcing the Navi to leave the Omaticaya Hometree and relocate.

2. Do you think illness imposes a circular time or linear time for the patient?

    a. What types of illness make patients perceive time more as circular time? Why?

    b. What types of illness make patients perceive time more as linear time? Why?

    c. Do you think physicians and patients may have different perceptions of time? In what ways?

3. Looking at your personal or your family's illness experiences, do you/they have any event that was incorporated into a transformative story – an automythology – that allows that patient to re-orient their life meanings and worldviews?

    a. In what ways were the stories transformative? What are the values and worldviews that are reshaped as a result of the illness event?

    b. Do they conform to the cultural expectations of the society or community that the patient belongs to? In what ways?

4. Do you think there are illness stories and experiences that one would have a difficult time sharing in your community? What are they? Why are they "unappreciated," "ignored," or "disdained" in your community?

5. Do you think your religion or spirituality helps you cope with your illness? In what ways?

    a. Do you think the coping strategies embraced by your religious or spiritual views are compatible or appreciated by the field of medicine?

    b. If you are an atheist, do you think such attitudes influence your coping strategies in an illness event? In what ways?

6. Do you and your family engage in joint storytelling? What kinds of stories are they?

    a. Why do you think people try to co-tell a story?

    b. In what ways are those stories "performed" (as opposed to being "factual")?

    c. Do you think there are values, principles, or moral claims in those stories?

7. What can be a "symbol" in a person's illness experience?

    a. Identify examples of a symbol in a particular context. Can a symbol be an object? A physical scar? A specific experience? A statement?

    b. Explain why it is a symbol? In other words, what are the meanings it carry beyond its form (e.g., symptoms or physical experiences)?

    c. How does the symbol help the patient connect their personal experiences to the values of the Mythic Connection world?

C. References

Atkinson, D. J., & Field, D. F. (Eds.). (2013). *New dictionary of Christian ethics & pastoral theology*. InterVarsity Press.

Bakhtin, M. M. (1981). *The dialogic imagination: Four essays by M. M. Bakhtin* (M. Holquist & C. Emerson, Trans.). University of Texas Press.

Barnes, M. (Director). (2009). *Doctors' diaries*. [DVD]. PBS. https://www.pbs.org/wgbh/nova/doctors/program.html

Batt, S. (2003). *Patient no more: The politics of breast cancer*. Spinifex Press.

Bormann, E. G. (1985). Symbolic convergence theory: A communication formulation. *Journal of Communication, 35*(4), 128–138.

Bourgois, P. (1998). The moral economies of homeless heroin addicts: Confronting ethnography, HIV risk, and everyday violence in San Francisco shooting encampments. *Substance Use & Misuse, 33*(11), 2323–2351.

Bridgeman, L. (2017). Embodying Islam: The political, social and spiritual use of the body in performative practice. *Performing Islam, 6*(2), 123–154.

Brody, H. (1994). "My story is broken; can you help me fix it?": Medical ethics and the joint construction of narratives. *Literature and Medicine, 13*(1), 79–92.

Brown, M. H. (1985). That reminds me of a story: Speech action in organizational socialization. *Western Journal of Speech Communication, 49*(1), 27–42.

Bury, M. (1982). Chronic illness as biographical disruption. *Sociology of Health & Illness, 4*(2), 167–182.

Bussing, A., Abu-Hassan, W. M., Matthiessen, P. F., & Ostermann, T. (2007). Spirituality, religiosity, and dealing with illness in Arabic and German patients. *Saudi Medical Journal, 28*(6), 933–942.

Büssing, A., Michalsen, A., Balzat, H.-J., Grünther, R.-A., Ostermann, T., Neugebauer, E. A. M., & Matthiessen, P. F. (2009). Are spirituality and religiosity resources for patients with chronic pain conditions? *Pain Medicine, 10*(2), 327–339.

Bute, J. J., & Vik, T. A. (2010). Privacy management as unfinished business: Shifting boundaries in the context of infertility. *Communication Studies, 61*(1), 1–20.

Cameron, J. (Director). (2009). *Avatar*. [Film]. Lightstorm Entertainment, Dune Entertainment, & Ingenious Film Partners.

Campbell, J. (2004). *Pathways to bliss: Mythology and personal transformation* (D. Kudler, Ed.). New World Library.

Carricaburu, D., & Pierret, J. (1995). From biographical disruption to biographical reinforcement: The case of HIV-positive men. *Sociology of Health & Illness, 17*(1), 65–88.

Charmaz, K. (1987). Struggling for a self: Identity levels of the chronically ill. In J. A. Roth & P. Conrad (Eds.), *Research in the sociology of health care: The experience and management of chronic illness* (Vol. 6, pp. 283–321). JAI Press.

Charmaz, K. (1991). *Good days, bad days: The self in chronic illness and time*. Rutgers University Press.

Charmaz, K. (1994). Identity dilemmas of chronically ill men. *Sociological Quarterly, 35*(2), 269–288.

Charmaz, K. (1999). Stories of suffering: Subjective tales and research narratives. *Qualitative Health Research, 9*(3), 362–382.

Charmaz, K. (2002). Stories and silences: Disclosures and self in chronic illness. *Qualitative Inquiry, 8*(3), 302–328.

Collins, A. Y. (Ed.). (1986). *Semeia 36: Early Christian apocalypticism: Genre and social setting*. Scholars Press.

Collins, J. J. (2014). What is apocalyptic literature? In J. J. Collins (Ed.), *The Oxford handbook of apocalyptic literature* (pp. 1–16). Oxford University Press.

De Cillis, M. (2013). *Free will and predestination in Islamic thought: Theoretical compromises in the works of Avicenna, al-Ghazali and Ibn 'Arabi.* Routledge.

Eliade, M. (1959). *The sacred and the profane: The nature of religion* (W. R. Trask, Trans.). Harcourt.

Fadiman, A. (1997). *The spirit catches you and you fall down: A Hmong child, her American doctors, and the collision of two cultures.* Farrar, Straus and Giroux.

Fischer, P., Ai, A. L., Aydin, N., Frey, D., & Haslam, S. A. (2010). The relationship between religious identity and preferred coping strategies: An examination of the relative importance of interpersonal and intrapersonal coping in Muslim and Christian faiths. *Review of General Psychology, 14*(4), 365–381.

Flood-Grady, E., & Koenig Kellas, J. K. (2019). Sense-making, socialization, and stigma: Exploring narratives told in families about mental illness. *Health Communication, 34*(6), 607–617.

Frank, A. W. (2013). *The wounded storyteller: Body, illness, and ethics* (2nd ed.). University of Chicago Press.

Gadamer, H.-G. (2005). *Truth and method* (J. Weinsheimer & D. G. Marshall, Trans.; 2nd rev. ed.). Continuum. (Original work published 1960)

Habermas, J. (1985). *The Theory of Communicative Action: Lifeworld and System, a critique of functionalist reason* (T. McCarthy, Trans.; 3rd ed., Vol. 2). Beacon. (Original work published 1981)

Hastings, A. C., Fadiman, J., & Gordon, J. S. (2018). *Health for the whole person: The complete guide to holistic medicine.* Routledge. (Original work published 1980)

Hjelmblink, F., & Holmstrom, I. (2006). To cope with uncertainty: Stroke patients' use of temporal models in narratives. *Scandinavian Journal of Caring Sciences, 20*(4), 367–374.

Hsieh, E. (2004). Stories in action and the dialogic management of identities: Storytelling in transplant support group meetings. *Research on Language and Social Interaction, 37*(1), 39–70.

Hsieh, E., Ju, H., & Kong, H. (2010). Dimensions of trust: The tensions and challenges in provider-interpreter trust. *Qualitative Health Research, 20*(2), 170–181.

Istoft, B. (2010). Avatar fandom as nature-religious expression? *Journal for the Study of Religion, Nature & Culture, 4*(4), 394–413.

Kaiser, K. (2008). The meaning of the survivor identity for women with breast cancer. *Social Science & Medicine, 67*(1), 79–87.

King, S. (2004). Pink Ribbons Inc: Breast cancer activism and the politics of philanthropy. *International Journal of Qualitative Studies in Education, 17*(4), 473–492.

Kirmayer, L. (2001). Cultural/variations in the clinical presentation of depression and anxiety: Implications for diagnosis and treatment. *Journal of Clinical Psychiatry, 62*(Suppl. 13), 22–30.

Kirmayer, L. J., & Young, A. (1998). Culture and somatization: Clinical, epidemiological, and ethnographic perspectives. *Psychosomatic Medicine, 60*(4), 420–430.

Klein, W. (2013). *Time in language.* Routledge. (Original work published 1994)

Kleinman, A. (2004). Culture and depression. *New England Journal of Medicine, 351*(10), 951–953.

Kocnig Kellas, J., & Trees, A. R. (2006). Finding meaning in difficult family experiences: Sense-making and interaction processes during joint family storytelling. *Journal of Family Communication, 6*(1), 49–76.

Kong, H. (2016). *Finding peace in life's unexpected journey: The process of grieving and identity transformation for mothers of children with Down syndrome* [Dissertation, University of Oklahoma]. Norman, OK. https://hdl.handle.net/11244/34679

Kong, H., & Hsieh, E. (2012). The social meanings of traditional Chinese medicine: Elderly Chinese immigrants' health practice in the United States. *Journal of Immigrant and Minority Health, 14*(5), 841–849.

Kramer, E. M. (2013). Hermeneutics: The world as conversation. In C. McIlwain (Ed.), *Philosophy, method, and cultural criticism* (pp. 13–36). Hampton.

Leeming, D. A. (2010). *Creation myths of the world: An encyclopedia* (2nd ed.). ABC-CLIO.

Lévi-Strauss, C. (1978). *Myth and meaning*. University of Toronto Press.

Lo, M.-C.M., & Bahar, R. (2013). Resisting the colonization of the Lifeworld? Immigrant patients' experiences with co-ethnic healthcare workers. *Social Science & Medicine, 87*(Suppl. C), 68–76.

Makoul, G. (Director). (2004). *Sharon: Living with dying*. [eVideo]. Center for Communication & Medicine, Northwestern University.

Manoogian, M. M., Harter, L. M., & Denham, S. A. (2010). The storied nature of health legacies in the familial experience of type 2 diabetes. *Journal of Family Communication, 10*(1), 40–56.

McAdams, D. P. (1993). *The stories we live by: Personal myths and the making of the self.* Guilford Press.

McMahan, I. (2017, May 11). *An ACL injury is no longer a career killer, but can athletes ever truly be the same?* The Guardian. https://www.theguardian.com/sport/2017/may/11/acl-injuries-sports-athletes-careers

Meraviglia, M. G. (1999). Critical analysis of spirituality and its empirical indicators: Prayer and meaning in life. *Journal of Holistic Nursing, 17*(1), 18–33.

Miller, P. J., Hengst, J., Alexander, K., & Sperry, L. L. (2000). Versions of personal storytelling/versions of experience: Genres as tools for creating alternate realities. In K. S. Rosengren & C. N. Johnson (Eds.), *Imagining the impossible: Magical, scientific, and religious thinking in children* (pp. 212–246). Cambridge University Press.

Mishler, E. G. (1984). *The discourse of medicine: Dialectics of medical interviews*. Ablex.

Möller, H.-G. (1999). Zhuangzi's "Dream of the Butterfly": A Daoist interpretation. *Philosophy East and West, 49*(4), 439–450.

Morris, D. (1994). *The human zoo*. Vintage. (Original work published 1969)

Moules, N. J. (2002). Hermeneutic Inquiry: Paying heed to history and Hermes; An ancestral, substantive, and methodological tale. *International Journal of Qualitative Methods, 1*(3), 1–21.

Munn, N. D. (1992). The cultural anthropology of time: A critical essay. *Annual Review Of Anthropology, 21*, 93–123.

Niesiolowski-Spano, L., & Laskowski, J. (2016). *The origin myths and holy places in the old testament: A study of aetiological narratives*. Routledge.

PBS. (2001). *Transcripts: Survivor MD: Hearts and minds.* http://www.pbs.org/wgbh/nova/transcripts/2808hearts.html

PBS. (2009). *Doctors' Lives videos*. https://www.pbs.org/wgbh/nova/doctors/lives.html

Pitaloka, D., & Hsieh, E. (2015). Health as submission and social responsibilities: Embodied experiences of Javanese women with type II diabetes. *Qualitative Health Research, 25*(8), 1155–1165.

Putnam, L. L. (1982). Paradigms for organizational communication research: An overview and synthesis. *Western Journal of Communication, 46*(2), 192–206.

Quave, C. L., & Pieroni, A. (2005). Ritual healing in Arbëreshë Albanian and Italian communities of Lucania, Southern Italy. *Journal of Folklore Research, 42*(1), 57–97.

Rasmussen, D. M. (2012). *Mythic-symbolic language and philosophical anthropology: A constructive interpretation of the thought of Paul Ricœur.* Springer.

Rimmon-Kenan, S. (2002). The story of "I": Illness and narrative identity. *Narrative, 10*(1), 9–27.

Roe, D., & Davidson, L. (2005). Self and narrative in schizophrenia: Time to author a new story. *Med Humanit, 31*(2), 89–94.

Rohlof, H. G., Knipscheer, J. W., & Kleber, R. J. (2014). Somatization in refugees: A review. *Social Psychiatry and Psychiatric Epidemiology, 49*(11), 1793–1804.

Sadati, A. K., Lankarani, K. B., Gharibi, V., Fard, M. E., Ebrahimzadeh, N., & Tahmasebi, S. (2015). Religion as an empowerment context in the narrative of women with breast cancer. *Journal of Religion and Health, 54*(3), 1068–1079.

Secrist, E. S., Bhat, S. B., & Dodson, C. C. (2016). The financial and professional impact of anterior cruciate ligament injuries in National Football League athletes. *Orthopaedic Journal of Sports Medicine, 4*(8), Article 2325967116663921. https://doi.org/10.1177/2325967116663921

Sideris, L. H. (2010). I see you: Interspecies empathy and avatar. *Journal for the Study of Religion, Nature & Culture, 4*(4), 457–477.

Siegel, T. (Director). (1984). *Between two worlds: The Hmong shaman in America.* [Film]. Collective Eye Films.

Siegel, T. (Director). (2001). *The split horn: Life of a Hmong shaman in America.* [Film]. Collective Eye Films.

Smilansky, S. (2012). A problem about the morality of some common forms of prayers. *Ratio, 25*(2), 207–215.

Swidler, A. (2003). *Talk of love: How culture matters.* University of Chicago Press.

Tan, C. D. (2018). "I'm a normal autistic person, not an abnormal neurotypical": Autism Spectrum Disorder diagnosis as biographical illumination. *Social Science & Medicine, 197*, 161–167.

Thomas-MacLean, R. (2004). Understanding breast cancer stories via Frank's narrative types. *Social Science & Medicine, 58*(9), 1647–1657.

Todres, L., Galvin, K., & Dahlberg, K. (2007). Lifeworld-led healthcare: Revisiting a humanising philosophy that integrates emerging trends. *Medicine, Health Care and Philosophy, 10*(1), 53–63.

Varagur, K. (2017, March 16). *Mother Teresa was no saint.* HuffPost. https://www.huffpost.com/entry/mother-teresa-was-no-saint_b_9470988

Waitzkin, H., & Magana, H. (1997). The black box in somatization: Unexplained physical symptoms, culture and narratives of trauma. *Social Science & Medicine, 45*(6), 811–825.

Yoshida, K. K. (1993). Reshaping of self: A pendular reconstruction of self and identity among adults with traumatic spinal cord injury. *Sociology of Health & Illness, 15*(2), 217–245.

Zhuangzi. (2013). *The complete works of Zhuangzi* (B. Watson, Trans.). Columbia University Press.

4

Cultural Consciousness III

Perspectival Thinking and the Emergence of Modern Medicine

Chapter 4 examines the emergence of modern medicine as a result of Perspectival Thinking. We will first examine the cultural consciousness of Perspectival Thinking by comparing and contrasting it with Magic Consciousness and Mythic Connection. We will then review the history of modern medicine to examine how Perspectival Thinking shapes the nature and the dominant worldview of medicine today. By recognizing that medicine itself is a form of culture, we will examine how medicine creates, enforces, and maintains its social order and meanings through the educational process of a health professional.

I. Perspectival Thinking and Dissociation

A. Perspectival Thinking: Meanings Dependent on Perspective

In the **Theory of Dimensional Accrual and Dissociation**, Eric Kramer and colleagues have argued that different structures of cultural consciousness (i.e., Magic Consciousness, Mythic Connection, and Perspectival Thinking) entails different dimensional worldviews (Kramer, 2013; Kramer & Ikeda, 1998). In the idolic world of Magic Consciousness (i.e., the one-dimensional world), one is indistinguishable and inseparable from the rest of the world. Magic Consciousness is timeless and pre-spatial. Past and future as well as close and far are merged into one. Meanings are inherent in all things.

In the symbolic world of Mythic Connection (i.e., the two-dimensional world), one begins to separate from the world, developing some sense of polarities (e.g., good-evil, yin-yang) but striving to create coherence of meanings to their world. Although there is a sense of time, time is circular and revolving. Space emerges as individuals recognize that meanings and "things" are not the same – symbols are needed to create the necessary connection between them. Communities engage in storytelling to develop shared meanings and identities.

In the signalic world of **Perspectival Thinking** (i.e., the three-dimensional world), the world is characterized by a complete fragmentation and dissociation. This shift from mythic polarity to perspectival fragmentation, from compassion to objective disinterest, and from collectivism to individualism is evident in all modes of life, including religion. Both magical ritual and mythological prayer are communal activities involving the full participation of everyone in the group. For instance, the Western teleological notion of judgment day initially meant a time when all the dead would be judged together at the end of time. However, with the emergence of perspectivity, religion, like all other civilizational expressions, mutated so that the individual deathbed judgment and private confession emerged. As Max Weber (1905–1920/2002) noted, modern Christianity even embraced private property economics in a symbiotic fashion. A measure of piety is personal wealth. In prosperity theology (also known as prosperity gospel), God blesses faithful individuals with worldly positions, giving them personal fortunes of material wealth (Lee, 2007). In politics, the perspectival is manifested as the principle of individual civil liberties and the political behavior of "one man, one vote." Economically, perspectivism appears as intense privatization. Modern philosophies are obsessed with the individual, with existential crisis, identity crisis, and the Other. Dissociation is the emerging sense that the world is made up of discrete things such as atoms and molecules. Each unit stands on its own. This attitude perceives humans as independent individuals.

Individuals become increasingly dissociated and alienated with the world in psyche, time, and space. Perspectival Thinking is obsessed with standardization and precision, emphasizing the need for increasingly "correct" measurement, consistency, and mechanism. For example, time is no longer adequate to be measured by seasons, months, days, hours, or even seconds. In the 1960s, recognizing that earth was not a very good timekeeper for the definition of the second, researchers invented the atomic clock, which would allow for the redefinition of a second in 1967 (Grandjean, 1988; see Figure 4.1). The atomic clock has become the standard tool for modern scientific timekeeping, achieving estimated uncertainty of 1 nanosecond (1 billionth of a second) or an uncertainty of one second in 30 million years (Piester et al., 2008). The obsession with precision motivates specialization. The "reality" of the world is no longer part of us or what we can connect through our senses. Instead, reality is an aggregation of objects that exist outside of us, independent of our senses, observations, and feelings. As a result, in a Perspectival Thinking consciousness, measurement (i.e., the perspective/tool through which reality is measured) defines our reality. Things become the sum of their measures in standardized units of space and time. Even water, a seemingly stable, single "thing," includes components of different chemical elements and minerals and can entail different PH levels. Thus, not all waters are the same.

Things no longer hold inherent meanings. Rather, they are simply objects to be further analyzed and identified. Kramer & Ikeda (1998) explained,

> As dimensional awareness accrues, dissociation increases with countless consequences such as an increasing sense of isolation, a metaphysical denial of meaning, an increasing manipulation of a fragmented world which enables technical acuity, and a hyper-valuation of disinterest. In the modern world everything is in need of "improvement" and "development" in accord with linear progressivism. And the best way to solve problems is to first fragment them into smaller parts. Hence, the essence of reductionism and perspective. (p. 39)

Reality through measurements becomes "real." We have become accustomed to a reality defined by our measurements. For example, although statistics is not a true science but

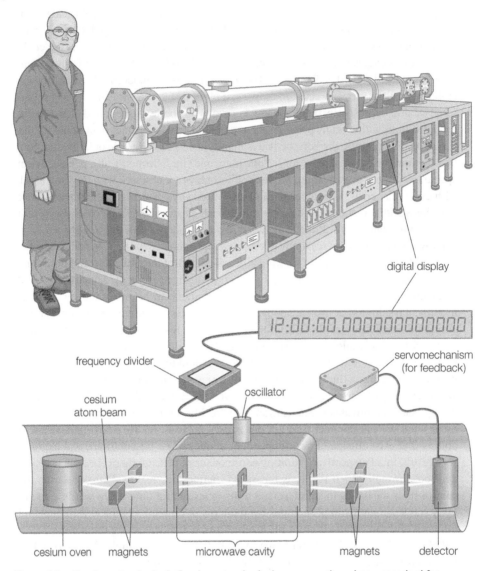

digital display

12:00:00.000000000000

frequency divider

servomechanism
(for feedback)

cesium
atom beam

oscillator

cesium oven   magnets   microwave cavity   magnets   detector

Figure 4.1 Caesium atomic clock. Caesium atomic clocks serve as the primary standard for the definition of the second in the International System of Units.

a form of measurement for mathematical probabilities, one does not question the "reality" of 3.24 (with a margin of error ±.01) members for the family size in the United States, even though in reality there cannot be a "real" .24 person (U.S. Census Bureau, 2019). We make decisions about social policies and government spending based on the projected life expectancy in 2060 (i.e., 81.6–87.1 and 76.9–83.7 years for native-born females and males in the United States) without questioning the various factors that may make such prediction inaccurate (e.g., geopolitical disabilities or climate crises; Medina et al., 2019). Reality is reduced to what is measurable and if something cannot be measured, it does not exist.

What is measurable is equated to what is real. When revealing the result of her genetic ancestry testing, Oprah Winfrey announced to audiences in Jonesburg, South Africa, "I always wondered what it would be like if it turned out I am a South African, [because] I feel so at home here ... Do you know that *I actually am one*? I went in search of my roots and had my DNA tested, and *I am a Zulu*" (emphasis added; Yang, 2007, p. 32). Senator Elizabeth Warren, faced with questions about her claim of Native American ancestry, took a DNA test to show that she had Native American ancestry 6 to 10 generations in the past (Scher, 2019). Oprah can discern her ancestry story through her skin color and Warren has family stories of Native American heritage; nevertheless, they relied on the genetic information obtained through laboratory testing to present the irrefutable "truth" of what they really are.

In the Perspectival Thinking world, we believe that truths are objective and verifiable facts. However, genetic researchers are aware that the genetic database can have a significant impact on the validity of ancestry testing (e.g., geographic locations, race, and migration patterns; Resnick, 2019; Yang, 2007). For example, due to the lack of representation of minorities in genetic databases, minorities' testing results are much vaguer (Resnick, 2019). In a later DNA test, it turned out that Oprah's ancestry is more likely to be with the Kpelle of Liberia and that she is also 5% Asian and 8% Native-American (Yang, 2007)! Does that mean that Oprah is also Asian and Native American? What does it mean when researchers claim that identical twins do not have identical DNA (O'Connor, 2008)? In other words, despite the presumptive belief that genetic ancestry testing is "precise," "objective," and "verifiable," and thus "accurate," the tool (i.e., the genetic ancestry testing) is only as accurate and reliable as its perspective allows. When one steps outside of the particular perspective, the reality proposed by the "measurement" can be problematic, inadequate, or unjust. In the wake of their announcement, Oprah and Warren also faced challenges against their claims, questioning whether their DNA, a seemingly irrefutable, objective form of evidence, is the appropriate measure for one's heritage or identity.

Because reality is limited to the perspective adopted, one's interpretation of reality is also limited to the tools and languages that define that reality. A controversial study relevant to Māori Australians was the "warrior gene" hypothesis, proposed by a genetic study conducted in New Zealand. Māori is the indigenous Polynesian people of New Zealand, who originated and migrated from eastern Polynesia arriving in New Zealand in several waves of canoe voyages between 1250 and 1300. A genetic epidemiologist, Rod Lea, presented his research findings at a genetic conference in Australia, noting that Māori men were twice as likely as European men to carry a monoamine oxidase (MOA), the "warrior gene" (Lea & Chambers, 2007). At the time, the findings were not unique since multiple genetic studies have linked MOA to addictive behaviors (Perbal, 2013). However, by coining the concept of a "warrior gene" and attributing it to the Māori people, Lea and his research team emphasized that the gene may contribute to Māori people's risk-taking behaviors, propensity for violence (e.g., domestic abuse), and lack of self-control (e.g., alcoholism). Lea explained that the gene may have contributed to positive aspects of Māori people's survival and successful voyages. However, Lea also hypothesized, "I think there is a link, it definitely predisposes people to be more likely to be criminals and engage in that type of behaviour as they grow older" (Perbal, 2013, p. 384). Māori leaders were outraged and criticized the statement for reinforcing stereotypes and discrimination against Māoris. Others raised concerns about pathologizing Māori's sociocultural problems, which effectively made being a Māori a "disease" and lead to additional discrimination and disparities by insurance companies (Hook, 2009).

Reflective methods and experiences are essential to Perspectival Thinking. Nietzsche (1962/2012) argues that experiences of "oneness of all things," a "mystical" experience, is a result of human intuition; however, "scientific reflection" can provide "means" that allow individuals to articulate the intuited and/or mystical experiences through words and concepts (Krebbs, 1997). Meanings in Perspectival Thinking are dependent on the perspectives one takes (Haynes, 2000). As such, Perspectival Thinking is intensely narrow and specific to the particular perspective one chooses to take. Diverging perspectives may lead to irreconcilable differences and realities.

As a result, the challenge in a technically advanced world of Perspectival Thinking is to recognize that precision does not necessarily define reality, truth, or justice. In Olympic swimming events, time is measured to two decimal places of a second. In the 2016 Olympic 100-meter butterfly final, Michael Phelps tied with two other swimmers – Laszlo Cseh of Hungary and Chad le Clos of South Africa – for silver at 51.14 seconds (see Figure 4.2). The officials could have broken the tie by comparing their times by one additional decimal place. However, an Olympic standardized pool tolerates differences up to three centimeters between pool lanes. In a thousandth of a second, Phelps's pace would allow him to travel a bit under 3 mm (Parr, 2016). In other words, the differences may come down to a fresh coat of paint or a slightly protruding tile. Recognizing that they were able to measure time better than they measure the pool length, the officials acknowledged that a three-way tie was necessary (Griswold, 2016).

Although one may be quick to think that Magic Consciousness is more primal and uncivilized than Perspectival Thinking, it is important to know that the accrual or

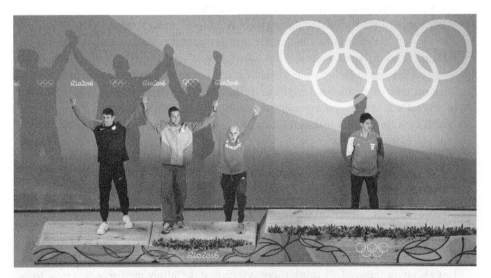

Figure 4.2 Three silver medalists for the men's 100 m butterfly final of the Rio 2016 Olympic Games. Joint silver medalists, Michael Phelps of United States, Chad Guy Bertrand le Clos of South Africa, Laszlo Cseh of Hungary and gold medalist Joseph Schooling of Singapore celebrate on the podium during the medals ceremony. *Source:* Richard Heathcote/Getty Images

adding up of dimensions is not a simple unilinear and irreversible process. Perspectival Thinking is not necessarily "better" or "more advanced" than Magic Consciousness. Rather, they represent different ways of conceptualizing realities, resulting in corresponding and variable worldviews, values, and principles. Perspectival Thinking can become problematic, deficient, and dangerous, legitimizing bias, prejudice, and even discrimination as in the case of "warrior genes" for the Māori people. After all, adopting a perspective means discriminating against all other perspectives.

B. Perspectival Thinking in Western History

The emergence of the worldview of Perspectival Thinking has occurred twice in western history. First calumniating with Aristotle who might be called the first modern thinker and then reemerging again as dominant after the European Renaissance (essentially the rebirth of Aristotelianism). The perspectival world is three-dimensional. The retrograde from Aristotelian classical Greco-Roman thinking to a predominantly mythic worldview lasted for over one thousand years and it can be exemplified and evinced in many ways. One is the disappearance of three-dimensional sculpture during this period. Studies in the physical sciences, medicine, mathematics, and logic largely disappeared to be replaced by grammarians and theologians. Literacy plummeted and libraries filled with the pagan writings of antiquity were deliberately destroyed. The universities were closed, and scholars fled the rise of persecution at the hands of Christian zealots and leaders such as the Christian emperor Justinian. The original Platonic Academy where many classical scholars studied, including Cicero, was closed in 88 BC due to the First Mithridatic War. It was reopened as the Neoplatonic Academy but then was destroyed in 529 AD. The study of mathematics, natural philosophy, logic and dialectics would disappear except when used in very limited ways by Christian apologists such as Tertullian and Thomas Aquinas.

It was more than a thousand years after the fall of Plato's Academy that Donatello unveiled his marble statue of David in 1409 and a later bronze David in 1444. These were the first freestanding sculptures made in Europe since the fall of Pagan Rome. Preoccupation with perspective and depth space erupts during the Renaissance, marking an essential quality of the era. Global, spatial exploration was launched. Cartography was reborn. Galileo turned the telescope skywards to explore the heavens. Pythagorean geometry reemerged. Leon Alberti published his work *De Pictura* (1435) on accurately depicting depth space, an effort culminating in Leonardo da Vinci's codification of geometric perspective a few decades later.

This rebirth demonstrates that worldviews do not unfold in only one direction. Magic Consciousness, Mythic Connection, and Perspectival Thinking do not occur in linear order. Societies can retrograde. Unilinear "progress" is not assumed by the Theory of Dimensional Accrual and Dissociation (Kramer, 2013; Kramer & Ikeda, 1998). Pure notions of progress (without ambivalence) are presumed in *only* the three-dimensional world of Perspectival Thinking. The perspectival world is a world obsessed with space, change, and "progression," including new declarations for social mobility, trade, and innovative thinking. People begin to be seen as mutable and no longer predestined by their blood heritage (e.g., royalty by blood as Magic Consciousness). Education, the effort to improve people's minds reemerges with notions of individualism and democratizing meritocracy.

II. Medicine as Culture

A. Emergence of Modern Medicine

1. Medicine in the Worlds of Magic Consciousness and/or Mythic Connection

Medicine has a long history of being infused with Magic Consciousness and Mythic Connection. In Chapter 3, we explored how the meaning-rich Lifeworld (see Chapter 3) derives, invokes, and sustains meanings through contexts that are grounded in everyday life (i.e., Magic Consciousness and Mythic Connection). In ancient worlds as well as many cultures today, medicine and medical practices remain an essential resource and they generate meaning as part of the Lifeworld. In ancient times, the medical systems of the Near East (i.e., Egypt, Syria, Mesopotamia, and Babylonia) combined theology and healing. The emblem of medicine (see Figure 4.3) in the United States incorporates symbols rooted in ancient Greek, including the caduceus[1] (i.e., a symbol of the Greek god) and the snakes (i.e., a symbol of renewal due to the sloughing of its skin; see Figure 4.4). Magic and mythic priest-physicians diagnose patients by assessing how divine displeasure, transgressions of various kinds, or magical forces have caused various symptoms (Bynum, 2008). Healing temples of the Greek god of Medicine, Asclepius, were run by resident priests who received patients and interpreted illnesses based on patients' reported dreams. Patients' illness bridges individuals' secular world with supernatural forces and the divine, requiring the intervention of **magico-religious medicine.** Magico-religious medicine believes that causes of diseases are attributed to supernatural beings or forces

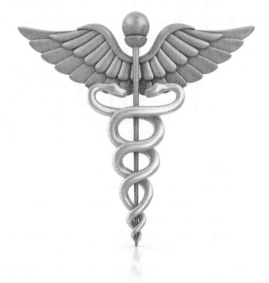

Figure 4.3 Caduceus. Caduceus is often used as a symbol of medicine, especially in the United States. *Source:* pagadesign/Getty Images

---

[1] The caduceus is the traditional symbol of Hermes and features two snakes winding around a winged staff. It is often mistakenly used as a symbol of medicine instead of the Rod of Asclepius, especially in the United States.

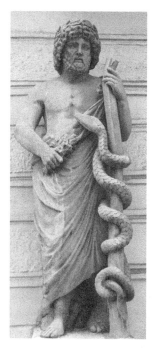

Figure 4.4 Greek God Asclepius. The Rod of Asclepius s a serpent-entwined rod wielded by the Greek god Asclepius, a deity associated with healing and medicine. *Source:* Zwiebackesser / Depositphotos

(e.g., evil spirits or angered gods). Prayers, incantations, purifications, sacrifices, exorcism as well as holy items (e.g., religious relics) are often employed to cure illnesses.

Due to the transformative powers of healing, medicine is often intertwined with Magic Consciousness and Mythic Connection. Many researchers have found that healing played an essential role in early Christianity (Ferngren, 1992). Most miracles involve healing, raising the dead, restoring mobility, regaining eyesight, among others. In the healing traditions of Judaism and the late Hellenistic world, there were competing modes of healing, including miracle cures, magic, and medicine (Kee, 1988). In the Gospels and the New Testament, Jesus and his disciples also used prayers to achieve healing through miracles (i.e., through "appeal to, and subsequent action by the gods"). Examples of magic are also abundant as Jesus casts out demons by his command (e.g., Mark 1:25; 5:8) or through physical touch (e.g., Mark 1:31; 6:16; Kee, 1988).

It is beyond the scope of this book to explore the definitive boundaries between magic, religion, and medicine. Although magico-religious medicine is rooted in the cultural structures of Magic Consciousness and/or Mythic Connection, the specific boundaries between Magic Consciousness and Mythic Connection may be dependent on how the specific cures are employed and interpreted. For example, Magic Consciousness is evoked when a person uses prayers in the sense of chanting and incantation or believing that a holy relic has inherent healing powers for its holders; in contrast, Mythic Connection dominates when a patient uses prayers to appeal to God and hope for corresponding intervention or assumes that holy relics allows a person to be favored by Gods (but does not have inherent power in itself). If one loses a magic relic, one has lost the magic. The object and its power are identical. The same is true of mystical healers, shaman, and those with "the gift." They are special people and their gift cannot be learned or transferred. Their supernatural powers are not arbitrary or replaceable. Their power is inherent in them and so they are often identified as children by others with supernatural powers or are known members of a bloodline of those with supernatural powers. When they die, parts of their bodies may become talisman and relics that contain supernatural power. Magic is nontransferable, irreplaceable, and not arbitrary. If a true holy relic such as an actual piece of the cross or the bone of a holy saint is lost, something irreplaceable is lost. Their supernatural power is gone. By contrast, if one loses a mythic symbol such as a crucifix, one does not lose god because it is not literally God. Yet ambiguously, it is not totally arbitrary either. One would not mistake a golf club for a crucifix. A crucifix, though not magical, entails strong emotional attachment. If it is lost, God is not lost.

It is essential to recognize that imbuing Magic Consciousness and Mythic Connection in the meanings and practice of medicine is not only prevalent in the ancient world but also in the modern world. The practices of Vodou in Haitian communities (Vonarx, 2011), the charms and holy items sold by *Brujos* (wizards) in Mexican herb markets (Ugent, 2000), and the adoption of faith healing and ritual healing in many parts of the world, including the United States (McGuire, 1988; Offit, 2015), are all examples of medical practices that are infused with Magic Consciousness and/or Mythic Connection. Modern industrial societies are not purely perspectival or scientific. A recent survey found that healing prayers are highly prevalent among U.S. adults: 78.8% reported having prayed for self (lifetime prevalence = 78.8%), 87.4% prayed for others, 54.1% asked asking for prayer, 26.1% used laying-on-of-hands technique to treat another person, and 53.0% participated in a prayer group (Levin, 2016; see Figure 4.5). Magic Consciousness and Mythic Connection are fundamental to the use and acts of healing prayers. They are not limited to the ancient world or people with superstitious beliefs. Nevertheless, although such cultural perspectives are common even in today's world, it is crucial to recognize that without Perspectival Thinking, there is no modern medicine.

2. Medicine in the World of Perspectival Thinking

Under Perspectival Thinking, nothing is sacred. All "things" are just things to be studied, examined, and analyzed. The **System** in Habermas' Theory of Communicative Action imposes a calculated, impersonal, purposeful rationality that is devoid of sentimentality or morality. Habermas (1981/1985) argued that the world of the System involves a purposeful, instrumental understanding of the social world. Within the

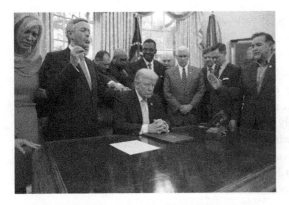

Figure 4.5 Laying-on-of-hands. On September 1, 2017, religious leaders prayed with President Donald Trump after he signed a proclamation for a national day of prayer to occur on Sunday, September 3, 2017, in the Oval Office of the White House in Washington. *Source:* AP photos

System, actions are oriented to achieve the success defined by relevant technical considerations. The System does not consider morality, nor does it hold sentimental values for things. Rather, the System operates through technocratic and impersonal rationality, demanding all that is involved to be subjected to its standards and perspectives. The System is best reflected in the emergence of modern medicine as technical interests are embraced through scientific attitudes where researchers and practitioners aim to develop abstract rules applicable irrespective of contexts.

In the Perspectival Thinking world, things are arbitrary, replicable, and transferable. According to science, knowledge requires replication (Schmidt, 2009). If a claim (e.g., the ability to perform cold fusion) cannot be replicated, it is not true knowledge. It does not matter who formulates the theory or who tests it. The only judge is empirical outcomes. Either the theory is true or false and even if a super famous person supports the theory, an unknown researcher can challenge the theory and demand that everyone see how it is supposed to work so they can independently test it. We do not take anyone's word at face value in science. All theories are contingent on testing (National Academies of Sciences, Engineering, and Medicine, 2019).

For instance, in the Perspectival Thinking world, physicians cannot claim that only they can cure cancer due to their own unique supernatural abilities. In the Perspectival Thinking world, knowledge can be transferred to anyone, they do not have to have special powers of a bloodline. And anyone of any gender, age, race, ethnicity can make discoveries and inventions. Anyone can become a doctor. All they have to do is study the techniques to develop the knowledge and skill that will enable them to heal. If a doctor dies, she does not take with her a special power or knowledge because in the Perspectival Thinking world, knowledge exists as a shared set of testable claims, reviewed by other independent experts, recorded, and shared. This sharing has enabled profound advances in science and medicine. In the past, sorcerers, wizards, witches, and necromancers kept their techniques secret and so they could not be tested, replicated, or executed by others. When they died, their secrets died with them unless they passed them on to a trusted apprentice. This was meant to keep the power of the magic. But science is an open book. Science is democratic and relies on the free marketplace of ideas. Anyone can make claims, and anyone can challenge them. Claims must be published (shared). Claims that cannot be reliably established do not count as knowledge but instead as private opinions and guesses.

The emergence of modern medicine is inseparable from the rise of rationalism and empiricism, both can be traced back to ancient Greece (Bluhm & Borgerson, 2011). **Rationalism** in medicine emphasizes "the importance of empirical investigation into basic mechanisms of disease" (Bluhm & Borgerson, 2011, p. 204). Hippocrates, a Greek physician of the Age of Pericles, emphasized the importance of uncovering the mecha nisms of disease. Hippocratic physicians identified problems and reason through the effects of various treatments by grounding their analysis on their knowledge of physiology, anatomy, and other basic sciences (Bluhm & Borgerson, 2011). Reflecting on the rise of medical education and medical research after World War II, Newton (2001) explained, "The orthodoxy of modern medicine is rationalist; a large majority of physicians within academic medical centers and in practice are subspecialists who are experts in a particular set of diseases and focus on particular organ systems or diseases." A rationalist approach believes that the understanding of *basic mechanisms of disease* should guide all clinical decisions.

Empiricism in medicine focuses on "whether something works, regardless of causes of mechanisms" (Bluhm & Borgerson, 2011, p. 204), emphasizing on the outcomes of patients. The primary interest of empiricists is in identifying the best treatment for a condition rather than understanding the cause of the disease. Empiricists embrace *observations* of individual cases rather than abstractions and general medical theories. Their practices are based on their experiences and knowledge of past observations, progressions of symptoms, and distinctions between individuals cases (Newton, 2001). Clinical epidemiology best reflects the tradition of empiricism in medicine, arguing that *data obtained from the specific patients*, rather than theoretical tangents or general clinical experiences, should guide treatment decisions at bedside (Bluhm & Borgerson, 2011).

It is important to note that rationalism and empiricism in medical literature do not correspond to the classic philosophical accounts of these terms (Bluhm & Borgerson, 2011). For example, Hume (1748/2007) viewed rationalism as *demonstrative reasoning*, a deductive reasoning method that focuses on the logical relationship between ideas; in contrast, empiricism was conceptualized as *factual reasoning*, an inductive process that draws on apparently reasonable but not logically certain conclusions based on the available and incomplete evidence (Millican, 2007). However, in medicine, the underlying cause of disease and the proposed treatments are often intertwined and inseparable.

Although rationalism and empiricism approaches can be complementary, the tensions between these two approaches in medicine can explode around specific clinical controversies (Newton, 2001). For example, cardiologists in the early 1990s continue to prescribe calcium-channel blockers, because it was "*biologically plausible* that calcium-channel blockers were better than beta-blockers" despite the initial evidence of clinical trials that calcium-channel blockers not only does not improve but can worsen patients' outcomes (Newton, 2004, p. 139). Surgeons may overlook clinical guidelines and other sources of evidence because they are more confident in their own judgments (Kitto et al., 2007). In other words, a provider with rationalist approaches may provide treatment that works in "theory" despite little clinical evidence to support the decision.

In contrast, a provider adopting empiricist approaches may provide treatments that are effective despite little knowledge about why the treatment was effective. Although such an approach may appear "unscientific," patients who face significant ambiguity and uncertainty in the diagnosis of their illness (e.g., burnout, fibromyalgia, chronic fatigue syndromes, and multiple chemical sensitivity) often need to rely on an empiricist approach to alleviate their suffering because a rationalist approach can result in denying the legitimacy of their illnesses due to a lack of biological facts (Dumit, 2006; Engebretsen, 2018; Nettleton et al., 2005). Similarly, rheumatologists often assist patients in identifying practical and effective ways to manage their musculoskeletal pain despite challenges in identifying the cause of the pain (Rice & Pisetsky, 1999). More recently, researchers have argued that focusing on patients' experiences with symptoms (e.g., number and frequency of symptoms), rather than the underlying biological or psychological diagnosis, are essential to address the suffering of patients with medically unexplained symptoms (Dusenbery, 2018; Rosendal et al., 2017).

Evidence-based medicine, a paradigm shift in clinical care that emerged in the early 1990s, is a response in addressing the tensions between rationalism and empiricism in medicine. "Evidence-based medicine de-emphasizes intuition, unsystematic clinical experience, and pathophysiologic rationale as sufficient grounds for clinical decision making and stresses the examination of evidence from clinical research" (Evidence-Based Medicine Working Group, 1992, p. 2420). By defining evidence-based medicine as "the conscientious, explicit, and judicious use of current best evidence in making decisions about the care of individual patients," physicians' practice integrates "individual clinical expertise with the best available external clinical evidence from systematic research" (Sackett et al., 1996, p. 71). In short, although evidence-based medicine fits squarely in the empiricism tradition of medicine by focusing on patient outcomes, the meticulously regulated and supervised process of clinical trials and research reflects rationalist approaches to medicine as researchers investigate the basic mechanisms of disease (Bluhm & Borgerson, 2011; Kelly & Moore, 2012).

Within the cultural perspectives of Perspectival Thinking, nothing is too sacred to be challenged or questioned. Rather than considering human bodies or certain diseases to be sacred and thus beyond the scrutiny of medicine, human bodies are dissected, experimented, and studied in the name of science (Roach, 2003). Practitioners reject metaphysical speculation, supernatural forces, and superstition. They argue that evidence must be gathered and analyzed through unbiased experiments, and findings to be examined and evaluated by the larger scientific communities (Goldenberg, 2006). Seen from the tensions between Magic Consciousness, Mythic Connection, and Perspectival Thinking, the conflicts between men of science (e.g., Galileo, Newton, and Darwin) and the Church are inevitable because the conflicts are not simple differences of opinions but fundamental, incompatible worldviews of cultures *and* realities. By emphasizing that "facts" are the only standards to adjudicate between competing standards of clinical practices or scientific beliefs, evidence-based medicine is construed to adopt transparent, neutral, objective, and universal standards (Goldenberg, 2006). Evidence-based medicine is the embodiment of Perspectival Thinking in medicine.

B. The Voice of Medicine and the Medical Gaze

Influenced by Habermas' conceptualization of the System, Mishler (1984) found that health care providers often structure their narratives and understanding through the **Voice of Medicine**, which is oriented to and framed by the biomedical framework. The Voice of Medicine involves a technical understanding of health and illness that defines and controls the scope of a providers' work. Patients' individual and subjective experiences are ignored or suppressed in provider-patient interactions as their illness narratives are forced into the structured, routinized, and standardized terms defined by the biomedicine. Physicians actively frame and reframe a patient's illness narratives and subjective experiences through the Voice of Medicine. A patient's narratives of numbness in the leg are construed to be unhelpful, insufficient, or irrelevant unless such his experiences can be categorized into "meaningful" terms in clinical medicine (See Chapter 3). Patients struggle to fit their everyday, subjective, and unique experiences into the neatly framed and tightly controlled Voice of Medicine. For example, when describing his frustration in explaining his symptoms to the doctor, a patient commented,

There's a fuzzy feeling. And the doctor looks at you and goes, "So what do you mean?" It's like a whoosh. "Describe whoosh." And I told her, "I feel poopy." I mean, that's how I feel but what's the medical terminology for that? (Brashers et al., 2006, p. 29)

Both "whoosh" and "poopy" are real and meaningful experiences for the patient, but in the world of the Voice of Medicine, they become meaningless and out-of-place. This is true when fellow patients may share the same experiences or side effects of medicine, and thus sharing a similar Lifeworld. The world of System and the Voice of Medicine deny such an individualized understanding of illness and require a standardized frame of health, bodies, and experiences. From this perspective, the Voice of Medicine is more than a passive linguistic or cultural resource for individual patients to adopt. Rather, it imposes a strict framework that dictates individuals' experiences and assesses the appropriateness of behaviors. In fact, a patient who can structure their experiences through the Voice of Medicine is more likely to obtain necessary or desired resources.

The imposition of frames of the System in healthcare settings is unrelenting. All participants of the System are subject to the Voice of Medicine, including that of the doctors. In *The Birth of the Clinic*, Michel Foucault (1973) argued that the training of physicians (e.g., autopsy and anatomy) in the late 18th century created a radical shift in medicine that fundamentally changed how health care providers came to view their patients. Foucault proposed that the **medical gaze** permeated through the discursive practices and professional practices of medicine, resulting in a changed relationship of man to himself – we allow ourselves to become an *object* of science. By adopting an "objective" and scientific undertone in the discourse of medicine, the medical System hides its power, appearing to assume a posture of a neutral, disinterested observer of individuals' health and illnesses. Human bodies and experiences are objectified, medicalized, and pathologized. Medical textbooks begin to be organized in organs and organ systems, and physicians' diagnoses involve identifying the localization, site, and origin of illnesses (see Figure 4.6). Whereas in the early 18th century, a physician may ask "what's the matter with you?" to start her diagnostic task, assuming that the patient's experience is best understood as a whole – a holistic approach to health and illness rooted in Hippocratic medicine; a physician in the late 18th century would instead ask, "where does it hurt?" A patient's Lifeworld is no longer incorporated in a physician's medical inquiry (Gray & Gunderman, 2016). Their bodies are conceptually dissected into specific organs and body parts, each with its unique physiology and course of treatment.

Modern medicine becomes increasingly fragmented and specialized because the medical community believes that specialization was necessary to achieve the rigorous observations required to expand medical knowledge (Weisz, 2003). Medical specialists in certain areas have basically no patient contacts (e.g., radiology and pathology) or brief patient contact (e.g., surgery, anesthesiology, and emergency medicine; Lefevre et al., 2010; Totman, 2015). In other words, patients' Lifeworld may have little impact on these medical specialists' practice. In Fadiman's (1997) investigative report, *The Spirit Catches You and You Fall Down*, an emergency care physician who worked on Lia, a patient with life-threatening conditions, for more than twelve hours straight without realizing that the patient was a girl. Fadiman (1997) concluded, "Here was American medicine at its worst and its best: the patient was reduced from a girl to

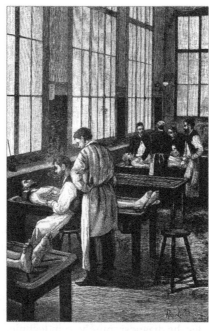

Figure 4.6 Autopsy training. Through autopsy training, medical students learn to adopt the medical gazev toward human bodies, a clinical, objective, and impersonal understanding of health and illness. A medical student explained his transformation, "Now I'm learning, actually, what it is that's going on inside. I'm familiar with it, I've seen it. It's now part of my world" (Barnes, 2009, 7:10). *Source:* ilbusca/Getty Images

an analyzable collection of symptoms, and the physician, thereby able to husband his energies, succeeded in keeping her alive" (p. 147). A patient's illness is detached from a patient's Lifeworld experiences and situated in clinical terms within different components of a patient's body.

Several studies also found interpreters in provider-patient interactions often favored physicians' Voice of Medicine, rather than patients' Lifeworld (Bolden, 2000; Elderkin-Thompson et al., 2001). In one of our studies, an interpreter explained her enforcement of Voice of Medicine: "[I have a patient who] is a talker, you know. And every time, the doctor asked a question, he would ask a yes or no question or just a short answer, and she answers it and then, after that, she tries to say different things. ... What do I do? I just control it. I mean, I said, 'Excuse me, please just answer the question.' [...The doctor] was not interested in this, you know?" (Hsieh & Kramer, 2012, p. 160). Leanza and colleagues even found that physicians interrupted patients' Voice of the Lifeworld significantly more with a trained interpreter than with a bilingual family member who served as an interpreter (Leanza et al., 2010).

The medical gaze is unforgiving, demanding all are subject to its System to give in to its framework of understanding and standards of professionalism. Many early researchers equated physicians' roles and narratives with the System and the Voice of Medicine, as they imposed medical gaze onto the patients' Lifeworld experiences. For example, Waitzkin (1991) argued that physicians often act as agents of social control, using discursive practices (e.g., interjecting questions, interrupting patient's talk, or changing topics) to reinforce the power of physicians and the medical System.

Individuals' Lifeworld experiences are at the mercy of the medical gaze, demanding patients' compliance with norms of appropriate behaviors and narratives within the medical system.

C. Professionalism versus Natural Attitude

The medical gaze subjects all within the medical system to its control. Although researchers initially theorized the medical gaze and Voice of Medicine in terms of its effects and control over the patient, researchers later recognized that *everyone* in the medical system is subject to the demands of the medical gaze, including the doctors. Physicians' training often socialized them to adopt the views of the medical gaze, to become the enforcer of the System, speaking as the Voice of Medicine. For example, when medical students present their cases during the morning reports, they are socialized to display a professional identity. Faculty physicians evaluate their performance based on conciseness, relevance, smoothness of delivery, and mastery of technical language (Gross et al., 1999). When students deviate from the biomedical framework to include the Voice of the Lifeworld (i.e., the biopsychosocial model that recognizes emotional, social, and contextual factors as relevant to identifying, understanding, and treating illness), faculty members often respond by reinforcing the Voice of Medicine: telling students to "consider the diagnosis purely from technical evidence rather than from information contributed by the patient" (Apker & Eggly, 2004, p. 422).

Medical students' emotional socialization into the field of medicine is an excellent example of the tensions between the System and the Lifeworld. Various studies have found that although students enter medical schools expressing more empathy and compassion, such attitudes are significantly reduced by the third year, only to be replaced by cynicism (Underman & Hirshfield, 2016). The groundbreaking work by Renée Fox (1988) on medical education found that medical students learn and adopt **detached concern**, the combination of "the counterattitudes of detachment and concern to attain the balance between objectivity and empathy expected of mature physicians in the various kinds of professional situations they encounter" (p. 56). Fox argued that the autopsy training requires students to develop detached concern in emotionally charged situations so that they can normalize the handling and cutting of naked, dead bodies. The sterility of the room and the covering of the face and genitals allowed the students to assume a "scientific orientation," focusing on the pathology and anatomy of the autopsy. Hafferty (1988) argued that anatomy lab was essential for medical students to learn the "feeling rules" – detaching their fear, anxiety, and disgust from their judgment about patient care because that is what professionalism demands of physicians.

Based on their ethnographic work, Smith and Kleinman (1989) concluded, "Because we associate authority in this society with an unemotional persona, affective neutrality reinforces professionals' power and keeps clients from challenging them," professionalism in medicine means physicians are expected to adopt emotional detachment, paternalism, and restricted communication with patients (p. 56; see also Borgstrom et al., 2010). "A detached, clear and rational approach both benefits the patient most and best befits the profession as a whole"(Borgstrom et al., 2010, p. 1332).

The paradigm of emotional detachment as a necessity for medical professionals is not limited to physicians. The medical gaze objectifies interpreters. Interpreters are often

conceptualized as instruments in the process, providing one-to-one machine-like interpretation, without influencing the content or process of provider-patient interactions
(Hsieh & Kramer, 2012). Interpreters talked about their role as robots or machines, functioning with great precision without getting emotionally involved. To be professional
requires them to disown their human presence and their own voice. They only speak
when others speak. An interpreter argued, "If you want to keep your job, you want to
become – really, a kind of robot" (Hsieh, 2008, p. 1371). Interpreters neutrality is enacted
through their impartiality (e.g., "I interpret everything."), invisibility (e.g., "I try to be
faceless." or "I am the voice.")' and the lack of personal opinions or judgment (e.g., "I
don't think;" Hsieh, 2009). In other words, interpreters were trained to believe that they
should not be seen as, nor should they try to be, a "person" during medical encounters.

But we are not robots. Healthcare providers cannot be robots. Physicians have their
own Lifeworld. Lifeworld is where the physicians and patients can connect at an interpersonal level in the social world. We cannot pluck ourselves out of the social world.
Husserl (1948/1975) proposed that the **natural attitude** is how we experience the
world. Natural attitude represents our unquestioned, normative frame of mind in the
taken-for-granted world of everyday life. We experience things, including emotions,
identities, and self, as they are. It is the opposite of Perspectival Thinking, which
requires critical thinking and an attitude to dissect, analyze, and bracket our Lifeworld.
The natural attitude precedes any critical analysis of who we are and why we do certain things and feel certain ways. When we are in our Lifeworld, we don't analyze or
question why we are happy or sad. We just feel that way. Scheper-Hughes (1992, p. 28)
commented, "We cannot rid ourselves of the cultural self we bring with us into the
field any more than we can disown the eyes, ears, and skin through which we take in
our intuitive perceptions about the new and strange world we have entered." In other
words, we cannot "objectively" interpret or understand the world as our subjectivity is
embedded in our consciousness.

It is the challenges and inability to completely rid ourselves from our natural attitude, and thus our Lifeworld, that healthcare providers find themselves in a bind and
contemplate a new paradigm of professionalism in medicine. When asked about how
her training shaped her understanding of her role and performance as an interpreter,
an interpreter said in frustration:

> "We learned that we don't have to talk to patients. We learned that. We are not
> allowed, right? I don't like that. I can tell you, 'It's not right.' *We are not robots.
> We have training; I know why we are here. But I say that because it's not true, I
> am not a robot.*" [emphasis added] (Hsieh, 2008, p. 1367)

When asked about challenges faced by medical professionals, a physician responded,

> "In medicine we face a difficult balance. We have a professional duty to the
> patient and their families. However, we are also individuals and carry with us
> our own experiences... *We cannot be automatons, suppressing our experiences,
> nor is it good for clinical practice. Combining professional and personal aspects
> brings humanity where it matters most.*" [emphasis added] (Borgstrom et al.,
> 2010, p. 1334)

When we witness others' suffering, we cannot help but feel – feeling empathic to their struggles and pain. As healthcare providers witness patients' illness experiences, they cannot escape their natural attitude of shared consciousness of being human (see also Kramer & Hsieh, 2019).

If everyone, including healthcare providers, patients, and even interpreters, has his/ her own Lifeworld, how can they enter the field of medicine, assume a desirable identity, adopt appropriate behaviors in the System – without ridding themselves the "cultural self that we bring with us" (Scheper-Hughes, 1992, p. 28)? Increasingly, emerging values for the new paradigm of professionalism in medicine mean that physicians are encouraged to replace their detached concerns with **empathy** (Halpern, 2001). Empathy is not just an attitude. Rather, empathy is a "psychological process that encompasses a collection of affective, cognitive, and behavioral mechanisms and outcomes in reaction to the observed experiences of another" (Larson & Yao 2005, p. 1102). Medical schools now recognize that empathy is an essential part of medical education and a critical component in the provider-patient relationship (Batt-Rawden et al. 2013). Physicians are encouraged to engage with patients' emotions, adopt a patient-centered approach, and maintain open communication (Borgstrom et al. 2010). Physicians are encouraged to see interpreters as collaborators and partners, rather than as passive instruments to relay information from one language to another, in providing culturally appropriate and sensitive care that meets the patients' emotional needs (Gutierrez et al. 2019; Hsieh & Kramer 2012).

The effort to promote the new patient-centered paradigm is not without resistance. Physicians reported struggles to balance the tensions between the old and new paradigms of professionalism and clinical care (Borgstrom et al. 2010). Larson and Yao (2005) noted that empathy in clinical settings should be understood as **emotional labor**, requiring health care providers to actively manage the experience and display of emotions to present a desirable identity. Researchers have cited the negative consequences (e.g., emotional exhaustion, compassion fatigue, and burnout) of healthcare professionals' emotional labor (Figley, 1995; Marshall & Kasman, 1980; Theodosius, 2008). Interpreters' close identification with the patients' shared cultural, sociopolitical, ethnic, geopolitical, or life histories can contribute to feelings of being overwhelmed by the emotional effects of their interpreting tasks (Green et al., 2012; Johnson et al., 2009). Teegen and Goennenwein (2002) found 20% of interpreters for refugees experienced some level of posttraumatic stress disorders. When examining the interrelationship between empathy, communication, and burnout, Miller et al. (1988) found that when medical professionals hold higher levels of empathic concern, they are more likely to be communicatively responsive to patients (i.e., responding to patients' distress effectively and appropriately). Communicative responsiveness, however, is a predictor for the onset of burnout, which can ultimately lead to emotional exhaustion and reduced commitment to the job. As a result, medical professionals may "find it necessary to develop a stance in which concern for another can be held independent of emotional involvement" (Miller et al., 1988, p. 262).

Emotional contagion, a form of empathic response, involves sharing and experiencing the emotion of another person (i.e., "catching" the emotion of another). People catch the emotions of others all the time, in all societies. Hatfield et al. (2011) argued that as social beings, we share *primitive emotion contagion*, a building block of human connection that allows us to connect with others by sharing and understanding the feelings of each other. We consciously and subconsciously attend to the constant stream of moment-to-moment reactions, often unaware of, or even surprised by, how we "catch" the emotion of others (Parkinson, 2011). Emotional contagion acts as our natural attitude, working at the level of Magic Consciousness – often occurring "automatically and outside of awareness" (Parkinson, 2011, p. 436). This is not a planned process or a deliberate attempt to "share" another's emotion. When a kid's shrieking cry in pain makes a mom start crying, her experience of pain is not a simple "understanding" of her kid's pain. She feels her kid's pain. The kid's pain is inseparable and indistinguishable from her own pain. At the moment of emotional contagion, they are one.

Because emotional contagion can induce such intense feelings, it is often found to be one of the strongest predictors for burnout, emotional exhaustion, and reduced occupational commitment for medical professionals (Miller et al., 1988). Emotional contagion makes the labor of emotion work so much harder. It is estimated that 28.8% of resident physicians experience depression (Mata et al., 2015). Compared to the general population, male and female physicians are 41% and 127%, respectively, more likely to commit suicide (Schernhammer, 2005; Schernhammer & Colditz, 2004). In short, medical professionals have begun to recognize that detached concern is problematic and ineffective care to address patients' experiences of health and illness. In addition, they also realize that a complete immersion of patients' Lifeworld is not the solution (Goldman et al., 2015). A clinical psychologist explained, "Once you are in the shoes of your patient, you cannot possibly be of any help ... because he has been in his shoes all along, and obviously not done too well" (Malakh-Pines et al., 1981, p. 55).

The delicate balance between providing empathy to facilitate patient-centered care and maintain sufficient detachment to avoid potential burnout is essential to patients' quality of care as well as providers' well-being. More recently, researchers have proposed the practice of **mindfulness** for medical professionals as a way to maintain the balance between the Voice of the Lifeworld and the Voice of Medicine (Epstein, 1999), a very perspectival dichotomy that does not exist in magic or mythic worlds. Because of the modern stress on being objective, the problem of emotional attachment has become salient just as the issue of communication emerges only when people feel they are not communicating. To address this problem of emotional dissociation and detachment that characterized modern society, experts have turned to the notion of mindfulness.

Mindfulness encourages physicians to become more self-aware, identifying their values and connect with what is most meaningful in their work. Mindfulness allows physicians to fill the gaps between their knowledge of medicine, their personal values, and the actions to take. Epstein (1999) argued that when physicians are aware of their core values, they can be more empathic, compassionate, and altruistic (if these are their core values and motives which are in fact enshrined in the Hippocratic Oath): "To be empathic, I must *witness* and *understand* the patient's suffering and my reactions to the patient's suffering to distinguish the patient's experience from my own. Then I can *communicate* my understanding and be compassionate, to use my presence to relieve suffering and to put the patient's interests first" [emphasis added] (p. 836). Mindfulness training for medical students has been found to have significant and durable improvements in burnout, mood disturbance, and empathy (Krasner et al., 2009).

Witnessing provides a new perspective for healthcare providers to orient their roles in clinical settings that counters the unrelenting and impersonal pressure of the medical gaze. By constructing their presence as a "witness" to patients' suffering, which requires attentive listening to patients' life stories, medical students learn to reconcile their personal perspectives of the Lifeworld with the Perspectival Thinking of the medical gaze (Davenport, 2000). Their presence as a witness gives "voice" to patients' struggles. "We are not going to fix [the failing social system that contributed to patients' suffering], but we're going to bear witness," a medical student explained (Davenport, 2000, p. 316). The act of witnessing transforms the "reality" of the provider-patient interaction. Providers are no longer passive actors under the Perspectival Thinking of the medical gaze. Instead, providers become a symbol, highlighting a *moral* reflection of their presence in patients' illness journey. Providers were thus able to resist the impersonal Perspectival Thinking of the medical gaze by envoking moral claims through Mythic Connection (Borkan et al., 2001). Their presence is symbolic in resisting the objectification of patients by "bearing witness" to their suffering. More importantly, rather than a complete refusal or denial of the medical gaze, witnessing allows providers to reconcile their professional duties with their Lifeworld. Witnessing affords providers a sense of agency yet requires them to submit to the medical gaze. In other words, providers' witnessing under the Mythic Connection worldview finds a way to co-exist with the Perspectival Thinking of the medical gaze – strengthening the sustainability and stability of a neutral but empathic healthcare provider.

It's important to note that mindfulness, sometimes called **clinical empathy**, is not the same as layman's understanding of everyday empathy, especially in the form of emotional contagion. It is a controlled exercise and management of emotions. From this perspective, mindfulness is a Perspectival Thinking approach to emotions. Although the physician is able to see their own, and (some of) the patient's Lifeworld, and the corresponding values, the physician is also simultaneously contemplating the best way to achieve the goals of ethical, appropriate, and optimal care. To excel at mindful practice, a healthcare provider needs to be able to see and appreciate different perspectives and different needs; at the same time, s/he also needs to adopt a sense of clinical detachment that subordinates his own interests and values to that of the patients.

Physician altruism requires the medical professionals to identify and appreciate all the values and priorities involved (including his own and others' Lifeworlds as well as that of the System's structural imperatives) *and* exercise his choice and/or control to achieve what is right and just. For example, a physician may recognize a hospital's and his own economic interests for profit but chooses to support the patient for limited treatment in response to her religious beliefs. In other words, this is a combined result when a person understands and appreciates *all* the cultural perspectives, including Magic Consciousness, Mythic Connection, and Perspectival Thinking. More importantly, the physician's decision or action is situated in contexts (e.g., interpersonal, institutional, and legal contexts) rather than to be dictated by a specific cultural perspective (e.g., Magic Consciousness, Mythic Connection, or Perspectival Thinking).

In summary, in Chapter 4, we have explored how Perspectival Thinking shapes the emergence and rise of modern medicine. In early studies of the Voice of Medicine, researchers often equated physicians' talk as the Voice of Medicine. The Voice of Medicine and the medical gaze subject patients' illness and experiences to tightly controlled and limited frames of biomedicine. Despite their natural attitudes and Lifeworld, healthcare providers cannot escape the impositions of Perspectival Thinking of medicine in their practice and performance. However, medical communities increasingly have acknowledged the potentials of compromised care and found strategies to resist such pressures. Mindfulness, witnessing, clinical empathy, and physician altruism all require providers to recognize and accommodate various perspectives from different parties (e.g., health institutions, patients, and family members) while navigating the terrain of western biomedicine. This requires providers to develop cultural perspectives that go beyond the Perspectival Thinking of the medical gaze and modern medicine – an integral worldview, which we will explore more in Chapter 5.

IV. Additional Resources

A. Key Terms and Theories

Theory of Dimensional Accrual and Dissociation
Perspectival Thinking
magico-religious medicine
modern medicine
System (in Habermas' Theory of Communicative Action)
rationalism (in medicine)
empiricism (in medicine)
evidence-based medicine
Voice of Medicine
medical gaze
detached concern
natural attitude
empathy
emotional labor
emotional contagion
mindfulness (for physician training)
witnessing
clinical empathy
physician altruism

B. Discussion Questions

1. Can you provide examples in modern society that show we hold Perspectival Thinking? Explain why it constitutes Perspectival Thinking.
2. Explain and give examples of the Voice of Medicine.
   a. In what ways are patients' Lifeworld experiences frustrated by the Voice of Medicine?
   b. As physicians learn the Voice of Medicine, do you think they can continue to maintain their Voice of the Lifeworld?
   c. Does healthcare providers' voice of the Lifeworld make them better or worse healthcare providers? Why?
3. When visiting a physician, do you have expectations about how they should display their emotions? What are they?
   a. Are their situations that you expect an emotional display? In emergency care? When disclosing bad news?

b. Do you think you have different expectations for different medical specialties?
c. Among the different ways we have talked about physicians' emotional display (e.g., empathy, witnessing, and mindfulness), which one do you like more? Why?

In *Doctors' Diaries*, a PBS documentary that follows young medical students' journey to become "real" doctors, a medical resident, Jane Liebschutz, was initially fascinated by the medial complexity of a patient's heart surgery. But Jane herself was unable to maintain the Voice of Medicine when her *own* Lifeworld experiences and interactions with the patient became salient and overwhelming. Jane started the scene by showing excitement to participate in a complex surgery led by a surgeon and Dr. Johnson, a senior physician.

JANE: Okay. I think being in the operating room is one of the most vintense experiences one can ever have. Having your hand on a case and actually helping when you feel needed is probably among the top 10 experiences to have in the world. What's happening is they're taking some vein from his leg, and then some other vessels that are in the chest wall, and connecting them up to where the coronary arteries are, which give the heart blood. Where would you see the R.V. from here?

DR. JOHNSON: This is the R.V. That's the anterior R.V.

JANE: This is the anterior R.V.?

DR. JOHNSON: Yep.

JANE: Wow. That is really cool.

DR. JOHNSON: The chest is a great place to see anatomy. Let's wait and see what happens here.

JANE: Do you understand what's happening right now? His heart isn't working, and Dr. Johnson is pumping, he's actually pumping the heart himself. There's no ... the heart's failed. It's not, it's not working. So that's what's happening right now, as we speak.

[minutes later]

JANE: Oh, god, this is terrible. I feel like I'm bad luck or something.

DR. JOHNSON: Oh, come on.

JANE: I can't believe it. I told this guy he was going to do fine.

SURGEON: ... conduit. We did okay with not having any conduit.

DR. JOHNSON: I don't know what more I can do.

JANE: That's it?

DR. JOHNSON: Yeah.

SURGEON: That's it.

JANE: Oh, my god.

SURGEON: 11:37.

JANE (CRYING): I'm sorry. I know, I just ...

DR. JOHNSON: The responsibility we have now is to kind of keep a calm head and help the family understand it. I feel the way you feel, but I can't go up to them like that.

JANE: Well, I wasn't going to go up to them. It's funny. I've never really had a patient that I've gotten to know who's died. And here it just happened.

DR. JOHNSON: I know. Sure, sure.

JANE: It's like a bad dream or something. Like, "Let this be over already." He was going to wear his kilt. I don't know. I'm sorry. I shouldn't be ... I don't ...

DR. JOHNSON: No, no, no. You're attached in a way that is perfectly appropriate. But you have to understand all kinds of other things. Like, from the start of this operation, he could have, from the aorta, he could have had a stroke, and he never would have worn his kilts again. You know, it would have even been worse.

JANE: I know. And I also know he wouldn't have lived with his arteries like that anyway.

DR. JOHNSON: Oh no, he was ... he couldn't do anything.

JANE: I know that. I'm not ... I know that. But it's so hard to watch it.

DR. JOHNSON: But see, that's where you ... that's the physician part. I know.

1. Can you identify when Jane speaks in the Voice of Medicine? When? Why are these examples of the Voice of Medicine?
2. Can you identify when Jane speaks in the Voice of the Lifeworld? When? Why are these examples of the Voice of the Lifeworld?
3. Did Jane's Voice of Medicine and Voice of the Lifeworld conflict with one another? How did she manage the tensions?
4. How did Dr. Johnson respond when Jane spoke in the Voice of the Lifeworld? What does it mean to be a physician, a professional, to Dr. Johnson?

C. References

Apker, J., & Eggly, S. (2004). Communicating professional identity in medical socialization: Considering the ideological discourse of morning report. *Qualitative Health Research*, *14*(3), 411–429.

Barnes, M. (Director). (2009). *Doctors' diaries*. [DVD]. PBS. https://www.pbs.org/wgbh/nova/doctors/program.html

Batt-Rawden, S. A., Chisolm, M. S., Anton, B., & Flickinger, T. E. (2013). Teaching empathy to medical students: An updated, systematic review. *Academic Medicine*, *88*(8), 1171–1177.

Bluhm, R., & Borgerson, K. (2011). Evidence-based medicine. In F. Gifford (Ed.), *Philosophy of medicine* (pp. 203–238). Elsevier.

Bolden, G. B. (2000). Toward understanding practices of medical interpreting: Interpreters' involvement in history taking. *Discourse Studies*, *2*(4), 387–419.

Borgstrom, E., Cohn, S., & Barclay, S. (2010). Medical professionalism: Conflicting values for tomorrow's doctors. *Journal of General Internal Medicine*, *25*(12), 1330–1336.

Borkan, J., Reis, S., & Medalie, J. (2001). Narratives in family medicine: Tales of transformation, points of breakthrough for family physicians. *Families, Systems, & Health*, *19*(2), 121–134.

Brashers, D. E., Rintamaki, L. S., Hsieh, E., & Peterson, J. L. (2006). Pragma-dialectics and self-advocacy in physician-patient interactions. In P. Houtlosser & A. van Rees (Eds.), *Considering pragma-dialectics* (pp. 23–34). Erlbaum.

Bynum, W. (2008). *The history of medicine: A very short introduction*. Oxford University Press.

Davenport, B. A. (2000). Witnessing and the medical gaze: How medical students learn to see at a free clinic for the homeless. *Medical Anthropology Quarterly, 14*(3), 310–327.

Dumit, J. (2006). Illnesses you have to fight to get: Facts as forces in uncertain, emergent illnesses. *Social Science & Medicine, 62*(3), 577–590.

Dusenbery, M. (2018). *Doing harm: The truth about how bad medicine and lazy science leave women dismissed, misdiagnosed, and sick.* HarperOne.

Elderkin-Thompson, V., Silver, R. C., & Waitzkin, H. (2001). When nurses double as interpreters: A study of Spanish-speaking patients in a US primary care setting. *Social Science & Medicine, 52*(9), 1343–1358.

Engebretsen, K. M. (2018). Suffering without a medical diagnosis. A critical view on the biomedical attitudes towards persons suffering from burnout and the implications for medical care. *Journal of Evaluation in Clinical Practice, 24*(5), 1150–1157.

Epstein, R. M. (1999). Mindful practice. *JAMA, 282*(9), 833–839.

Evidence-Based Medicine Working Group. (1992). Evidence-based medicine: A new approach to teaching the practice of medicine. *JAMA, 268*(17), 2420–2425.

Fadiman, A. (1997). *The spirit catches you and you fall down: A Hmong child, her American doctors, and the collision of two cultures.* Farrar, Straus and Giroux.

Ferngren, G. B. (1992). Early Christiantiy as a religion of healing. *Bulletin of the History of Medicine, 66*(1), 1–15.

Figley, C. R. (Ed.). (1995). *Compassion fatigue: Coping with secondary traumatic stress disorder in those who treat the traumatized.* Brunner-Routledge.

Foucault, M. (1973). *The birth of the clinic.* Vintage Books.

Fox, R. C. (1988). *Essays in medical sociology: Journeys into the fields* (2nd, enlarged ed.). Transaction Books.

Goldenberg, M. J. (2006). On evidence and evidence-based medicine: Lessons from the philosophy of science. *Social Science & Medicine, 62*(11), 2621–2632.

Goldman, M. L., Shah, R. N., & Bernstein, C. A. (2015). Depression and suicide among physician trainees: Recommendations for a national response. *JAMA Psychiatry, 72*(5), 411–412.

Grandjean, F. (1988). Time: Its history and measurement billions of years within a nanosecond. In G. J. Long & F. Grandjean (Eds.), *The time domain in surface and structural dynamics* (pp. 7–17). Springer.

Gray, B. R., & Gunderman, R. B. (2016). Lessons of history: The medical gaze. *Academic Radiology, 23*(6), 774–776.

Green, H., Sperlinger, D., & Carswell, K. (2012). Too close to home? Experiences of Kurdish refugee interpreters working in UK mental health services. *Journal of Mental Health, 21*(3), 227–235.

Griswold, A. (2016, August 13). *The simple reason why swimmers keep tying for Olympic medals.* Quartz. https://qz.com/757794/the-simple-reason-why-swimmers-keep-tying-for-olympic-medals

Gross, C. P., Donnelly, G. B., Reisman, A. B., Sepkowitz, K. A., & Callahan, M. A. (1999). Resident expectations of morning report: A multi-institutional study. *Archives of Internal Medicine, 159*(16), 1910–1914.

Gutierrez, A. M., Statham, E. E., Robinson, J. O., Slashinski, M. J., Scollon, S., Bergstrom, K. L., Street, R. L., Parsons, D. W., Plon, S. E., & McGuire, A. L. (2019). Agents of empathy: How medical interpreters bridge sociocultural gaps in genomic sequencing disclosures with Spanish-speaking families. *Patient Education and Counseling, 102*(5), 895–901.

Habermas, J. (1985). *The theory of communicative action: Lifeworld and system, a critique of functionalist reason* (T. McCarthy, Trans.; 3rd ed., Vol. *2*). Beacon. (Original work published 1981)

Hafferty, F. W. (1988). Cadaver stories and the emotional socialization of medical students. *Journal of Health and Social Behavior, 29*(4), 344–356.

Halpern, J. (2001). *From detached concern to empathy: Humanizing medical practice.* Oxford University Press.

Hatfield, E., Rapson, R. L., & Le, Y.-C. L. (2011). Emotional contagion and empathy. In J. Decety & W. Ickes (Eds.), *The social neuroscience of empathy* (pp. 19–30). MIT Press.

Haynes, J. D. (2000). *Perspectival thinking: For inquiring organisations.* Informing Science Press.

Hook, G. R. (2009). "Warrior genes" and the disease of being Māori. *Mai Review, 2*, 1–11. http://www.review.mai.ac.nz/mrindex/MR/article/view/222/243.html

Hsieh, E. (2008). "I am not a robot!" Interpreters' views of their roles in health care settings. *Qualitative Health Research, 18*(10), 1367–1383.

Hsieh, E. (2009). Bilingual health communication: Medical interpreters' construction of a mediator role. In D. E. Brashers & D. J. Goldsmith (Eds.), *Communicating to manage health and illness* (pp. 135–160). Routledge.

Hsieh, E., & Kramer, E. M. (2012). Medical interpreters as tools: Dangers and challenges in the utilitarian approach to interpreters' roles and functions. *Patient Education and Counseling, 89*(1), 158–162.

Hume, D. (2007). *An enquiry concerning human understanding* (P. Millican, Ed.). Oxford University Press. (Original work published 1748)

Husserl, E. (1975). *Experience and judgment: Investigation in a genealogy of logic* (J. S. Churchill & K. Ameriks, Trans.). Northwestern University Press. (Original work published 1948)

Johnson, H., Thompson, A., & Downs, M. (2009). Non-Western interpreters' experiences of trauma: The protective role of culture following exposure to oppression. *Ethnicity & Health, 14*(4), 407–418.

Kee, H. C. (1988). *Medicine, miracle and magic in New Testament times.* Cambridge University Press.

Kelly, M. P., & Moore, T. A. (2012). The judgement process in evidence-based medicine and health technology assessment. *Social Theory & Health, 10*(1), 1–19.

Kitto, S., Villanueva, E. V., Chesters, J., Petrovic, A., Waxman, B. P., & Smith, J. A. (2007). Surgeons' attitudes towards and usage of evidence-based medicine in surgical practice: A pilot study. *ANZ Journal of Surgery, 77*(4), 231–236.

Kramer, E. M. (2013). Dimensional accrual and dissociation: An introduction. In J. Grace & E. M. Kramer (Eds.), *Communication, comparative cultures, and civilizations* (Vol. 3, pp. 123–184). Hampton.

Kramer, E. M., & Hsieh, E. (2019). Gaze as embodied ethics: Homelessness, the other, and humanity. In M. J. Dutta & D. B. Zapata (Eds.), *Communicating for social change* (pp. 33–62). Palgrave Macmillan.

Kramer, E. M., & Ikeda, R. (1998). Understanding different worlds: The theory of dimensional accrual/dissociation. *Journal of Intercultural Communication, 1*(2), 37–51.

Krasner, M. S., Epstein, R. M., Beckman, H., Suchman, A. L., Chapman, B., Mooney, C. J., & Quill, T. E. (2009). Association of an educational program in mindful communication with burnout, empathy, and attitudes among primary care physicians. *JAMA, 302*(12), 1284–1293.

Krebbs, R. S. (1997). Criticism and perspectivism: The transition between Nietzsche's two truths. *The European Legacy, 2*(2), 388–393.

Larson, E. B., & Yao, X. (2005). Clinical empathy as emotional labor in the patient-physician relationship. *JAMA, 293*(9), 1100–1106.

Lea, R. A., & Chambers, G. (2007). Monoamine oxidase, addiction, and the "warrior" gene hypothesis. *New Zealand Medical Journal, 120*(1250), Article U2441.

Leanza, Y., Boivin, I., & Rosenberg, E. (2010). Interruptions and resistance: A comparison of medical consultations with family and trained interpreters. *Social Science & Medicine, 70*(12), 1888–1895.

Lee, S. (2007). Prosperity theology: T.D. Jakes and the gospel of the almighty dollar. *Cross Currents, 57*(2), 227–236.

Lefevre, J. H., Roupret, M., Kerneis, S., & Karila, L. (2010). Career choices of medical students: A national survey of 1780 students. *Medical Education, 44*(6), 603–612.

Levin, J. (2016). Prevalence and religious predictors of healing prayer use in the USA: Findings from the Baylor Religion Survey. *Journal of Religion and Health, 55*(4), 1136–1158.

Malakh-Pines, A., Aronson, E., & Kafry, D. (1981). *Burnout: From tedium to personal growth*. Free Press.

Marshall, R. E., & Kasman, C. (1980). Burnout in the neonatal intensive care unit. *Pediatrics, 65*(6), 1161–1165.

Mata, D. A., Ramos, M. A., Bansal, N., Khan, R., Guille, C., Di Angelantonio, E., & Sen, S. (2015). Prevalence of depression and depressive symptoms among resident physicians: A systematic review and meta-analysis. *JAMA, 314*(22), 2373–2383.

McGuire, M. B. (1988). *Ritual healing in suburban America*. Rutgers University Press.

Medina, L., Sabo, S., & Vespa, J. (2019, April 19). *Living longer: Historical and projected gains to life expectancy, 1960–2060*. United States Census Bureau. https://www.census.gov/library/working-papers/2019/demo/paa19_medina_sabo.html

Miller, K. I., Stiff, J. B., & Ellis, B. H. (1988). Communication and empathy as precursors to burnout among human service workers. *Communication Monographs, 55*(3), 250–265.

Millican, P. (2007). Introduction. In D. Hume, *An enquiry concerning human understanding* (p. ix-lvi). Oxford University Press.

Mishler, E. G. (1984). *The discourse of medicine: Dialectics of medical interviews*. Ablex.

National Academies of Sciences, Engineering, and Medicine. (2019). *Reproducibility and replicability in science*. National Academies Press.

Nettleton, S., Watt, I., O'Malley, L., & Duffey, P. (2005). Understanding the narratives of people who live with medically unexplained illness. *Patient Education and Counseling, 56*(2), 205–210.

Newton, W. (2001). Rationalism and empiricism in modern medicine. *Law and Contemporary Problems, 64*(4), 299.

Newton, W. P. (2004). Whose evidence anyway? A perspective on what different doctors mean by "proof." In W. Rosser, D. C. Slawson, & A. F. Shaughnessy (Eds.), *Information mastery: Evidence-based family medicine* (2nd ed., pp. 139–146). BC Decker.

Nietzsche, F. (2012). *Philosophy in the tragic age of the Greeks* (M. Cowan, Trans.). Regnery. (Original work published 1962)

O'Connor, A. (2008, March 11). *The claim: Identical twins have identical DNA*. The New York Times. https://www.nytimes.com/2008/03/11/health/11real.html

Offit, P. (2015). *Bad faith: When religious belief undermines modern medicine*. Basic Books.

Parkinson, B. (2011). Interpersonal emotion transfer: Contagion and social appraisal. *Social and Personality Psychology Compass, 5*(7), 428–439.

Parr, A. (2016, August). *Olympic measurements*. University of Cambridge. https://nrich.maths.org/12815

Perbal, L. (2013). The "warrior gene' and the Maori people: The responsibility of the geneticists. *Bioethics, 27*(7), 382–387.

Piester, D., Bauch, A., Breakiron, L., Matsakis, D., Blanzano, B., & Koudelka, O. (2008). Time transfer with nanosecond accuracy for the realization of International Atomic Time. *Metrologia, 45*(2), 185–198.

Resnick, B. (2019, May 23). *The limits of ancestry DNA tests, explained*. Vox. https://www.vox.com/science-and-health/2019/1/28/18194560/ancestry-dna-23-me-myheritage-science-explainer

Rice, J. R., & Pisetsky, D. S. (1999). Pain in the rheumatic diseases: Practical aspects of diagnosis and treatment. *Rheumatic Disease Clinics of North America, 25*(1), 15–30.

Roach, M. (2003). *Stiff: The curious lives of human cadavers*. W. W. Norton.

Rosendal, M., Olde Hartman, T. C., Aamland, A., van der Horst, H., Lucassen, P., Budtz-Lilly, A., & Burton, C. (2017). "Medically unexplained" symptoms and symptom disorders in primary care: Prognosis-based recognition and classification. *BMC Family Practice, 18*, Article 18. https://doi.org/10.1186/s12875-017-0592-6

Sackett, D. L., Rosenberg, W. M. C., Gray, J. A. M., Haynes, R. B., & Richardson, W. S. (1996). Evidence based medicine: What it is and what it isn't. *BMJ, 312*(7023), 71–72.

Scheper-Hughes, N. (1992). *Death without weeping: The violence of everyday life in Brazil*. University of California Press.

Scher, B. (2019, August 27). *'Pocahontas' could still be Elizabeth Warren's biggest vulnerability*. Political Magazine. https://www.politico.com/magazine/story/2019/08/27/pocahontas-elizabeth-warrens-biggest-vulnerability-227912

Schernhammer, E. (2005). Taking their own lives – The high rate of physician suicide. *New England Journal of Medicine, 352*(24), 2473–2476.

Schernhammer, E. S., & Colditz, G. A. (2004). Suicide rates among physicians: A quantitative and gender assessment (meta-analysis). *American Journal of Psychiatry, 161*(12), 2295–2302.

Schmidt, S. (2009). Shall we really do it again? The powerful concept of replication is neglected in the social sciences. *Review of General Psychology, 13*(2), 90–100.

Smith, A. C., & Kleinman, S. (1989). Managing emotions in medical school: Students' contacts with the living and the dead. *Social Psychology Quarterly, 52*(1), 56–69.

Teegen, F., & Goennenwein, C. (2002). Posttraumatic stress disorder of interpreters for refugees. *Verhaltenstherapie and Verhaltensmedizin, 23*(4), 419–436.

Theodosius, C. (2008). *Emotional labour in health care: The unmanaged heart of nursing*. Routledge.

Totman, A. (2015). *Roamap to choosing a medical specialty: Questions to consider*. Stanford School of Medicine Academic Advising and the Office of Medical Student Wellness. http://med.stanford.edu/md/student-affairs/student-wellness/_jcr_content/main/panel_builder_2/panel_1/download_1095234323/file.res/Roadmap%20to%20Choosing%20a%20Medical%20Specialty%20.pdf

U.S. Census Bureau. (2019). *Families and households*. https://www.census.gov/topics/families/families-and-households.html

Ugent, D. (2000). Medicine, myths and magic the folk healers of a Mexican market. *Economic Botany, 54*(4), 427–438.

Underman, K., & Hirshfield, L. E. (2016). Detached concern?: Emotional socialization in twenty-first century medical education. *Social Science & Medicine, 160*, 94–101.

Vonarx, N. (2011). Haitian vodou as a health care system: Between magic, religion, and medicine. *Alternative Therapies in Health and Medicine, 17*(5), 44–51.

Waitzkin, H. (1991). *The politics of medical encounters: How patients and doctors deal with social problems.* Yale University Press.

Weber, M. (2002). *The Protestant ethic and the "spirit" of capitalism and other writings* (P. Baehr & G. C. Wells, Eds. & Trans.). Penguin. (Original work published 1905–1920)

Weisz, G. (2003). The emergence of medical specialization in the nineteenth century. *Bulletin of the History of Medicine, 77*(3), 536–575.

Yang, A. (2007). Is Oprah Zulu? Sampling and seeming certainty in DNA ancestry testing. *CHANCE, 20*(1), 32–39.

5

Cultural Consciousness IV

Integral Fusion and Health Professionals in Healthcare Settings

In Chapter 5, we propose that an Integral Fusion worldview, one that fuses the cultural perspectives of Magic Consciousness, Mythic Connection, and Perspectival Thinking, provides cultural actors the flexibility and sustainability necessary to cope with dynamic and emergent challenges in their social world. We will first explore the process of and tensions in cultural fusion as cultural participants reconcile different, if not competing or conflicting, worldviews. Using physicians as an example, we will then explore the variety of cultural perspectives and worldviews that may challenge physicians' biomedical training, a Perspectival Thinking worldview. Finally, we will discuss how cultural fusion can address potential conflicts and tensions in a healthcare team and facilitate provider-patient communication.

I. Integrated Worldviews: Cultural Fusion as Process

A. Fusion Means Integration, Not Unlearning

1. Accrual of Cultural Dimensions

Although one-dimensional Magic Consciousness, two-dimensional Mythic Connection, and three-dimensional Perspectival Thinking are distinctive worldviews, the accrual of dimensions – that they add up – means that the "past" is not gone but is present while being reshaped by additional dimensions. The rebirth of Aristotelianism demonstrates that dimensions of cultural consciousness accrue or add up which means that "previous" dimensions are presumed and even depended upon by "higher" dimensionality (see Chapter 4). In the Theory of Dimensional Accrual and Dissociation, Kramer and Ikeda (1998) explained, "As dimensions of awareness increase the total is different from the sum of parts. The whole exhibits synergy. The whole is more than the sum of parts" (p. 43). Although the signalic world of Perspectival Thinking exhibits extreme dissociation and alienation, Magic Consciousness and Mythic Connection are not all lost in the perspectival world.

The modern world of Perspectival Thinking tends to emphasize and to be prejudiced toward rational spatial thinking and independent individualism. Yet it has strong veins of magic idolic and mythic symbolic forms of communication and emotional valences running through it. The predominantly modern perspectival person is still driven and defined by grand stories (i.e., culture as myth) and may still exhibit

Rethinking Culture in Health Communication: Social Interactions as Intercultural Encounters, First Edition. Elaine Hsieh and Eric M Kramer.
© 2021 John Wiley & Sons, Inc. Published 2021 by John Wiley & Sons, Inc.

obsessive passion and identification for things, including science and medicine. The drive and desire to become a scientist and/or physician, to endure the hardships of years of academic training and even economic costs, is rooted in a deep faith that one can achieve an identity that in the eyes of others has status, value, and may even invoke admiration (Chen, 2018). The *push* to be rational, logical, and objective is itself rooted in Magic Consciousness. Such efforts to change the way individuals and society view the world and solve problems are rooted in a passion and belief system (Stengers, 1993/2000). Progress is seen as something good and what we all should want and strive for. Science, as chemist Michael Polanyi (1946/1964) stated, is a passion, an ambition, an enduring dream to achieve a greater understanding of the universe and to serve humanity. He noted that if scientists really took a totally disinterested view of the universe, they would have no focus. Humans are not satisfied with how things are. Human culture, including art and science, is the compilation of artifacts and efforts to alter nature (Kramer et al., 2014). The obsession and pursuit of the best measure/tool/solution in a Perspectival Thinking world can, in fact, result in Mythic Connection with the measure/tool/solution as symbolic expressions or even Magic Consciousness as the measure/tool/solution becomes identical with the definition of the phenomenon investigated (the thing becomes the sum of measures).

When reviewing Kuhn's (1962/2012) work, *The Structure of Scientific Revolutions*, Maier and Shibles (2010) explained, "Kuhn showed how scientists, and by extension also medical researchers, are captivated by their paradigms such that they are not open to alternative ideas. He even argues that prevailing paradigms can hold us captive and turn scientific thinking into fashionable models and dogma. *When metaphors are taken literally, it turns metaphor into myth, delusion, and dogma. Perspectival thinking is lost*" [emphasis added] (p. 3). When individuals no longer adopt a reflexive attitude about their perspectives but become "true believers" of their perspective, they have shifted away from the signalic world of Perspectival Thinking and entered the symbolic world of Mythic Connection and/or the idolic world of Magic Consciousness.

2. Cultural Fusion Creates Integral Fusion Worldviews

The word fuse is derived from the Proto-Indo-European root gheu- meaning "to pour." Fusion means to blend. **Cultural fusion** is the process of intercultural encounters (Kramer, 2019). As individuals encounter different worldviews, the differences force them to reflect on their own and others' cultural worlds. As Eric Kramer (2017) explained,

> Ultimately the Other demonstrates the arbitrariness of my world. But that does not negate my world including its enduring net of conventions. Fear of the Other need not dominate our comportment. In fact, the Other can encourage my devotion to and preservation of my worldview identified via the difference enabled by the existence of the Other, while also appreciating and borrowing from the world of the Other – cultural fusion. (p. 249)

The understanding of cultural fusion is similar to what Lull (2000) called **transculturation**, "a process whereby cultural forms literally move through time and space where they interact with other cultural forms and settings, influence each other, produce new forms, and change the cultural settings" (p. 242), resulting in "cultural hybrids – the fusing of cultural forms" (p. 243). The outcome of cultural fusion is identical to neither "parent" culture. It is a new form with elements of the original sources still evident and operant.

Cultural fusion incorporates the fusional aspects of information sharing and the process of integration between individuals from different communities. **Integration** means that different ideas, people, processes come together and form innovative and creative ensembles that are *different* from all the sources yet contain aspects of them all. Similarly, Rogers (2006) explained that integration involves "internalization of some or all the imposed culture without (complete) displacement or erasure of native culture and identity" (p. 481). As one acquires different cultural worldviews and blends them, the resulting worldview is **Integral Fusion** – a *new* cultural perspective that is influenced by all cultural perspectives but also unique in its blending of cultures (Kramer, 2000). As a worldview, Integral Fusion is a result of cultural fusion *without* the erasure of the original cultural self (Kramer, 1997, 2000, 2008). Through contact, new forms (of music, cuisine, art, literature, science, history, fashion, business models, etc.) proliferate. This is aperspectival because it is both intentional and unintentional (without directional intent). This is what Hans-Georg Gadamer (1960/2005) means when he states that all communication constitutes a threat to equilibrium – but without such challenges, there is no change, including what one might deem social progress or personal growth.

Some researchers have used the term, **third culture**, to illustrate cultural sojourners' blending of cultural perspectives that are distinctive from the original cultures (e.g., Casmir, 1993; Moore & Barker, 2012). However, the term, third culture, suggests a uniformity and finality of the process of cultural blending. We believe that not all Asians who grow up in the United States with their first-generation immigrant parents share the same "third-culture." Rather, although these Asian Americans may share common experiences as second-generation immigrants, their Integral Fusion can entail unique perspectives that are *situated in* and *evolve with* their personal experience, social network, geographic location, socioeconomic status, and other factors. An Integral Fusion worldview involves the *continuing interplay* between an individual and her lived environment.

What we now understand about evolution is that no single species evolves without communication with the environment. What this means is that the entire environment is a complex web of interconnections. Each species impacts other species within the environment either directly or indirectly. This is what is meant by eco-logic, the way species as well as living and nonliving aspects of an environment, such as rivers, soil, sunlight, form a complex community. An **ecologic approach** (also called systems approach) focuses on "the interfaces and communication processes" that take place within a System (i.e., the ecological structure; Auerswald, 1968). By recognizing that a System is sustained by the communications among parts of a system and between systems, ecological approaches adopt a holistic and nonexclusive view to communications, emphasizing agency, interdependence, and interplay of cultural participants and the System (and subsystems). An ecological approach, thus, embraces the evolving and dynamic nature of cultural participants' interactions as they work to create, maintain, and co-exist in a sustainable and evolving System (Odum, 1998).

What we now understand is that removing just one species from a community will impact all the others (Kramer et al., 2014). Similarly, by adding a new species, the

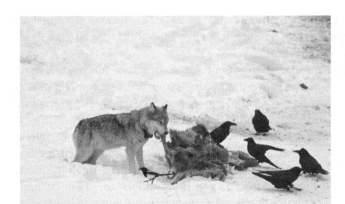

Figure 5.1 Gray wolf at Yellowstone. The introduction of gray wolves resulted in the rippling effects of a transformed ecological system at the Yellowstone National Park. *Source:* James Hager/Age Fotostock

community is altered. A famous example is the 1995/1996 reintroduction of gray wolves into Yellowstone National Park after a 70-year absence. During the first 15 years after wolf reintroduction, researchers found significant recovery in the Yellowstone ecosystem (Ripple & Beschta, 2012). Although the elk population decreased, beavers and bison numbers increased. There are also significant changes in plant species, including aspen, cottonwoods, and willows, restoring forests. Renewed canopies create homes for other plant species. The whole ecosystem was changed (see Figure 5.1). Species evolve together, not separately. When one changes, the effects reverberate throughout the ecosystem, prompting behavioral and biological changes across the system.

This is also true of cultural systems and their interface with exogenous physical systems. Cultures find solutions to problems and the problems vary depending on whether they exist on a semiarid high plateau or in a tropical rain forest; whether they have perennially hostile relations with neighboring groups or live isolated on an island. Cultures are systems that exist within larger systems and they also interact with each other sharing solutions and sometimes falling into competition for scarce resources. There are several channels of communication and interaction with the physical and cultural environment. And the consequences are multidirectional, not unidirectional as in simple assimilation. This multiplex of churning information and adjustments (adaptations) constitutes pan-evolution.

In human communities, we see the same sort of **pan-evolutionary** connectivity (i.e., changes in one can lead to changes in all others that are connected in the system). But here, we are talking not about biological but instead cultural interaction. The process is very similar. The impact of foreign ideas and ways is not correlated with quantity either. If just one Asian family moves into a town and opens a restaurant, everyone in the community is impacted by having an instant increase in the choice of cuisine. If a musician moves into a town dominated by coalminers, then he or she may find themselves in great demand for teaching the children of the town musical skills. Though the music they bring with them may initially be well received, over time their neighbors may convince them to take up tunes the local folks know and enjoy. Even the maintenance of their instrument may be altered by limitations in the types of wood readily available in their newly adopted home. The point here is that *diversity enriches communities*. Diversity is stimulating, disequilibrating. Although conservative tendencies may see such uncertainty only leading to anxiety, it also leads to all new things (innovation, optimism, curiosity, and discovery). It is a catalyst for experimentation and innovation. The people who bring different ideas, values, and perspectives to a System can be at an advantage as part of host societies as they are now co-cultural. (Also see discussions of *medical pluralism and co-cultural groups* in Chapter 6). They have the ability to transition between cultures and cultural worlds.

The encounters of different cultural worldviews can be an intense and complicated process. It is not always pleasant. Evolution can occur in abrupt mutational ways. In a very short time, for instance, the "English invasion" of rock and roll bands in the 1960s profoundly altered American popular culture, music, trends, even political outlooks. The Beatles refused to perform in the segregated South until venues opened their doors to all races of young fans ("The Beatles Banned Segregated Audiences, Contract Shows," 2011). And the results are never static. Culture is alive and evolving. But evolution does not mean cultures are moving toward some final goal when they can then stop. Evolution in biology and culture never ends. New forms of life and culture are constantly emerging.

Nevertheless, when cultures encounter one another, they often react with some resistance. It takes time to integrate new cultural forms, values, beliefs, motives, and expectations. The rate of integration varies from culture to culture. Every technology brings with it beliefs, motives, expectations. New technologies and techniques very often displace old ones that may have very different ontological and cosmological assumptions. For example, technology in *genetics* (i.e., the study of the genes people inherit at birth) and *genomics* (i.e., the study of mutations in genes) leads to the new field of *precision medicine*, an approach "for disease treatment and prevention that takes into account individual variability in genes, environment, and lifestyle for each person" (U.S. National Library of Medicine, n.d., para. 1). By tackling health and illness at a genetic level and a personalized approach, precision medicine transformed fundamental assumptions of the "old" medicine, which focused on external threats (e.g., germs and virus) and demographic risk factors (e.g., gender and age). Precision medicine, a field that would not have existed without genetics, changed the way we think about illness and how people can be ill. In addition, the same practice/technology may hold very different meanings for people in different cultures. When Louis Brown, the world's first "test tube baby" conceived through in vitro fertilization (IVF), was born on July 25, 1978, not everyone embraced the now-common procedures for couples with infertility concerns. Although some new media celebrated the good news, there were also plenty of doom-laden warnings accusing doctors of "playing God" and creating "Frankenbabies"(Mroz, 2017). Do IVF and other reproductive technologies erode our respect for the universe? Does it matter if a human baby is conceived naturally or artificially? Does the purpose (e.g., helping loving couples struggling with infertility or creating future organ donors) or process (e.g., the success rate of healthy babies) matter? Ethics and morality are common battlegrounds when cultures collide (Kass & Wilson, 1998). Integrating such differing worldviews begins with recognizing their existence and the validity they hold for people.

Individuals may strategically adopt an Integral Fusion worldview, aiming to maximize their resources and survival. For example, a Hmong immigrant arriving in the

United States may be quick to get a driver's license to improve their mobility but resist western biomedicine for illness management (Fadiman, 1997). To avoid becoming homeless, Khmer refugees were found to "fake blindness and madness in their clinic examinations, creating dysfunctioning bodies/minds" in order to obtain welfare support in the United States but also rely on traditional healers for treatment (Ong, 1995, p. 1254). Individuals' strategic and intentional applications of different worldviews can lead to frustration and resentment of the host society (Fadiman, 1997), resulting in tensions in intercultural encounters. Forced compliance (e.g., compelled assimilation) tends to lead to cognitive dissonance and resistance (Festinger & Carlsmith, 1959) as well as emotional or affective dissonance (Olusanya, 2016), which can be more intransigent. The results of cultural fusion experiments are not always "good." Some mixtures of music and food never find an enthusiastic audience. Sometimes we demand more, and sometimes no more.

Cultural fusion is an *organic* process shaped by multiple factors. All in a community participate in the experimental process of cultural fusion by embracing or rejecting certain beliefs, attitudes, behaviors, or practices. Individuals' efforts to incorporate other cultural elements and practices may face backlash in society. When Kim Kardashian West promoted and applied for trademarks for a line of shapewear called, "Kimono," she explained, "I understand and have deep respect for the significance of the kimono in Japanese culture" and the clothing line was "a nod to the beauty and details that goes [sic] into a garment" (Friedman, 2019). #KimOhNo, a hashtag, quickly made the rounds on social media, along with protests and petitions against Kim Kardashian West's cultural appropriation of Kimono. The process of cultural fusion can involve strong emotions, tensions, and resistance.

B. Yoga in School: Tensions between and Fusions of Competing Worldviews

Because health and illness are fundamental human conditions, they are always intertwined with cultural values and practices. The cultural consciousness of individuals' diverse worldviews can lead to drastically different interpretations of reality. For example, do you think yoga is a good physical exercise? Is it an exercise for relaxation and mindfulness? Is it okay to teach yoga to school children? In recent years, public schools face increasing pressure from some groups to ban yoga from the physical exercise curriculum (Brown, 2019).

A report at *The Atlantic* stated:

> In 2016, an elementary school in Cobb County, Georgia, became the subject of heated controversy after introducing a yoga program. Parents' objections to the yoga classes – on the grounds that they promoted a non-Christian belief system – were vociferous enough to compel the district to significantly curtail the program, removing the "namaste" greeting and the coloring-book exercises involving mandalas. A few years before that, a group of parents sued a San Diego County school district on the grounds that its yoga program promoted Eastern religions and disadvantaged children who opted out. (Wong, 2018, para. 3)

Would learning yoga's positions and movements makes a person less Christian because it promotes non-Christian beliefs and Eastern philosophy (see Figure 5.2)? Is making the Namaste gesture a greeting like saying "hello," or does it transform a person into a different reality when people "place the hands together at the heart chakra, close the eyes, and bow the head" (Geno, 2018, "How to Make the Namaste Gesture" section)? Is coloring a mandala an exercise of patience and fine motor skills or does it teach children "about life being cyclical and every circle is unending, every circle has a center and humans too must find their center in their inner selves" (Brown, 2019, p. 97)?

In the signalic world of Perspectival Thinking, yoga is merely a physical exercise and coloring mandalas is just an artistic expression, mechanisms through which one can improve children's bodies and minds. A review of clinical studies found when compared to other forms of exercise, yoga is equal or superior in lowering blood pressure, improving mood and anxiety, strengthening the immune system, and even in reducing the side-effects of chemotherapy (Ross & Thomas, 2010). Other studies have also found that coloring mandalas, a reasonably complex geometric pattern, can induce a meditative state, reduce anxiety, and improve perseverance (See Figure 5.3; Curry & Kasser, 2005; Eaton & Tieber, 2017; van der Vennet & Serice, 2012). The National Institutes of Health listed yoga as a complementary health approach that is *scientifically* proven to improve both physical and psychological well-being in both healthy and diseased populations (National Center for Complementary and Alternative Medicine, 2018).

However, just as the Muslim performance of prayer (i.e., Salat) represents the Mythic Connection for the complete surrender and submission to Allah, can a person perform Namaste or color mandalas without embodying the corresponding cultural consciousness? Both performing yoga and coloring mandalas have been promoted as **mindfulness** activities. (Note: the mindfulness in this Chapter should not be

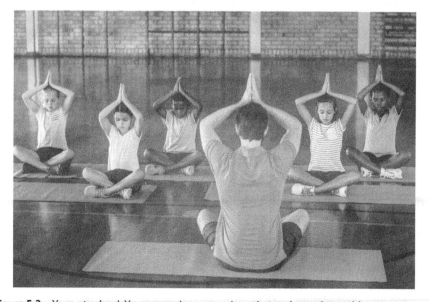

Figure 5.2 Yoga at school. Yoga poses have meanings that go beyond stretching your muscles – it's a way to connect your body, mind, and spirit with the world. *Source:* Wavebreak Media Ltd/123RF

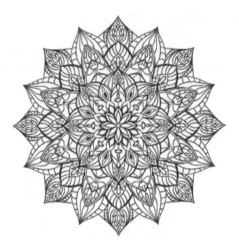

Figure 5.3 Mandala. Psychological studies show that coloring mandalas have the same effect as that of meditation.

understood as the clinical empathy, also called mindfulness, in physician training discussed in Chapter 4). Kabat-Zinn (2013) defined mindfulness as "the awareness that arises by paying attention on purpose, in the present moment, and nonjudgmentally" (p. xxxv). Bishop et al. (2004) defined mindfulness as a mode of awareness that involves self-regulation of attention to achieve a non-elaborative awareness of present experiences. In both definitions, the emphasis on focusing and opening one's mind to the awareness of the present suggests a cultural consciousness different from Perspectival Thinking. Perspectival Thinking is analytical and methodical. It fragments time, space, and identities into ever smaller, independent units. In contrast, mindfulness activities encourage individuals to open and focus one's awareness on the here and now (i.e., time disappears) and open oneself to all the senses as a whole (e.g., senses are synthesized, not fragmented). When describing the meanings of greeting one another with the Namaste gesture, Geno (2018) explained,

> Namaste allows two individuals to come together energetically to a place of *connection* and *timelessness*, free from the bonds of ego-connection. If it is done with deep feeling in the heart and with the mind surrendered, a deep union of spirits can blossom. [emphasis added] (para. 7)

In American yoga culture, the Sanskrit salutation Namaste is often translated as "the Divine in me bows to the Divine in you," "the light in me honors the light in you," "obeisance to you," or "reverence to you" (Brown, 2019, p. 74). Such a practice aims to encourage a sense of connection to the larger world. If a person performs Namaste with Mythic Connection, she expresses her desire and effort to abandon her ego and connect with the other. If a person performs Namaste with Magic Consciousness, she literally is connected to the other as the gesture is completed (see Figures 5.4 and 5.5). Abandoning one's ego and surrendering one's mind to another fellow human being (not God) is unthinkable in many religions – nevertheless, such an attitude is promoted in Eastern religions and philosophies, including Buddhism, because all beings are equal.

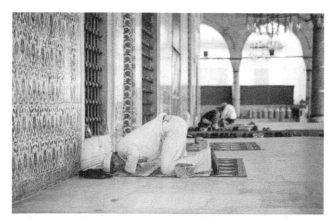

Figure 5.4 Salat. Salat is a Muslim ritual prayer to be performed five times a day. It is a physical, mental, and spiritual act of worship. *Source:* Cielo De La Paz / EyeEm/Getty Images

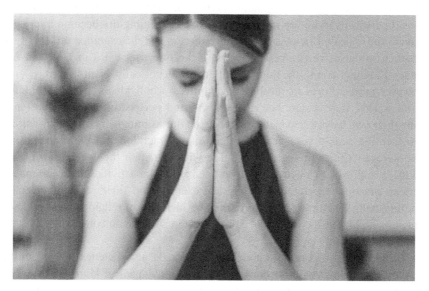

Figure 5.5 Namaste. Namaste is usually spoken with a slight bow and hands pressed together, palms touching and fingers pointing upwards, thumbs close to the chest. *Source:* ammentorp/123RF

When India's Prime Minister, Narenda Modi, a Hindu nationalist, tried to make yoga compulsory for all school-aged children in 2014, India's Muslim, Sikh, and Christian minorities protested (Brown, 2019). Brown (2019) explained, "Muslim spokespersons object that Sūrya Namaskāra 'requires a person to bow to the Sun God.' A Muslim mother of school-aged children, Amina Begum, explained in 2016: 'Islam being a monotheistic religion doesn't allow followers to bow before anyone except Allah. We don't like our kids following this routine in their schools. Surely, there are other neutral forms of exercises which can benefit children?'" (p. 65). Examining how mindfulness is understood as a secular or religious activity in the West, Stratton (2015) noted that some religious groups, particularly "Fundamentalist and Evangelical Christians," may find "mind-emptying" practices as introductions of "explicitly non-Christian spiritual influences" and avoid "any meditation beyond explicitly Christian prayer-based forms" (p. 106). Because religiosity requires individuals to embrace non-Perspectival Thinking worldviews, it is not surprising that other religious groups are quick to see and protest the potential impact when children are exposed to symbols that may connect them to other cultural worldviews that are incompatible with their Mythic Connection or Magic Consciousness worlds.

The rise of global controversies about including yoga as part of a physical education curriculum for school-aged children highlights how intense conflicts and emotions among the cultural participants can result when worldviews collide. This is true even when both cultures adopt Mythic Connection, as the symbols, values, and appropriate forms of connection are still different in two cultures. They may even be mutually excluding if their doctrines explicitly claim their path as the exclusive path of righteous thinking and behaving. Under such late-mythic constructs (such as monotheism), there can only be one "right" way. As spatial thinking intensifies, magic wholeness begins to fragment. Mythic polarity increasingly hardens into (defines) perspectival duality until compromise and ambiguity become impossible as seen in the logical principles of noncontradiction and the excluded middle. A single path to progressive (utopian) salvation, the one true word of God and law, excludes all others as unholy. Fundamentalism, categorically, is intolerant.

However, most cultures are flexible and adaptive. As individuals encounter different cultural worlds, they accumulate different cultural perspectives and dimensions – finding their own ways to navigate and reconcile the seemingly incompatible cultural terrains. In the case of yoga in the United States, practitioners have proposed new forms of yoga: "Christian yoga," yoga fused with Christian theology (Brown, 2018; Jain, 2017), and "American yoga," yoga branded as secular activities to "accommodate American practitioners' interest in physical exercise and their religious diversity" (Coskuner-Balli & Ertimur, 2017, p. 130). Such blending of religious and/or secular worldviews highlights the process of cultural fusion with the outcome being an active Integral Fusion worldview.

Nevertheless, it is important to note that individuals' and societies' acts of cultural fusion are still fraught with tensions. For example, Evangelical Marcia Montenegro commented, "'Christian Yoga' is an oxymoron. ... Just as there is no Christian Ouija board and no Christian astrology, so there is no Christian Yoga that is either truly Yoga or truly Christian" (Brown, 2019, p. 59). In recent years, memories of cultural imperialism and fears of assimilation and exploitation of marginalized and colonized cultures often emerge as charges of cultural appropriation (Brown, 2018; Rogers, 2006). Communication professor Richard Rogers (2006) explained, "**Cultural appropriation**, defined broadly as the use of a culture's symbols, artifacts, genres, rituals, or technologies by members of another culture, is *inescapable* when cultures come into contact, including virtual or representational contact" [emphasis added] (p. 474). Nevertheless, concerns about "(in)voluntariness, (in)equality, (im)balance, and (im)purity" may make some forms of cultural appropriation (e.g., cultural exploitation or cultural dominance) more problematic than others (e.g., transculturation; Rogers, 2006, p. 499).

In summary, cultural fusion is an inescapable process whenever different cultural consciousness structures encounter one another. Although cultural participants may be more willing to embrace differences in some areas (e.g., fashion or music), they may also express intense resistance in others (e.g. religion). Because health and illness are often intertwined with cultural worldviews, examples of tensions between and fusion of competing cultural worldviews are prevalent in health contexts. Using the introduction of yoga to school-aged children as an example, we demonstrated that the same act may have drastically different meanings in "reality" for individuals with different cultural worldviews. The success of intercultural encounters relies on the participants' ability to understand, appreciate, and negotiate such diverging worldviews.

II.   Physicians as Cultural Groups: Physicians' Integral Fusion Worldviews

In Chapter 2, we laid out four primary ways that scholars have conceptualized the meanings and functions of culture. In Chapters 3 and 4, we explored how patients' Voice of the Lifeworld and providers' Voice of Medicine may represent different ways of understanding the world, resulting in challenges to provider-patient communication. In the literature of health communication, provider-patient encounters are often conceptualized as interpersonal communication in health contexts – we assume that providers and patients are from the same culture because they live in the same community and speak the same language. However, given what we have learned so far, can we reconsider provider-patient interactions as intercultural encounters?

Diversity is essential to the strength and health of a system, allowing the System to be adaptive and responsive to challenges (Gelfand et al., 2017). Historically, the medical literature presumes that clinicians are neutral professionals who are trained to follow guidelines based on objective, evidence-based biomedicine and are unaffected by their own personal variables and/or prejudice (both enabling and limiting; Berger, 2008). However, cultural variance "adds" to one's cultural dimensions (e.g., scope of understanding). When encountering a new culture, it is important to consider the variety of cultural dimensions and worldviews that may shape the physicians' Integral Fusion worldviews.

A.   Culture as Ethnic/Racial and Gender Group

There remain significant demographic disparities in the healthcare industry. Both faculty members in medical school and the workforce of active physicians are predominately White and male (Association of American Medical Colleges, 2019). According to the 2019 report of the Association of American Medical Colleges (AAMC), among active physicians, 56.2% identified as Non-Hispanic White, 17.1% as Asian, 5.8% as Hispanic, 5.0% as Black or African American, 0.3% as Native American, and 13.7% reported Unknown. In contrast, among the U.S. population, 60.4% identified as Non-Hispanic White, 5.9% as Asians, 18.3% as Hispanic/Latino, 13.4% as Black, and 1.3% as Native American (U.S. Census Bureau, 2018). Black, Hispanic, and Native American physicians are significantly underrepresented in a wide range of medical specialties.

The literature suggests that a physician's race and ethnicity can contribute to different clinical practices and communicative behaviors. Physicians' practices of end of life care mirror the preferences of the ethnic or racial group that they identified with (Mebane et al., 1999). Asian-American primary care residents are least likely to address cervical cancer; in contrast, African-American residents are most likely to do so (Arredondo et al., 2003). A national survey of primary care physicians found physicians' race/ethnicity contributed to significant variation in treatment recommendations for depression, anxiety, and medically unexplained symptoms (Lawrence et al., 2015).

In addition, there is a global trend in recruiting and retaining physicians from other countries (Ranasinghe, 2015). *One in four* physicians in the United States and Canada are **international medical graduates** (IMG; i.e., physicians who received their medical school education outside of the United States or Canada; Hart et al., 2007; Ranasinghe, 2015; Tsugawa et al., 2017). The leading source countries for IMGs include India, the Philippines, Pakistan, and Mexico (not including U.S. citizens who received medical education abroad). More than 20 million Americans live in areas where at least half of the physicians are IMGs (American Immigration Council, 2018). These physicians, who also are cultural sojourners, may face unique challenges in providing culturally sensitive care to patients in the host society (Liao, 2017; Michalski et al., 2017; Skjeggestad, Gerwing, & Gulbrandsen, 2017; Tsugawa et al., 2017). Recognizing the differences between their cultural worldviews, social norms, and provider-patient relationship/hierarchy, international physicians acknowledged that their patients may perceive their own behaviors to be "strange" and "different," making the interaction "not very comfortable" (Dorgan et al., 2009, p. 1570).

There are also significant gender differences. Among active physicians in 2018, 64.1% are male, 35.8% are female, and .2% unknown (Association of American Medical Colleges, 2019). Although female physicians are well-represented in pediatric care (75%), obstetrics and gynecology (85%), family medicine (58%), and psychiatry (57%), these are the only specialties that women are well-represented in (Dusenbery, 2018; Vassar, 2015). Dusenbery (2018) explained, "There remain large segments of medicine where women are vastly outnumbered: women make up about a quarter of emergency medicine physicians, neurologists, and anesthesiologists; less than 20% of general surgeons; 12% of cardiologists; 7% of urologists; and less than 5% of orthopedic surgeons" (p. 9). The gender disparities among medical professionals are also reflected in the demographics of faculty members in medical school (Association of American Medical Colleges, 2019), their tenure and promotion records (Carr et al., 2017), records of grants and academic awards (Silver et al., 2017), and compensations (Dusenbery, 2018; Read et al., 2018).

B. Culture as Speech Community

Traditionally, although patients are often viewed as diverse populations, the literature has generally conceptualized physicians as a *single* cultural group, trained professionals who speak the Voice of Medicine (Apker & Eggly, 2004; Timmermans & Alison, 2001). In a study about communication patterns of primary care physicians in the United States, researchers found that the biomedical model is prevalent in physicians' communicative patterns, accounting for 85% of provider talk (Roter et al., 1997). More specifically, Roter et al. (1997) found five distinct communication patterns: (a) "narrowly biomedical," characterized by closed-ended medical questions and biomedical talk occurring (32% of visits); (b) "expanded biomedical," characterized by a restricted pattern but with moderate levels of psychosocial discussion (33%); (c) "biopsychosocial," reflecting a balance of psychosocial and biomedical topics (20%); (d) "psychosocial," characterized by psychosocial exchange (8%); and (e) "consumerist," characterized primarily by patient questions and physician information giving (8%). Although all physicians used more than one pattern during a visit, more than half of the 127 physicians used one pattern for the majority of the visit, often favoring either "narrowly biomedical" or "expanded biomedical" (Roter et al., 1997).

However, rather than assuming that physicians are one speech community, the literature suggests that not all physicians share the same communicative patterns. For example, when comparing the communicative patterns of primary care physicians, Bensing et al. (2003) found that 46% of the U.S. physicians' communicative patterns were biomedically intensive; in contrast, 18% of the Dutch physicians' talk was in the same category; in contrast, 50% of Dutch physicians' talk was categorized as socioemotional style, whereas only 10% of the U.S. physicians' talk was socioemotional. The differences in the United States and Dutch physicians' communication patterns influenced the *content* of provider-patient communication, including the focus on instrumental and affective behaviors (Bensing et al., 2003). Bensing et al. (2003) argued that the differences may reflect the countries' differences in "medical training and philosophy, health care system characteristics, and cultural values and expectations relevant to the delivery and receipt of medical services" (p. 335). It is likely that medical training and healthcare system characteristics are themselves derivative of more fundamental cultural values and expectations.

Several studies have identified *gender* as a factor for physicians' communicative styles. A study of Japanese primary care physicians found that female physicians substantially modified their communication behaviors based on patient gender and male physicians did not (Noro et al., 2018). Compared to male physicians, female physicians adopt more patient-centered communication, have longer office visits, and are more likely to discuss complementary and alternative medicine (Kurtz et al., 2003; Roter et al., 2002).

It is also possible that different *medical specialties* may adopt different communicative patterns. For example, internal medicine physicians asked more biomedical questions while family practice physicians were more likely to engage in psychosocial discussions and provide emotional support (Paasche-Orlow & Roter, 2003). A study of Malaysian physicians found that oncologists' communicative patterns exhibited the highest level of patient centeredness (Chan & Ahmad, 2012). Obstetricians and gynecologists have the second highest level, followed by primary care physicians, and surgeons have the lowest level of patient-centered communication (Chan & Ahmad, 2012). Among fourth-year medical students, demographic characteristics that are associated with more patient-centered attitudes included female gender, European-American ethnicity, and career interests in primary care (Haidet et al., 2002).

C. Culture as Worldview

Traditionally, researchers have argued that the *medical gaze* is the viewpoint adopted by physicians as they pathologize human bodies and (bio)medicalize issues of health and illness (See Chapter 4 for review of the medical gaze; Clarke et al., 2003). The

medicalization of human experiences means that the particular experience/problem "is defined in medical terms, described using medical language, understood through the adoption of a medical framework, or 'treated' with medical intervention" (Conrad, 2007, p. 5). For example, researchers have argued that childbirth and pregnancy are areas that have been deliberately and methodically medicalized, resulting in a 97–99% hospital birth rate (Barker, 1998; Cahill, 2001). Although gravity enhancing positions (e.g., squatting) may be most natural in facilitating women giving birth, birthing women were instead placed in reclining horizontal positions in elevated beds in order to help physicians better control and view of the birthing process (i.e., the viewpoint shifts from the mother to the physician, and hence, the medical gaze). With increasing medical specialization, technicalities, and monitoring devices, women have less and less control over the process and procedure of giving birth (Crossley, 2007). The medicalization of human conditions has redefined our lived experiences. Surgical options for beauty (e.g., weight loss surgery for obesity and cosmetic surgery for better pictures on social media), hormonal therapies for the aging (e.g., testosterone treatment for men and estrogen replacement treatment for women), therapies for relationships and love (e.g., counseling and sex therapy), and medications for mood fluctuation (e.g., treatment for unhappiness and bipolar disorder) have not only shaped physicians' approach to human suffering but also our expectations for everyday life (Dworkin, 2001; Earp et al., 2015; Lee & Mysyk, 2004; Zola, 1991).

The literature suggests that *religion* may also shape providers' worldviews, resulting in differences in providers' delivery of care (Bateman & Clair, 2015). Religious worldviews differ from the biomedical worldview of Perspectival Thinking because religions inherently entail values and decision-making about life and death (and thus, health and illness) that involve Mythic Connection and/or Magic Consciousness. Religion imposes moral judgments on actions while the perspectival biomedical worldview focuses on operational material outcomes. Religion asks, "is it morally right," while operational biomedicine asks, "does it work?" As a result, physicians' religious attitudes were found to influence their practice in areas that often generate deep moral controversy, including end-of-life care (e.g., withholding or withdrawing life support) and reproductive medicine (e.g., abortion, emergency contraception, assisted reproductive technologies, and treatment in cases of unavoidable pregnancy loss).

Conscientious refusal is defined by healthcare providers' refusal to provide medical services or goods, including medication and information, due to their religious, moral, philosophical, or ethical beliefs. In end-of-life care, physicians who report to be non-religious "were more likely than others to report having given continuous deep sedation until death, having taken decisions they expected or partly intended to end life, and to have discussed these decisions with patients judged to have the capacity to participate in discussions" (Seale, 2010, p. 677). In contrast, compared to physicians with low religiosity, highly religious physicians are 4.2 times more likely to object to physician-assisted suicide and 2.6 times more likely to object to terminal sedation (Curlin et al., 2008). Compared to physicians of other religious faiths, Catholic physicians are 2.8 times more likely to object to withdrawing life support, which may reflect the Catholic doctrine of prohibiting actions intended to shorten life (Curlin et al., 2008). In fact, *religious intensity* is the strongest predictor for whether a physician believes that they are never obligated to do what they personally believe to be wrong. Catholic and Orthodox physicians are most likely to hold such beliefs (Lawrence & Curlin, 2009). The most religious physicians are more likely than the least religious physicians to support refusing to accommodate a patient's request (Brauer et al., 2016). Physicians who are more religious are also more likely to recommend chemotherapy and less likely to recommend hospice for patients with advanced illness (Frush et al., 2018). In fact, Frush et al. (2018) fount that physicians' religious intensity was a stronger predictor for treatment recommendations for advanced cancer care than patient deposition (e.g., age and preferences).

The literature also suggests that physicians may hold different worldviews as a result of their *medical specialties*. Because different medical specialties often hold different emphases on biological and psychological bodies, it is only natural that medical specialties may impact providers' diagnosis and treatment decisions. The differences in worldviews between medical specialties are most salient when there is no clear clinical evidence for recommended procedures. For example, women with silicone breast implants reported a wide range of complex and debilitating symptoms. Physicians often struggled to make sense of these patients' symptoms. Zimmermann (1998) discussed the experiences of Sheila, a breast implant patient diagnosed with chronic fatigue syndrome and other immunological disorders:

> [When she approached physicians] with her symptoms, they ruled out only the conditions and diseases that they were equipped to understand within their fields of specialization – her gynecologist believed Sheila had a reproductive problem, her endocrinologist checked for a hormonal imbalance, and her neurologist ordered a brain scan hoping to understand why she was experiencing cognitive difficulties. The inability of these doctors to understand Sheila's health troubles outside the narrow scope of their own medical specialties resulted in their belief that Sheila's problem must be psychological, not physical. (p. 133)

Specialization is a prominent characteristic of the modern perspectival worldview. Fragmentation of knowledge enhances deeper but narrower expertise. This has both good and bad consequences.

Vanderford and Smith (1996) found that when faced with the uncertainty of symptoms and diagnosis, different specialists held different beliefs about the safety of silicone gel breast implants. "The rheumatologists we interviewed had seen cases that convinced them that implants were potentially harmful at least to some women. The plastic surgeons repeatedly referred to the absence of scientific data showing a danger. The family physician and gynecologists had not seen patients with problems and were inclined to discount the claims of danger" (Vanderford & Smith, 1996, p. 102). Whereas plastic surgeons see concrete problems, have clear procedures to follow, and can see how successful their interventions have been, rheumatologists often work with vaguer symptoms for a longer period of time, helping their patients manage, rather than cure, the illness. Vanderford & Smith (1996) concluded:

> Plastic surgeons and rheumatologists practice medicine differently, particularly in how they proceed in the face of uncertainty. They regarded case examples as playing different roles in medical knowledge. They differed in their reaction to

the cases of a number of patients they saw in common. This difference about the usefulness of cases accounts for much of their difference in medical judgment. (p. 107)

Similarly, in the case of localized prostate cancer, although the literature does not have evidence to suggest whether radiation therapy or surgery is the superior primary therapy, urologists and radiologists overwhelmingly recommended treatment that they themselves deliver and believed that their treatment was better than other alternatives (Fowler et al., 2000; Kim et al., 2014). In fact, the physician that a patient sees matters far more for treatment recommended than the patients' preferences – if he sees an oncologist, he is likely to be treated with chemotherapy; if he sees a surgeon first, he is more likely to receives a prostatectomy (Sommers et al., 2008).

D. Culture as a Living Process

We want to emphasize that the biomedical worldview in Western medicine is pervasive and dominant. Despite the earlier discussions about alternative worldviews that physicians may adopt, there are also studies that found that clinicians' religious beliefs, religiosity, specialty, or age do *not* impact their decision-making in a variety of contexts, including end-of-life care (Burns et al., 2001). In other words, as we examine the various ways through which culture and cultural views can influence physicians' practices and decision-making, we believe that physicians do not always "prioritize" different worldviews, allowing one to replace another (e.g., assimilation). Rather, physicians may develop an Integral Fusion worldview that fuses various aspects of their cultural worlds (as in the case of *witnessing*, see Chapter 4). Not all physicians develop an Integral Fusion worldview as some may be more comfortable to allow a specific worldview to dominate healthcare processes and clinical practices. Nevertheless, given the inescapability of other competing worldviews (e.g., ethnicity/race/gender, religion, and medical specialty), the fact that we "cannot rid ourselves of the cultural self we bring with us" (Scheper-Hughes, 1992, p. 28), and the expected performance of biomedical professionals in healthcare settings, it is likely that physicians need to actively consolidate and reconcile the tensions in diverging cultural values and worldviews.

For example, compared to less religious Muslim physicians, American Muslim physicians who read the Quran every day are more likely to recommend the tubal ligation and procedures that are judged to be normatively prohibited by Islamic law (Mahdi et al., 2016). Mahdi et al. (2016) argued that these highly religious physicians may feel more comfortable in recommending these decisions because their daily readings allowed them to derive ethical teachings from scriptural sources and interpret a variety of verses to be in accordance with the procedure. Similarly, Lawrence and Curlin (2009) found that while 78% of primary physicians agreed with the statement that "A physician should never do what he or she believes is morally wrong, no matter what experts say," 57% also agreed with the statement "Sometimes physicians have a professional ethical obligation to provide medical services even if they personally believe it would be morally wrong to do so" (p. 1278).

How do healthcare providers reconcile the tensions between their right to exercise conscientious refusal as a religious person with their professional duty to provide care? Despite strong and prevalent support among physicians' for their right to exercise conscientious refusal, a study of 2,000 U.S. physicians found that the majority (57%) of physicians agreed that "physicians have a professional duty to *refer* patients for all legal medical services for which the patients are candidates, even if the physician believes that such a referral is immoral" (Combs et al., 2011, p. 398).

Although women over 17 years and older can purchase emergency contraception at U.S. pharmacies without a prescription, many studies have reported that most Catholic hospitals in the United States do not provide emergency contraception even to rape victims (Wicclair, 2011). A study found that while none of the 30 non-Catholic hospitals surveyed prohibited staff from discussing emergency contraception with rape victims, 12 of the 28 Catholic hospitals in the study had such a policy and seven of the Catholic hospitals also prohibited physicians from prescribing emergency contraception even if patients asked for it (Smugar & Spina, 2000). In Catholic hospitals that explicitly prohibit physicians from discussing or prescribing emergency contraception for rape victims, physicians were found to "tell victims that they have a policy prohibiting discussion of emergency contraception," refer the victims to another provider where the information would be provided, invite rape counselors to the emergency to provide such information, or just discuss the information despite hospital policy (Smugar & Spina, 2000, p. 1373).

In short, physicians' Integral Fusion worldviews allow them to reconcile differences and tensions between different cultural worlds that they encounter and affiliate with. When asked to provide services that violate the moral principles of their religious worldviews of Mythic Connection or Magic Consciousness, physicians may develop new understandings of the religious texts to realign their religious beliefs with professional duties or compartmentalize their worldviews through strategic actions (e.g., referring patients to a willing physician to protect patient autonomy while refusing medical services to protect their faith and identity).

III. Implication for the Delivery of Care

A. Culture in Interprofessional Health Teams

By examining the complexity of physicians' cultural perspectives, we aim to demonstrate the variety of worldviews that can shape a provider's clinical practice. Such complexity and diversity of cultural perspectives are also exhibited by other types of healthcare providers, including nurses, technicians, social workers, and patient advocates, among others. The Perspectival Thinking in modern medicine, motivated by the desire for precision, is reflected in the increasing specialization and fragmentation of medicine. However, patients' illness experiences and symptoms are intertwined. For example, a patient with cancer is also likely to experience depression, oral complications, and cardiovascular complications as a result of cancer therapy (Caruso et al., 2017; Epstein et al., 2012; Yeh & Bickford, 2009). As a result, throughout the illness event, a cancer patient is likely to receive care from various specialists such as an oncologist, a mental health specialist, a dentist, a cardiologist as well as attention from nurses, imaging technicians, pharmacists, and other health professionals. It is not surprising to imagine how a patient may be confused by and frustrated about managing different aspects of his or her health in an illness event.

Interprofessional health teams first emerged as a solution in the 1970s in response to the increasing pressure of specialization in medicine and the dangers of fragmenting patients' illness experiences (Schmitt et al., 2013). An interprofessional health team is defined as "health professionals who are working together to achieve positive patient outcomes" (Weiss et al., 2016, p. 6). Training for interprofessional health teams is now considered an essential part in many fields, including medicine, nursing, pharmacy, dentistry, social work, and allied health. Conflicts within an interprofessional health team can disrupt teamwork, compromise patient care, reduce team members' job satisfaction and well-being, and increase overall healthcare costs (Brown et al., 2011; Cullati et al., 2019; Pavlish et al., 2014). Examining these challenges through the perspectives of cultural fusion provides opportunities to anticipate areas of tension and identify possible solutions.

First, an interprofessional health team, by definition, involves differences of (cultural) perspectives and, thus, is inherently disposed to manifest differences and the co-existence of meanings and realities (Burns et al., 2001; Skjørshammer, 2001). For example, in the contexts of end-of-life care, a physician's clinical decisions reflect a balancing act between resource allocation (for other patients), family members' potential conflicts of interest, patients' preference, and their own values (Oberle & Hughes, 2001). In contrast, nurses can experience distress if they believe that "doctors too often act on their own values, rather than those of the patients and families" (Oberle & Hughes, 2001, p. 711), resulting in suboptimal care (e.g., delayed or insufficient disclosure). In their analysis of nurse-physician conflicts in end-of-life care, Oberle and Hughes (2001) concluded, "Doctors and nurses are confronted with different problems and ask different questions in the *same* care situation" [emphasis added] (p. 714). The different perspectives reflect the health professionals' diverse understanding of their "moral identities": what does it mean to be a good nurse or a good physician (Pavlish et al., 2014)?

Traditionally, to resolve conflicts in interprofessional health teams, **medical dominance** allows physicians to exert power in clinical settings over other health professionals, displacing others' perspectives. Medical dominance is often embedded in organizational structures, allowing the culture of medicine to exert power over other professions (e.g., nursing and pharmacy). For example, a nurse reported that after discussing end-of-life options with a severely ill patient, a physician reprimanded her by saying, "It was not your responsibility or business to discuss that with my patient" (Pavlish et al., 2014, p. 133). Nurses reported that some physicians and nurse managers "jump down [their] throat," "slap [them] around," or "dismiss [them]" when they raised ethical questions that challenged physicians' clinical practice in end-of-life care (Pavlish et al., 2014, p. 133). Similarly, due to medical dominance, interpreters may feel that while they are a part of the health care process and team, "[they are] also somewhat peripheral to the process, playing an auxiliary or supporting role" (Hsieh & Kramer, 2012, p. 161). Feeling being treated as marginal to the process, interpreters may actively silence their own and patients' voice (Hsieh & Kramer, 2012).

Medical dominance is likely to create frustrations for non-physicians. For example, compared to physicians, nurses are more likely to report difficulties to voice their opinions, be less satisfied with the quality of collaboration and communication, and feel that disagreements are not appropriately resolved in interprofessional teams (Thomas et al., 2003). Interpreters reported frustration and helplessness when providers' lack of communicative competence lead to substandard care (Hsieh, 2006, 2007). Nevertheless, as other health professionals (e.g., nurses and pharmacists) have increasingly expanded their roles and services into areas traditionally performed by physicians, the interprofessional health team is becoming the norm. "Medical dominance grounded in the medical gaze has been dislocated and relocated in a *democratizing* of medical practice" [emphasis added] (Bleakley, 2013, p. 27), promoting dialogue and collaboration between different professionals to reconcile differences (i.e., a process of cultural fusion). This is because interprofessional teamwork often requires team members to collaborate on certain tasks while making independent decisions on others (MacNaughton et al., 2013). Thus, successful collaborations require team members to develop strategies to identify and negotiate **taskwork** (i.e., the functions that individuals must perform to accomplish the team's objective; MacNaughton et al. 2013).

Second, relying on role boundaries to avoid conflict is likely to be ineffective unless the healthcare team is able to generate an Integral Fusion approach to illness management that encourages discussion, negotiation, and compromise from team members to achieve mutually agreeable goals (see also Hsieh, 2016). **Role boundaries** suggest that each professional has specific, territorial claim and *exclusive* control over the process of healthcare delivery. For example, nurses expect physicians to know what to do whenever problems arise and physicians expect nurses to just follow their orders. We may expect interpreters to limit their expertise in language and culture and physicians to focus on medicine in interpreter-mediated medical encounters. However, in medical practice, the boundaries between what is medical (biological or psychological), social, cultural, linguistic, moral, and ethical are not always clear. These boundaries are dynamic and shifting. They often reflect a variety of cultural perspectives and situational contexts, such as team providers' specialties (e.g., mental health, oncology, or nursing), clinical experiences, gender, issues emerging during medical consultation (e.g., routine checkup vs. disclosure of bad news), and/or a patient's background (e.g., cultural specific needs). In addition, unlike the clarity and certainty that the medical gaze would like to project, uncertainty is prevalent and unavoidable in modern medicine and medical practices (Han et al., 2011; Niland & Lyons, 2011; see also Chapter 9). A rigid adherence to preconceived role boundaries is likely to lead to individuals who have less power (e.g., nurses) in an interprofessional team to avoid communication in an effort to minimize conflicts (Skjørshammer, 2001) or to adopt *covert* strategies to circumvent physicians' control and institutional rules (Beagan & Ells, 2009; Hsieh, 2006, 2010). Nevertheless, both strategies fail to address the underlying disagreement in the health professionals' perceived realities and perspectives, increasing risks of compromised care, failed teamwork, and ethical conflicts.

Finally, as we consider the variety and diversity presented by the cultural perspectives of interprofessional team members, it is important to remember that despite these differences, the team members likely share significant agreement and similarities in their understanding of care (Levorato et al., 2001). For example, Burns et al. (2001) found that nearly two-thirds of pediatric critical care physicians and nurses express views on end-of-life care in strong agreement with consensus positions on these issues adopted by national professional organizations. As a healthcare team, all team members assumed a pre-determined objective of providing optimal care to improve patient outcomes. The shared objective provides opportunities for healthcare professionals to reconcile their diverging perspectives through open communication. Rather than allowing these (moral) disagreements to progress into irreconcilable ethical conflicts, Pavlish et al. (2014) argued that interprofessional health teams should form **moral communities** that encourage timely, respectful conversations about moral perspectives and responsibilities among all team members. Moral communities highlight the process of cultural fusion within the healthcare team. Moral communities are characterized by respectful team relationships, timely communication, ethics-minded leadership, readily available ethics resources, and provider awareness and willingness to use ethics resources. As all members are "encouraged to illuminate ethical concerns and grapple with them in a manner that promotes trust, shared understanding, and mutual respect," team members can identify their shared values and goals in patient care (Pavlish et al., 2014, p. 138).

Cultural fusion does not mean that all conflicts between team members can be eliminated. An ethicist explained, physicians need to accept that "sometimes the result you like will not happen … that what you believe with all your heart is wrong, someone else cannot accept as wrong. There can simply be moral disagreement, and people can base it on very sound values and good moral reasoning" (Pavlish et al., 2014, pp. 133–134). Developing and identifying an Integral Fusion worldview among health team members and patients can encourage individuals to adopt a more flexible and inclusive stance toward their own and others' perspectives. In fact, in our study about provider-interpreter collaboration, we found:

> To achieve optimal care, providers are willing to compromise on certain issues as they recognize gains in other areas. For example, an assertive male family interpreter who makes decisions for the female patient may not meet a provider's desire for patient autonomy, but many providers also recognize such practices as cultural norms. They argue that insisting on a professional interpreter and excluding the male family relative in the interpreter-mediated encounter may, in fact, create patient anxiety and distrustful relationships. When they recognize interpreters' familiarities in the clinical knowledge and procedures, they welcome interpreters' active involvement during the encounter (e.g., checking understanding or reminders of missed topics). In other words, our findings suggest that there are situations in which providers do not expect complete control over the process and content of the provider-patient interaction. When specific criteria are met, they are willing to accept and, in fact, welcome interpreters' active involvement in the communicative process. (Hsieh, 2016, p. 234)

An Integral Fusion worldview does not mean a complete elimination of differences. Integrating perspectives does not mean eliminating perspectives (i.e., forced compliance). Each individual's perspective endures, but a shared worldview also emerges. The Integral Fusion worldview materializes through the team's shared objectives. As a moral community, the team provides the flexibility, ambiguity, and respectfulness necessary to embrace shared values. More importantly, because differences in team members' individual (or initial) perspectives are recognized and embraced, such differences provide the valuable diversity that enables the team to respond to a wide range of complex issues in illness management.

B. Implications for Provider-Patient Communication

Although healthcare providers are exposed to and trained in the biomedical worldview of Perspectival Thinking, they also are affiliated with and may identify with other cultural worldviews that have been demonstrated to influence their communicative behaviors and clinical practices. Nevertheless, patients and providers often downplay and even are unaware of how their culture and ethnicity can shape provider-patient interactions (Scholl et al., 2011). Ignoring the diversity of their cultural perspectives and assuming that providers are always neutral "mechanics" poses a significant risk to the quality and process of care.

However, it is important that we do not stop at acknowledging providers' complex Integral Fusion worldviews but also situate them in provider-patient interactions. The literature has highlighted the significance of the *interplay* between providers' and patients' demographics (and worldviews). Like interprofessional health teams, providers and their patients may need to negotiate and formulate a shared, Integral Fusion worldview to achieve optimal care. Providers' clinical practice and treatment bias may be a result of their patients' demographics and expectations. For example, patients are more likely to perceive physicians who prescribe an active mode of treatment as having a higher epistemic authority than physicians who give a passive recommendation – a phenomenon called **medical expertise bias** (Stasiuk et al., 2016). As a result, in response to a patient's bias, a provider may choose to recommend a more active or aggressive treatment, not for medically necessary reasons but to secure the patient's trust. Studies also suggest that patients may have different expectations for their physicians' communicative patterns. Levinson et al. (1997) found that in primary care, physicians who adopt other-oriented communication patterns and spend more time with their patients are less likely to have received malpractice claims; in contrast, a surgeon's communicative patterns and duration of visits do not predict their likelihood of receiving a malpractice claim. However, another study suggests that surgeons with a tone of voice that shows high dominance and low concern/anxiety are more likely to have malpractice claims than surgeons who do not have those vocal tones (Ambady et al., 2002). It is possible that patients hold different expectations for their family physicians and surgeons. In addition, because a visit with a surgeon is usually brief and limited to a specific period of time (e.g., a few weeks), a patient may not be sensitive to a surgeon's communicative patterns or duration of visits but instead base their judgement on whether the surgeon's tone of voice expresses dominance or lack of concern.

Some studies also have suggested that **demographic concordance** between physicians and patients has a positive effect on provider-patient interactions and quality of care. For example, African American, Asian American, and Hispanic patients rated their physicians, their medical care, and overall satisfaction higher when they shared the same race with their physicians (LaVeist & Nuru-Jeter, 2002). Patients seeing physicians of their own race rated their physicians' decision making styles as more participatory (Cooper-Patrick et al., 1999). Compared to racially discordant patients, patients in racially concordant provider-patient interactions were found to receive more information and to be more active in provider-patient communication (Gordon et al., 2006). Although only 10% of patients in a survey reported a preference for a physician of their own race, in practice, minority patients appear to actively seek care from a racially concordant physician, with a quarter of Blacks and Hispanics and nearly one-half of Asian patients reporting to have a physician of their own race/ethnicity (Saha et al., 2003). Patient-provider gender concordance has been found to have a positive impact on cancer screening (Malhotra et al., 2017). A review of the effect of gender concordance in medical encounters found that the effects were real but "typically small in magnitude" (Street, 2002, p. 205).

A key to a cultural fusion approach and an Integral Fusion worldview to the understanding of health and medicine is to recognize that the complexity and interplay of diverging perspectives and factors in healthcare settings. For example, Street et al. (2007) adopted an ecological approach to examine providers' communication styles and concluded, "Not only were physicians' communication behaviors linked to their perceptions of patients, both were influenced by a variety of factors, the most powerful being the patient's communication, the patient's ethnicity, and the physicians' orientation to the doctor-patient relationship" (p. 594). Despite studies that show positive effects of demographic concordance between patients and physicians, researchers have also found that patient-centered communication style has a significant effect in mitigating racial and cultural differences between providers and patients: "all immigrant racial/ethnic groups preferred providers who listened, spent enough time, and explained things well" (Chu et al., 2019, p. 5; see also Street et al., 2008). In fact, Saha et al. (2003) found that "patient-physician race concordance was *not* associated with better patient-physician interactions or with greater physician cultural sensitivity" [emphasis added] (p. 1716). Instead, health literacy was found to be a significant factor in the quality of provider-patient interaction, patient satisfaction, and use of health services (for more on health literacy, see Chapter 7; Saha et al., 2003). A review of a large-scale national survey between 2003–2010 identified a disconcerting finding: Hispanic patients seen by Hispanic providers received breast and colorectal cancer screening at significantly lower rates than Hispanic patients seen by non-Hispanic providers (Malhotra et al., 2017). Recognizing that influences of gender are situated in sociocultural and interpersonal contexts, Street (2002) argued that "gender may influence provider-patient interaction to the extent that it can be linked to the interactants' goals, skills, perceptions, emotions, and the way the participants adapt to their partner's communication" (p. 201).

In conclusion, a cultural fusion approach recognizes and embraces differences of perspectives. An Integral Fusion worldview finds common ground that allows all perspectives to co-exist, finding strength in their diversity *and* tensions. This is particularly important in health contexts as medicine inherently and paradoxically is fused with uncertainty. Even when all people can agree that no "futile" treatment can be offered, individuals' understanding of "futility" can be significantly different. Mebane et al. (1999) explained,

> The futility of any particular therapy is often based on an individual's life experiences. For some people, "futility is decided by rational, somewhat scientific, means based on a statistical probability of survival." For many groups with a history of oppression, their belief in "overcoming the odds" may make any conceivable chance of a good outcome a desirable option. Many individuals exhibit "less aversion." (pp. 585–586)

An Integral Fusion worldview encourages cultural participants to recognize, communicate, and negotiate their perspectives so that a mutually agreeable common ground can be identified. The success is dependent on the System structure and cultural participants' willingness to engage, coordinate, and collaborate with one another (see also Dialogic Spaces are Essential in Chapter 14).

IV. Additional Resources

A. Key Terms and Theories

cultural fusion
transculturation
integration
Integral Fusion worldview
third culture
ecological approach
pan-evolution
mindfulness (as meditation activities)
cultural appropriation
international medical graduates
medicalization
conscientious refusal
interprofessional health team
medical dominance
taskwork
role boundaries
moral community
medical expertise bias
demographic concordance

B. Discussion Questions

1. Do you think performing yoga can change people's cultural consciousness, making them embrace Eastern religions and lose their Christian or Muslim identity?
    a. Do you think playing American football will make a person learn about American values? What are they? What are the specific behaviors or practices in American football that may make a person embrace specific cultural values?
2. In addition to the example of teaching school-aged children yoga, can you identify any other examples of cultural fusion in your community?
    a. Do you like such forms of cultural fusion? Why or why not?
    b. Do you think there are people who are concerned about this fusional process? Why? Can you use the framework of cultural consciousness to explain their concerns?
    c. Do you think people would feel highly emotional about the resulting Integral Fusion worldview? Why or why not?

3. In addition to the different factors discussed in this Chapter, what other factors may influence a physician's (cultural) perspective?
   a. Would you prefer to have a doctor who shares the same race or gender with you? Are there other things that you think it'd be a plus to have in common with your doctor?
   b. Do you have different expectations for doctors in different specialties? Why?
   c. Looking at your own beliefs and attitudes, can you tell whether you are closer to Magic Consciousness, Mythic Connection, or Perspectival Thinking? Why?
   d. Do you think your own demographic characteristics play a role in your attitudes? Why?
4. If some cultural differences cannot be reconciled, what do you think about the following scenarios?
   a. What do you think about physicians or nurses refusing to provide medical services by asserting conscientious refusal?
   b. If you are a physician who works in a Catholic hospital that prohibits employees from discussing emergency contraception with victims, what would you do and why?
   c. Do you think it is acceptable, appropriate, or necessary for Catholic hospitals to prohibit employees from discussing emergency contraception to rape victims? How about underage kids? Or adults?
   d. Would it be okay for parents to refuse life-saving medical treatment for their kids by asserting religious beliefs?

C. References

Ambady, N., LaPlante, D., Nguyen, T., Rosenthal, R., Chaumeton, N., & Levinson, W. (2002). Surgeons' tone of voice: A clue to malpractice history. *Surgery*, *132*(1), 5–9.

American Immigration Council. (2018). *Foreign-trained doctors are critical to serving many U.S. communities.* https://www.americanimmigrationcouncil.org/sites/default/files/research/foreign-trained_doctors_are_critical_to_serving_many_us_communities.pdf

Apker, J., & Eggly, S. (2004). Communicating professional identity in medical socialization: Considering the ideological discourse of morning report. *Qualitative Health Research*, *14*(3), 411–429.

Arredondo, E. M., Pollak, K. I., Costanzo, P., McNeilly, M., & Myers, E. (2003). Primary care residents' characteristics and motives for providing differential medical treatment of cervical cancer screening. *Journal of the National Medical Association*, *95*(7), 576–584.

Association of American Medical Colleges. (2019). *Diversity in medicine: Facts and figures 2019.* https://www.aamc.org/data-reports/workforce/report/diversity-medicine-facts-and-figures-2019

Auerswald, E. H. (1968). Interdisciplinary versus ecological approach. *Family Process*, *7*(2), 202–215.

Barker, K. K. (1998). A ship upon a stormy sea: The medicalization of pregnancy. *Social Science & Medicine*, *47*(8), 1067–1076.

Bateman, L. B., & Clair, J. M. (2015). Physician religion and end–of–life pediatric care: A qualitative examination of physicians' perspectives. *Narrative Inquiry in Bioethics*, *5*(3), 251–269.

Beagan, B., & Ells, C. (2009). Values that matter, barriers that interfere: The struggle of Canadian nurses to enact their values. *Canadian Journal of Nursing Research, 41*(1), 86–107.

The Beatles banned segregated audiences, contract shows. (2011, September 18). BBC News. https://www.bbc.com/news/entertainment-arts-14963752

Bensing, J. M., Roter, D. L., & Hulsman, R. L. (2003). Communication patterns of primary care physicians in the United States and the Netherlands. *Journal of General Internal Medicine, 18*(5), 335–342.

Berger, J. T. (2008). The influence of physicians' demographic characteristics and their patients' demographic characteristics on physician practice: Implications for education and research. *Academic Medicine, 83*(1), 100–105.

Bishop, S. R., Lau, M., Shapiro, S., Carlson, L., Anderson, N. D., Carmody, J., Segal, Z. V., Abbey, S., Speca, M., Velting, D., & Devins, G. (2004). Mindfulness: A proposed operational definition. *Clinical Psychology: Science and Practice, 11*(3), 230–241.

Bleakley, A. (2013). The dislocation of medical dominance: Making space for interprofessional care. *Journal of Interprofessional Care, 27*(Suppl. 2), 24–30.

Brauer, S. G., Yoon, J. D., & Curlin, F. A. (2016). US primary care physicians' opinions about conscientious refusal: A national vignette experiment. *Journal of Medical Ethics, 42*(2), 80–84.

Brown, C. G. (2018). Christian yoga: Something new under the sun/son? *Church History, 87*(3), 659–683.

Brown, C. G. (2019). *Debating yoga and mindfulness in public schools: Reforming secular education or reestablishing religion?* University of North Carolina Press.

Brown, J., Lewis, L., Ellis, K., Stewart, M., Freeman, T. R., & Kasperski, M. J. (2011). Conflict on interprofessional primary health care teams – Can it be resolved? *Journal of Interprofessional Care, 25*(1), 4–10.

Burns, J. P., Mitchell, C., Griffith, J. L., & Truog, R. D. (2001). End-of-life care in the pediatric intensive care unit: Attitudes and practices of pediatric critical care physicians and nurses. *Critical Care Medicine, 29*(3), 658–664.

Cahill, H. A. (2001). Male appropriation and medicalization of childbirth: An historical analysis. *Journal of Advanced Nursing, 33*(3), 334–342.

Carr, P. L., Gunn, C., Raj, A., Kaplan, S., & Freund, K. M. (2017). Recruitment, promotion, and retention of women in academic medicine: How institutions are addressing gender disparities. *Women's Health Issues, 27*(3), 374–381.

Caruso, R., Nanni, M. G., Riba, M., Sabato, S., Mitchell, A. J., Croce, E., & Grassi, L. (2017). Depressive spectrum disorders in cancer: Prevalence, risk factors and screening for depression: A critical review. *Acta Oncologica, 56*(2), 146–155.

Casmir, F. L. (1993). Third-culture building: A paradigm shift for international and intercultural communication. *Annals of the International Communication Association, 16*(1), 407–428.

Chan, C. M. H., & Ahmad, W. A. W. (2012). Differences in physician attitudes towards patient-centredness: Across four medical specialties. *International Journal of Clinical Practice, 66*(1), 16–20.

Chen, I. (2018, October 14). *Coming to terms with six years in science. Obsession, isolation, and moments of wonder.* STAT. https://www.statnews.com/2018/10/14/phd-six-years-scientific-research

Chu, J., Wang, N., Choi, Y. S., & Roby, D. H. (2019). The effect of patient-centered communication and racial concordant care on care satisfaction among U.S. immigrants. *Medical Care Research and Review.* https://doi.org/10.1177/1077558719890988

Clarke, A. E., Shim, J. K., Mamo, L., Fosket, J. R., & Fishman, J. R. (2003). Biomedicalization: Technoscientific transformations of health, illness, and U.S. biomedicine. *American Sociological Review, 68*(2), 161–194.

Combs, M. P., Antiel, R. M., Tilburt, J. C., Mueller, P. S., & Curlin, F. A. (2011). Conscientious refusals to refer: Findings from a national physician survey. *Journal of Medical Ethics, 37*(7), 397–401.

Conrad, P. (2007). *The medicalization of society: On the transformation of human conditions into treatable disorders.* Johns Hopkins University Press.

Cooper-Patrick, L., Gallo, J. J., Gonzales, J. J., Vu, H. T., Powe, N. R., Nelson, C., & Ford, D. E. (1999). Race, gender, and partnership in the patient-physician relationship. *JAMA, 282*(6), 583–589.

Coskuner-Balli, G., & Ertimur, B. (2017). Legitimation of hybrid cultural products: The case of American yoga. *Marketing Theory, 17*(2), 127–147.

Crossley, M. L. (2007). Childbirth, complications and the illusion of 'choice': A case study. *Feminism & Psychology, 17*(4), 543–563.

Cullati, S., Bochatay, N., Maître, F., Laroche, T., Muller-Juge, V., Blondon, K. S., Junod Perron, N., Bajwa, N. M., Viet Vu, N., Kim, S., Savoldelli, G. L., Hudelson, P., Chopard, P., & Nendaz, M. R. (2019). When team conflicts threaten quality of care: A study of health care professionals' experiences and perceptions. *Mayo Clinic Proceedings: Innovations, Quality & Outcomes, 3*(1), 43–51.

Curlin, F. A., Nwodim, C., Vance, J. L., Chin, M. H., & Lantos, J. D. (2008). To die, to sleep: US physicians' religious and other objections to physician-assisted suicide, terminal sedation, and withdrawal of life support. *American Journal of Hospice and Palliative Medicine, 25*(2), 112–120.

Curry, N. A., & Kasser, T. (2005). Can coloring mandalas reduce anxiety? *Art Therapy, 22*(2), 81–85.

Dorgan, K. A., Lang, F., Floyd, M., & Kemp, E. (2009). International medical graduate–patient communication: A qualitative analysis of perceived barriers. *Academic Medicine, 84*(11), 1567–1575.

Dusenbery, M. (2018). *Doing harm: The truth about how bad medicine and lazy science leave women dismissed, misdiagnosed, and sick.* HarperOne.

Dworkin, R. W. (2001). The medicalization of unhappiness. *Public Interest,* (144), 85–99.

Earp, B. D., Sandberg, A., & Savulescu, J. (2015). The medicalization of love. *Cambridge Quarterly of Healthcare Ethics, 24*(3), 323–336.

Eaton, J., & Tieber, C. (2017). The effects of coloring on anxiety, mood, and perseverance. *Art Therapy, 34*(1), 42–46.

Epstein, J. B., Thariat, J., Bensadoun, R.-J., Barasch, A., Murphy, B. A., Kolnick, L., Popplewell, L., & Maghami, E. (2012). Oral complications of cancer and cancer therapy. *CA: A Cancer Journal for Clinicians, 62*(6), 400–422.

Fadiman, A. (1997). *The spirit catches you and you fall down: A Hmong child, her American doctors, and the collision of two cultures.* Farrar, Straus and Giroux.

Festinger, L., & Carlsmith, J. M. (1959). Cognitive consequences of forced compliance. *Journal of Abnormal & Social Psychology, 58*(2), 203–210.

Fowler, J., Floyd, J., McNaughton Collins, M., Albertsen, P. C., Zietman, A., Elliott, D. B., & Barry, M. J. (2000). Comparison of recommendations by urologists and radiation oncologists for treatment of clinically localized prostate cancer. *JAMA, 283*(24), 3217–3222.

Friedman, V. (2019). *Kim Kardashian West and the Kimono controversy.* The New York Times, ST6. https://nyti.ms/2NivfIE

Frush, B. W., Brauer, S. G., Yoon, J. D., & Curlin, F. A. (2018). Physician decision-making in the setting of advanced illness: An examination of patient disposition and physician religiousness. *Journal of Pain and Symptom Management, 55*(3), 906–912.

Gadamer, H.-G. (2005). *Truth and method.* (J. Weinsheimer & D. G. Marshall, Trans.; 2nd rev. ed.). Continuum. (Original work published 1960)

Gelfand, M. J., Harrington, J. R., & Jackson, J. C. (2017). The strength of social norms across human groups. *Perspectives on Psychological Science, 12*(5), 800–809.

Geno, R. (2018, November 12). *The meaning of "Namaste."* Yoga Journal. https://www.yogajournal.com/practice/the-meaning-of-quot-namaste-quot

Gordon, H. S., Street, R. L., Jr., Sharf, B. F., & Souchek, J. (2006). Racial differences in doctors' information-giving and patients' participation. *Cancer, 107*(6), 1313–1320.

Haidet, P., Dains, J. E., Paterniti, D. A., Hechtel, L., Chang, T., Tseng, E., & Rogers, J. C. (2002). Medical student attitudes toward the doctor–patient relationship. *Medical Education, 36*(6), 568–574.

Han, P. K. J., Klein, W. M. P., & Arora, N. K. (2011). Varieties of uncertainty in health care: A conceptual taxonomy. *Medical Decision Making, 31*(6), 828–838.

Hart, L. G., Skillman, S. M., Thompson, M., Hagopian, A., & Konrad, T. R. (2007). International medical graduate physicians in the United States: Changes since 1981. *Health Affairs, 26*(4), 1159–1169.

Hsieh, E. (2006). Conflicts in how interpreters manage their roles in provider-patient interactions. *Social Science & Medicine, 62*(3), 721–730.

Hsieh, E. (2007). Interpreters as co-diagnosticians: Overlapping roles and services between providers and interpreters. *Social Science & Medicine, 64*(4), 924–937.

Hsieh, E. (2010). Provider-interpreter collaboration in bilingual health care: Competitions of control over interpreter-mediated interactions. *Patient Education and Counseling, 78*(2), 154–159.

Hsieh, E. (2016). *Bilingual health communication: Working with interpreters in cross-cultural care.* Routledge.

Hsieh, E., & Kramer, E. M. (2012). Medical interpreters as tools: Dangers and challenges in the utilitarian approach to interpreters' roles and functions. *Patient Education and Counseling, 89*(1), 158–162.

Jain, A. R. (2017). Yoga, Christians practicing yoga, and God: On theological compatibility, or is there a better question? *Journal of Hindu-Christian Studies, 30*(1), 46–52.

Kabat-Zinn, J. (2013). *Full catastrophe living: Using the wisdom of your body and mind to face stress, pain, and illness.* Random.

Kass, L., & Wilson, J. Q. (1998). *The ethics of human cloning.* AEI Press.

Kim, S. P., Gross, C. P., Nguyen, P. Y., Smaldone, M. C., Thompson, R. H., Shah, N. D., Kutikov, A., Han, L. C., Karnes, R. J., Ziegenfuss, J. Y., & Tilburt, J. C. (2014). Specialty bias in treatment recommendations and quality of life among radiation oncologists and urologists for localized prostate cancer. *Prostate Cancer and Prostatic Diseases, 17*(2), 163–169.

Kramer, E. M. (1997). *Modern/postmodern: Off the beaten path of antimodernism.* Praeger.

Kramer, E. M. (2000). Cultural fusion and the defense of difference. In M. K. Asante & J. E. Min (Eds.), *Socio-cultural conflict between African and Korean Americans* (pp. 182–223). University Press of America.

Kramer, E. M. (2008). Theoretical reflections on intercultural studies: Preface. In S. M. Croucher, *Looking beyond the hijab* (pp. ix-xxxix). Hampton.

Kramer, E. M. (2017). Cassirer as revolutionary: Semiotics as embodied worldview appreciating the other in ourselves. *American Journal of Semiotics, 33*(3-4), 233–332.

Kramer, E. M. (2019). Cultural fusion theory. In J. F. Nussbaum (Ed.), *Oxford research encyclopedia of communication.* Oxford University Press. https://doi.org/10.1093/acrefore/9780190228613.013.679

Kramer, E. M., Adkins, G., Kim, S. H., & Miller, G. (2014). *Environmental communication and the extinction vortex: Technology as denial of death.* Hampton.

Kramer, E. M., & Ikeda, R. (1998). Understanding different worlds: The theory of dimensional accrual/dissociation. *Journal of Intercultural Communication, 1*(2), 37–51.

Kuhn, T. S. (2012). *The structure of scientific revolutions.* (4th ed.). University of Chicago Press. (Original work published 1962)

Kurtz, M. E., Nolan, R. B., & Rittinger, W. J. (2003). Primary care physicians' attitudes and practices regarding complementary and alternative medicine. *The Journal of the American Osteopathic Association, 103*(12), 597–602.

LaVeist, T. A., & Nuru-Jeter, A. (2002). Is doctor-patient race concordance associated with greater satisfaction with care? *Journal of Health and Social Behavior, 43*(3), 296–306.

Lawrence, R. E., & Curlin, F. A. (2009). Physicians' beliefs about conscience in medicine: A national survey. *Academic Medicine, 84*(9), 1276–1282.

Lawrence, R. E., Rasinski, K. A., Yoon, J. D., & Curlin, F. A. (2015). Physician race and treatment preferences for depression, anxiety, and medically unexplained symptoms. *Ethnicity & Health, 20*(4), 354–364.

Lee, S., & Mysyk, A. (2004). The medicalization of compulsive buying. *Social Science & Medicine, 58*(9), 1709–1718.

Levinson, W., Roter, D. L., Mullooly, J. P., Dull, V. T., & Frankel, R. M. (1997). Physician-patient communication: The relationship with malpractice claims among primary care physicians and surgeons. *JAMA, 277*(7), 553–559.

Levorato, A., Stiefel, F., Mazzocato, C., & Bruera, E. (2001). Communication with terminal cancer patients in palliative care: Are there differences between nurses and physicians? *Supportive Care in Cancer, 9*(6), 420–427.

Liao, D. (2017). *The invisible other in cross-cultural care: International medical graduates/nonnative physicians in provider-patient interactions* [MA Thesis, University of Oklahoma]. Norman, OK. https://hdl.handle.net/11244/50781

Lull, J. (2000). *Media, communication, culture: A global approach.* Columbia University Press.

MacNaughton, K., Chreim, S., & Bourgeault, I. L. (2013). Role construction and boundaries in interprofessional primary health care teams: A qualitative study. *BMC Health Services Research, 13*, Article 486. https://doi.org/10.1186/1472-6963-13-486

Mahdi, S., Ghannam, O., Watson, S., & Padela, A. I. (2016). Predictors of physician recommendation for ethically controversial medical procedures: Findings from an exploratory national survey of American Muslim physicians. *Journal of Religion and Health, 55*(2), 403–421.

Maier, B., & Shibles, W. A. (2010). *The philosophy and practice of medicine and bioethics: A naturalistic-humanistic approach.* Springer.

Malhotra, J., Rotter, D., Tsui, J., Llanos, A. A. M., Balasubramanian, B. A., & Demissie, K. (2017). Impact of patient–provider race, ethnicity, and gender concordance on cancer screening: Findings from medical expenditure panel survey. *Cancer Epidemiology Biomarkers & Prevention, 26*(12), 1804–1811.

Mebane, E. W., Oman, R. F., Kroonen, L. T., & Goldstein, M. K. (1999). The influence of physician race, age, and gender on physician attitudes toward advance care directives and preferences for end-of-life decision-making. *Journal of the American Geriatrics Society, 47*(5), 579–591.

Michalski, K., Farhan, N., Motschall, E., Vach, W., & Boeker, M. (2017). Dealing with foreign cultural paradigms: A systematic review on intercultural challenges of international medical graduates. *PLoS One, 12*(7), Article e0181330. https://doi.org/10.1371/journal.pone.0181330

Moore, A. M., & Barker, G. G. (2012). Confused or multicultural: Third culture individuals' cultural identity. *International Journal of Intercultural Relations, 36*(4), 553–562.

Mroz, J. (2017). *Scattered seeds: In search of family and identity in the sperm donor generation.* Basic Books.

National Center for Complementary and Alternative Medicine. (2018, October 31). *Yoga.* https://nccih.nih.gov/health/yoga

Niland, P., & Lyons, A. C. (2011). Uncertainty in medicine: Meanings of menopause and hormone replacement therapy in medical textbooks. *Social Science & Medicine, 73*(8), 1238–1245.

Noro, I., Roter, D. L., Kurosawa, S., Miura, Y., & Ishizaki, M. (2018). The impact of gender on medical visit communication and patient satisfaction within the Japanese primary care context. *Patient Education and Counseling, 101*(2), 227–232.

Oberle, K., & Hughes, D. (2001). Doctors' and nurses' perceptions of ethical problems in end-of-life decisions. *Journal of Advanced Nursing, 33*(6), 707–715.

Odum, E. (1998). *Ecological vignettes: Ecological approaches to dealing with human predicaments.* Harwood Academic Publishers.

Olusanya, O. (2016). *Emotions, decision-making and mass atrocities: Through the lens of the macro-micro integrated theoretical model.* Routledge.

Ong, A. (1995). Making the biopolitical subject: Cambodian immigrants, refugee medicine and cultural citizenship in California. *Social Science & Medicine, 40*(9), 1243–1257.

Paasche-Orlow, M., & Roter, D. (2003). The communication patterns of internal medicine and family practice physicians. *The Journal of the American Board of Family Practice, 16*(6), 485–493.

Pavlish, C., Brown-Saltzman, K., Jakel, P., & Fine, A. (2014). The nature of ethical conflicts and the meaning of moral community in oncology practice. *Oncology Nursing Forum, 41*(2), 130–140.

Polanyi, M. (1964). *Science, faith and society.* University of Chicago Press. (Original work published 1946)

Ranasinghe, P. D. (2015). International medical graduates in the US physician workforce. *The Journal of the American Osteopathic Association, 115*(4), 236–241.

Read, S., Butkus, R., Weissman, A., & Moyer, D. V. (2018). Compensation disparities by gender in internal medicine. *Annals of Internal Medicine, 169*(9), 658–661.

Ripple, W. J., & Beschta, R. L. (2012). Trophic cascades in Yellowstone: The first 15 years after wolf reintroduction. *Biological Conservation, 145*(1), 205–213.

Rogers, R. A. (2006). From cultural exchange to transculturation: A review and reconceptualization of cultural appropriation. *Communication Theory, 16*(4), 474–503.

Ross, A., & Thomas, S. (2010). The health benefits of yoga and exercise: A review of comparison studies. *The Journal of Alternative and Complementary Medicine, 16*(1), 3–12.

Roter, D. L., Hall, J. A., & Aoki, Y. (2002). Physician gender effects in medical communication: A meta-analytic review. *JAMA, 288*(6), 756–764.

Roter, D. L., Stewart, M., Putnam, S. M., Lipkin, M., Jr., Stiles, W. B., & Inui, T. S. (1997). Communication patterns of primary care physicians. *JAMA, 277*(4), 350–356.

Saha, S., Arbelaez, J. J., & Cooper, L. A. (2003). Patient–physician relationships and racial disparities in the quality of health care. *American Journal of Public Health, 93*(10), 1713–1719.

Scheper-Hughes, N. (1992). *Death without weeping: The violence of everyday life in Brazil.* University of California Press.

Schmitt, M. H., Gilbert, J. H. V., Brandt, B. F., & Weinstein, R. S. (2013). The coming of age for interprofessional education and practice. *The American Journal of Medicine, 126*(4), 284–288.

Scholl, J. C., Wilson, J. B., & Hughes, P. C. (2011). Expression of patients' and providers' identities during the medical interview. *Qualitative Health Research, 21*(8), 1022–1032.

Seale, C. (2010). The role of doctors' religious faith and ethnicity in taking ethically controversial decisions during end-of-life care. *Journal of Medical Ethics, 36*(11), 677–682.

Silver, J. K., Slocum, C. S., Bank, A. M., Bhatnagar, S., Blauwet, C. A., Poorman, J. A., Villablanca, A., & Parangi, S. (2017). Where are the women? The underrepresentation of women physicians among recognition award recipients from medical specialty societies. *PM&R, 9*(8), 804–815.

Skjeggestad, E., Gerwing, J., & Gulbrandsen, P. (2017). Language barriers and professional identity: A qualitative interview study of newly employed international medical doctors and Norwegian colleagues. *Patient Education and Counseling, 100*(8), 1466–1472.

Skjørshammer, M. (2001). Co-operation and conflict in a hospital: Interprofessional differences in perception and management of conflicts. *Journal of Interprofessional Care, 15*(1), 7–18.

Smugar, S., & Spina, B. J. (2000). Informed consent for emergency contraception: Variability in hospital care of rape victims. *American Journal of Public Health, 90*(9), 1372–1376.

Sommers, B. D., Beard, C. J., D'Amico, A. V., Kaplan, I., Richie, J. P., & Zeckhauser, R. J. (2008). Predictors of patient preferences and treatment choices for localized prostate cancer. *Cancer, 113*(8), 2058–2067.

Stasiuk, K., Bar-Tal, Y., & Maksymiuk, R. (2016). The effect of physicians' treatment recommendations on their epistemic authority: The medical expertise bias. *Journal of Health Communication, 21*(1), 92–99.

Stengers, I. (2000). *The invention of modern science* (D.W. Smith, Trans.). University of Minnesota Press. (Original work published 1993)

Stratton, S. P. (2015). Mindfulness and contemplation: Secular and religious traditions in Western context. *Counseling and Values, 60*(1), 100–118.

Street, R. L. (2002). Gender differences in health care provider–patient communication: Are they due to style, stereotypes, or accommodation? *Patient Education and Counseling, 48*(3), 201–206.

Street, R. L., Gordon, H., & Haidet, P. (2007). Physicians' communication and perceptions of patients: Is it how they look, how they talk, or is it just the doctor? *Social Science & Medicine, 65*(3), 586–598.

Street, R. L., Jr., O'Malley, K. J., Cooper, L. A., & Haidet, P. (2008). Understanding concordance in patient-physician relationships: Personal and ethnic dimensions of shared identity. *Annals of Family Medicine, 6*(3), 198–205.

Thomas, E. J., Sexton, J. B., & Helmreich, R. L. (2003). Discrepant attitudes about teamwork among critical care nurses and physicians. *Critical Care Medicine, 31*(3), 956–959.

Timmermans, S., & Alison, A. (2001). Evidence-based medicine, clinical uncertainty, and learning to doctor. *Journal of Health and Social Behavior, 42*(4), 342–359.

Tsugawa, Y., Jena, A. B., Orav, E. J., & Jha, A. K. (2017). Quality of care delivered by general internists in US hospitals who graduated from foreign versus US medical schools: Observational study. *BMJ, 356*, Article j273. https://doi.org/10.1136/bmj.j273

U. S. Census Bureau (2018). *QuickFacts: United States.* https://www.census.gov/quickfacts/fact/table/US/PST045218

U.S. National Library of Medicine. (n.d.). *What is precision medicine?* https://medlineplus.gov/genetics/understanding/precisionmedicine/definition/

van der Vennet, R., & Serice, S. (2012). Can coloring mandalas reduce anxiety? A replication study. *Art Therapy, 29*(2), 87–92.

Vanderford, M. L., & Smith, D. H. (1996). *The silicone breast implant story: Communication and uncertainty.* Erlbaum.

Vassar, L. (2015, February 18). *How medical specialties vary by gender.* AMA. https://www.ama-assn.org/residents-students/specialty-profiles/how-medical-specialties-vary-gender

Weiss, D., Tilin, F. J., & Morgan, M. A. J. (2016). *The interprofessional health care team: Leadership and development.* (2nd ed.). Jones & Bartlett Learning.

Wicclair, M. R. (2011). Conscientious refusals by hospitals and emergency contraception. *Cambridge Quarterly of Healthcare Ethics, 20*(1), 130–138.

Wong, A. (2018, September 20). *Why schools are banning yoga.* The Atlantic. https://www.theatlantic.com/education/archive/2018/09/why-schools-are-banning-yoga/570904

Yeh, E. T. H., & Bickford, C. L. (2009). Cardiovascular complications of cancer therapy. *Incidence, Pathogenesis, Diagnosis, and Management, 53*(24), 2231–2247.

Zimmermann, S. M. (1998). *Silicone survivors: Women's experiences with breast implants.* Temple University Press.

Zola, I. K. (1991). The medicalization of aging and disability. *Advances in Medical Sociology, 2*, 299–315.

6

Culture and Health Behaviors

Culture Assumptions in Health Theories and Practices

In previous chapters, we have explored how fundamental differences in cultural understanding can lead to significant differences in our worldviews, values, and the realities we live in. We will now explore how these cultural perspectives can bring insights into our understanding of health behaviors.

In Chapter 6, we will first review three major theories that are common in health campaigns and follow by an analysis of the underlying assumptions held by the theories. We will then explore how certain common values that are prevalent and fundamental to medicine and healthcare delivery in the West (e.g., informed consent, patient autonomy, and self-determinism) are also cultural products, which may create tensions and ethical dilemmas when patients and providers do not share the same cultural values.

I.   Theories about Health Behaviors

Theories are valuable in understanding a social phenomenon because they represent researchers and practitioners' efforts to crystallize a complex process through a systematic framework. In other words, "A **theory** is a set of interrelated concepts, definitions, and propositions that present a systematic view of events or situations by specifying relations among variables, in order to explain and predict the events or situations" (Glanz et al., 2008, p. 26). After a theory is developed, researchers can apply the theory in different contexts to examine the validity and reliability of the theory, the findings of which can provide insights into whether and how to modify the theory in order to better conceptualize the issue of interest.

In this section, we will cover: (a) The Health Belief Model (HBM) and (b) The Theory of Reason Action (TRA)/Theory of Planned Behavior (TPB). These are major theories for behavioral change that have been widely adopted in health campaigns and interventions for decades. They remain popular today. Each theory adopted a different approach to understanding and incorporating culture in its theoretical framework. As we review the major constructs of these theories, it will be helpful to consider how and why the theorists adopted these theoretical lenses to understand health behaviors and behavioral change in health contexts.

Rethinking Culture in Health Communication: Social Interactions as Intercultural Encounters,
First Edition. Elaine Hsieh and Eric M Kramer.
© 2021 John Wiley & Sons, Inc. Published 2021 by John Wiley & Sons, Inc.

A. Health Belief Model (HBM)

The Health Belief Model (HBM) is one of the first health theories that explain individuals' health behaviors and provides a conceptual framework for health interventions (Skinner et al., 2015). It is also one of the most widely used health theories, spawning tens of thousands of health education and health research projects and publications. HBM was initially developed during the 1950s by researchers in the U.S. Public Health Services to explain why people fail to participate in preventive care even though such services are readily available.

HBM is a form of value-expectancy theory. In particular, HBM assumes that individuals (a) *value* avoiding illness/getting well, and (b) *expect* that certain health actions may prevent (or ameliorate) illness (Skinner et al., 2015). Since the 1950s, HBM has evolved significantly to include several key concepts that explain and predict whether or not individuals may take specific health actions to achieve a specific health outcome (see Figure 6.1). The specific constructs are:

- *Perceived Threats.* Perceived Threats includes two components: perceived susceptibility and perceived severity.
  - *Perceived susceptibility.* If a person believes that she has a high chance of experiencing the illness condition, she is more likely to take the health action to avoid contracting the illness.
  - *Perceived severity.* If a person believes that the consequences of the illness condition or health outcome are serious, she is more likely to take actions to avoid the consequences.
- *Perceived benefit.* If a person believes that taking health action can reduce risks (i.e., susceptibility) or negative consequences (i.e., severity), she is more likely to adopt the advised action.
- *Perceived barrier.* If a person believes that there are high barriers (e.g., tangible challenges and psychological costs) to adopt the advised action, they are less likely to adopt the health action.
- *Cues to action.* Certain incidents and events that prompt a person to adopt the advised action.
- *Self-efficacy.* The stronger a person believes that she has the ability to adopt the advised action, the more likely she will take the health action. Self-efficacy was not explicitly incorporated into the early formulation of HBM, which focused on one-time, preventive health action (e.g., getting a vaccine shot).

Reviews of several decades of studies have noted that overall the effects of HBM constructs are small but generally hold a stronger effect for one-time, preventive health behaviors (e.g., vaccination and illness screening) than for maintenance behaviors (e.g., treatment adherence; Carpenter, 2010; Harrison et al., 1992; Janz & Becker, 1984). Among all the constructs, perceived barrier is the most powerful predictor across all studies and health behaviors, followed by perceived benefits (Champion & Skinner, 2008). Although some studies found that perceived severity is the weakest construct (Harrison et al., 1992; Janz & Becker, 1984), others suggested that perceived susceptibility is the weakest one (Carpenter, 2010).

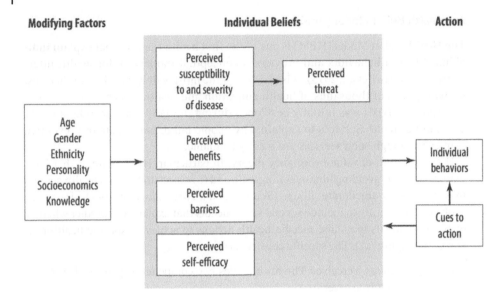

Figure 6.1 The Health Belief Model. *Source:* Adapted from Skinner, C. S., Tiro, J., & Champion, V. L. (2015). The Health Belief Model. In K. Glanz, B. K. Rimer, & K. Viswanath (Eds.), Health behavior and health education: Theory, research, and practice (5th ed., pp. 75–94). Wiley

1. **Underlying Assumptions of HBM**

The intuitive nature of HBM makes it one of the most popular models for health interventions: individuals are conceptualized as rational thinkers who are motivated to adopt health behaviors that allow them to achieve the desired outcome based on a cost-benefit analysis. Such findings are consistent with the conceptual framework of a value-expectancy theory: a person is likely to adopt a behavior if they value the outcome and expect that adopting the behavior is likely to result in the desired outcome.

Despite its title of the "health belief" model, HBM does not directly address how individuals formulate the beliefs about their expectations (i.e., perceived threat, benefits, and barrier). As a psychological model, HBM focuses on individual traits and fails to consider the systematic impacts of social norms or peer influences. Researchers have suggested that demographic (e.g., age, gender, and ethnicity), sociopsychological (e.g., social network and education levels), and structural (e.g., socioeconomic status and geographic locations) variables may shape individuals' understanding of the key HBM constructs. By recognizing that these "modifying" factors can shape individuals' beliefs, researchers implicitly incorporate cultures in the analysis and assessment of health beliefs. Nevertheless, these "other variables" have not been officially incorporated into HBM.

2. **Understanding HBM through Cultural Perspectives**

Although culture has been indirectly incorporated into the assessment of health beliefs in HBM through the recognition of modifying factors, such an approach fails to recognize the complexity of cultures in health contexts and can confound the interrelationships of these modifying factors. When taking cultural perspectives into consideration, the modifying factors do not simply moderate the intensity of constructs of HBM. Rather, they can fundamentally change the meanings and implications of the constructs.

Our health beliefs are often shaped by multiple, competing cultural systems. For example, how can we predict or influence the health behaviors of a religious, young person who is also an ethnic minority? African Americans are often found to hold strong religious and spiritual beliefs, which guide their health behaviors and decision-making (Johnson et al., 2005). One study suggests that belief in the superiority of spiritual or religious intervention by a higher power through prayer or laying-on-of-hands compared to medical treatment may contribute to African American women delaying care-seeking, resulting in advanced-stage breast cancer at diagnosis (Mitchell et al., 2002). Such an understanding of "preferred" intervention is not based on a simple cost-benefit analysis of the effectiveness of a medical treatment or existence of barriers (i.e., Perspectival Thinking). Rather, by choosing to rely on religious and spiritual beliefs, African American women actively make identity and moral claims (e.g., recognizing one's life purpose and destiny; defining character and acting within subjectively meaningful moral principles) of their struggles (Mattis, 2002). Nevertheless, religious and spiritual beliefs do not dictate African American women's health behaviors (Gullatte et al., 2010). African American women who had told a person about their breast symptoms were more likely to seek medical care sooner than those who had disclosed their breast symptoms only to God (Gullatte et al., 2010). Gullatte et al. (2010) concluded:

> [African American] women's decisions regarding whether and when to seek medical care after self-discovery of a breast symptom are complex. Religious and spiritual beliefs are important factors in their initial response to finding a symptom, but it appears that additional factors, such as their willingness to share their symptom with a person and receive support, are also important in the decision making for seeking medical care. (p. 70)

Such an understanding of health behaviors and health decision-making also highlights why HBM is likely to be a model that is a better fit for one-time health behaviors, rather than long-term health maintenance. The initial formulation of HBM centers on swaying individuals' decision-making by shaping their cost-benefit analysis of medical efficacy, a highly perspectival way of thinking by weighing benefits and barriers to determine the decision to take. However, for complex health behaviors (e.g., cancer treatment seeking and treatment adherence), individuals' decision-making and meaning-making can include a wide range of factors (e.g., identity construction, morality claim, and interpersonal networks) that can have a stronger effect than medical efficacy. These factors can involve Magic Consciousness (e.g., whatever happens to me is God's will) or Mythic Connection (e.g., the illness presents opportunities for me to show my devotion to God through prayers). For example, Hmong parents who are concerned about their daughter's epilepsy may feel conflicted about ridding the illness completely when epilepsy is perceived as a gift from God and signs of the blessed life of becoming a shaman (Fadiman, 1997). Pitaloka and Hsieh (2015) found that some Javanese women view their diabetes as punishment from God. One woman said, "I never talk to my family about my disease. People in my village think that diabetes is a curse. According to villagers, you get diabetes because you committed many sins in your life. I got divorced from my husband, and I don't want people in my village think that I got diabetes because of my divorce" (Pitaloka & Hsieh, 2015, p. 1161). When an illness is considered a punishment for past sins, one is unlikely to seek active treatment to ameliorate the physical illness. Rather, a spiritual approach for the physical illness would be necessary as a patient explained, "I don't want people to visit me in the hospital and cry. I'm so prepared for this, and I feel I'm strong! I resign my fate to God" (Pitaloka & Hsieh, 2015, p. 1161). In these situations, it is not the case that the patient is unaware of the perceived susceptibility or perceived severity of their deteriorating health. Patients recognize that they have diabetes, a life-long illness with potentially devastating implications to their physical health, mobility, and overall well-being. Nevertheless, because they viewed the illness as an embodiment of God's will rather than a personal failure to manage an appropriate level of blood sugar, they interpret their suffering as cues to action to accept fate (e.g., lessons to submit themselves to God's will) and validate their faith (e.g., diabetes as a test of spiritual strength) rather than an urgent call to seek biomedical care (Pitaloka & Hsieh, 2015).

Without accounting for these powerful motivators and cultural perspectives, healthcare providers may be at a loss to explain why a person may refuse to seek care even when she recognizes the medical efficacy of the proposed treatment.

B. Theory of Reasoned Action (TRA) and Theory of Planned Behaviors (TPB)

The Theory of Reasoned Action (TRA) and the Theory of Planned Behavior (TPB) are theoretical frameworks that identify "key behavioral, normative, and control beliefs affecting behaviors" (Montaño & Kasprzyk, 2008, p. 76; See Figure 6.2). By noting that behavioral intentions are the best predictors of behavioral performance, they proposed that behavioral intentions are shaped by:

- *Attitude.* Attitude is shaped by individuals' *behavioral belief* (i.e., the belief about outcomes or attributes of performing the behavior) and *evaluations of behavioral outcomes* (i.e., whether such an outcome is desirable).
- *Subjective Norm.* Subjective norm is shaped by individuals' *normative beliefs* (i.e., whether the referent individuals approve or disapprove of the action) and *motivation to comply* (i.e., the degree to which one is motivated to comply with the referents).
- *Perceived Control* (TPB only). In later studies, researchers recognized that Attitudes and Subjective Norms (both are key constructs under TRA) may be insufficient to predict behavior performance if the person does not have volitional control over the behavior. As a result, researchers added a third construct, *Perceived Control*, to TRA and created the theory of TPB. Under TPB, perceived control is shaped by *control beliefs* (i.e., a person's assessment of the facilitators and barriers to behavior performance) and *perceived power* (i.e., their self-efficacy and the impact of each control factor to facilitate or inhibit the behavior).

In recent years, theorists of TRA/TPB have proposed an Integrative Model of Behavioral Prediction that includes background influences (e.g., past behavior, personality, and medial exposure) and environmental factors to TRA/TPB to create a more comprehensive theoretical framework (for detailed discussions, see Fishbein, 2008). One of the factors included in the background factors is culture, noting that culture can influence

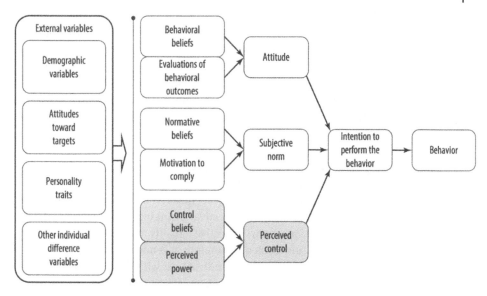

Figure 6.2 Theory of Reasoned Action and Theory of Planned Behavior. The unshaded boxes show the TRA; the entire figure shows the TPB. *Source:* Adapted From Montaño, D. E., & Kasprzyk, D. (2015). Theory of Reasoned Action, Theory of Planned Behavior, and the Integrated Behavioral Model. In K. Glanz, B. K. Rimer, & K. Viswanath (Eds.), Health behavior and health education: Theory, research, and practice (5th ed., pp. 95-124). Wiley

individuals' behavioral, subjective, and normative beliefs. The pathways and processes of these additional factors in shaping individuals' health decision making, however, are less defined than the key constructs of TRA/TPB.

Finally, because TRA/TPB beliefs include both individual and normative components, several studies have examined different weights in belief types placed in individualistic and collectivistic cultures. For example, a study found that Americans (i.e., an individualist culture) may be more likely to adopt behavioral change when persuasive messages target personal behavioral belief (e.g., seeking professional mental health care is good); in contrast, Thai people (i.e., a collectivist culture) are more likely to adopt behavior change when persuasive messages address their normative beliefs (e.g., my supportive others believe that seeking mental health care is good; Christopher et al., 2006). Whereas U.S. teachers' behavioral, normative, and control beliefs are all effective predictors on whether they would refer students with ADHD to healthcare providers, South Korean teachers' decisions are influenced by their normative and control beliefs (but not behavioral beliefs; Lee, 2014). In other words, depending on cultural emphasis on specific types of beliefs, "a behavior that is attitudinally driven in one culture or population may be normatively driven in another" (Fishbein, 2008, p. 839).

1. Underlying Assumptions of TRA/TPB

Although culture was conceptualized as a factor of background influences in the integrative model, TRA/TPB's original approach to culture can be understood in a more nuanced and sophisticated manner. Unlike HBM, which assumes that individuals are rational thinkers in weighing the cost-benefit in adopting a health behavior, TRA/TPB do not assume that individuals act in a way that is based on beliefs that are "rational, logical, or correct by some objective standards" (Montaño & Kasprzyk, 2015, p. 103). For example, although people with mental illness may not necessarily be able to think rationally, interventions that targeted their TRA beliefs have been found to change their behavioral intention, resulting in behavioral change (Blank & Hennessy, 2012). The emphasis of noting that individuals' behavioral, normative, and control beliefs are not formulated through "objective standards" is an important one as it recognizes the complexity of cultural perspectives.

2. Understanding TRA/TPB through Cultural Perspectives

"Objective standards" is purely a phenomenon of Perspectival Thinking. Believing that an "objective" reality can be verified and recognized as the "accurate" truth without bias is a deeply held belief of the Perspectival Thinking worldview. For Magic Consciousness or Mythic Connection, "objective" reality does not exist, in part, because the subject is not yet fully evident. Therefore, it is not a driving issue to verify whether one's understanding is accurate. Individuals with Magic Consciousness accept the world as is. Individuals with Mythic Connection believe that there exists a "reality" that they may not necessarily appreciate or comprehend but should nevertheless follow. By proposing that individuals are *rational actors* whose *reasoned actions* are motivated by their subjective understanding of their beliefs, TRA/TPB provides a way to incorporate Magic Consciousness and Mythic Connection into their key constructs. A person who believes that receiving blood will demonstrate her distrust of God's grace (i.e., behavioral belief), make him appear weak among his peers (i.e., normative belief), or is not her decision to make (i.e., control belief), she will act "rationally" to refuse a blood transfusion even if such belief is unsound or inaccurate by an objective standard.

In addition, because cultures may weigh different types of beliefs with varying degrees of importance, it is possible that certain beliefs are of little importance for specific behaviors. Fishbein (2008) explained,

> [O]ne or another of the 3 factors (attitude, norm, or perceived behavioral control) may not carry any significant weight in the prediction of intention. When this happens, it merely indicates that for the particular behavior and population under investigation, the factor in question is not an important consideration in the formation of intentions. ... [I]nterventions that are successful in one culture or population may be a complete failure [sic] in another. (p. 839)

From this perspective, TRA/TPB provides considerable flexibility in addressing cultural differences in health behaviors.

In summary, when considering how culture can be understood in TRA/TPB, there are two possibilities. First, TRA/TPB recognizes that individuals' sense-making (through their cultural lens) needs not to be judged against an objective standard to shape their health behaviors. Second, TRA/TPB recognizes that not all cultures place the same weigh on different beliefs for all behavior, resulting in different motivators and predictors for behavioral change. Because Magic Consciousness, Mythic Connection, and Perspectival Thinking creates different meanings, relationships, and obligations for individuals' beliefs and health behaviors, successful health campaigns require individuals to understand and respond to participants' cultural perspectives accordingly (see also Chapter 13).

II. Underlying Assumptions in Health Services

Cultural systems often encompass values that compete, if not conflict, with one another. Although we often think of the healthcare system as a coherent cultural system (e.g., the Voice of Medicine), it is important to remember that conflicts and challenges to provide effective and appropriate care often arise from differences in cultural values even within the same system. In the following section, we will examine some of the fundamental values of western medicine and consider the interrelationships and tensions between these values.

Although HBM and TRA/TPB have adopted different approaches in conceptualizing individuals' health behaviors and health decision making, as theories developed in the West, they also shared some fundamental assumptions that are inherent in the Western cultural understanding of effective and appropriate provider-patient interactions. For example, both models assume that individuals' health behaviors are shaped by the *individuals'* decision-making. Whether it's influenced by a cost-benefit analysis or behavioral intentions, both HBM and TRA/TPB focused on influencing "the person of interest" to change the person's health behavior. Such approaches rest on the assumption of individualism.

A. Assumptions about Patient Needs: Patients as Independent Actors

Individualism has deep roots in western cultures. Some of the features of individualism include an emphasis on one's autonomy and personal goals and a focus on individual emotions, values and thoughts, rather than those of the in-group (Lewandowska-Tomaszczyk & Wilson, 2019). The Perspectival Thinking that emerged during the Classical Greek and Roman period and again during the Renaissance has led to the burgeoning of modern medicine: understanding health and illness through objective, scientific observations along with the freedom of inquiry spawning experimentation. To the early natural philosopher/scientist, nothing was sacred. Dissecting human bodies, for instance, was not a spiritual issue but a necessity for learning (Roach, 2003). Individual curiosity was pitted against collective authority, in the form of religious power. At the same time, Perspectival Thinking also facilitates the growth of individualism, which sets the foundation for medical ethics. "From the outset, the conceptual framework of bioethics has accorded paramount status to the value-complex of individualism, underscoring the principles of individual rights, autonomy, self-determination and their legal expression in the jurisprudential notion of privacy" (Fox, 1990, p. 206).

Patient autonomy sets the foundational value in western medicine, establishing the standards for quality care (e.g., patient-centered care) and legal practices (e.g., informed consent) in healthcare settings. Patient autonomy in health contexts is most salient in understanding that patients should be allowed or enabled to make autonomous decisions about their health care, emphasizing the concept of

self-determinism: a patient's role as a decision-maker about their own bodies and their fate (Entwistle et al., 2010).

In 2001, the Institute of Medicine set **Patient-Centered Care** (PCC) to be one of its core aims to improve the quality of care, noting that patients should be informed decision-makers in their care (Institute of Medicine, 2001). Since then, various studies have connected PCC to the process and outcomes of healthcare delivery, noting its positive impacts on patient satisfaction and well-being (Kupfer & Bond, 2012; Rathert et al., 2013). PCC's focus on engaging the patient as an informed decision-maker is a response to an earlier medical model in which providers assume a controlling role in a patient's healthcare experiences (Barry & Edgman-Levitan, 2012).

In the United States, patient autonomy emerged in the 1960s in response to the overall atmosphere of anti-paternalism (Maclean, 2009; Rothman, 2001). As a result, an ideal patient is constructed as an informed patient who is capable and willing to assume all responsibilities in their illness events (Kapp, 2007). By focusing on a patient's agency and individuality, PCC is conceptualized as "the experience (to the extent the informed, individual patient desires it) of transparency, individualization, recognition, respect, dignity, and choice in all matters, without exception, related to one's person, circumstances, and relationships in health care" (Berwick, 2009, p. 560). PCC aims to provide care that "is respectful of and responsive to individual patient preferences, needs, and values, and ensuring that patient values guide all clinical decisions" (Institute of Medicine, 2001, p. 40).

The emphasis on respecting patient-autonomy and self-determinism is also reflected in the practice of informed consent, a legal right of patients protected by the courts. In the leading court holding for the legal significance of informed consent, the court explained that the purpose of **informed consent** is to protect "the prerogative of every patient to chart his [sic] own course and to determine what action he [sic] will take" (*Scott v. Bradford*, 1979, para. 14). The *Scott* court explained, "Anglo-American law starts with the premise of thoroughgoing self-determination, each man [sic] considered to be his [sic] own master. ... The doctrine of informed consent arises out of this premise" (para. 9–10). The notion that a patient is actively engaged in decision-making is consistent with the image of the ideal patient in PCC: The legal practice of informed consent protects patient autonomy through protecting a patient's right to choose. In short, by operationalizing informed consent as individuals' exercise of patient autonomy and self-determinism, western medicine has embedded individualism in its vision of best practices.

B. Health Decisions as Social Decisions

Under the traditional conceptualization of informed consent, patients are conceptualized as independent decision-makers who are able and willing to choose the healthcare options that best meet their needs. Recognizing that patients cannot make meaningful decisions without sufficient and accurate information, the legal standard of informed consent requires providers' full disclosure of information that is relevant to a patients' decision-making, including relevant risks and conflicts of interest. Nevertheless, the strong emphasis on patient's agency and independence (i.e., self-determinism) fails to recognize the interactive and dynamic nature of health-decision making. Even in the most individualistic, perspectival world, few people make health decisions in isolation from sociocultural contexts or interpersonal influences. The current assumptions about informed consent in western medicine create challenges and barriers to healthcare delivery.

1. The Collaborative Nature of Health Decision-Making

First, by viewing patients as decision-makers and providers as information providers, the practice of informed consent overlooks the collaborative nature of health decision-making. In addition to situations in which patient autonomy can be questioned or compromised (e.g., cognitive impairment), researchers have argued that the singular focus on protecting patients' autonomous decision-making during informed consent can be problematic because it fails to recognize the interactive and relational nature of health decision-making (Entwistle et al., 2010). Patient preferences are not without limits: "For some decisions, there is one clearly superior path, and patient preferences play little or no role – a fractured hip needs repair, acute appendicitis necessitates surgery, and bacterial meningitis requires antibiotics" (Barry & Edgman-Levitan, 2012, p. 780). Because medicine is expert knowledge, relying solely on patient autonomy to guide decision-making can create tensions in power balance and decisional authority in the provider-patient relationship.

As a result, rather than expressly disagreeing or overruling a patient's preference which gives the impression of **medical paternalism** (i.e., physicians know best what is in the best interests of patients because of their medical expertise; Kilbride & Joffe, 2018), a healthcare provider may strategically frame or disclose certain information to influence patient's decision-making. In an observational study, a provider successfully persuaded a 75-year-old patient to abandon her initial preference for surgery by providing extensive details about the surgery (e.g., touching a patient's body as she identified the long incision line and named the organs that she will remove, and later drew an anatomical chart with various organs to be identified in red crayon), concluding that the patients' preference for a "big" surgery with serious and uncertain consequences was actually an unsavory, if not unwise, "gamble" (Hsieh et al., 2016). However, as soon as the patient chose the providers' recommended nonsurgical option, the provider quickly accepted the patient's decision without engaging in the corresponding pros and cons. The provider's increasing disclosure about surgical risk was used to manipulate the patient's decision-making, a direct threat to self-determinism. In recent years, some providers have argued that such "**nudging**" is necessary "to steer people's choices in directions that will improve their own welfare" (Sunstein & Thaler, 2003, p. 3), which can be particularly important when medical knowledge and expertise are increasingly specialized (Munoz et al., 2015). Others, however, have argued that provider nudging is medical paternalism and a direct threat to patient autonomy (Simkulet, 2018). Providers' nudging behaviors during the informed consent process highlight the tensions between provider expertise and patient preferences and have raised concerns about medical paternalism (Ploug & Holm, 2015).

Medical communities struggle to find the balance in avoiding medical paternalism and protecting patient autonomy. One of the solutions proposed is **shared decision-making**, which gained traction in the 1980s and remains the preferred model for provider-patient interactions (Kilbride & Joffe, 2018). In shared decision-making, "both parties share information: the clinician offers options and describes their risks and benefits, and the patient expresses his or her preferences and values. Each participant is thus armed with a better understanding of the relevant factors and shares responsibility in the decision about how to proceed" (Barry & Edgman-Levitan, 2012, p. 781). This is particularly helpful when "more than one reasonable path forward exists (including the option of doing nothing, when appropriate), and different paths entail different combinations of possible therapeutic effects and side effects. ... In such cases, patient involvement in decision-making adds substantial value" (Barry & Edgman-Levitan, 2012, p. 780). In addition, despite the availability of, and easy access to, health information and services for patients to research symptoms and order laboratory/genetic tests, patients will continue to rely on providers for "advice, procedural expertise, and access to restricted medical services" (Kilbride & Joffe, 2018, p. 1974). Successful shared decision-making, thus, relies on individuals' ability to communicate and coordinate their needs and expertise.

In summary, informed consent as a legal standard and medical practice in western medicine overlooks the collaborative nature of health decision-making. A patient's ability to exercise effective and meaningful autonomy to achieve a desirable outcome is dependent on a provider's ability to not only provide sufficient and accurate information but also to situate the information in social contexts, incorporating the patient's unique needs and perspectives.

2. Cultural Functions and Meanings of Information

Second, the diverging functions and meanings of information in different cultural perspectives can lead to provider-patient conflicts during the informed consent process. Fundamental to the practice of informed consent in western medicine is the belief that "knowledge is power." In Perspectival Thinking, information is dissociated from interpersonal contexts. Information, thus, becomes a "thing," something external to individuals' identities or sociocultural contexts. Accurate information is viewed as the only path to "truth" and "reality" (singular and positively knowable). It is empowering. As a result, western patients feel that only when they were given the truth (i.e., accurate and full information) are they empowered to make decisions. Such a belief is so strong that one study found that U.S. physicians had a consistent pattern of telling children about their cancer diagnosis (i.e., 65% always told the child; less than 1% rarely or never told): Even children should be entitled to the information to have an "accurate" understanding of what is going on with their bodies and fate (Parsons et al., 2007). In contrast, the same study found Japanese physicians had greater variability in their patterns of telling (with only 9.5% always telling, 34.5% rarely or never telling).

The difference in physicians' normative disclosure is due to different cultural perspectives about the meanings and functions of information. Perspectival Thinking encourages individuals to take an objective, analytical approach to information. The perspectival world is **visio-centric**, meaning that it is dominated by spatial thinking (Kramer, 1997; Kramer & Ikeda, 2000). Transparency, the clarity of vision and understanding, is a major presumption of western perspectival culture. All information should be shared. And it is why science, the demand for objective referees, and total disclosure of experimental procedures and results have made for great advances in knowledge (National Academies of Sciences, Engineering, and Medicine, 2019). This virtue of openness impacts all aspects of western culture from businesses being required to publish honest annual reports for the public to read, to voters having access to important background information of political candidates, and to healthcare patients to participate in decision-making. To be enfranchised is the essence of the democratic ethos and what the famous theorist of science Karl Popper (1945/2013) called the "open society." Corruption happens when people hide the truth. Western people prefer the truth, even when it is bad news and/or inconvenient because without the truth, we cannot make informed decisions.

In cultures with less of a democratic ethos and dedication to an open society, power is less equally distributed because knowledge is power, and knowledge is hoarded. Strict criteria justifying the withholding of information tends to be to protect innocent people, victims of crimes, and national security (e.g., medical paternalism to protect patients). A strength of western civilization has been its reluctance to tolerate secrets and lies. Record-keeping is extensive in the perspectival world. Falsified records, be they personal resumes or official state reports, are strongly stigmatized if not criminalized. Neither democracy nor science can function without free speech and open access to information (National Academies of Sciences, Engineering, and Medicine, 2019; Post, 2011). This is why the first public libraries and universities were invented in the perspectival world during the Renaissance and greatly expanded after the Enlightenment (Harris, 1999). Although this may sound all good to an American reader who is themselves more or less dominated by the perspectival consciousness structure, this push toward individualism, independence, and free-will has produced negative effects. The all-inclusive wholeness of the Magic Consciousness world and the community ties of the Mythic Connection world are evaporating leaving a world of all-against-all where the individual is personally and solely responsible for all their successes and failures.

Nevertheless, we all rely on the sustaining efforts of others to make our modern world work. Sharing is also curtailed by an extreme emphasis on private property. Hence, homeless people live next to skyscrapers where individuals of immense wealth reside. Community is curtailed by an extreme emphasis on privacy so that we no longer know our neighbors. You cannot be your "brother's keeper" if you don't know your brother or sister and their problems. Personal rights and liberties can conflict with the need to listen and submit to expert authority. Individuals now go to doctors and argue with them basing on things they personally read on the Internet. Empiricism, believing only what one has direct, personal experience with, can exaggerate biases rather than enhance rational problem-solving.

Due to the Perspectival Thinking worldview, over 90% of U.S. adults believe that withholding discussions about poor prognosis is an unacceptable way to maintain hope (Apatira et al., 2008). In fact, most U.S. children and adolescents with cancer also believe that they have a "right" to know and indicate preferences of knowing about their diagnosis (Kelly et al., 2017). U.S. physicians are also influenced by their own sense of responsibility for telling children about their cancer diagnosis (Parsons et al., 2007). Individuals of Perspectival Thinking typically associate information, good or bad, as empowering their decision-making process.

In contrast, under the Mythic Connection and Magic Consciousness, information-giving is more than just "receiving information." Mythic Connection may construe that truth-telling can take away a person's hope, resulting in a shortened life. For example, whereas European-Americans and African-Americans are more likely to view truth-telling as empowering, enabling the patient to make choices (i.e., Perspectival Thinking), Korean-Americans and Mexican-Americans are more likely to see truth-telling as cruel, and even harmful, to patients (Blackhall et al., 2001). For patients from certain cultures, to inform someone about their poor prognosis takes away their hope. One Korean patient explained, "I don't want to know about my impending death... without hope, one cannot live... So anyone who says that she or he wants to know about having a disease is out of their minds because the knowing itself is painful. If the patients have more stress, their lives are shortened" (Blackhall et al., 2001, p. 65). Myth as an alternative story to reality can be distracting and comforting. Myth offers an imagined self without disease.

Alternatively, Mythic Connection can also attach new meanings to "truth-telling" in end-of-life contexts that orient cultural participants to "proper" behaviors. For example, in the movie *The Farewell* (Wang, 2019), when a Chinese-American child challenged the family's decision of not informing her grandmother about the devastating prognosis of cancer, her father responded, "You want to tell Nai Nai (note: grandma) the truth because you feel too much responsibility carrying it. If you tell her, then you don't have to feel guilty anymore. We're not telling her because it is *our responsibility to carry this emotional burden* for her." Rather than denying or challenging the "truth" of the diagnosis, the father transformed the act of end-of-life truth-telling from an impersonal disclosure to facilitate decision making to a loving act of bearing the burden for one's loved ones, a task too challenging to a person who is selfish or weak. Thus, in the context of end-of-life disclosure, one can argue that individualistic cultures may create myths about empowerment and self-determinism for the *individual* patients; in contrast, collectivistic cultures create myths about the shared burden and love for *all* that is involved in a patient's illness event. The same act, depending on the culture, entail different meanings and realities (Xue et al., 2011).

Magic Consciousness may construct truth-telling as imposing a death sentence, setting a timed clock or a powerful curse, on a person's life (Bowman, 1997; Rolland, 1999). Christoph Wilhelm Hufeland (1762–1832), a noted physician in Jena and Berlin, once stated, "To prophesy death is to cause it" (Lee & Wu, 2002, p. 534). A Korean American elderly explained, "Since I am over 70 years old, I may die in the near future, but I don't want to know when I will die because that would be like having a death sentence" (Berkman & Ko, 2010, p. 248). Bioethicists have noted that the cultural differences in understanding the meanings and functions of truth-telling of poor prognosis can make the practice of informed consent not only problematic but also "unethical" (de Pentheny O'Kelly et al., 2011; Pergert & Lützén, 2012).

Because cultural practices are always loaded with values and morality claims, it is important to recognize that cultural actors in these scenarios do not simply view these as differences in cultural practices. In fact, in some ways, one can argue that even under Perspectival Thinking, individuals can develop Mythic Connection about their practice and morality claims. For example, when asked to find a way to balance family's desire to shield bad news from the patient and truth-telling to a dying patient, a physician responded, "When I was in medical school, it was driven home to us that autonomy was the lynchpin concept. You're destroying my moral compass" (Solomon, 1997, p. 90). The way the physician describes the practice of truth-telling and patient autonomy is *not* Perspectival Thinking, which often is reflected in an objective, non-emotional understanding of its cultural worldviews. Instead, the physician has developed a Mythic Connection about his practice of informed consent that connects his professional identity and moral character to his ability and willingness to give a patient the "truth" even if the patient's family resists such practices. Is truth-telling a fatalistic prognosis heroic or wicked? It depends on who is receiving the information and the worldviews involved.

In summary, a cultural approach to healthcare delivery can be more complicated than simply recognizing that patients and physicians do not share the same cultural views. It is also more nuanced than identifying differences in cultural patterns. The traditional approach to cultures is to think of culture as being a somewhat static entity in which a person is born or socialized into the culture and stays in the culture forever (e.g., a Chinese versus an American versus a German person). In contrast, we argue that cultures can be more nuanced and fluid. Informed consent and end-of-life disclosure are challenging tasks because of the different meanings and functions of information. Even for physicians who adopt a Perspectival Thinking approach, they can, at the same time, develop Mythic Connection that connects their moral character to the practice of truth-telling. This is the complexity of cultural fusion. Individuals develop layers of understanding of health practices, recognizing the differences of meanings in cultural perspectives and navigating the different cultural norms to achieve their individual preferences.

III. Informed Consent in Medicine

A. Informed Consent in Ethical and Legal Contexts

Informed consent is an essential element in western medicine. However, the practice of informed consent has become increasingly rigid as it embodies the philosophy of medical ethics, practice guidelines of healthcare delivery, and legal actions of malpractice claims. A landmark case in delineating providers' duty of disclosure took place in 1972 with the District of Columbia Circuit Court's opinion in *Canterbury v. Spence*. Although recognizing that provider disclosure and patient consent may be "two sides of the same coin" (*Canterbury v. Spence*, 1972, p. 780), the court distinguished the two by pointing out that "vital inquiry on duty to disclose relates to the physician's performance of an obligation, while one of the difficulties with analysis in terms of 'informed consent' is its tendency to imply that what is decisive is the degree of the patient's comprehension" (p. 780). The *Canterbury* court held that the physician breached his duty when he failed to disclose sufficient information about a risky and invasive diagnostic procedure.

When considering the provider disclosure, the *Canterbury* court noted that "the focus of attention is more properly upon the nature and *content* of the physician's divulgence than the patient's understanding or consent" [emphasis added] (p. 780). The scope of providers' disclosure must be "measured by the patient's needs" (p. 786). Because the purpose of provider disclosure is to provide "information material to the [patient's] decision," "the test for determining whether a particular peril must be divulged is its materiality to the patient's decision: all risks potentially affecting the decision must be unmasked" (pp. 786–787). Such an emphasis on patients' needs and decision-making inevitably heighten the tensions between the underlying principle of self-determinism and the court's desire to avoid interfering with clinical practice. However, the *Canterbury* court's holding stopped short in assessing a patient's actual needs for meaningful decision-making. Instead, the court adopted an *objective reasonable patient standard*, requiring providers to disclose information that would be material to a reasonable person in the patient's position (i.e., a fictitious "reasonable patient"). By raising policy concerns of protecting providers from "the patient's hind-sight and bitterness" and placing factfinders in search of a "speculative answer to a hypothetical question" (p. 791), the court concluded, "the physician discharges the duty [to disclose] when he makes a reasonable effort to convey sufficient information although the patient, without fault of the physician, may not fully grasp it" (p. 780). The objective reasonable patient standard, thus, centers on the sufficiency of informa-tion (i.e., the content) as opposed to the patient's actual understanding.

The *Canterbury* court rejected the reasonable physician standard (i.e., "what infor-mation a reasonable, prudent physician would have disclosed to the patient under similar circumstances") and adopted a patient-oriented standard measured by what is a "reasonable disclosure" under the circumstances would be material to a reasonable patient. However, the focus on the content of disclosure, rather than patients' prefer-ence or understanding, as a legal standard of informed consent can motivate providers to engage in complex considerations of ethical and cross-cultural care. In addition, researchers and practitioners have raised concerns about the current practice of informed consent in healthcare settings.

First, rather than incorporating measures to check a patient's understanding, the current legal standards of informed consent focus on providers' disclosure of risk: assuming that physicians' disclosure would automatically translate into patients' understanding. An argument fundamental to the courts' reasoning for the informed consent is that sufficiency of information is a prerequisite of a patient's ability to exer-cise self-determinism through informed consent. However, various studies have debunked such a direct, linear relationship between decision-making and sufficiency of information (Brashers et al., 2002). More information does not necessarily facilitate decision-making or allow a patient to be more informed (Laidsaar-Powell et al., 2013). Patients may feel overwhelmed in processing information and paralyzed for decision-making when there is "too much information, contradictory information, too much medical jargon, too much information at one time, and insufficient time to absorb the information" (Berger, 2003, p. 747). A review of 103 clinical trials between 1980–2013 found that the proportion of participants in clinical trials who understood different components of informed consent varied from 52.1% to 75.8% (Tam et al., 2015). Focusing on the content (and quantity) of information overlooks the purpose it aims to serve: self-determinism. Beauchamp and Childress (2009) explained, "The element of understanding emphasizes that while disclosure is an element of informed consent, disclosure to the patient without patient understanding is not sufficient" (p. 124).

Second, by focusing on full disclosure of risk, various researchers have raised con-cerns about the **nocebo effect** of informed consent (Cohen, 2014; Wells & Kaptchuk, 2012). Nocebo effect is the mirror-phenomenon of the placebo effect: As patients are informed about the relevant risks and possible negative outcomes, they may experi-ence corresponding symptoms or experience their symptoms in higher intensity. One study found that compared to research participants who were not given information about potentials of gastrointestinal side-effects, the participants who did receive such information were six times more likely to withdraw from a research study because of subjective, minor gastrointestinal symptoms (Myers et al., 1987). In a study using beta-blocker to treat patients who were newly diagnosed with cardiovascular disease, 3.1% of men reported erectile dysfunction (ED) when they were not told the drug's name. Comparatively, 15.6% reported ED when they were told the drug's name but not the risk of ED, and 31.2% when they were told both the drug name and the risk of ED (Silvestri et al., 2003). Researchers concluded, "For some kinds of side effects, disclosing a possible adverse event significantly increases the probability of such an event occurring" (Silvestri et al., 2003, p. 37).

Third, because the legal standard of informed consent centers on the sufficiency (as opposed to the appropriateness) of provider disclosure, it provides openings for coercion – a direct threat to patient autonomy. For example, a provider may purposefully increase disclosure about surgical risks to manipulate a patient's decision making as in the case of provider nudging discussed earlier. Similarly, the recent rise in states' regulations on provider disclosure for patients seeking abortions is couched under the concept of informed consent. For example, South Dakota now requires physicians to state that abortion will "terminate the life of a whole, separate, unique, living human being" (S.D. Codified Law, 2012). Oklahoma law prohibits a medical provider from performing an abortion unless she first performs an ultrasound, "display[ing] the ultrasound images so that the pregnant woman may view them" (Okla. Stat. tit. 63, 2004), and provides a verbal description thereof. Although these compelled disclosure statutes claim their legitimacy through the process of informed consent, many have raised concerns about the coercive nature of the disclosure. In his concurring opinion, Justice Blackmun analogized for such requirements that require "a visual preview of an operation to remove an appendix," which he argued "plays no part in a physician's securing informed consent to an appendectomy," and "does not constructively inform" medical decision-making (*Planned Parenthood of Southeastern Pennsylvania v. Casey*, 1992, p. 937). A literature review concluded, "Empirical clinical research demonstrates that our current legal concepts of informed consent are at odds with not only modern medical practice, but also individual autonomy rights. As a result, legal scholars should rethink current informed consent laws." (King & Moulton, 2006, p. 491)

B. Individual Preferences and Cultural Norms

Individuals' understanding of health practices is grounded in their cultural norms and is interactively negotiated during a medical encounter. When individual preferences are consistent with normative practices, provider-patient communication and collaboration works seamlessly. For example, In the West, because the individualist cultures place emphasis on patient autonomy and self-determinism, providers, patients, and family members can all appreciate full disclosure of information for illness management (Blackhall et al., 2001). Studies done in Western cultures found that adolescents want to hear complete prognostic information early or in tandem with their parents (Rosenberg et al., 2017). In addition, they are capable of thoughtful and mature decision making and want to be involved in decisions related to their care (Rosenberg et al., 2017).

Different cultures, however, may impose different cultural norms and expectations for decision-making in health contexts. For example, communication beliefs, religious practices, and varying family structures are common themes of cultural influences on Asian families' decisions concerning the disclosure of cancer diagnosis of their children (Thibodeaux & Deatrick, 2007). Systematic reviews suggest **collusion** (i.e., a cultural practice in which family members request withholding information from the patient) is common in regions where families, rather than individual patients, are considered the central unit of medical decision-making (Yeung, 2017). Culturally based family preferences for collusion regarding a diagnosis of cancer is common all over the world, including Asia, Africa, Europe, and the Middle East (Rosenberg et al., 2017).

The differences in cultural preferences should not be understood as rigid expectations of cultural practices. For example, prior to the shift from medical paternalism to patient-centered care in the 1960s, nondisclosure of physicians is not uncommon in the United States: In 1961, 88% of physicians did not practice disclosure (Oken, 1961); by 2008, 98% of health care providers believe that disclosure is an ethical and practical imperative (Daugherty & Hlubocky, 2008). Comprehensive reviews of disclosure patterns in Middle Eastern cultures (e.g., Egypt, Iran, Israel and Palestine, Jordan, Lebanon, Kuwait, Pakistan, Saudi Arabia, Turkey, and the United Arab Emirates) found that preferences for (non)disclosure are shaped by a wide range of factors, including: countries, patients' age, providers' specialties and experiences, family beliefs, and the manner in which the information is disclosed (Rosenberg et al., 2017).

In other words, although it is important to recognize that cultural norms provide providers insights about behavioral patterns, one must also recognize that individuals, regardless of whether they are from individualist or collectivist cultures, may have preferences that are not necessarily the same as the larger cultural norms. For example, socioeconomic class, education level, and neighborhood environment may be better predictors than racial or ethnic identities of individuals' health behaviors and health outcomes (Browning et al., 2003; Kaufman et al., 1997; Sudano & Baker, 2006). The tensions between individual preferences and the normative practices of a specific healthcare setting can become salient, if not contentious, when they conflict with one another. For example, some adolescents may believe that they have a "right" to know about their cancer prognosis but would prefer not to know about the information or to have family members to filter the information for them (Kelly et al., 2017; Pousset et al., 2009). A cultural approach to health communication requires providers to be sensitive to the larger cultural patterns and be attentive to the patient's unique needs.

In recent years, the rise of **cultural relativism** has fostered tolerance of diverse beliefs and behaviors by withholding judgment on foreign cultural practices and behavioral norms. By noting that different societies have different normative practices and moral standards and that one culture's values are not inherently better than others, a cultural relativist approach encourages healthcare providers to accommodate patients' needs without imposing judgments or condemnation. Although this approach can be helpful in educating providers to avoid bias or discrimination, it is inadequate to address issues of a universal truth and reality (e.g., universal human rights) or obviously problematic cultural practices (e.g., female genital mutilation). Rosenberg et al. (2017) concluded that cultural relativism "does not justify assumptions that all individuals within a single culture share the same values, nor does it demand that clinicians sacrifice their own codes of conduct out of cultural respect" (p. 1113).

To be clear, we are not advocating that informed consent should be abandoned or that individual agency restricted. The respect and emphasis on patients' autonomous, independent decision-making have been the cornerstone of western medicine. Rather, we argue that healthcare providers should be sensitive to their own cultural norms and values, recognize potential differences with other cultures, and be attentive to patients' individual needs. This is a fluid, interactive understanding of culture as it dynamically emerges in provider-patient interactions. At the same time, healthcare professionals and experts are increasingly coping with dis- and misinformation channeled to their patients. Successful provider-patient interactions are not dependent on providers' willingness to embrace patients' preferences unconditionally but on providers' and patients' willingness and ability to share their understandings and negotiate a mutually acceptable strategy to manage their differences.

C. Health Practices as Cultural Practices

Health practices are cultural practices. As we make sense of our everyday life, our understanding of information, behaviors, and motivations are embedded in cultural contexts. So are our theories that are developed to explain health behaviors.

We examined three dominant theories of health behaviors, which guide the design and execution of health campaigns. The theories have proven to be effective depending on the nature and characteristics of the particular health intervention. The theories, however, entail cultural assumptions that are not readily apparent to the casual observer. The theories all assume that the best way to influence a person's health behavior is to influence the person's attitudes and thinking about the specific behaviors. They assume that individuals have agency to make decisions and to change their behaviors. Although TRA/TPB consider the influences of a person's social networks, it still centers on the individuals' perception of the network's preferences, norms, and beliefs, rather than the actions that may be taken by the network to manipulate or control a person's health behaviors.

It is from this perspective that we want to highlight the limitations of these theories. Though they are meaningful and effective, they have incorporated cultural assumptions of individualism, patient autonomy, and self-determinism. These cultural assumptions are intuitive and taken-for-granted. Yet few would acknowledge that these are culturally-based theories. But they are. To adopt a cultural approach means that we begin by acknowledging our own cultural perspectives (Dutta & de Souza, 2008), recognizing how our perspectives can limit our worldviews.

In this Chapter, we used informed consent as an example to delineate the complexities and interrelationships of cultural assumptions and individual understandings. Informed consent is a good example for such a purpose because this is a taken-for-granted cultural practice in healthcare settings that few in the United States would ever challenge its appropriateness or effectiveness. Nevertheless, once we begin to consider informed consent as a cultural practice and situate the practice in different cultural perspectives, it becomes obvious why such a taken-for-granted practice can ignite intense conflicts between providers and patients.

Informed consent highlights the difference in cultural perspectives. It also begs the question of what it means to be informed and the value of information and source credibility. For example, under Perspectival Thinking, physicians may argue that informed consent constitutes the necessary precondition for a patient to exercise autonomy and self-determinism. In contrast, family members' may believe that informing the patient about his poor prognosis is cruel (e.g., hearing the news can take diminish a person's hope and chance of survival; i.e., Mythic Connection) and can result in real harm (as the words are said, the harm is done; i.e., Magic Consciousness).

Informed consent also shows that individuals can adopt multiple cultural perspectives (i.e., Integral Fusion) at the same time. For example, by constructing informed consent as an ethical imperative rather than a necessary practice, a physician transforms a Perspectival Thinking phenomenon that stresses individualism to enhance patient autonomy to a Mythic Connection of identity and morality. Failure to achieve full disclosure to a patient threatens both the patient's and the physician's identities. As such, informed consent becomes a cultural instrument, carrying the cultural meanings of ethical behaviors and morality claims.

Informed consent involves variations of understandings and practices within "cultural norms." For example, even though Middle Eastern cultures generally involve family members in health decision making, researchers have found variations of cultural practices and patterns caused by a wide range of factors (Rosenberg et al., 2017). Even in the United States where most patients and physicians agree that patients have a right to know, many patients hold different expectations and preferences about whether family members should filter the information for them (Brashers et al., 2002; Kelly et al., 2017). The variations of cultural expectations can evolve in response to temporal changes and ideological shifts as observed in the United States, Lebanon, and Saudi Arabia (Rosenberg et al., 2017).

In short, by conceptualizing informed consent as a cultural practice, researchers and practitioners are freed from a static, rigid understanding of health practice. As researchers recognize the complex meanings of patient autonomy in different cultures (Ishikawa & Yamazaki, 2005; Rosenberg et al., 2017), a new approach to medical ethics is emerging: informed consent is best practiced and understood within sociocultural, historical, and economic contexts (Rosenberg et al., 2017; Stevenson, 2016; Yeung, 2017). In other words, informed consent is not "context-free" as Perspectival Thinking would have portrayed. If being objective means transcending and abandoning cultural situatedness, then informed consent can never be objective. Rather, it is a process and a product negotiated through collaborative efforts between the providers and patients to achieve shared decision-making within the Lifeworld. The Voice of Medicine does not exist in a vacuum. It is a cultural propensity and exists within living cultural contexts. Treatments are conditioned on availability, affordability, cultural imperatives, expertise, and other contextual factors. Such an understanding presents providers and patients discursive space to share their cultural perspectives and meanings and to acknowledge potential differences in other areas (e.g., cultural and interpersonal contexts, among others). Negotiation among "equals" and discursive space are phenomena of Perspectival Thinking. This Chapter has shown that the ability and desire for negotiation is both a virtue and a challenge.

In summary, conceptualizing health practices as cultural practices is to recognize the complexity and diversity of cultural perspectives. It does not necessarily take the form of cultural relativism. Rather, it acknowledges the variations as well as fusions of cultural perspectives of individuals and within cultures. It is a fluid and flexible approach to address individuals' health practices.

IV. Additional Resources

A. Key Terms and Theories

theory
Health Belief Model

perceived threat
    perceived susceptibility
    perceived severity
perceived benefit
perceived barrier
cues to action
self-efficacy
Theory of Reasoned Action
    attitude
    behavioral belief
    evaluation of behavioral outcome
    subjective norm
    normative belief
    motivation to comply
Theory of Planned Behavior
    perceived control
    control belief
    perceived power
patient autonomy
self-determinism
Patient-Centered Care
informed consent
medical paternalism
nudging
shared decision-making
visio-centrism
nocebo effect
collusion
cultural relativism

B. Discussion Questions

1. What is a theory? Why is theory helpful to researchers and practitioners in addressing health-related issues or health interventions?

2. Using diabetes management as an example, please explore how the following people may have different understandings about the following constructs of HBM: (a) perceived susceptibility, (b) perceived severity, (c) perceived benefit, (d) perceived barrier, (e) cues to action, and (f) self-efficacy.

   a. A U.S. physician who believes in science
   b. A Native American from a community where 60% of the adult population have diabetes and youth aged 10-19 are 9 times is more likely to be diagnosed with diabetes than a non-Hispanic White
   c. A religious Indonesian woman who lives in extreme poverty

3. The Integrative Model of Behavioral Prediction proposes that culture can influence individuals' behavioral, subjective, and normative beliefs. Using cervical cancer as an example, explore how different cultural approaches (i.e., Magic Consciousness,

Mythic Connection, and Perspectival Thinking) may lead to different behavioral claims for (a) behavioral, (b) subjective, and (c) normative beliefs.

4. Do you think there are differences between medical paternalism and nudging? What are they? Can an ethical line be drawn? How? How can we respect healthcare providers' medical authority without compromising patients' decision-making?

    a. How can reliance on the merit-based expertise of a healthcare provider aid in patient decision-making?

    b. How can a healthcare provider encourage communication, including sharing fears, doubts, and questions, about diagnoses and prognoses?

    c. Should family and friends be invited to participate in such information-sharing conversations? Should clergy?

    d. Would it be comforting to you to have a trusted friend or family member present to also evaluate the information (two heads being better than one)? Or would you prefer privacy?

5. What are your beliefs about informed consent? Would you like to know all relevant information before making a health decision? Based on your answers, can you tell what kind of cultural perspectives you hold?

6. What do you think about healthcare providers' or legislators' use of informed consent to influence individuals' health decision-making? What are the pros and cons of such practices?

C. References

Apatira, L., Boyd, E. A., Malvar, G., Evans, L. R., Luce, J. M., Lo, B., & White, D. B. (2008). Hope, truth, and preparing for death: Perspectives of surrogate decision makers. *Annals of Internal Medicine*, *149*(12), 861–868.

Barry, M. J. & Edgman-Levitan, S. (2012). Shared decision making – The pinnacle of patient-centered care. *New England Journal of Medicine*, *366*(9), 780–781.

Beauchamp, T. L., & Childress, J. F. (2009). *Principles of biomedical ethics* (6th ed.). Oxford University Press.

Berger, K. (2003). Informed consent: Information or knowledge? *Medicine and Law*, *22*(4), 743–750.

Berkman, C. S., & Ko, E. (2010). What and when Korean American older adults want to know about serious illness. *Journal of Psychosocial Oncology*, *28*(3), 244–259.

Berwick, D. M. (2009). What 'patient-centered' should mean: Confessions of an extremist. *Health Affairs*, *28*(4), w555– w565.

Blackhall, L. J., Frank, G., Murphy, S., & Michel, V. (2001). Bioethics in a different tongue: The case of truth-telling. *Journal of Urban Health*, *78*(1), 59–71.

Blank, M. B., & Hennessy, M. (2012). A reasoned action approach to HIV prevention for persons with serious mental illness. *The ANNALS of the American Academy of Political and Social Science*, *640*(1), 173–188.

Bowman, K. (1997). *Chinese canadian attitudes toward end of life decisions* (Publication Number 0-612-27879-4) [Dissertation, University of Toronto]. Toronto, Ontario. https://tspace.library.utoronto.ca/bitstream/1807/10753/1/NQ27879.pdf

Brashers, D.E., Goldsmith, D. J., & Hsieh, E. (2002). Information seeking and avoiding in health contexts. *Human Communication Research*, *28*(2), 258–271.

Browning, C. R., Cagney, K. A., & Wen, M. (2003). Explaining variation in health status across space and time: Implications for racial and ethnic disparities in self-rated health. *Social Science & Medicine, 57*(7), 1221–1235.

Canterbury v. Spence, 464 F. 2d 772 (D.C. Cir. 1972). https://www.courtlistener.com/opinion/304903/jerry-w-canterbury-v-william-thornton-spence-and-the-washington hospital

Carpenter, C. J. (2010). A meta-analysis of the effectiveness of Health Belief Model variables in predicting behavior. *Health Communication, 25*(8), 661–669.

Champion, V. L., & Skinner, C. S. (2008). The Health Belief Model. In K. Glanz, B. K. Rimer, & K. Viswanath (Eds.), *Health behavior and health education: Theory, research, and practice* (4th ed., pp. 45–65). Jossey-Bass.

Christopher, M. S., Skillman, G. D., Kirkhart, M. W., & D'Souza, J. B. (2006). The effect of normative and behavioral persuasion on help seeking in Thai and American college students. *Journal of Multicultural Counseling and Development, 34*(2), 80–93.

Cohen, S. (2014). The nocebo effect of informed consent. *Bioethics, 28*(3), 147–154.

Daugherty, C. K., & Hlubocky, F. J. (2008). What are terminally ill cancer patients told about their expected deaths? A study of cancer physicians' self-reports of prognosis disclosure. *Journal of Clinical Oncology, 26*(36), 5988–5993.

de Pentheny O'Kelly, C., Urch, C., & Brown, E. A. (2011). The impact of culture and religion on truth telling at the end of life. *Nephrology Dialysis Transplantation, 26*(12), 3838–3842.

Dutta, M. J., & de Souza, R. (2008). The past, present, and future of health development campaigns: Reflexivity and the critical-cultural approach. *Health Communication, 23*(4), 326–339.

Entwistle, V. A., Carter, S. M., Cribb, A., & McCaffery, K. (2010). Supporting patient autonomy: The importance of clinician-patient relationships. *Journal of General Internal Medicine, 25*(7), 741–745.

Fadiman, A. (1997). *The spirit catches you and you fall down: A Hmong child, her American doctors, and the collision of two cultures.* Farrar, Straus and Giroux.

Fishbein, M. (2008). A reasoned action approach to health promotion. *Medical Decision Making, 28*(6), 834–844.

Fox, R. C. (1990). The evolution of American bioethics: A sociological perspective. In G. Weisz (Ed.), *Social science perspectives on medical ethics* (pp. 201–217). Springer.

Glanz, K., Rimer, B. K., & Viswanath, K. (2008). Health behavior and health education: Theory, research, and practice. In K. Glanz, B. K. Rimer, & K. Viswanath (Eds.), *Health behavior and health education: Theory, research, and practice* (4th ed., pp. 23–40). Jossey-Bass.

Gullatte, M. M., Brawley, O., Kinney, A., Powe, B., & Mooney, K. (2010). Religiosity, spirituality, and cancer fatalism beliefs on delay in breast cancer diagnosis in African American women. *Journal of Religion and Health, 49*(1), 62–72.

Harris, M. H. (1999). *History of libraries of the Western world* (4th ed.). Scarecrow Press.

Harrison, J. A., Mullen, P. D., & Green, L. W. (1992). A meta-analysis of studies of the Health Belief Model with adults. *Health Education Research, 7*(1), 107–116.

Hsieh, E., Bruscella, J., Zanin, A., & Kramer, E. M. (2016). "It's not like you need to live 10 or 20 years": Challenges to patient centered care in gynecologic oncologist-patient interactions. *Qualitative Health Research, 26*(9), 1191–1202.

Institute of Medicine. (2001). *Crossing the quality chasm: A new health system for the 21st century*. National Academy Press.

Ishikawa, H., & Yamazaki, Y. (2005). How applicable are western models of patient-physician relationship in Asia?: Changing patient-physician relationship in contemporary Japan. *International Journal of Japanese Sociology, 14*(1), 84–93.

Janz, N. K., & Becker, M. H. (1984). The Health Belief Model: A decade later. *Health Education Quarterly, 11*(1), 1–47.

Johnson, K. S., Elbert-Avila, K. I., & Tulsky, J. A. (2005). The influence of spiritual beliefs and practices on the treatment preferences of African Americans: A review of the literature. *Journal of the American Geriatrics Society, 53*(4), 711–719.

Kapp, M. B. (2007). Patient autonomy in the age of consumer-driven health care: Informed consent and informed choice. *Journal of Legal Medicine, 28*(1), 91–117.

Kaufman, J. S., Cooper, R. S., & McGee, D. L. (1997). Socioeconomic status and health in blacks and whites: The problem of residual confounding and the resiliency of race. *Epidemiology, 8*(6), 621–628.

Kelly, K. P., Mowbray, C., Pyke-Grimm, K., & Hinds, P. S. (2017). Identifying a conceptual shift in child and adolescent-reported treatment decision making: "Having a say, as I need at this time." *Pediatric Blood & Cancer, 64*(4), Article e26262. https://doi.org/10.1002/pbc.26262

Kilbride, M. K., & Joffe, S. (2018). The new age of patient autonomy: Implications for the patient-physician relationship. *JAMA, 320*(19), 1973–1974.

King, J. S., & Moulton, B. W. (2006). Rethinking informed consent: The case for shared medical decision-making. *American Journal of Law & Medicine, 32*(4), 429–501.

Kramer, E. M. (1997). *Modern/postmodern: Off the beaten path of antimodernism*. Praeger.

Kramer, E. M., & Ikeda, R. (2000). The changing faces of reality. *Keio Communication Review, 22*, 79–109.

Kupfer, J. M., & Bond, E. U. (2012). Patient satisfaction and patient-centered care: Necessary but not equal. *JAMA, 308*(2), 139–140.

Laidsaar-Powell, R. C., Butow, P. N., Bu, S., Charles, C., Gafni, A., Lam, W. W. T., Jansen, J., McCaffery, K. J., Shepherd, H. L., Tattersall, M. H. N., & Juraskova, I. (2013). Physician–patient–companion communication and decision-making: A systematic review of triadic medical consultations. *Patient Education and Counseling, 91*(1), 3–13.

Lee, A., & Wu, H. (2002). Diagnosis disclosure in cancer patients – when the family says "no!". *Singapore Medical Journal, 43*(10), 533–538.

Lee, J.-Y. (2014). Predictors of teachers' intention to refer students with ADHD to mental health professionals: Comparison of U.S. and South Korea. *School Psychology Quarterly, 29*(4), 385–394.

Lewandowska-Tomaszczyk, B., & Wilson, P. A. (2019). Wellbeing and collective identity in polish and english contexts. In B. Lewandowska-Tomaszczyk (Ed.), *Contacts and contrasts in cultures and languages* (pp. 193–219). Springer.

Maclean, A. (2009). *Autonomy, informed consent and medical law: A relational challenge*. Cambridge University Press.

Mattis, J. S. (2002). Religion and spirituality in the meaning-making and coping experiences of African American women: A qualitative analysis. *Psychology of Women Quarterly, 26*(4), 309–321.

Mitchell, J., Lannin, D. R., Mathews, H. F., & Swanson, M. S. (2002). Religious beliefs and breast cancer screening. *Journal of Women's Health, 11*(10), 907–915.

Montaño, D. E., & Kasprzyk, D. (2008). Theory of reasoned action, theory of planned behavior, and the integrated behavioral model. In K. Glanz, B. K. Rimer, & K. Viswanath (Eds.), *Health behavior and health education: Theory, research, and practice* (4th ed., pp. 67–96). Jossey-Bass.

Montaño, D. E., & Kasprzyk, D. (2015). Theory of reasoned action, theory of planned behavior, and the integrated behavioral model. In K. Glanz, B. K. Rimer, & K. Viswanath (Eds.), *Health behavior and health education: Theory, research, and practice* (5th ed., pp. 95–124). Wiley.

Munoz, R., Fox, M., Gomez, M., & Gelfand, S. (2015). Evidence-based nudging: Best practices in informed consent. *American Journal of Bioethics, 15*(10), 43–45.

Myers, M. G., Cairns, J. A., & Singer, J. (1987). The consent form as a possible cause of side effects. *Clinical Pharmacology and Therapeutics, 42*(3), 250–253.

National Academies of Sciences, Engineering, and Medicine. (2019). *Reproducibility and replicability in science.* National Academies Press.

Oken, D. (1961). What to tell cancer patients: A study of medical attitudes. *JAMA, 175*(13), 1120–1128.

Okla. Stat. tit. 63 § 1-738.3d (2004). https://law.justia.com/codes/oklahoma/2014/title-63/section-63-1-738.3d

Parsons, S. K., Saiki-Craighill, S., Mayer, D. K., Sullivan, A. M., Jeruss, S., Terrin, N., Tighiouart, H., Nakagawa, K., Iwata, Y., Hara, J., Grier, H. E., & Block, S. (2007). Telling children and adolescents about their cancer diagnosis: Cross-cultural comparisons between pediatric oncologists in the US and Japan. *Psycho-Oncology, 16*(1), 60–68.

Pergert, P., & Lützén, K. (2012). Balancing truth-telling in the preservation of hope: A relational ethics approach. *Nursing Ethics, 19*(1), 21–29.

Pitaloka, D., & Hsieh, E. (2015). Health as submission and social responsibilities: Embodied experiences of Javanese women with type II diabetes. *Qualitative Health Research, 25*(8), 1155–1165.

Planned Parenthood of Southeastern Pennsylvania v. Casey, 505 U.S. 833 (1992). https://www.oyez.org/cases/1991/91-744

Ploug, T., & Holm, S. (2015). Doctors, patients, and nudging in the clinical context—four views on nudging and informed consent. *American Journal of Bioethics, 15*(10), 28–38.

Popper, K. R. (2013). *The open society and its enemies.* Princeton University Press. (Original work published 1945)

Post, R. (2011). Participatory democracy and free speech. *Virginia Law Review, 97*(3), 477–490.

Pousset, G., Bilsen, J., De Wilde, J., Benoit, Y., Verlooy, J., Bomans, A., Deliens, L., & Mortier, F. (2009). Attitudes of adolescent cancer survivors toward end-of-life decisions for minors. *Pediatrics, 124*(6), e1142–e1148.

Rathert, C., Wyrwich, M. D., & Boren, S. A. (2013). Patient-centered care and outcomes: A systematic review of the literature. *Medical Care Research and Review, 70*(4), 351–379.

Roach, M. (2003). *Stiff: The curious lives of human cadavers.* W. W. Norton.

Rolland, J. S. (1999). Families and genetic fate: A millennial challenge. *Families, Systems, & Health, 17*(1), 123–132.

Rosenberg, A. R., Starks, H., Unguru, Y., Feudtner, C., & Diekema, D. (2017). Truth telling in the setting of cultural differences and incurable pediatric illness: A review. *JAMA Pediatrics, 171*(11), 1113–1119.

Rothman, D. J. (2001). The origins and consequences of patient autonomy: A 25-year retrospective. *Health Care Analysis, 9*(3), 255–264.

S.D. Codified Law § 34-23A-10.1(1)(b)-(c) (2012). https://law.justia.com/codes/south-dakota/2011/title34/chapter23a/34-23a-101

Scott v. Bradford, 606 P.2d 554 (Supreme Court of Oklahoma 1979). https://law.justia.com/cases/oklahoma/supreme-court/1979/48164.html

Silvestri, A., Galetta, P., Cerquetani, E., Marazzi, G., Patrizi, R., Fini, M., & Rosano, G. M. C. (2003). Report of erectile dysfunction after therapy with beta-blockers is related to patient knowledge of side effects and is reversed by placebo. *European Heart Journal, 24*(21), 1928–1932.

Simkulet, W. (2018). Nudging, informed consent and bullshit. *Journal of Medical Ethics, 44*(8), 536–542.

Skinner, C. S., Tiro, J., & Champion, V. L. (2015). The Health Belief Model. In K. Glanz, B. K. Rimer, & K. Viswanath (Eds.), *Health behavior and health education: Theory, research, and practice* (5th ed., pp. 75–94). Wiley.

Solomon, M. Z. (1997). From what's neutral to what's meaningful: Reflections on a study of medical interpreters. *Journal of Clinical Ethics, 8*(1), 88–93.

Stevenson, S. A. (2016). Toward a narrative ethics: Indigenous community-based research, the ethics of narrative, and the limits of conventional bioethics. *Qualitative Inquiry, 22*(5), 365–376.

Sudano, J. J., & Baker, D. W. (2006). Explaining US racial/ethnic disparities in health declines and mortality in late middle age: The roles of socioeconomic status, health behaviors, and health insurance. *Social Science & Medicine, 62*(4), 909–922.

Sunstein, C. R., & Thaler, R. H. (2003). Libertarian paternalism is not an oxymoron. *The University of Chicago Law Review, 70*(4), 1159–1202.

Tam, N. T., Huy, N. T., Thoa, L. T. B., Long, N. P., Trang, N. T. H., Hirayama, K., & Karbwang, J. (2015). Participants' understanding of informed consent in clinical trials over three decades: Systematic review and meta-analysis. *Bulletin of the World Health Organization, 93*(3), 186–198H.

Thibodeaux, A. G., & Deatrick, J. A. (2007). Cultural influence on family management of children with cancer. *Journal of Pediatric Oncology Nursing, 24*(4), 227–233.

Wang, L. (Director). (2019). The farewell. [Film]. A24.

Wells, R. E., & Kaptchuk, T. J. (2012). To tell the truth, the whole truth, may do patients harm: The problem of the nocebo effect for informed consent. *American Journal of Bioethics, 12*(3), 22–29.

Xue, D., Wheeler, J. L., & Abernethy, A. P. (2011). Cultural differences in truth-telling to cancer patients: Chinese and American approaches to the disclosure of 'bad news.' *Progress in Palliative Care, 19*(3), 125–131.

Yeung, C. W. (2017). The ethics of collusion and nondisclosure in cancer care: A perspective from professional psychology. *Professional Psychology: Research and Practice, 48*(1), 46–53.

7

Health Literacy

Cultural Approaches to Health Behaviors and Decision-Making

Chapter 7 examines health literacy and social determinants of health as a field of study, focusing on how their emergence and development are shaped by sociocultural and sociopolitical forces. Then, adopting a critical stance toward this field, we will explore how the field of health literacy and social determinants of health may have oversimplified, if not ignored, the roles and functions of culture in shaping individuals' health behaviors and societal responses to health policies. Recognizing that cultural worldviews and values are reflected and embodied in hieratical priorities, we will examine how hidden cultural values have shaped our understanding of health literacy and the social determinants of health.

I. The Shifting Fields of Health Literacy

A. What is Health Literacy?

Literacy as a theoretical concept and measurement has changed significantly over the years. For example, in the mid-1800s and through the mid-1930s, the U.S. Census Bureau asked individuals whether they can read or write in any language to assess whether they are literate or not (Berkman et al., 2010). At the time, literacy was understood as a *binary* assessment of whether an individual was able to read and write texts. Literacy assessments traditionally centered on individuals' competency with printed materials (Kirsch & Guthrie, 1977). However, such an approach fails to address the significant variations in individuals' literacy levels. It also fails to assess whether a person's literacy level accurately reflects her ability to navigate everyday tasks. The report of the Committee on Reading concluded that despite the decline of illiteracy levels, many individuals living in the United States continue to have severe reading problems (Carroll & Chall, 1975). As a result, researchers have proposed the concept of **functional literacy**, which focuses on the "levels of skills that individuals or populations need in order to complete some specific real-life reading task" (Kirsch & Guthrie, 1977). Literacy centers on a fixed-level, text-oriented, universal assessment of individuals' skills to read and write; in contrast, functional literacy does not limit itself to specific sets of skills but emphasizes individuals' ability to navigate real-life challenges in their everyday life (e.g., having the skills necessary to obtain food, shelter, clothing, and health care; Kirsch & Guthrie, 1977). Advancing from the

Rethinking Culture in Health Communication: Social Interactions as Intercultural Encounters, First Edition. Elaine Hsieh and Eric M Kramer.

task-oriented view of functional literacy, the National Literacy Act of 1991 defines literacy as "the ability to read, write, and speak in English, and compute and solve problems at levels of proficiency necessary to function on the job and in society, to achieve one's goals, and develop one's knowledge and potential." ("The National Literacy Act of 1991," 1991§3). Literacy is no longer understood as an abstract, fixed level of individual capacity to be measured (see Figure 7.1). Rather, it is conceptualized as a set of problem-solving skills that are socially-oriented, culturally-sensitive, and goal-driven.

Health literacy first emerged as a field of research in the late 1980s. It was heavily influenced by the research on functional literacy. Researchers were quick to recognize that individuals' educational attainment was not an accurate or consistent indicator of their ability to navigate the complexity of everyday tasks (Kirsch et al., 1993). As a result, it is necessary to develop a meaningful definition and measurement of health literacy to assess individuals' ability to navigate health information. An early definition proposed by the Ad Hoc Committee on Health Literacy for the Council on Scientific Affairs of the American Medical Association focused on individuals' ability to "perform basic reading and numerical tasks required to function in the healthcare environment" (American Medical Association, 1999, p. 553). Such a definition views health literacy as a fixed level of skills held by individuals.

By the early 2000s, various government agencies had proposed a more dynamic, interactive conceptualization of health literacy. For example, the Institute of Medicine adopted the definition developed for the National Library of Medicine and used by Healthy People 2010, defining health literacy as "the degree to which individuals have the capacity to obtain, process, and understand basic information and services needed to make appropriate health decisions" (Nielsen-Bohlman et al., 2004, p. 32). Based on a review of 17 explicit definitions of health literacy in published studies, Sørensen et al. (2012) concluded that a common characteristic of the definitions was their focus on "*individual skills* to obtain, process and understand health information and services necessary to make appropriate health decisions" [emphasis added] (p. 3).

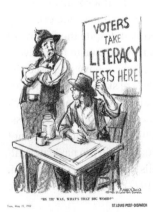

Figure 7.1 Literacy test. During the 1950s–1960s, literacy tests were the most prevalent and most effective mechanism of political exclusion to reinforce racial discrimination and disenfranchise African Americans. In recent years, legal scholars have raised concerns about the economic, social, and political exclusion of minorities through felon disenfranchisement laws (Goldman, 2004). *Source:* St. Louis Post-Dispatch/The Library of Congress

In the same review, Sørensen et al. (2012) also noted that there was an emerging trend to move beyond an individual focus and consider health literacy "as an interaction between the demands of health systems and the skills of individuals" (p. 3). This trend continues. For example, Healthy People 2030, proposed two health literacy concepts: (a) **personal health literacy:** the degree to which individuals have the ability to find, understand, and use information and services to inform health-related decisions and actions for themselves and others, and (b) **organizational health literacy:** the degree to which organizations equitably enable individuals to find, understand, and use information and services to inform health-related decisions and actions for themselves and others (Office of Disease Prevention and Health Promotion, 2020a, "How does Healthy People define health literacy?" section). This approach recognizes that individuals' health literacy level is not static as a fixed skill to be identified. Rather, health literacy is conceptualized as a dynamic set of skills that are situated in contexts (e.g., interpersonal, organizational, environmental, and cultural contexts).

Low health literacy is a prevalent problem in the United States, where more than one-third of the English-speaking population and half of the Spanish-speaking population struggle with it (Kutner et al., 2006). Health literacy is critical to individuals' illness experience: Low health literacy is linked to negative impacts on individuals' health statuses, treatment adherence, health outcomes, and communications with healthcare providers (Michielutte et al., 1999). Researchers have concluded that people with inadequate health literacy have poorer health, less knowledge about their medical conditions and treatments, less understanding and use of preventive services, poor communication with providers, and higher health care costs (American Medical Association, 1999; Berkman et al., 2004; Nielsen-Bohlman et al., 2004).

B. A Model of Health Literacy

Nutbeam (2000) proposed a **model of health literacy** that includes three levels of health literacy: (a) functional health literacy (i.e., communication of information); (b) interactive health literacy (i.e., development of personal skills); and (c) critical health literacy (i.e., personal and community empowerment). These are conceptualized as different levels of knowledge and skills that progressively support greater patient autonomy and personal empowerment for health decision-making and health management (Nutbeam, 2009).

Functional Health Literacy focuses on basic reading and writing skills that allow individuals to understand and apply health information (e.g., having an accurate understanding of health risks and navigating the health system). Nutbeam argued that traditional health campaigns focused on improving individuals' functional literacy or limiting their negative impacts, and conceptualizing individuals' low health literacy as a risk factor to health outcomes (Nutbeam, 2008). Echoing the literature on functional literacy, many "screening aids" have been developed to help clinicians to identify individuals with low health literacy. For example, the Rapid Estimate of Adult Literacy in Medicine (REALM) measures a patient's ability to pronounce common medical words and lay terms for body parts and illnesses (e.g., behavior, exercise, menopause, rectal, antibiotics; Agency for Healthcare Research and Quality, 2016; Davis et al., 1993). The Test of Functional Health Literacy in Adults (TOFHLA) used multiple-choice questions to assess individuals' ability to identify missing words in sentences common in healthcare settings (e.g., I agree to give correct information to _____ if I can receive Medicaid: a. hair; b. salt; c. see; d. ache; Nielsen-Bohlman et al., 2004; Parker et al., 1995). Researchers have criticized how these commonly used health literacy measurement tools have failed to accurately and comprehensively assess individuals' health literacy because they focus only on individuals' overall capacity (Baker, 2006).

Rather than viewing health literacy as a risk factor for individuals' health management, Nutbeam (2008) argued that essential to the conceptualization of health literacy is that it is socially situated and interactively managed: From a public health perspective, health literacy can be an asset, something to be built on to improve individuals' health outcome and overall well-being. The World Health Organization (WHO) noted that "health literacy means more than being able to read pamphlets and make appointments. By improving people's access to health information and their capacity to use it effectively, health literacy is critical to empowerment"(Nutbeam, 1998, p. 10).

Interactive health literacy involves increasing advanced cognitive and literacy skills that allow individuals to interact with health providers to obtain, process, and apply information to meet their needs. Interactive health literacy extends beyond individuals' use of printed materials and recognizes individuals' communicative abilities to manage their healthcare needs. From this perspective, Baker's (2006) "health-related oral literacy" (i.e., ability to orally communicate about health) or skills such as listening and vocal fluency noted by Paasche-Orlow and Wolf (2007) should be understood as individuals' interactive health literacy.

Because interactive health literacy recognizes that individuals' health literacy is socially situated, the focus of the intervention centers on helping targeted individuals to develop personal and social skills to achieve their desired outcome. For example, rather than simply relying on "just say no" as a campaign slogan, researchers have advocated **Life Skills Training** (LST) that help individuals to develop specific self-management and social skills that aim to "enhance personal and social competence and to decrease motivations to use drugs and vulnerability to [the] social influences that support drug use" (Botvin & Griffin, 2004, p. 216). Reviews of LST campaigns found consistent reductions in smoking, alcohol use, and marijuana use of 50% or more in students receiving the LST program relative to controls, as well as reductions in illicit drug use and improvements in a host of important risk and protective factors for adolescent drug abuse (Botvin & Griffin, 2004).

Because of the prevalence of low health literacy in patient populations, researchers have recommended physicians adopt specific communicative strategies to ensure effective understanding and appropriate decision-making. Chung et al. (2016, p. 147) proposed the following strategies:

1. using plain "living room" language with avoidance of medical jargon;
2. using "chunk and check" – delivering information in small amounts and checking for understanding;
3. using pictures, drawings, models, and demonstration to supplement verbal communication;
4. using written information to supplement verbal messages, incorporating written handouts as part of verbal counseling by pointing, circling, and highlighting key points on the page; and
5. using teach-back and show-back: asking patients and parents to repeat their understanding in their own words or through demonstration.

Critical health literacy entails the more advanced cognitive skills to critically analyze information to exert control over one's life, emphasizing the ultimate objectives of patient autonomy and empowerment. Chinn (2011) proposed that critical health literacy involves three domains of interconnected skills: (a) the critical analysis of information, (b) understanding of the social determinants of health, and (c) engagement of collective action. Whereas the first domain still centers on skills and capacities held by individuals, the second and third domains move beyond the individual-level understanding to incorporate community- and system-levels considerations for health literacy (and its corresponding interventions).

The critical analysis of information requires individuals to assess the source, credibility, reliability, and validity of the information. Rather than emphasizing the traditional emphasis of a biomedical model of health knowledge and health information, researchers have argued that critical health literacy takes the perspectives of the individuals (as opposed to the System). For example, Rubinelli et al. (2009) argued, "'critical' health literacy reflects the individual's capacity to contextualize health knowledge for his or her own good health, to decide on a certain action after a full appraisal of what that specific action means for them 'in their own world'" (p. 309). In other words, critical health literacy is "internalized" and "integral to the lived experience of the person" (Rubinelli et al., 2009, p. 309). Critical health literacy requires individuals to not just understand the health information (e.g., what is good for them) but also contextualize the message (and information-seeking behaviors) in a way that is meaningful to them. From this perspective, health literacy is no longer a risk factor to be assessed on a spectrum (i.e., a Perspectival Thinking perspective). Rather, health literacy becomes a resource for people to create meanings for their everyday life (i.e., a Mythic Connection perspective). A person who has high critical health literacy is able to draw from various resources to support health decisions that makes their life more meaningful.

II. The Individual-System Interactions of Health Literacy

For the second and third domains of critical health literacy proposed by Chinn (2011), we decided to set off a new section because these two other domains highlight system-level issues that are traditionally not addressed in the health literacy literature, particularly when health literacy is conceptualized as individual-level skills. These two domains have been shaped by the recent development of health literacy research and have even emerged as a new field of research themselves.

A. Social Determinants of Health

Chinn (2011) argued that the expanded definitions of health literacy include an understanding of social determinants of health. **Social determinants of health** (SDH) are "the conditions in the environments where people are born, live, learn, work, play, worship, and age that affect a wide range of health, functioning, and quality-of-life outcomes and risks" (Office of Disease Prevention and Health Promotion, 2020b) and the fundamental drivers of these conditions (World Health Organization, 2019). Examples of SDH include employment conditions, social exclusions, gender equity, globalization, and urbanization. Healthy People 2030 proposes five domains of SDH:

(a) economic stability, (b) education access and quality, (c) health care access and quality, (d) neighborhood and built environment, and (e) social and community context (Office of Disease Prevention and Health Promotion, 2020a; for more on Health People, see page 329). By situating health literacy in the contexts of SDH, we begin to recognize that health decisions are not context-free considerations. Rather, individuals' decisions are deliberate choices made in response to the contexts that define their health experiences.

For example, individuals' seemingly unhealthy, risky, or self-destructive behaviors may entail important functions for identity performance and relational maintenance. An ethnographic study of homeless heroin addicts found that they frequently engage in needle sharing practices, which allow them to maintain their "dope fiend" identities, communicate mutual bonding, and demonstrate trust in their fragile social network (Bourgois, 1998). Many homeless women choose to remain in an abusive, exploitative relationship with a male partner, considering it as a rational strategy to maintain stability and companionship in street life (Bourgois et al., 2004). Whereas such decisions would be easily categorized as self-destructive behaviors, these actions represent "positive" meanings (e.g., bonding, trust, and stability) that can be necessary to the homeless individuals' survival on the street. Similarly, non-dominant (ethnic) minorities often actively engage in risky health behaviors in their everyday life (e.g., smoking, alcohol consumption, sexual risk behaviors, overeating, and unsafe driving habits) to exert agency and to resist (and protest) against structural injustice (Factor et al., 2011; Factor et al., 2013). As such, these risky health behaviors become an important resource for minorities to develop a sense of control and resilience in a potentially hostile environment.

In early 2000, researchers began to report a group of HIV-negative gay men who called themselves "bug chasers." They actively engaged in unprotected sex with HIV-positive or potentially positive gay men with the explicit aim to become infected with HIV (Moskowitz & Roloff, 2007). Some bug chasers viewed such actions as a "politically charged" action against the larger, homophobic culture that discriminates and stigmatizes gay men (Gauthier & Forsyth, 1999). Others talked about bug chasing as an active strategy to manage their fear and uncertainty, finding relief when they are diagnosed HIV-positive and thus, affirm their gay identity and community membership. From this perspective, the act of bug chasing takes on new meanings through Mythic Connection. Although such actions may appear irrational and incomprehensible to outsiders, for gay men who struggle with social stigma and instability, these risky health behaviors become political actions that decry the social injustice and empowers them to affirm their destiny and biography as gay men (Sheon & Crosby, 2004).

By recognizing individuals' health literacy is situated in sociocultural, sociopolitical, and socioeconomic environments, policymakers, and researchers have identified innovative ways to improve public health. For example, rather than focusing on poor people's diet and obesity as a result of low health literacy for nutrition, recent studies have explored the structural (and paradoxical) connections between poverty and obesity (Dinour et al., 2007). Researchers found poor families often struggle with food insecurity despite efforts to reduce food waste (e.g., cooking new dishes from leftovers) and grow vegetables to supplement their diets (Buck-McFadyen, 2015). By recognizing poverty can reduce individuals' ability for cognitive control (Spears, 2011), some researchers have argued that overeating is an adaptive behavior to food insecurity, allowing individuals to obtain high energy-density (but low nutritional value) food at low costs and to survive cycles of unpredictable food insecurity (Stinson et al., 2018). In addition, researchers have found that individuals who experience increased worry, powerlessness, and low social status are more likely to adopt overeating behaviors and develop weight gain (Dinour et al., 2007). Finally, people experiencing food insecurity were found to adopt practices that pose food safety risks, including removing spoiled sections, slime, mold, and insects from food; eating other people's leftovers; and, eating meat found as roadkill (Kempson et al., 2002). As a result, solutions to food insecurity should not be limited to increasing health literacy of individuals to choose healthy food because such an approach fails to recognize the myriads of SDH that shapes individuals' diet and eating behaviors.

B. Health Literacy as a Coordinated Achievement

The third domain of health literacy involves a coordinated effort, such that network members are collaborators in information management (see Brashers et al., 2002; Brashers et al., 2004). Health literacy is not a set of skills and competencies of an isolated patient, but a set of different skills and resources that can be coordinated between patients and their supportive others. Research on uncertainty and self-management for chronic illness, for example, has suggested that illness events often require the patient and his or her supportive others to coordinate their management of information and resources (Brashers et al., 2004; Gallant, 2003). A person may be too distressed to obtain and use illness-related information, and may, therefore, rely on his or her relational partner to learn the latest treatment options, communicate with providers, and make treatment decisions. Brashers and colleagues (2004) argued that supportive others "*can be sources of information..., collaborators in information gathering, and evaluators of information, or they can serve as buffers against information.* [emphasis added] They also facilitate information management by encouraging development of information-seeking and decision-making skills" (p. 324). The knowledge and ability to manage the illness event, thus, is coordinated between various individuals rather than independently possessed by an isolated patient.

Individuals can rely on others for advice, medical expertise, and information management skills that they may not possess themselves. Individuals then have the ability to achieve optimal coping and positive outcomes through appropriate and effective (a) appraisals of event tasks, skills, and resources, and social support needed for illness management, (b) communication and negotiation of one's appraisals and/or needs with others, and (c) coordination with others in executing information and illness management behaviors. This ability is not limited to the patient but also includes the patients' supportive others. The supportive others defined here include all individuals who are involved in a patient's illness event at family, community, and systems levels.

Health literacy, from this perspective, includes both cognitive and social components as a skill set. It is about problem-solving: Individuals will manage their illness successfully if they have abilities to accurately identify the problem (i.e., appraisal) and generate adaptive strategies (i.e., coping) to meet the challenges (Glasgow et al., 2004). It is important to point out that appraisal and coping are theoretically distinct concepts: **Appraisal** is about the cognitive process aim at evaluation; in contrast, **coping** focuses on the execution of appraisals, including cognitive and behavioral strategies, meant to manage illness and its effects.

1. Patient Empowerment for Optimal Coping and Outcomes

Patient empowerment is an underlying value of health literacy (Speros, 2005). The patients' perspective is privileged in the sense that optimal coping and positive outcomes are viewed from the *patients'* perspective, addressing the patients' primary concerns for their illness events (Zubialde & Aspy, 2001). They are not necessarily the best health outcomes. Although health care systems tend to view the quality of healthcare in terms of the efficiency and accuracy of diagnosis and treatments, patients have a much more complex understanding of the quality of care (Zubialde & Mold, 2001). Individuals may make health-related decisions that are critical to other areas in their lives and improve their quality of life overall, although they may not be beneficial to health (Lloyd et al., 2005). For example, a person may choose to keep a demanding job, although it interferes with the treatment regimen, perhaps because he or she needs the money or because of the identity concern of not appearing weak or disabled.

Because successful illness management is a coordinated and collaborative accomplishment of the patient and his or her supportive others, it is important that the supportive others also have high health literacy for illness management. For example, providers can help patients to identify and prioritize various tasks in achieving health goals that are meaningful to patients (Zubialde & Mold, 2001). When a physician is able to help a patient "to *understand* the situation, *appreciate* the risks and benefits of the available options, *use reasoning* to arrive at a sound decision, and *communicate* the decision to others" (Mold, 2006, p. 1209), regardless whether the decision was agreeable to the physician, the patient may have reached his or her optimal coping and positive outcomes. A physician's health literacy is based on his or her ability to communicate, negotiate, and coordinate with the patient in the appraisal and coping process. In other words, although the patients' point of view is privileged, the success of health literacy is dependent on the supportive others' ability to influence, sometimes through negotiation, the patients' appraisal and coping processes.

2. Evolving Abilities Situated in Illness Experiences

The temporal aspect of illness management requires individuals to develop different skills for illness management and learn to coordinate with others efficiently and appropriately. For example, a patient has different informational needs and relies on different individuals at different phases of an illness event (Rutten et al., 2005). Researchers also have noted that patients' coping strategies evolve over time and can shift from less adaptive to more adaptive coping strategies (Reeves et al., 1999). Patients with chronic illnesses also develop the ability to appraise uncertainty and trust different individuals for different needs (Brashers et al., 2000). Researchers found that patients have clinically significant improvements in HbA_{1c} levels, systolic and diastolic blood pressures, aspirin use, and weight within one year of a new diagnosis of diabetes (O'Connor et al., 2006). From this perspective, one may suggest that as an individual becomes more familiar with the needs in the illness event, he or she will develop higher health literacy for issues related to illness experiences.

Some studies suggest, however, that other factors may lead to deterioration in illness management. In a large-scale study, in a two-year period, 10.8% of the patients who originally had good diabetes control crossed over to poor control and 38.7% of the patients who originally had poor control crossed over to improved control (Weiner & Long, 2004). In addition, compared with Whites, Blacks were 1.76 times as likely to switch from good to poor control and only 0.56 times as likely to switch from poor to good control. To develop effective interventions, researchers need to identify the factors that may make patients become more (or less) appropriate and effective in assessing their needs, identifying the skills and resources needed, and soliciting support from the person that best meets their needs.

III.   Rethinking Health Literacy through the Lenses of Culture

If personal health literacy is "the ability to find, understand, and use information and services to inform health-related decisions and actions for themselves and others" (Office of Disease Prevention and Health Promotion, 2020a, "How does Healthy People define health literacy?" section), how can we understand health literacy through the lenses of culture? How does health literacy operate through Magic Consciousness, Mythic Connection, Perspectival Thinking, or Integral Fusion?

A.   Health Literacy is Inherently Perspectival

It should not be a surprise to find that health literacy, as a theoretical concept, fits naturally to the western understanding of medicine and medical ethics. The pursuit of knowledge and self-determinism is pervasive in how the medical profession and society assess the quality of care and patient-provider communication. At its core, especially at the initial conceptualization of the phenomenon, the literature of health literacy envisions a "perfect" patient who is well-read and knowledgeable, not afraid to and capable of pursuing information needed, and willing to take responsibility for the decision made. This is clearly a perspectival understanding of information and human decision-making. The patient is capable of obtaining, processing, and understanding objective information to make neutral decisions that best meet the goals of his or her health management. Such an understanding is likely to misconstrue minority and marginalized groups' perspectives, whose approaches to and use of health information are likely to be less individualistic or perspectival.

Traditionally, health literacy as a theoretical concept is also text-oriented. For example, Baker (2006) recognized that health-related oral literacy can be a distinct concept but wondered if the concept would be too intertwined to the health-related print health literacy to warrant a different, independent measurement. Even when oral communicative competence is incorporated into a dimension of health literacy, the information exchange envisioned often centers on a provider-patient pair. For example, Paasche-Orlow and Wolf (2007) argued that providers need to learn how to "communicate in plain terms to confirm important items in a patient's history and evaluate patient comprehension of important action items" (p. S22). In addition to "avoiding medical jargon[s]," it may be helpful to use "pictures, multimedia, and decision aids" (Paasche-Orlow & Wolf, 2007, p. S22).

The perspectival, individualistic, and text-oriented view of health literacy is a product of a western society where there is a strong middle class. To have high health literacy, a person (a) needs to be well-educated so that they have the ability to scrutinize information for its accuracy and (b) live in a community that has abundant access to high-quality health information. However, we know that minority and marginalized populations already experience disparities in other areas of life (e.g., education and socioeconomic status) and face other challenges and barriers that are likely to contribute to their different patterns of information management.

Different cultures do not see information nor decision-making the same way. The differences can lead to significant disparities for minority and marginalized populations. For example, the federal government learned that it was necessary to adopt different enrollment interventions for different ethnic groups for the Patient Protection and Affordable Care Act (2010; i.e., ACA; Obamacare). The ACA first opened for enrollment on October 1, 2013. The federal government set up the Health Insurance Marketplace (i.e., a.k.a. the Health Insurance Exchange), a website (https://www.healthcare.gov) that allowed people without health care insurance to find information about health insurance options and also purchase health care insurance. By March 2014, researchers found that although many people were comfortable and enthusiastic about participating in the ACA through the Marketplace, Hispanic populations were enrolling at a rate slower than other under-insured populations. Researchers identified two major causes for the enrollment lags for the Hispanic populations.

1. Minority Groups' Historical Distrust of Healthcare Authorities

Researchers first pointed to the historical events and reasons for the mistrust between marginalized populations and governments on the issues of health and medicine (Molina, 2017). Health research has demonstrated that minorities often have a lower level of trust for governments and healthcare providers than other groups. In a national survey, a researcher found that African Americans, Hispanics, and Asians are more likely than Whites to perceive that: (a) they would have received better medical care if they belonged to a different race/ethnic group; and (b) medical staff judges them unfairly or treats them with disrespect based on race/ethnicity and how well they speak English (Johnson et al., 2004). Minorities' distrust of government and healthcare providers not only reflects their marginalized status in society, but often reflect the chronic struggle and tumultuous histories they share with the dominant groups.

Medicine and medical professionals have not been neutral in the history of minority health and healthcare. In the late 1890s, social Darwinism provided new fuel for racism in the United States, arguing that primitive peoples could not be assimilated into a complex, White civilization (Brandt, 1978). Brandt (1978) observed, "Physicians studying the effects of emancipation on health concluded almost universally that freedom had caused the mental, moral, and physical deterioration of the black population" (p.21). Under the practice of eugenics for "race betterment" and the umbrella of public health concerns, various states in the United States passed **sterilization laws** that mandated **forced sterilization** of three categories of people between the early 1920s to late 1960s: idiots, morons, and imbeciles. Although idiots were clinically defined as people who were mentally defective with a mental age of no more than 35 months, morons or imbeciles were more porous categories, often including individuals who experienced significant social disadvantages and disparities – such as "prostitutes, orphans, depressives, vagrants, petty criminals, schizophrenics, dyslexics, feminists, rebellious adolescents – anyone, in short, whose behaviors, desires, choices, or appearance fell outside the accepted norm" (Mukherjee, 2016, p. 79). As a result, the majority of the individuals who were subjected to the government-enforced sterilization were poor women, with women of color and immigrants being sterilized at a significantly higher rate than native-born, middle-class White women (Kline, 2005; Stern, 2016; see Figure 7.2).

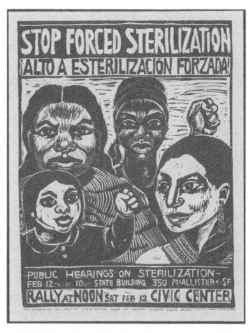

Figure 7.2 Poster of public hearings on forced sterilization. A "stop forced sterilization" poster published by San Francisco Poster Brigade in 1977. *Source:* Romero, Rachael / The Library of Congress

The **Tuskegee Syphilis Study** conducted by the U.S. Public Health Services (USPHS) remains a haunting memory for minorities. Between 1932–1972, USPHS conducted experiments in Macon County, Alabama, to determine the natural course of untreated, latent syphilis in African American males (Centers for Disease Control and Prevention, 2015). Researchers told the participants that they were being treated for "bad blood" and never informed them that they had syphilis (Centers for Disease Control and Prevention, 2015). When penicillin became widely available by the early 1950s as a highly effective treatment for syphilis, the men *did not receive treatment*. On several occasions, USPHS even sought to prevent treatment. Over the 40-year period, "of about 600 Alabama Black men who originally took part in the study, 200 or so were allowed to suffer the disease and its side effects without treatment, even after penicillin was discovered as a cure for syphilis. Treatment then probably could have saved or helped" (Heller, 2017, para. 7). An investigatory panel issued a report in 1972, noting that at least 28 (but maybe as many as 100+) died as a direct result of advanced syphilitic lesions. The penal concluded that the study was "ethically unjustified" and that penicillin should have been given to the research participants (Brandt, 1978). On May 16, 1997, President Clinton issued a formal apology to the surviving participants and the living relatives of the non-surviving participants. President Clinton further commented, "To our African American citizens, I am sorry that your federal government orchestrated a study so clearly racist. That can never be allowed to happen again" (White House, 1997, para. 10; see Figure 7.3).

Sexually Transmitted Disease Experiments in Guatemala mark an even darker history of the violation of human rights and medical ethics by U.S. medical researchers. Overall, 5000+ research participants representing many vulnerable populations in

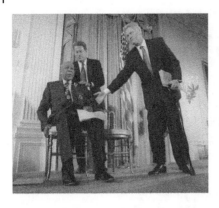

Figure 7.3 Tuskegee apology. President Clinton and Vice President Al Gore, back, help Herman Shaw, 94, a Tuskegee Syphilis Study victim, during a news conference Friday, May 16, 1997. Making amends for a shameful U.S. experiment, Clinton apologized to Black men whose syphilis went untreated by government doctors. *Source:* AP Photo

Guatemalans, including children, orphans, and child/adult prostitutes, Guatemalan Indians, leprosy patients, mental patients, prisoners, and soldiers, were experimented on (Rodriguez & García, 2013). Between 1946–1948, U.S. medical researchers funded by the National Institutes of Health, with the cooperation of Guatemalan authorities, *intentionally infected* at least 1308 research participants with sexually transmitted diseases, including syphilis, gonorrhea, and chancroid, without their knowledge or consent (Rodriguez & García, 2013). Many were left untreated for over half a century. On October 1, 2010, President Obama apologized to the Guatemalan president and reaffirmed the United States' commitment to "ensure that all human medical studies conducted today meet exacting US and international legal and ethical standards" (White House, 2010, para. 1).

The abhorrent treatment of minorities and marginalized groups has not been limited to the distant past. The **HIV Discordant Couples Study in Haiti** also raised significant ethical concerns. Between 1985–2005, researchers from Cornell Medical College ran a U.S. government-funded grant at an AIDS research clinic in Port-au-Prince, Haiti, exploring whether uninfected partners of HIV+ patients can develop "natural immunity" that can be made into a vaccine when they continue to be exposed to the virus through unprotected sex (Daniels, 2000). The uninfected Haitian research participants were minimally informed about the risks of unprotected sex with an HIV+ partner. Experts agreed that if the research were done in the United States, the physicians would be obligated to prescribe antiretroviral drugs and deliver more effective counseling against unprotected sex (Bernstein, 1999). Marc Fleisher, an outside member of the Cornell committee for human subject research, commented, "It's like, since we're making this a better place, we're going to exploit it in a way we could never get away with in the United States" (Bernstein, 1999, para. 9).

In summary, in contrast to the Whites' expectation of the presumed trustworthiness of a governmental health campaign or healthcare providers, minorities and immigrants have *learned* from past experiences that health interventions and government-sanctioned medical projects may pose serious threats to their interests and well-being. For the victims of these minority marginalized populations, their surviving relatives, and even community at large, these events are not simply forgotten and forgiven when a president apologizes, or court settlements are reached.

These events take on new meanings through the contexts of Mythic Connection, highlighting the strained relationships and exploitable status minorities hold in a society. The stories and cautionary tales are handed down through the generations. For example, the Tuskegee study has become a collective trauma for the African American community, calling out lessons to be learned and never forgotten (Reverby, 2012). Although in the Tuskegee study, Black men were not intentionally infected with syphilis but were left untreated or undertreated, the persistent belief that Black men were deliberately infected convincingly enforces and transforms the study into a powerful metaphor of racism and the danger of government-sponsored healthcare (i.e., a belief persists through Mythic Connection; Reverby, 2001). Such collective memories speak to and reinforce minority groups' fears of organized genocide (Gamble, 1997) – echoing a not-so-distant memory of the forced sterilization of women of color. When reflecting on the legacy of the Tuskegee study, Lorene Cary (1992), a *Newsweek* contributing editor, eloquently stated:

> We Americans continue to value the lives and humanity of some groups more than the lives and humanity of others. That is not paranoia. It is our historical legacy and a present fact; it influences domestic and foreign policy and the daily interaction of millions of Americans. ... It is no longer true that an African-American's life can be bought outright; and U.S. laws no longer allow token penalties for the murder of a Black person. But it is true that African-American life in the United States has long been, and is still, devalued. The fact is, to quote Gwendolyn Brooks's poem: "We die soon." (p. 23)

From this perspective, can we really say that minorities have "low" health literacy *because* they do not trust healthcare providers? Or should we begin to reconsider how different groups may (and to their benefit to) rely on different sources of information for health decision-making?

As we reflect on what the tests of health literacy measure and how low health literacy is often correlated with minorities, it is helpful to consider the lessons we learned about the evolution and emerging understanding of general IQ tests, a test of "intelligence" that often tracks along racial lines (Kramer & Johnson, 1997). As Mukherjee (2016) explained:

> Tests that are explicitly designed to capture variance in abilities will likely capture variance in abilities – and these variations may well track along racial lines. But to call the score in such a test "intelligence," especially when the score is uniquely sensitive to the [cultural] configuration of the test, is to insult the very quality it sets out to measure. (p. 349)

In other words, when we allow ourselves to reconsider the meanings of low health literacy as indicated by many of the available tests of health literacy, it is important for researchers and health practitioners to recognize a low score in a test of health literacy does not mean that the patients are stupid or less educated. Rather, a low score of health literacy may suggest that the test-takers employ different modes of speaking, understanding, thinking, and communication than the test-makers.

2. Cultural Preferences for Sources of Health Information

To further explain Hispanic populations' under-enrollment in the ACA, researchers have pointed to the different ways minorities seek and use information for health decision-making. Schembri and Ghaddar (2018) explained, "Hispanic consumers are highly dependent on trust relationships with friends and family, with a strong familial network interwoven throughout the community. Hispanic professionals within the Hispanic community are trusted professionals and especially so with many local professionals being friends and family" (p. 150). Based on an analysis of a national survey, Smith (2011) concluded, "Hispanic persons are more likely than other race/ethnicities to get health information from family and friends and Whites are more likely than other race/ethnicities to obtain health information from healthcare providers" (p. 203). To a certain degree, the uneasy histories of minority groups' experiences with healthcare authorities and the government help explain their preferences for different sources of information for health-decision making.

For example, by examining women's experiences with infertility problems, Bell (2014) found that women of high socioeconomic status seek health information through support groups, physicians, and the Internet; in contrast, women of low socioeconomic status do not discuss their health problems with peers for fear of social stigma and lack access to and distrust physicians. A national survey found that individuals with low socioeconomic status reported less confidence to obtain information, less likely to trust a health care provider, and less likely to trust the Internet (Richardson et al., 2012). Compared to Whites and Hispanics, Blacks place significantly more trust for health information disseminated by religious organizations and leaders (Asare et al., 2018; Richardson et al., 2012). One study concluded that culturally sensitive intervention strategies are necessary for Haitians with low health literacy because they "placed greater trust in family and friends and religious organizations and leaders" (as opposed to healthcare providers) as sources of information about health or health or medical topics (Lubetkin et al., 2015, p. 447). The differences in patterns of information-seeking and information sharing should not be simply attributed to individuals' health literacy or lack thereof. Rather, we should reconsider the complexity and interrelationships between the implicit cultural construction of health literacy.

In a perspectival culture, health information is a neutral resource to facilitate a patient's autonomy and decision-making; in contrast, in cultures with predominantly Magic Consciousness or Mythic Connection views, information carries symbolic meanings. The meanings are not simply carried by the content of the information but also by the process of information management (e.g., how a person seeks information; the types of information sought; and the ways that the information is communicated) within cultural contexts. In a review of 46 studies that examined physician disclosure of advanced life-limiting illnesses, researchers found that physicians from Anglo-Saxon cultures mostly believe that patients should be informed; in contrast, most physicians from non-Anglo Saxon countries are less likely to offer poor prognosis (Hancock et al., 2007). In Span, Italy, Greece, and as many other collective cultures (e.g., Saudi Arabia, Egypt, Japan, and China), physicians often disclose poor prognosis to family members before informing the patient, following the family's requests for information management rather than disclosing bad news directly to the patient (Mystakidou et al., 2004). Even when patients wish to know about their diagnosis, they may prefer receiving only basic (rather than extensive) information, using euphemistic language (to soften the blow), hearing it from specific persons (e.g., physician, nurse, or family members), and maintaining hope (Mystakidou et al., 2004). In other words, the information management of illness disclosure is dependent on the cultural considerations of appropriate place, time, process (e.g., who should do the disclosure), and purpose (e.g., maintaining hope).

Anthropologist Edward T. Hall (1976) introduced the concepts of low-context cultures and high-context cultures, noting their significant differences in domains of communication patterns. For example, Native Americans, East Asian (e.g., Chinese, Korean, Japanese, Taiwanese cultures), Eastern Mediterranean (e.g., Greeks, Turks, and Arabs), and Latin American cultures (which reflects a fusion of Iberian and Indian traditions) are all high context cultures, with languages that involve high ambiguity of messages or have grammatical structures that cultivate ambiguity (Andersen et al., 2003; Lim, 2003). In contrast, Western cultures (e.g., German, Switzerland, Denmark, Canada, and the United States) are low-context cultures (Andersen et al., 2003).

In **low-context cultures**, individuals are individualistic and rely heavily on elaborate texts (i.e., the literal message) of the information exchanged to derive meanings. Western medicine is also a low-context culture (i.e., the Voice of Medicine; see Chapter 4). Low-context cultures are inclined to Perspectival Thinking. Meanings in low-context communication are explicit (i.e., what is said is what is meant; objective facts conveyed), rather than inferred. Meanings of the information exchanged does not rely on the interactants' understanding of their identities, personal histories, or communicative contexts. The success of low-context communication relies on individuals' ability to include detailed, precise content in the message itself. Low-context communicators tend to view themselves as open and direct. Low-context communicators generate extensive and detailed explanations of phenomena and events. They fill libraries with books of law, science, philosophy, and then add commentaries upon commentaries, parsing words and meanings. And they tend to talk more than high-context communicators. This is because low-context communicators do not presume much from the context; in contrast, high context communicators infer much meaning from the context, including who, what, and when things are being conveyed. As a consequence, low-context communicators literally use many more words to convey their intent than relatively high context communicators who assume much from the whole of the relationship. Low-context perspectival communicators fragment meaning to enhance precision; in contrast, high context communicators use fewer words and are more comfortable with ambiguity and generalizations (Kramer, Callahan, & Zuckerman, 2013; McLain et al., 2015).

The striving for "clarity" is manifested by a low tolerance for ambiguity among low-context communicators and a higher tolerance for ambiguity among high context communicators (Kramer et al., 2013). For high context magic and mythic communicators (i.e., high context communicators), the avalanche of words, jargon, and complex explanations offered by medical professionals in an effort to fully inform patients and clarify (disambiguate) diagnoses and prognoses may be bewildering if not frightening. Fragmentation (including measurement) creates precision limiting tolerances and uncertainty in machine tooling and also in other perspectival processes, including descriptive and explanatory talk itself. But for magic and mythic people, more words and more parsing of meanings is not always helpful. It may even give them a sense that things are utterly determined (rather than indeterminate) and therefore hopeless. Magic Consciousness and Mythic Connection rely more on touch than dissociated examination via various scopes and other visual enhancements. Perspectival Thinking people tend to concentrate on the words in manuals and books; in contrast, people with Magic Consciousness and/or Mythic Connection concentrate on how the words are spoken (an emotional dimension) as well as nonverbal gestures (ritualistic and normative). The simple raising of a hand can express a powerful message to a magic or mythic person whereby perspectival people tend to want more information to determine more precisely what the gesture means.

In **high-context cultures**, individuals are collective-oriented. High-context cultures are more inclined to inhabit Magic Consciousness or Mythic Connection. The interactants rely on the cultural and mutually shared understandings inherently pre-established contextually (e.g., shared relationships, identities, personal histories, and gender) as well as nonverbal communication to interpret meanings conveyed. Stories and metaphors are common features of high-context communication. It is important to know that high-context communication is not less effective than low-context communication despite the fact that it does not rely on explicit, detailed messages for effective communication. High-context communication can be just as effective and can even carry richer implications for participants' identities and relationships because it operates in a more holistic fashion incorporated context into text prior to fragmentation. The success of high-context communication relies on participants' familiarity and ability to apply inferences through cultural norms and expectations.

The more Magic Consciousness and Mythic Connection are part of the communication ecology, the more disclosure practices and information management in health contexts are fused with meanings about identity and relationships. For example, in Chinese culture, if a son fails to assume the responsibilities of information management for the patient (e.g., seeking information about treatment options or concealing information from the patient), he may face public criticism that he is an inadequate son (Muller & Desmond, 1992). On the other hand, if a Chinese father gives permission to his son to take over the responsibilities of information management and to be a proxy decisionmaker (e.g., making decisions about treatments), the father is demonstrating his commitment to and trust for his family and community (Ellerby et al., 2000). Rees and Bath (2000) found that when mothers with breast cancer withheld information from their daughters, it often was motivated by a desire to protect their daughters. Miller and Zook (1997) noted that (before the legalization of same-sex marriage,) AIDS patients' care partners negotiated and legitimized their roles by actively seeking information from physicians.

Information management in a family is not only just about patient autonomy but also about family members' identities as part of the family (Blackhall et al., 2001). Thus, in high-context communication, the patients and their support network engage in complex coordination of information management not only for illness management but also for identity performance and relationship maintenance. As such, the preferred health decision-making model for these cultures is the **family-centered model** (i.e., medical decisions are jointly determined by the patient and her support network; family-determinism), rather than the **patient autonomy model** (i.e., medical decisions is made solely by the patient; self-determinism). In the contexts of health literacy, this means that individuals from high-context cultures may purposefully rely on non-healthcare professionals (e.g., family members, friends, and religious leaders) for information-seeking and health decision-making as these actions are essential to their understanding, performance, and fulfillment of their social roles.

Tensions in clinical care arise when providers and patients have to communicate through their different preferences for high- v. low-context communication. For example, when a physician is focused on diagnosing the illness by narrowing the clinical talk to illness symptoms, a patient may feel that the physician is uninterested in his experiences when he wants to share stories that situate his illness experiences in the Lifeworld. "If clinicians, in their time-pressured clinics, try to 'speed things up,' high context communicators can easily feel intimidated and pressured and, in the face of overly direct communication, may fall silent or withdraw altogether" (Zwi et al., 2017, p. 67).

When applying the concepts of high- and low-contexts communication to health literacy, researchers have examined communication conflicts when providers and patients are from cultures that do not share the same levels of context (i.e., they are contextually "out-of-sync"). In a study examining interpreters' function as a cultural advocate to facilitate patients' communicative competence, an interpreter explained, "Now back home, a doctor is someone who has high social status. You wouldn't dare to argue with [the doctor] – whatever doctor say, you got to listen. So...they don't like talk, and whatever doctor says they will agree...whatever doctor think best" (Butow et al., 2012, p. 238). In other words, the interpreter recognized that the patient's low health literacy (e.g., lack of information-seeking behaviors) is not due to a lack of communicative skills or medical knowledge but an expected performance of the patient's cultural norms. For these patients, asking too many questions or even asking a physician for clarification would be considered disrespectful to the physicians' authority. In observational studies of Mandarin Chinese interpreters working in hospitals in the United States, Hsieh (2013) noticed that to enhance patients' communicative competence, interpreters often make inexplicit information explicit, elaborating on a speaker's comment to improve a patient's ability to request services, to understand medical procedures, and to engage in effective provider-patient interactions.

The differences are not limited to ethnic or national boundaries. Rather than viewing contextual communication in dichotomy (i.e., high versus low), researchers have argued that contextual communication should be viewed as a continuum from low to high context communicator style. Even within a single culture, some activities (e.g., beginning of a romantic relationship) or topics (e.g., death and dying) may involve communicative patterns with higher context than others activities or topics (e.g., medical history-taking). It certainly would be an awkward conversation for couples at an early stage of a relationship to talk about the state of the relationship (e.g., what the relationship will lead to) or relationship norms (e.g., how much time they spend with each other; Knobloch & Carpenter-Theune, 2004). In fact, Knobloch and Carpenter-Theune (2004) found that couples perceive most relationship damage when communicating about avoided topics at low levels of intimacy and adopt indirect, oblique, and evasive communicative strategies at moderate levels of intimacy. In other words, low-context communication at an early stage of a romantic relationship is not only dispreferred but can create barriers to relationship escalation.

In the healthcare contexts, compared to mundane, common illnesses (e.g., a cold or a broken leg), death and dying are often imbued with profound cultural meanings. Conversations regarding such topics often adopt a high-context communication style. In contrast, biomedicine is perspectival, adopting a low-context approach to illness. Miscommunication and conflicts can arise when physicians default to their comfortable norms of low-context communication in biomedicine while patients struggle to make sense of bad news through high-context communication (Hallenbeck, 2006).

B. Health Literacy as Integral Fusion

One of the most important issues when incorporating cultural perspectives into healthcare practices is recognizing the complexities of cultures. Beyond the differences between cultures, there are also differences within subgroups or for specific practices within a culture. Nevertheless, cultures are also flexible and adaptive. As the world becomes increasingly westernized and embraces biomedicine, we can also expect that a perspectival view of health literacy, including information-seeking and health decision-making, will be normalized in many high-context cultures. For example, a recent study on end-of-life care found that as Japanese Americans become more acculturated in the United States, their views shift toward western values on preferences for disclosure, willingness to forgo care, and attitudes for advanced care planning (Matsumura et al., 2002).

Integral Fusion contributes valuable insights into a cultural understanding of health literacy. Rather than conceptualizing individuals' health literacy as restricted to a fixed, cultural perspective (e.g., Magic, Mythic, or Perspectival views), an Integral Fusion approach recognizes that individuals' understanding of health literacy can be layered with different cultural meanings. For example, although we have cast biomedicine and health literacy primarily through Perspectival Thinking perspectives in this chapter, it is important to recognize that healthcare providers may also hold other cultural understandings of information-seeking that contain Magic Consciousness or Mythic Connection. Healthcare providers not only navigate through different cultural perspectives with their patients but also with themselves.

For example, Parsons et al. (2007) identified significant differences in U.S. and Japanese providers' communicative patterns about children's cancer diagnoses, although both practice western biomedicine. Whereas 65% of U.S. physicians reported to always tell children about their cancer diagnoses, only 9.5% of Japanese physicians reported the same. In fact, less than 1% of U.S. physicians reported rarely or never telling children about their cancer diagnoses; in contrast, 34.5% of Japanese physicians reported doing so. It is important to note that these communicative patterns are culturally situated and are driven by system norms, reflecting corresponding beliefs, ethics, and values. For example, whereas 92.8% of U.S. physicians believe that informing a child of a cancer diagnosis would not increase the parental burden, 43.5% of Japanese physicians believe that it would. Parsons et al. (2007) explained,

> US physicians endorsed the belief (completely agreed or generally agreed) that it is their responsibility to tell the child the cancer diagnosis (98%), that the child's knowledge enhances their participation in their care (99.1%), and that knowledge of the cancer diagnosis within the community would enhance the child's psychosocial support (98.3%). ... The pattern of response was significantly different ... for Japanese physicians for each of these variables. (p. 64)

It is also important to remember that parents and physicians in the United States do not always subscribe to such disclosure practices. Prior to 1960, both parents and physicians in the United States believed that children should not be informed about their cancer diagnoses (Chesler et al., 1986). The shift in U.S. physicians' and parents' attitudes further highlights the socially constructed nature of provider-patient interactions. In other words, what appears to be a universal value within western biomedicine (e.g., patients' right to information) is, in fact, a recently emerged social construct of the U.S. culture.

Our readers may be quick to notice that Japanese physicians' disclosure patterns are situated in their preference of high-context communication and a paternalistic, collectivistic, and family-oriented approach to pediatric care. Such attributions would be appropriate as their approach to family-decision making and non-disclosure of bad news can entail meanings generated through Mythic Connection (e.g., informing poor prognosis would take away a patient's hope) or Magic Consciousness (e.g., saying it make it so). However, it is important to always remember that practices in biomedicine can take on Mythic Connection or Magic Consciousness as well. As U.S. physicians reported that comprehensive disclosure is their "responsibility" (Parsons et al., 2007, p. 64) and failure to do so may destroy their "moral compass" (Solomon, 1997, p. 90), physicians have at the same time infused social values and moral principles with the act of illness disclosure, indicating a Mythic Connection. The meanings are dependent on the *social constructions* that sustain cultural worldviews.

As we travel between cultures, we inevitably accumulate cultural views that we encounter in our life journeys. **Medical pluralism** is defined as people adopting multiple healing practices even when biomedicine is available. Researchers first observed medical pluralism in minorities and migrants, who often travel between cultures. In particular, **co-cultural groups** (i.e., minority groups that are marginalized by dominant groups in society) often adopt the cultural repertoire of the dominant groups and, at the same time, retain their cultural perspectives and practices (Kramer, 2019; Orbe, 1997; Razzante & Orbe, 2018). To achieve optimal survival, co-cultural groups strategically shift between different cultural perspectives to cope with their marginalized status and limited resources. In the healthcare context, medical pluralism is prevalent in minority and marginalized populations. These groups do not simply abandon their cultural practices to embrace western biomedicine. Rather, they strategically incorporate different cultural practices to maximize their gain. For example, when examining international health interventions in Ethiopia, Carruth (2014) found that "despite rising demand for pharmaceuticals and diagnostic technologies, and even in the midst of different public health and humanitarian interventions" (p. 405), local communities continued to draw upon popular ideas about humoral flows, divine action, and spirit possession. Carruth (2014) explained, "Demands for therapeutic camel's milk, Qur'anic spiritual healing, herbal remedies, and other historically popular therapies continued, but were fundamentally shaped by people's *concurrent demands* for and understandings of diagnostic biotechnologies and pharmaceutical medications" [emphasis added] (p. 406). Similarly, a study of Aboriginals in Canada found that 30–40% of them consulted health providers in community health centers and hospitals but also accepted treatment from traditional healers (Kaufert, 1999).

As we travel across and between cultures, we do not simply choose to adopt one cultural perspective and abandon prior views, even when they may be incompatible with one another. Diverse cultural perspectives co-exist as our cultural repertoires, creating rich meanings for our social world. Recent literature on acculturation has demonstrated that individuals are unlikely to abandon their own cultural values once they become familiar with or even adaptive to the new cultural practices (Kramer, 2013; Wade et al., 2007). For example, even though acculturations of Japanese Americans would entail adopting U.S. norms, Japanese Americans continue to retain traditional Japanese attitudes that influence their end-of-life care and health decision-making (Matsumura et al., 2002).

Individuals tend to develop layers of consciousness and pluralistic approaches to managing different areas of life. In other words, time does not make a person forget or abandon his or her original cultural norms. Several studies have demonstrated that acculturation level does not predict individuals' health practices in abandoning prior health beliefs and health practices (Ma, 1999; Wade et al., 2007); rather, interactions between cultural systems allow individuals to develop multiple repertoires. For example, a Chinese patient may prefer to adopt a biomedical model for acute conditions but rely on traditional Chinese medicine for chronic illnesses (Chung et al., 2014). An American physician may welcome shamanistic practices for patients' spiritual well-being but feel strongly about ensuring accurate medication and dosing practices (Brown, 2009).

Individuals' strategic adherence to diverse medical systems may make them appear to have low health literacy. In the book *The Spirit Catches You and You Fall Down*, the western doctors were furious and shocked to realize that the dedicated, loving Hmong parents systematically underdosed their daughter's anticonvulsant drugs, which often resulted in serious and long-lasting side effects (Fadiman, 1997). As the child patient continued to have seizures caused by epilepsy, the frustrated doctors questioned that either the parents did not care or that they were too ignorant to understand the consequences of their actions. However, from the parents' perspectives, the medications were making their child sicker. The daughter's epileptic seizures suggested to them that she might "grow up to be a shaman, [because she had these spirits in her...] this was not so much a medical problem as it was a blessing" (Fadiman, 1997, p. 22). The parents' strategic dosing was intended to maintain the delicate balance of positive health status with the culturally valued status of a shaman (see Figure 7.4).

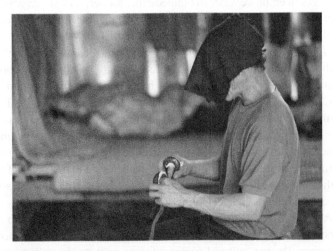

Figure 7.4 Hmong shaman during a ceremony. *Source:* Eric Lafforgue/agefotostock

Conceptualizing health literacy through cultural lenses does not mean that there are no standards for (high versus low) health literacy. Zarcadoolas et al. (2005) proposed that cultural literacy should be a domain of health literacy. **Cultural literacy** was defined as "the ability to recognize and use collective beliefs, customs, worldview and social identity in order to interpret and act on health information" (Zarcadoolas et al., 2005, p. 197). Can we establish standards to measure health literacy *and* to account for corresponding cultural perspectives? The challenges of adopting a medical pluralistic approach to an understanding of health literacy lie in the delicate balance of patient autonomy, patient empowerment, and "appropriate" health decision-making.

When considering how to best achieve ethical decision-making, Oppong (2019) argued that different cultures would likely have different manifestations of behavioral processes. In other words, "ethical decisions will be expected to vary across cultural space and even evolve with time" (Oppong, 2019, p. 21). Recognizing that different cultures can have different preferences of information management (e.g., information seeking) to achieve optimal health-decision making for the patient means that researchers and healthcare providers must suspend the common tendency to view other cultural practices as inferior or as instances of low health literacy. Abhijit Banerjee and Esther Duflo (2019), 2019 Nobel Prize winners in economics, explained:

> It is both patronizing and wrong-headed, in our view, to assume people must have screwed up just because we might have behaved differently. And yet society routinely overrules people's choices, especially if they are poor, supposedly for their own good, for instance when we give them food or food stamps rather than cash. We justify this on the grounds we know better what they really need. [...We] argue that the choices of the poor often make more sense than we give them credit for. (p. 100)

Within the health literacy literature, an ideal patient is envisioned to be someone who is able and willing to independently obtain, process, understand, and use basic information and services for health decision making. However, such an ideal is a product of western biomedicine, cultural influences, and economic affluence. It is important to avoid equating the ideal patient prescribed in the literature as a universal or transcendental model of an ideal patient in every culture. A cultural approach to health literacy recognizes that individuals' health decisions are bound by cultural contexts and the environment in which they are embedded. As such, whether a person has high health literacy or not is not necessarily dependent on the quantity or frequency of information-seeking. Rather, high health literacy is reflected when a person can effectively exercise the communicative skills needed to achieve their needs, including informational, interpersonal, and sociocultural objectives. As such, patients with high health literacy may require different communicative skills and have different communicative patterns depending on the contexts of the illness event.

IV. Additional Resources

A. Key Terms and Theories

literacy
functional literacy
health literacy
    personal health literacy
    organizational health literacy
functional health literacy
interactive health literacy
Life Skills Training (LST)
critical health literacy
social determinants of health
appraisal
coping
sterilization law
Tuskegee syphilis study
STD experiments in Guatemala
HIV discordant couples study in Haiti
low context cultures/communication
high context cultures/communication
family-centered model (of decision-making)
patient autonomy model (of decision-making)
medical pluralism
co-cultural groups
cultural literacy

B. Discussion Questions

1. Several definitions of health literacy are discussed in the chapter. Which one do you like best? Why?
2. Using an online search engine, can you find sample tests for the Rapid Estimate of Adult Literacy in Medicine (REALM) and The Test of Functional Health Literacy in Adults (TOFHLA)? Do you like these tests? Why or why not? Do they accurately measure our understanding of health literacy? What type of health literacy is measured?
3. Jose is a Spanish-speaking migrant agricultural worker. He woke up in the middle of the night, finding himself in a cold sweat, high fever, and severe cramps in his stomach. Please provide examples of the kinds of skills he should have for functional health literacy? How about interactive health literacy? Critical health literacy?
4. Using examples of social determinants of health (e.g., employment conditions, social exclusion, gender equity, globalization, and urbanization), please explain how these examples can shape a person's *critical* health literacy?

5. Please give examples of health behaviors that may first appear as poor or problematic to "outsiders" but are, in fact, adaptive and "rational" responses to a person's specific environment.
   a. Why are these behaviors considered problematic to the society of the System?
   b. Why are these behaviors "rational" to the individual?
6. Please define and give examples of low context communication and high context communication.
   a. Can you think of situations when you prefer low context communication? Why?
   b. Are there situations when you prefer high context communication? Why?
   c. What happens when people are mixing high with low context communicator styles and assumptions at the same time in the same conversation?
7. Do you engage in medical pluralism?
   a. How do you engage in medical pluralism? Can you offer some specific examples?
   b. Do you think they help you maintain your identity or relationships? Why?
   c. What kinds of people are more likely to adopt medical pluralism? Why?

C. References

Agency for Healthcare Research and Quality. (2016). *Health literacy measurement tools (revised)*. Retrieved August 8, 2020, from https://www.ahrq.gov/health-literacy/quality-resources/tools/literacy/index.html

American Medical Association (1999). Health literacy: Report of the Council on Scientific Affairs. *JAMA, 281*(6), 552–557.

Andersen, P. A., Hecht, M. L., Hoobler, G. D., & Smallwood, M. (2003). Nonverbal communication across cultures. In W. B. Gudykunst (Ed.), *Cross-cultural and intercultural communication* (pp. 73–90). Sage.

Asare, M., Peppone, L. J., Roscoe, J. A., Kleckner, I. R., Mustian, K. M., Heckler, C. E., Guido, J. J., Sborov, M., Bushunow, P., Onitilo, A., & Kamen, C. (2018). Racial differences in information needs during and after cancer treatment: A nationwide, longitudinal survey by the University of Rochester Cancer Center National Cancer Institute Community Oncology Research Program. *Journal of Cancer Education, 33*(1), 95–101.

Baker, D. W. (2006). The meaning and the measure of health literacy. *Journal of General Internal Medicine, 21*(8), 878–883.

Banerjee, A. V., & Duflo, E. (2019). *Good economics for hard times*. Public Affairs.

Bell, A. V. (2014). "I think about Oprah": Social class differences in sources of health information. *Qualitative Health Research, 24*(4), 506–516.

Berkman, N. D., Davis, T. C., & McCormack, L. (2010). Health literacy: What is it? *Journal of Health Communication, 15*(Suppl. 2), 9–19.

Berkman, N. D., DeWalt, D. A., Pignone, M. P., Sheridan, S. L., Lohr, K. N., Lux, L., Sutton, S. F., Swinson, T., & Bonito, A. J. (2004). *Literacy and health outcomes*. Agency for Healthcare Research and Quality, https://www.ncbi.nlm.nih.gov/books/NBK11942

Bernstein, N. (1999, June 6). *STRINGS ATTACHED – A special report.; For subjects in Cornell's Haiti study, free AIDS care has a price*. The New York Times. https://www.nytimes.com/1999/06/06/world/strings-attached-special-report-for-subjects-haiti-study-free-aids-care-has.html

Blackhall, L. J., Frank, G., Murphy, S., & Michel, V. (2001). Bioethics in a different tongue: The case of truth-telling. *Journal of Urban Health, 78*(1), 59–71.

Botvin, G. J., & Griffin, K. W. (2004). Life skills training: Empirical findings and future directions. *The Journal of Primary Prevention, 25*(2), 211–232.

Bourgois, P., & (1998). The moral economies of homeless heroin addicts: Confronting ethnography, HIV risk, and everyday violence in San Francisco shooting encampments. *Substance Use & Misuse, 33*(11), 2323–2351.

Bourgois, P., Prince, B., & Moss, A. (2004). The everyday violence of hepatitis C among young women who inject drugs in San Francisco. *Human Organization, 63*, 253–264.

Brandt, A. M. (1978). Racism and research: The case of the Tuskegee syphilis study. *Hastings Center Report, 8*(6), 21–29.

Brashers, D. E., Goldsmith, D. J., & Hsieh, E. (2002). Information seeking and avoiding in health contexts. *Human Communication Research, 28*(2), 258–271.

Brashers, D. E., Neidig, J. L., & Goldsmith, D. J. (2004). Social support and the management of uncertainty for people living with HIV or AIDS. *Health Communication, 16*(3), 305–331.

Brashers, D. E., Neidig, J. L., Haas, S. M., Dobbs, L. K., Cardillo, L. W., & Russell, J. A. (2000). Communication in the management of uncertainty: The case of persons living with HIV or AIDS. *Communication Monographs, 67*(1), 63–84.

Brown, P. L. (2009, September 20). *A doctor for disease, a shaman for the soul*. The New York Times, A20. http://www.nytimes.com/2009/09/20/us/20shaman.html

Buck-McFadyen, E. V. (2015). Rural food insecurity: When cooking skills, homegrown food, and perseverance aren't enough to feed a family. *Canadian Journal of Public Health, 106*(3), e140-e146.

Butow, P. N., Lobb, E., Jefford, M., Goldstein, D., Eisenbruch, M., Girgis, A., King, M., Sze, M., Aldridge, L., & Schofield, P. (2012). A bridge between cultures: Interpreters' perspectives of consultations with migrant oncology patients. *Supportive Care in Cancer, 20*(2), 235–244.

Carroll, J. B., & Chall, J. S. (1975). *Toward a literate society: The report of the Committee on Reading of the National Academy of Education*. McGraw-Hill.

Carruth, L. (2014). Camel milk, amoxicillin, and a prayer: Medical pluralism and medical humanitarian aid in the Somali Region of Ethiopia. *Social Science & Medicine, 120*(Suppl. C), 405–412.

Cary, L. (1992, April 6). Why it's not just paranoia: An American history of 'plans' for Blacks. *Newsweek, 119*(4), 23.

Centers for Disease Control and Prevention. (2015). *U.S. Public Health Service Syphilis Study at Tuskegee*. https://www.cdc.gov/tuskegee/index.html

Chesler, M. A., Paris, J., & Barbarin, O. A. (1986). "Telling" the child with cancer: Parental choices to share information with ill children. *Journal of Pediatric Psychology, 11*(4), 497–516.

Chinn, D. (2011). Critical health literacy: A review and critical analysis. *Social Science & Medicine, 73*(1), 60–67.

Chung, E. K., Siegel, B. S., Garg, A., Conroy, K., Gross, R. S., Long, D. A., Lewis, G., Osman, C. J., Jo Messito, M., Wade, R., Shonna Yin, H., Cox, J., & Fierman, A. H. (2016). Screening for social determinants of health among children and families living in poverty: A guide for clinicians. *Current Problems in Pediatric and Adolescent Health Care*, *46*(5), 135–153.

Chung, V. C. H., Ma, P. H. X., Lau, C. H., Wong, S. Y. S., Yeoh, E. K., & Griffiths, S. M. (2014). Views on traditional Chinese medicine amongst Chinese population: A systematic review of qualitative and quantitative studies. *Health Expectations*, *17*(5), 622–636.

Daniels, J. (2000). US funded AIDS research in Haiti: Does geography dictate how closely the United States government scrutinizes human research testing? *Albany Law Journal of Science and Technology*, *11*(1), 203–224.

Davis, T. C., Long, S. W., Jackson, R. H., Mayeaux, E. J., George, R. B., Murphy, P. W., & Crouch, M. A. (1993). Rapid estimate of adult literacy in medicine: A shortened screening instrument. *Family Medicine*, *25*(6), 391–395.

Dinour, L. M., Bergen, D., & Yeh, M.-C. (2007). The food insecurity–obesity paradox: A review of the literature and the role food stamps may play. *Journal of the American Dietetic Association*, *107*(11), 1952–1961.

Ellerby, J. H., McKenzie, J., McKay, S., Gariepy, G. J., & Kaufert, J. M. (2000). Bioethics for clinicians: 18. Aboriginal cultures. *Canadian Medical Association Journal*, *163*(7), 845–850.

Factor, R., Kawachi, I., & Williams, D. R. (2011). Understanding high-risk behavior among non-dominant minorities: A social resistance framework. *Social Science & Medicine*, *73*(9), 1292–1301.

Factor, R., Mahalel, D., Rafaeli, A., & Williams, D. R. (2013). A social resistance perspective for delinquent behaviour among non-dominant minority groups. *The British Journal of Criminology*, *53*(5), 784–804.

Fadiman, A. (1997). *The spirit catches you and you fall down: A Hmong child, her American doctors, and the collision of two cultures.* Farrar, Straus and Giroux.

Gallant, M. P. (2003). The influence of social support on chronic illness self-management: A review and directions for research. *Health Education & Behavior*, *30*(2), 170–195.

Gamble, V. N. (1997). Under the shadow of Tuskegee: African Americans and health care. *American Journal of Public Health*, *87*(11), 1773–1778.

Gauthier, D. K., & Forsyth, C. J. (1999). Bareback sex, bug chasers, and the gift of death. *Deviant Behavior*, *20*(1), 85–100.

Glasgow, R. E., Toobert, D. J., Barrera, M., Jr., & Strycker, L. A. (2004). Assessment of problem-solving: A key to successful diabetes self-management. *Journal of Behavioral Medicine*, *27*(5), 477–490.

Goldman, D. S. (2004). The modern-day literacy test: Felon disenfranchisement and race discrimination note. *Stanford Law Review*, *57*(2), 611–656.

Hall, E. T. (1976). *Beyond culture.* Anchor Books.

Hallenbeck, J. (2006). High context illness and dying in a low context medical world. *American Journal of Hospice and Palliative Medicine*, *23*(2), 113–118.

Hancock, K., Clayton, J. M., Parker, S. M., Wal der, S., Butow, P. N., Carrick, S., Currow, D., Ghersi, D., Glare, P., Hagerty, R., & Tattersall, M. H. (2007). Truth-telling in discussing prognosis in advanced life-limiting illnesses: A systematic review. *Palliative Medicine*, *21*(6), 507–517.

Heller, J. (2017, May 10). *AP was there: Black men untreated in Tuskegee syphilis study.* Associated Press. https://apnews.com/e9dd07eaa4e74052878a68132cd3803a

Hsieh, E. (2013). Health literacy and patient empowerment: The role of medical interpreters in bilingual health communication. In M. J. Dutta & G. L. Kreps (Eds.), *Reducing health disparities: Communication intervention* (pp. 41–66). Peter Lang.

Johnson, R. L., Saha, S., Arbelaez, J. J., Beach, M. C., & Cooper, L. A. (2004). Racial and ethnic differences in patient perceptions of bias and cultural competence in health care. *Journal of General Internal Medicine, 19*(2), 101–110.

Kaufert, J. M. (1999). Cultural mediation in cancer diagnosis and end of life decision-making: The experience of Aboriginal patients in Canada. *Anthropology & Medicine, 6*(3), 405–421.

Kempson, K. M., Keenan, D. P., Sadani, P. S., Ridlen, S., & Rosato, N. S. (2002). Food management practices used by people with limited resources to maintain food sufficiency as reported by nutrition educators. *Journal of the American Dietetic Association, 102*(12), 1795–1799.

Kirsch, I., & Guthrie, J. T. (1977). The concept and measurement of functional literacy. *Reading Research Quarterly, 13*(4), 485–507.

Kirsch, I., Jungeblut, A., Jenkins, L., & Kolstad, A. (1993). *Adult literacy in America: A first look at the findings of the National Adult Literacy Survey.* National Center for Education Statistics.

Kline, W. (2005). *Building a better race: Gender, sexuality, and eugenics from the turn of the century to the baby boom.* University of California Press.

Knobloch, L. K., & Carpenter-Theune, K. E. (2004). Topic avoidance in developing romantic relationships: Associations with intimacy and relational uncertainty. *Communication Research, 31*(2), 173–205.

Kramer, E. M. (2013). Dimensional accrual and dissociation: An introduction. In J. Grace & E. M. Kramer (Eds.), *Communication, comparative cultures, and civilizations* (Vol. 3, pp. 123–184). Hampton.

Kramer, E. M. (2019). Cultural fusion theory. In J. F. Nussbaum (Ed.), *Oxford research encyclopedia of communication.* Oxford University Press. https://doi.org/10.1093/acrefore/9780190228613.013.679

Kramer, E. M., Callahan, C., & Zuckerman, S. D. (2013). *Intercultural communication and global integration.* Kendall Hunt.

Kramer, E. M., & Johnson, L. J. (1997). A brief archaeology of intelligence. In E. M. Kramer (Ed.), *Postmodernism and race* (pp. 31–50). Praeger.

Kutner, M., Greenberg, E., Jin, Y., & Paulsen, C. (2006). *The health literacy of America's adults: Results from the 2003 National Assessment of Adult Literacy.* National Center for Education Statistics. http://nces.ed.gov/pubs2006/2006483.pdf

Lim, T.-S. (2003). Language and verbal communication across cultures. In W. B. Gudykunst (Ed.), *Cross-cultural and intercultural communication* (pp. 53–71). Sage.

Lloyd, C. E., Smith, J., & Weinger, K. (2005). Stress and diabetes: A review of the links. *Diabetes Spectrum, 18*(2), 121–127.

Lubetkin, E. I., Zabor, E. C., Isaac, K., Brennessel, D., Kemeny, M. M., & Hay, J. L. (2015). Health literacy, information seeking, and trust in information in Haitians. *American Journal of Health Behavior, 39*(3), 441–450.

Ma, G. X. (1999). Between two worlds: The use of traditional and Western health services by Chinese immigrants. *Journal of Community Health, 24*(6), 421–437.

Matsumura, S., Bito, S., Liu, H., Kahn, K., Fukuhara, S., Kagawa-Singer, M., & Wenger, N. (2002). Acculturation of attitudes toward end-of-life care. *Journal of General Internal Medicine, 17*(7), 531–539.

McLain, D. L., Kefallonitis, E., & Armani, K. (2015). Ambiguity tolerance in organizations: Definitional clarification and perspectives on future research. *Frontiers in Psychology, 6*, Article 344. https://doi.org/10.3389/fpsyg.2015.00344

Michielutte, R., Alciati, M. H., & El Arculli, R. (1999). Cancer control research and literacy. *Journal of Health Care for the Poor and Underserved, 10*(3), 281–297.

Miller, K., & Zook, E. G. (1997). Care partners for persons with AIDS: Implications for health communication. *Journal of Applied Communication Research, 25*(1), 57–74.

Mold, J. W. (2006). Facilitating shared decision making with patients. *American Family Physician, 74*(7), 1209–1210, 1212.

Molina, N. (2017). Why didn't more ethnic Mexicans sign up for Obamacare?: Examining public health's impact over one hundred fifty years. *American Journal of Medical Research, 4*(2), 20–46.

Moskowitz, D. A., & Roloff, M. E. (2007). The existence of a bug chasing subculture. *Culture, Health & Sexuality, 9*(4), 347–357.

Mukherjee, S. (2016). *The gene: An intimate history.* Scribner.

Muller, J. H., & Desmond, B. (1992). Ethical dilemmas in a cross-cultural context: A Chinese example. *Western Journal of Medicine, 157*(3), 323–327.

Mystakidou, K., Parpa, E., Tsilika, E., Katsouda, E., & Vlahos, L. (2004). Cancer information disclosure in different cultural contexts. *Supportive Care in Cancer, 12*(3), 147–154.

The National Literacy Act of 1991, Pub. L. 102–73 (1991). https://www.govinfo.gov/content/pkg/STATUTE-105/pdf/STATUTE-105-Pg333.pdf

Nielsen-Bohlman, L., Panzer, A. M., & Kindig, D. A. (Eds.). (2004). *Health literacy: A prescription to end confusion.* National Academies Press.

Nutbeam, D. (1998). Health promotion glossary. *Health Promotion International, 13*(4), 349–364.

Nutbeam, D. (2000). Health literacy as a public health goal: A challenge for contemporary health education and communication strategies into the 21st century. *Health Promotion International, 15*(3), 259–267.

Nutbeam, D. (2008). The evolving concept of health literacy. *Social Science & Medicine, 67*(12), 2072–2078.

Nutbeam, D. (2009). Defining and measuring health literacy: What can we learn from literacy studies? *International Journal of Public Health, 54*(5), 303–305.

O'Connor, P. J., Gregg, E., Rush, W. A., Cherney, L. M., Stiffman, M. N., & Engelgau, M. M. (2006). Diabetes: How are we diagnosing and initially managing it? *Annals of Family Medicine, 4*(1), 15–22.

Office of Disease Prevention and Health Promotion. (2020a, August 18). *Health literacy in Healthy People.* https://health.gov/our-work/healthy-people-2030/about-healthy-people-2030/health-literacy-healthy-people

Office of Disease Prevention and Health Promotion. (2020b). *Social determinants of health.* https://health.gov/healthypeople/objectives-and-data/social-determinants-health

Oppong, S. (2019). When the ethical is unethical and the unethical is ethical: Cultural relativism in ethical decision-making. *Polish Psychological Bulletin, 50*(1), 18–28.

Orbe, M. P. (1997). *Constructing co-cultural theory: An explication of culture, power, and communication.* Sage.

Paasche-Orlow, M. K., & Wolf, M. S. (2007). The causal pathways linking health literacy to health outcomes. *American Journal of Health Behavior, 31*(Suppl.), S19–S26.

Parker, R. M., Baker, D. W., Williams, M. V., & Nurss, J. R. (1995). The test of functional health literacy in adults: A new instrument for measuring patients' literacy skills. *Journal of General Internal Medicine, 10*(10), 537–541.

Parsons, S. K., Saiki-Craighill, S., Mayer, D. K., Sullivan, A. M., Jeruss, S., Terrin, N., Tighiouart, H., Nakagawa, K., Iwata, Y., Hara, J., Grier, H. E., & Block, S. (2007). Telling children and adolescents about their cancer diagnosis: Cross-cultural comparisons between pediatric oncologists in the US and Japan. *Psycho-Oncology, 16*(1), 60–68.

Patient Protection and Affordable Care Act, Pub. L. No. 111–148, 124 Stat. 119 (2010). https://www.govinfo.gov/content/pkg/PLAW-111publ148/pdf/PLAW-111publ148.pdf

Razzante, R. J., & Orbe, M. P. (2018). Two sides of the same coin: Conceptualizing dominant group theory in the context of co-cultural theory. *Communication Theory, 28*(3), 354–375.

Rees, C. E., & Bath, P. A. (2000). Meeting the information needs of adult daughters of women with early breast cancer: Patients and health care professionals as information providers. *Cancer Nursing, 23*(1), 71–79.

Reeves, P. M., Merriam, S. B., & Courtenay, B. C. (1999). Adaptation to HIV infection: The development of coping strategies over time. *Qualitative Health Research, 9*(3), 344–361.

Reverby, S. M. (2001). More than fact and fiction: Cultural memory and the Tuskegee syphilis study. *Hastings Center Report, 31*(5), 22–28.

Reverby, S. M. (2012). *Tuskegee's truths: Rethinking the Tuskegee syphilis study.* University of North Carolina Press.

Richardson, A., Allen, J. A., Xiao, H., & Vallone, D. (2012). Effects of race/ethnicity and socioeconomic status on health information-seeking, confidence, and trust. *Journal of Health Care for the Poor and Underserved, 23*(4), 1477–1493.

Rodriguez, M. A., & García, R. (2013). First, do no harm: The US sexually transmitted disease experiments in Guatemala. *American Journal of Public Health, 103*(12), 2122–2126.

Rubinelli, S., Schulz, P. J., & Nakamoto, K. (2009). Health literacy beyond knowledge and behaviour: Letting the patient be a patient. *International Journal of Public Health, 54*(5), 307–311.

Rutten, L. J., Arora, N. K., Bakos, A. D., Aziz, N., & Rowland, J. (2005). Information needs and sources of information among cancer patients: A systematic review of research (1980–2003). *Patient Education and Counseling, 57*(3), 250–261.

Schembri, S., & Ghaddar, S. (2018). The Affordable Care Act, the Medicaid coverage gap, and Hispanic consumers: A phenomenology of Obamacare. *Journal of Consumer Affairs, 52*(1), 138–165.

Sheon, N., & Crosby, G. M. (2004). Ambivalent tales of HIV disclosure in San Francisco. *Social Science & Medicine, 58*(11), 2105–2118.

Smith, D. (2011). Health care consumer's use and trust of health information sources. *Journal of Communication in Healthcare, 4*(3), 200–210.

Solomon, M. Z. (1997). From what's neutral to what's meaningful: Reflections on a study of medical interpreters. *Journal of Clinical Ethics, 8*(1), 88–93.

Sørensen, K., Van den Broucke, S., Fullam, J., Doyle, G., Pelikan, J., Slonska, Z., & Brand, H. (2012). Health literacy and public health: A systematic review and integration of definitions and models. *BMC Public Health, 12,* Article 80. https://doi.org/10.1186/1471-2458-12-80

Spears, D. (2011). Economic decision-making in poverty depletes behavioral control. *The B.E. Journal of Economic Analysis & Policy, 11*(1), Article 72. https://EconPapers.repec.org/RePEc:bpj:bejeap:v:11:y:2011:i:1:n:72

Speros, C. (2005). Health literacy: Concept analysis. *Journal of Advanced Nursing, 50*(6), 633–640.

Stern, A. M. (2016). *Eugenic nation: Faults and frontiers of better breeding in modern America.* University of California Press.

Stinson, E. J., Votruba, S. B., Venti, C., Perez, M., Krakoff, J., & Gluck, M. E. (2018). Food insecurity is associated with maladaptive eating behaviors and objectively measured overeating. *Obesity, 26*(12), 1841–1848.

Wade, C., Chao, M. T., & Kronenberg, F. (2007). Medical pluralism of Chinese women living in the United States. *Journal of Immigrant and Minority Health, 9*(4), 255–267.

Weiner, M., & Long, J. (2004). Cross-sectional versus longitudinal performance assessments in the management of diabetes. *Medical Care, 42*(2 Suppl.), II-34-II-39.

White House. (1997, May 16). *Presidential apology: Remarks by the President in apology for study done in Tuskegee.* Centers for Disease Control and Prevention. https://www.cdc.gov/tuskegee/clintonp.htm

White House. (2010, October 1). *Read-out of the President's call with Guatemalan President Colom.* Office of the Press Secretary. https://obamawhitehouse.archives.gov/the-press-office/2010/10/01/read-out-presidents-call-with-guatemalan-president-colom

World Health Organization. (2019). *Social determinants of health.* https://www.who.int/social_determinants/sdh_definition/en

Zarcadoolas, C., Pleasant, A., & Greer, D. S. (2005). Understanding health literacy: An expanded model. *Health Promotion International, 20*(2), 195–203.

Zubialde, J. P., & Aspy, C. B. (2001). It is time to make a general systems paradigm reality in family and community medicine. *Families, Systems, & Health, 19*(4), 345–359.

Zubialde, J. P., & Mold, J. W. (2001). Relational value: Bridging the worldview gap between patients and health systems. *Family Medicine, 33*(5), 393–398.

Zwi, K. J., Woodland, L., Kalowski, J., & Parmeter, J. (2017). The impact of health perceptions and beliefs on access to care for migrants and refugees. *Journal of Cultural Diversity, 24*(3), 63–72.

8

Group-Based Identities

Cultural Approaches to Social Stigma and Health Practices

Chapter 8 examines social stigma as a cultural structure to control and regulate both targeted groups and other members in a cultural system. By exploring the meanings and functions of social stigma in different cultural perspectives, we will investigate how such tensions can be resolved by the larger society through interventions in public health and health policy. Using veterans and LGBTQ individuals as examples of social groups, we will examine their experiences of and responses to social stigma. In addition, by examining how cultural perspectives shape their understanding and response to stigmatizing traits, we will examine why certain solutions and interventions are more effective than others.

I. Social Stigma and Health Behaviors

A. Social Stigma as Magic Consciousness

Magic Consciousness can be challenging to grasp as a theoretical concept, partly because we live in a highly perspectival culture – making it difficult to understand and recognize Magic Consciousness. At its core, Magic Consciousness is essential to one's very existence and life meanings. Magic Consciousness need not be "logical" in the sense of rationality through scientific means. Nevertheless, a person (or a group) is intensely emotionally invested in the maintenance, protection, and survival of the Magic Consciousness because it is the foundation of meanings and values of the person's (or the group's) existence. For a Jehovah's Witness who refuses life-saving blood transfusion or a Native American who risks sepsis by refusing to amputate a limb, learning more about the benefits of the proposed treatment or its positive outcomes would not change their minds. This is because they made these health decisions not because they lack the knowledge or do not have sufficient information to make the "right" choice. Rather, they know what they need to know already (i.e., what it takes to be a Native American with a good afterlife or to be a faithful Jehovah's Witness that is respected in his community). Their choice is not based on a cost-benefit analysis of the proposed treatment (i.e., Perspectival Thinking) but on their identities that are contingent upon following the corresponding Magic Consciousness. In addition, they would not have been aware that their decisions were based on Magic Consciousness – they are simply doing what is taken-for-granted.

Rethinking Culture in Health Communication: Social Interactions as Intercultural Encounters, First Edition. Elaine Hsieh and Eric M Kramer.
© 2021 John Wiley & Sons, Inc. Published 2021 by John Wiley & Sons, Inc.

Social stigma is one of the prime examples of how an individual (or society) constructs and maintains Magic Consciousness. In his seminal work, Goffman (1963/2009) argued that stigmas represent a unique relationship between individuals' attributes and negative stereotypes. Stigma links a person to an undesirable stereotype, reducing the person "from a whole and usual person to a tainted, discounted one" (Goffman, 1963/2009, p. 2). A stigmatized person experiences prejudice from others. **Prejudice** is "an aversive or hostile attitude toward a person who belongs to a group, simply because he belongs to that group, and is therefore presumed to have the objectionable qualities ascribed to the group" (Allport, 1958, p. 7). When concealed, the stigmatizing attribute remains "discrediting" and the person's identity is "discreditable;" however, once a person's stigmatizing attribute is known, the person's identity is permanently "discredited" to the ones who know the "truth" (Goffman, 1963/2009).

Goffman's (1963/2009) work on social stigma has inspired researchers from a wide range of disciplines to examine the nature, meaning, and functions of stigma in cultural systems. Illness as a deviation from a "normal" or "healthy" status is vulnerable to cultural attributions of stigma, resulting in individuals' experiences of marginalization and prejudice (Parsons, 1951). Stigma is the co-occurrence of labeling, stereotyping, separation, status loss, and discrimination in a context in which power is exercised (Link & Phelan, 2001). In other words, **public stigma** is the consequence when the power within a cultural system imposes stereotyping labels onto a specific group of people that results in the loss of status of the stigmatized group and, at the same time, approves (if not encourages) its cultural members to discriminate against the group. A stigmatized status can include a wide range of characteristics, including race/ethnicity, socioeconomic status (e.g., poverty and welfare recipients), illness status (e.g., HIV positive, leprosy, or mental illness), and personal traits (e.g., disability, obesity, and sexual orientations).

Stigma can occur "at the *individual* level (i.e., the unequal treatment that arises from membership in a particular social group) and at the *structural* level (i.e., societal conditions that constrain an individual's opportunities, resources, and well-being)" (Hatzenbuehler et al., 2013, p. e1). Researchers have found that social stigma has a profound impact on individuals' health and well-being, limiting one's access to resources (e.g., increased barriers to accessing social welfare or health facilities), shaping one's coping behaviors (e.g., social isolation), and impacting the quality of care (Stuber et al., 2008). For example, stigmatized individuals often *internalize* their experiences of stigma and accept the negative societal perceptions of one's stigmatized status (i.e., self-stigmatization or **self-stigma**). Self-stigma can result in loss of self-esteem and self-efficacy. For example, persons with schizophrenia and addiction issues have been found to reflect on their struggles with mental illness. One respondent reported, "Enjoying life is not possible if you do not believe that you even have a right to exist, let alone consider improving your self-esteem, which, in my experience, is one of most therapists' favorite topics" (Gallo, 1994, p. 409). A drug addict talked about feeling ashamed about his addiction, "At the end of the day, you've got to be happy with yourself and I'm not happy with myself, I don't look in the mirror and say I love myself, I don't even like myself, I self-loathe myself, I hate myself, I hate what I've done to myself and done to others by doing it to myself" (Matthews et al., 2017, p. 279). Reflecting on his relationships with the larger society, a homeless person explained:

I'm like, "Oh look at what they all have that I don't have." "Oh, look, normal people. Ohh." [laughs] Yeah, I've been getting a little bit bitter, I mean. I've already been excluded most of my life and now this is just one more stack against me that makes me even more excluded. You know, I'm just so sick of it. [laughs]. It's like I'm not a real person. (Kramer & Hsieh, 2019, p. 49)

In the movie, *Forrest Gump*, when Forrest first learned that he has a son, he emotionally and anxiously asks, "He's the most beautiful thing I've ever seen. But... is- is he smart? Or is he..." This was a powerful moment in the film because despite Forrest's triumph over his disabilities and his apparent financial, athletic, and even heroic successes, this was the first moment he publicly acknowledged that he is not "smart." As accomplished, optimistic, and naïve as he was, Forrest still internalized the social stigma of not being smart as the core aspect of his self-identity.

Stigmatized group members have also been found to experience an elevated level of stress in their everyday lives, resulting in a "corrosive influence on health" (Hatzenbuehler et al., 2013, p. e4). **Structural stigma** refers to the sociocultural structures that create systematic barriers and stigma against the targeted group. We will explore structural stigma more systematically in Chapter 14. In addition, according to Goffman (1963/2009), people who are associated with stigmatized individuals (e.g., friends and family members) can also experience **courtesy stigma** (i.e., stigma by affiliation). Family members of patients with HIV infection, schizophrenia, intellectual disabilities (e.g., Down syndrome and autism), and inherited disorders reported experiences of marginalization, including avoidance, hostile staring, and rude comments, from their communities (Ali et al., 2012; Angermeyer et al., 2003; Clarke, 2016; Gray, 2002). A review article found that in some non-western cultures (e.g., Arab, Bangladeshi, Pakistani, Indian, and Taiwanese cultures), family caregivers (usually mothers) are even marginalized *within* families after giving birth to a child with disabilities (Ali et al., 2012). Parents of children with autism reported that because their children failed to meet society's expectations, not only are their children stigmatized, they are also blamed for their lack of parental control (Gill & Liamputtong, 2011). From this perspective, a recipient of courtesy stigma may also incur additional social stigma targeting them (e.g., being a bad parent). Such additional stigma may be independent of their association with the stigmatized individuals.

Reflecting on the ways stigma is communicated, Smith (2007) argued that messages that stigmatize others have four attributes: They provide content cues (a) to distinguish people (i.e., identify or assign a mark/symbol that highlights their unique attributes), (b) to categorize these distinguished people as a separate social entity (i.e., labeling a group by its stigmatizing characteristics), (c) to link this distinguished group to physical and social peril (i.e., highlight dangers imposed by the group), and (d) to imply a responsibility of receiving the stigmatized status. Through communication, members of a community are motivated to enforce stigma (and the corresponding social order) within a network as they strengthen the bonds between in-group members.

In summary, social stigma highlights the demarcation of in-group and out-group membership. Once a person's stigmatizing trait is known, the stigmatized identity cannot be mitigated nor ignored – the identity is forever discredited, and the person is no longer viewed as an in-group member. The now (newly) stigmatized out-group member can be so "tainted" that even the in-group members who are affiliated with him or her will experience stigma by affiliation.

It is important to point out that not all social stigmas are a result of Magic Consciousness. For the same stigma, some may understand and enforce the stigma due to their cultural perspectives in Mythic Connection or Perspectival Understanding. Nevertheless, Magic Consciousness can be a powerful motivator for a society to encourage and promote a social stigma. Because social stigma is about a society (or a community) cultivating and imposing negative views of a particular group that results in discrimination against that particular group, why can we not simply tell the society to stop imposing these stigmatizing attitudes? Thornicroft et al. (2007) proposed that stigma involves the problem of knowledge (i.e., ignorance), attitude (i.e., prejudice), and behavior (i.e., discrimination). Can we educate members of society to make sure that they have accurate and sufficient knowledge so that they will stop stigmatizing a particular group? Believing that social stigma can be reduced or eliminated by "appropriate" knowledge is a product of Perspectival Thinking. Knowing HIV is mainly transmitted through unprotected sexual behaviors or sharing needles/ syringes does not necessarily eliminate one's fear or hostility about sharing the same living space with people with HIV. Knowing that LGBTQ is a biological condition that defines a person's sexual orientation does not necessarily reduce one's prejudice against people with LGBTQ status. Why? To think that providing a person with accurate knowledge will be sufficient to reduce stigma is a failure to recognize the possibilities of Magic Consciousness or Mythic Connection in supporting and maintaining these social stigmas.

B. Functions of Social Stigma

Social stigma is a powerful tool for social control. Bayer (2008) argued that although individual suffering and social inequity can be caused by stigma, there may be circumstances "when public health efforts that unavoidably or even intentionally stigmatize are morally defensible" (p. 471). Based on a review of 18 conceptual constructs of the literature on social stigma and prejudice, Phelan et al. (2008) concluded that social stigma and prejudice is a single phenomenon that is associated with three specific functions: (a) exploitation and domination (i.e., keeping people down); (b) norm enforcement (i.e., keeping people in); and (c) disease avoidance (i.e., keeping people away). At its core, social stigma functions through in-group and out-group distinctions. However, different cultural perspectives may have drastically different understandings about the distinctions between in- versus out-groups and the meanings of these functions.

1. From the Perspectives of Perspectival Thinking

For people with Perspectival Thinking, all three functions are a means to an end. The enforcement of social stigma is impersonal. Issues of morality and ethics are justified through the efficiency of the means in achieving desired ends. Under Perspectival Thinking, what is rational depends on wants and desires postulated as goals. Perspectival Thinking is not devoid of magic and mythic thinking. In fact, Magic Consciousness and Mythic Connection often endure and even motivate perspectival planning. The means to achieve those goals, which are rooted in emotional drives (wants, needs, and desires), are proposed and evaluated according to measures of achieving those goals and appear purely rational.

One of the worst episodes of social stigma in world history is the eugenics movements in the first half of the 20th century, particularly in Great Britain, the United States, and Germany (Kühl, 2002). Francis Galton (1883) coined the term **eugenics** by combining the Greek prefix *eu* – "good" with *genesis*: "good in stock, hereditarily endowed with noble qualities" (p. 24). For Galton, eugenics is "the betterment of the human race via artificial selection of genetic traits and directed breeding of human carriers" (Mukherjee, 2016, p. 72). The first eugenics sterilization legislation in the world was passed in 1907 by the state legislature in Indiana, allowing the use of involuntary sterilization to "prevent the procreation of confirmed criminals, idiots, imbeciles and rapists" (Hassenstab, 2014, p. 300; Medical Humanities-Health Studies Program, n.d.). In Nazi Germany in the 1940s, human eugenics was used to "justify grotesque experiments, culminating in confinement, sterilization, euthanasia, and mass murder" (Mukherjee, 2016, p. 13). In the United States, driven by "prejudiced notions of science and social control," federally-funded sterilization programs took place in 32 states throughout the 20th century (Ko, 2016).

In the United States, in a 1927 Supreme Court Case, *Buck v. Bell*, the State of Virginia won the case, by a vote of 8 to 1, to compel sterilization of Carrie Buck. Carrie's mother, Emmett Adaline Buck, was confined in the Virginia State Colony for life in 1920 after two doctors determined that she was "feebleminded" when she was arrested for vagrancy and/or prostitution. When Emmett was sent to the Colony, Carrie was placed in foster care, where she was raped and impregnated by her foster parents' nephew (see Figure 8.1). Carrie's daughter, Vivian Elaine, born in 1924, was placed in foster care. In Carrie's trial, a nurse claimed that both Emmett and Carrie

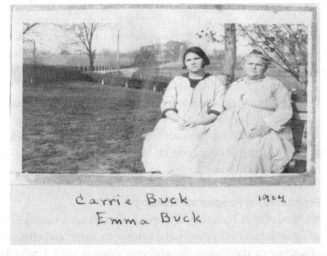

Figure 8.1 Carrie and Emma Buck at the Virginia Colony for Epileptics and Feebleminded. Carrie and Emma Buck in 1924, right before the *Buck v. Bell* trial, which provided the first court approval of a law allowing forced sterilization in Virginia. Courtesy of M.E. Grenander Department of Special Collections and Archives, University at Albany, SUNY. *Source:* Courtesy of M.E. Grenander Department of Special Collections and Archives, University at Albany, SUNY

were impulsive, irresponsible mentally, and "feebleminded." A social worker, who observed Carrie's daughter, explained that although it's difficult to assess an 8-month-old baby and she may be biased as a result of the trial of Carrie, "there is a look about it that is not quite normal, but just what it is, I can't tell" (Mukherjee, 2016, p. 82; see Figure 8.2). In the end, the Supreme Court held that Virginia's forced sterilization of Carrie was constitutional as Justice Holms concluded, "Three generations of imbeciles is enough" (*Buck v. Bell*, 1927, p. 207; see also Cohen, 2016). In other words, sterilization laws pertaining to the "feebleminded" were constitutional (Silver, 2004).

In the 1920s, "feeblemindedness" was regularly used by legislatures in the United States to legitimize government authority and to limit fundamental rights (e.g., due process, privacy, and reproductive rights) of a diverse group of men and women, "some with no mental illness at all – prostitutes, orphans, depressives, vagrants, petty criminals, schizophrenics, dyslexics, feminists, rebellious adolescents – anyone, in short, whose behavior, desires, choices, or appearance fell outside the accepted norm" (Mukherjee, 2016, p. 79). In the name of "science" and social Darwinism, scholars, scientists, government officials, and even judges all supported "racial betterment" through eugenics. Justice Stone explained, "Science has found and the law has recognized that there are certain types of mental deficiency associated with delinquency that are inheritable" (*Skinner v. Oklahoma*, 1942, p. 545). The Supreme Court decision in *Buck v. Bell* has had a lasting impact on sterilization laws in the United States, many of which were not repealed until the 1970s and 1980s (Silver, 2004). As of 2016, various states compelled sterilization of 60,000 to 70,000 individuals under these laws (Reilly, 1991; "The Supreme Court Ruling that Led to 70,000 Forced Sterilizations," 2016).

Eugenics movements in the United States provide excellent examples of the three functions of social stigma in a Perspectival Thinking culture. By identifying the specific traits and groups of people eligible for the enforcement of involuntary sterilization laws, a society effectively creates hierarchies between groups of people (i.e., exploitation and domination) and warns citizens about the dangers of and punishment for deviant, abnormal behaviors, which often are behaviors deemed undesirable by the authoritative powers (i.e., norm enforcement). Given the goal of attempting to overtly engineer a population of "better" individuals, eugenics appears to be a rational, dispassionate means, particularly if desired traits are believed to be predetermined by genetics. By highlighting that the bad traits (e.g., "feeblemindedness") are inheritable through genes, the government justified its violence and violation against these peoples' fundamental rights to ensure that its citizenship is healthy and untainted (i.e., disease avoidance).

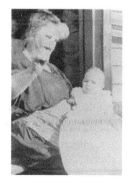

Figure 8.2 Mrs. Alice Dobbs, the foster mother of Carrie Buck's daughter Vivian, holds Vivian while flashing a coin past the baby's face, in a test to assess her intelligence. Because Vivian didn't follow the coin with her eyes, she was declared an imbecile. A. H. Estabrook, the person who initiated this test of the infant's intelligence and the photographer, took this picture the day before the *Buck v. Bell* trial in Virginia. Courtesy of M.E. Grenander Department of Special Collections, State University of New York at Albany. *Source:* Courtesy of M.E. Grenander Department of Special Collections, State University of New York at Albany.

The strong emotions evoked through social stigma are grounded in Magic Consciousness and, to a lesser degree, Mythic Connection. They do not exist under Perspectival Thinking. When Perspectival Thinking is taken to an extreme, a single perspective can be conflated with objective reality. It implies a hegemonic, authoritarian approach to reality. As Foucault (1966/2005) notes, this inflation of a single perspective to the totality of true objective reality is the essence of unequal power. When one perspective treated as the only "true" perspective, complexity and changes are lost. In other words, although Perspectival Thinking is not emotional or "superstitious," it does not mean that Perspectival Thinking is "better" or more "rational," "civilized," or "advanced."

As the readers can see that by arguing that science provides the objective and neutral evidence of "inheritable" traits, a society of Perspectival Thinking can easily embrace forced sterilization and even mass murder, including genocide of the groups of people who are reckoned via various operational instruments to be demonstrably inferior or dangerous (as so defined): the poor, the disabled, the mentally ill, criminals, indigenous people, and people of color (Black, 2012; Ko, 2016). A pure Perspectival Thinking view of eugenics considers selective breeding, sterilization, and killing of targeted groups as a mechanical process to achieve the desired objective of "race betterment." Such acts, though unfortunate, were considered effective and necessary to ensure the betterment of the human race.

2. From the Perspectives of Magic Consciousness and Mythic Connection

A closer examination of eugenics movements in the United States, however, suggests that for some people, their motivation is highly emotional and personal. Reflecting on the history of eugenics movements in the United States, Justice Marshall stated:

> [T]he mentally retarded have been subject to a "lengthy and tragic history" ... of segregation and discrimination that can only be called grotesque. ... Fueled by the rising tide of Social Darwinism, the "science" of eugenics, and the *extreme xenophobia* of those years, leading medical authorities and others began to portray the "feeble-minded" as a "menace to society and civilization ... responsible in a large degree for many, if not all, of our social problems." A regime of state-mandated segregation and degradation soon emerged that, in its virulence and bigotry, rivaled, and indeed paralleled, the worst excesses of Jim Crow. [emphasis added] (*City of Cleburne v. Cleburne Living Ctr.*, 1985, p. 461)

Researchers of eugenics movements in the United States have agreed that the rise of the movement is embedded in racism (Black, 2012; Kühl, 2002; Reilly, 2015). Mukherjee (2016) explained,

> Between 1890 and 1924, nearly 10 million immigrants – Jewish, Italian, Irish, and Polish workers – streamed into New York, San Francisco, and Chicago, packing the streets and tenements and inundating the markets with foreign tongues, rituals, and foods (by 1927, new immigrants comprised more than 40% of the populations of New York and Chicago). And as much as class anxiety had driven the eugenic efforts of England in the 1890s, "race anxiety" drove the eugenic efforts of Americans in the 1920s. (p. 82)

Xenophobia (i.e. an undue or excessive fear, hatred or dislike of strangers or foreigners) and racism necessitate a distinction of us versus "the Other." Viewing other races or new immigrants as pollutants or diseases that are threatening or even destroying the once harmonious balance of *our* society shifts the Perspectival Thinking into Mythic Connection and/or Magic Consciousness.

From this perspective, one can argue that exploitation and domination is a function adopted from a Perspectival Thinking perspective, but not for people with Magic Consciousness or Mythic Connection. This is because for people of Magic Consciousness and Mythic Connection, they do not think in terms of exploitation or domination. They simply believe that the hierarchy was just the way the world is meant to be (or God wants it to be). One of the best examples of such attitudes is described by Stephen Douglas in the famed Lincoln-Douglas debates in 1858 (see Figure 8.3):

> Douglas had nothing in particular against the Negro: "I would give him every right and every privilege which his capacity would enable him to enjoy." But that "capacity" was far below that of the white man, and "I am free to say to you, that ... this government of ours is founded on the white basis." For a white man to enslave a white man was a violation of the other white man's claim to freedom under the Constitution. But "a negro, an Indian, or any other man of an inferior race" belonged to an entirely different category; they could be enslaved without any violation of "free governments" because the American free government had never intended to include them. No "negro, descended from African parents" had moral, natural, or legal standing to plead for the protections the Constitution gave white people, any more than a horse, a cow, or a pig. (Guelzo, 2010, pp. 77–78)

For people with Magic Consciousness or Mythic Connection, their "discrimination" was not discriminatory per se. For people with Magic Consciousness, only the people in their communities are the true people because outsiders are not truly human. Magic people share a unified identity (and blood ties). Thus, for Douglas, it was perfectly natural and normal to think that although a White man cannot enslave another White man, such rules do not apply to outsiders, who are no different from stock animals. Magic Consciousness and Mythic Connection worldviews consider the denial of rights to "the Other" as part of the natural law. It was necessary to enforce the social (and natural) orders.

Under Magic Consciousness and Mythic Connection, order implies both social and natural categories of the sociocultural worldviews because the modern perspectival dichotomy of nature and culture does not yet dominate. Social implies convention. But if inequality is ordained by nature, there is no room for deviation. Norm enforcement and disease avoidance are often central functions for social stigma for Magic Consciousness and Mythic Connection. It is not "personal." It is simply the way things are, the "order of things," as Foucault (1966/2005) puts it. The "natural fact" is that the Other does not have the same rights, privileges, and responsibilities as myself and other members of my group. By constructing "the Other" as risks that threaten the survival of their cultures, magic and mythic peoples rely on social stigma to enforce central values and principles of their social worlds.

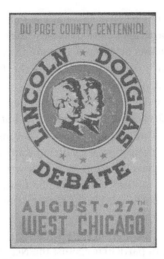

Figure 8.3 Poster of Lincoln-Douglas debate. The Lincoln–Douglas debates (also called The Great Debates of 1858) were a series of seven debates between Abraham Lincoln, the Republican Party candidate for the United States Senate from Illinois, and incumbent Senator Stephen Douglas, the Democratic Party candidate. At its core, the debates are about: What is the nature of the Union and how to best protect the interests of "We the People" in a free society? Lincoln took the Founding Fathers at their words, and invoked the Declaration of Independence, noting the Declaration "defined with tolerable distinctness in what they did consider *all men* created equal in certain inalienable rights, among which are life, liberty, and the pursuit of happiness. This they said, and this they meant" [emphasis added] (Lincoln & Douglas, 1860, p. 225). *Source:* The Library of Congress

For example, for many religious (and cultural/ethnic) groups, accepting or even acknowledging the existence or legitimacy of a person's LGBTQ status (i.e., lesbian, gay, bisexual, transgender, and queer) is fundamentally destabilizing to their faith. One study found that religious variables (e.g., religious affiliation and religiosity) have stronger effects than other demographic measures (e.g., gender, education, political ideology) on shaping individuals' attitudes about same-sex marriage (Olson et al., 2006). If one holds an anti-LGBTQ view as part of their Magic Consciousness for their collective identity with the group, then they will be highly motivated to eradicate any existence of LGBTQ presence (e.g., marginalizing LGBTQ members or even imposing death penalties) let alone making any accommodations or compromises to ensure LGBTQ members' equality in the society (Mogul et al., 2011; Ungar, 2000).

If a cultural group (or society) views certain illnesses as a punishment from God, then the cultural group as a whole may feel righteous and even empowered in their moral status as they punish and discriminate against others who are afflicted with the illness. For example, the Bible legitimizes social discrimination against people with leprosy: "Anyone with such a defiling disease must wear torn clothes, let their hair be unkempt, c cover the lower part of their face and cry out, 'Unclean! Unclean!' As long as they have the disease they remain unclean. They must live alone; they must live outside the camp" (*New International Version*, 1978/2011, Leviticus 13:45–46). The person with leprosy is expected to self-isolate from the larger society (i.e., live alone) and to claim a condemned status (i.e., cry out "unclean! unclean!" and wear "torn clothes"). To this day, there are still many (former) leprosy colonies in India, Brazil, and China, where people with leprosy are forced to live together due to government interventions and social/local pressures. From a Perspectival Thinking perspective, one may argue that the isolation is necessary due to the highly contagious nature of leprosy. However, Magic Consciousness does not justify its treatment to marginalized members through "logic" per se. Instead, a cultural group operating under Magic Consciousness simply accepts as normal and legitimate social discrimination because these groups of people are afflicted by supernatural forces or the larger universe. In contrast, under Mythic Connection, the persons are punished because they have "sinned" – a failure of their character and/or identity.

For people with Magic Consciousness or Mythic Connection, the stigmatized people are the "chosen ones." Marginalizing them is necessary to maintain the social values and moral standards (i.e., norm enforcement) and to keep "us" safe (i.e., disease avoidance). Accepting and legitimizing discrimination is essential to maintaining identity, the balance and harmony of the universe, and their social world.

In Amish communities, individuals who have committed serious offenses or who are seen as "kickin' up" trouble are usually met with the punishment of excommunication and shunning. Shunning is "a ritual of shaming that is used in public occasions and face-to-face interaction to remind the ostracized that they are outside the *moral order*" [emphasis added] (Kraybill, 2003, p. 16). Hurst and McConnell (2010) explained, "In theory, the system of excommunication and shunning illustrates that the authority of the church supersedes family ties. Family members are to shun their wayward relatives just as any other church member would; the baptismal water is expected to be thicker than blood" (p. 84). For a documentary about Amish people's shunning practice against people who have decided to leave their closed and tightly-knit communities, you may want to look up *The Amish: Shunned* (Wiser, 2014). The Magic Consciousness of Amish community/culture relies on connections to the church, rather than familial blood ties, as the criteria to distinguish insiders versus outsiders. Shunning, a communal act of excluding deviants, becomes a powerful tool of norm enforcement for both the ones that are shunned as well as those who stay within the community.

A critical element in these stigmatizing discourses is the cultural groups' concerns about how the stigmatized group, if left unchecked and unrestrained, may impose fundamental corruption and corrosion to the existence of their own cultural groups, values, or existence (i.e., disease avoidance). Similar processes have legitimized discrimination against various groups, including ethnic groups (e.g., Jewish; Isaac, 1964), personal traits (e.g., LGBTQ individuals; Kim, 2018), and illnesses (e.g., HIV; Kopelman, 2002). In a 2014 Supreme Court case, *Hobby Lobby* argued that when the Affordable Care Act requires all organizations to provide health insurance coverages that include four objectionable methods of contraception (i.e., two forms of morning-after pills and two types of intrauterine devices), its owners are forced to run their business in violation of "their religious beliefs and moral principles" because they believe that "human life begins at conception" and it is "against [their] moral conviction to be involved in the termination of human life" after conception, which they believe to be a "sin against God to which they are held accountable" (*Burwell v. Hobby Lobby Stores, Inc.*, 2014, p. 701). Magic Consciousness serves as the foundation of *Hobby Lobby*'s argument. They do not argue that these four methods of contraception are ineffective or harmful. Instead, the argument is highly personal (i.e., they will be held accountable by God if they provide access to contraceptives for their employees) and emotional (i.e., the government mandate requires them to commit immoral acts), highlighting the necessity to limit its employees' access to health resources despite its consequences for healthcare inequality. In her dissenting opinion, Justice Ginsburg raised concerns about how similar arguments may be used by commercial corporations to discriminate against race, religion, sex, or sexual orientation excused by and based on religious grounds (*Burwell v. Hobby Lobby Stores, Inc.*, 2014; Gasper, 2015).

As one considers the meanings, functions, and implications of social stigma, it is important to recognize that these cultural groups may sincerely believe that they do not "discriminate" or "hate" the stigmatized individuals. Their imposition of social stigma may not be a result of ignorance, which can be "fixed" by education. In fact, relying on education to eliminate social stigma reflects the western bias of Perspectival Thinking (Corrigan, 2018). Magic Consciousness is holistic and encompassing. The cultural groups may simply believe that such beliefs, acts, and practices are necessary because they are essential to the survival of their own cultural values and existence.

Finally, the general public is much more willing to accommodate and support individuals with physically-based stigma (e.g., blindness and Alzheimer's disease) than mental-behavioral stigma (e.g., HIV+, addiction, and obesity), which is often associated with individuals' perceived responsibility (Weiner et al., 1988). Because modern society highly aligns with a Perspectival Thinking worldview, many stigmatized groups have relied on biomedicalization of their experiences to circumvent the scrutiny of Magic Consciousness or Mythic Connection, which often emphasizes individual responsibilities and morality. By pathologizing and medicalizing their stigmatizing traits, stigmatized groups highlight their lack of control and minimize their responsibilities over their stigmatized status. Some examples of such efforts include the narratives of addiction as a brain disease (Berridge, 2017; Leshner, 1997) and sexual orientations as a result of genetic factors (Schüklenk et al., 1997). Such an approach to eliminate social stigma is highly perspectival, as the "deviant" and "abnormal" traits are objectified and pathologized. Although such an approach may be efficient in soliciting support to the stigmatized groups because they are no longer perceived to be responsible for their unfortunate status, it is important to point out that such an approach does not create a transformative environment for the stigmatized. It does not provide a sense of agency to empower stigmatized groups (Berridge, 2017). Such an approach does not demonstrate a society's willingness to understand the Other's perspectives: The society as a whole does not become more inclusive to "the Other" nor more empathetic to their suffering. In fact, ethicists have warned that such an approach can lead to science/medicine-based interventions to eliminate the undesirable genes (Schüklenk et al., 1997), echoing the not-so-distant memory of eugenics.

II. Managing Identities and Social Stigma

The literature on social stigma and health highlights that individuals' social identities are essential to their health behaviors as well as the communities' response to their struggles. A cultural approach to health and illness is to recognize the underlying cultural perspectives that influence individuals' health behaviors. In the following section, we reference two social groups, veterans and LGBTQ individuals, to illustrate how different cultural perspectives may lead to drastically different understandings of and responses to their health behaviors.

A. Veterans as a Social Group

1. Socialization for a Collective Identity

From ancient times, the military has been a critical part of society, defending its citizens against outsiders. According to National Center for Veterans Analysis and Statistics (2020), there were an estimated 19.2 million U.S. veterans (approximately 6% of the U.S. population) in 2019, among whom 10% were female. Roughly one in four veterans (i.e., 4.94 million) receives VA disability compensation. Over 47.1% of veterans are over age 65. The total number of U.S. veterans are expected to decline in the coming decades. The demographic profile of veterans is also expected to change dramatically between 2016 and 2045, with a higher percentage of female (18%), slightly younger, and racially and ethnically more diverse populations (Bialik, 2017).

Being a veteran is an identity of Magic Consciousness and/or Mythic Connection. Military socialization aims to transform new recruits from a civilian into a new identity that strongly identifies with the military community, creating a *disciplined body* capable of carrying out military labor and waging war on the enemy (Cooper et al., 2018). Military values, such as loyalty, integrity, courage, determination, and a commitment to duty, are not only aspired but *embodied* by soldiers and Marines (i.e., a person with Mythic Connection aspires to live by these values; a person with Magic Consciousness believe that *they* are the embodiment of these values). Failure to assimilate means the denial of membership. "Army of One." "Once a Marine, always a Marine." "Semper fidelis" (usually shortened to Semper Fi, meaning "always faithful" or "always loyal"). "Aut Vincere Aut Mors" (Latin for "conquer or die"). These slogans and mottos evoke a connected, shared identity. A ritual for Navy SEALs highlights the idolic Magic Consciousness and/or symbolic Mythic Connection of being one of "us" (see Figures 8.4 and 8.5):

> SEALs approach a gravesite one by one, remove the gold-colored pin from the left breast of their dress uniforms and pound them into the coffin of a fallen comrade. The living mourn, with the primary symbol of their brotherhood missing, to be replaced only after the dead have been buried.
>
> The dead take their comrades' SEAL pins with them to the grave.
>
> The pin is the most tangible sign of membership in a famously exclusive community: an eagle perched on a horizontal three-pronged trident, clutching a flintlock pistol, with an upright anchor nestled in the mix. They are symbols of the domains that comprise the SEAL acronym: Sea, Air and Land. (Ismay, 2019, para. 1–3)

Under Navy regulations, a SEAL's Trident can be taken if a commander loses "faith and confidence in the service member's ability to exercise sound judgment, reliability and personal conduct" (Phillipps, 2019 , para. 8). Thus, though one can easily purchase

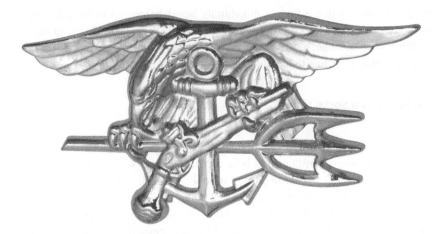

Figure 8.4 U.S. Navy Sea Air Land (SEAL) Trident badge. *Source:* Jason Meyer / Alamy Stock Photo

the pin online for $13.50, losing one's Trident is "tantamount to excommunication, being cast off to the hinterlands of the conventional Navy for reassignment" (Ismay, 2019, para. 8). For a SEAL, the pin is not a replaceable object (in Perspectival Thinking), but a symbol for an identity and values he honors (i.e., Mythic Connection). For some others, owning this pin or wearing the uniform means that he *is* a different category of person (i.e., Magic Consciousness). For a person with Magic Consciousness, there is no greater punishment than stripping a person's community membership, making him "the Other." To have the Trident removed can be an identity crisis for a SEAL. No mythic or magic interpretations can affect the impact of the loss. There is no "good way" to interpret or "spin" it.

2. Cultural Approaches to Mental Illness in Military Contexts

Recognizing the Magic Consciousness and/or Mythic Connection in a veteran's identity and worldview is essential in addressing veteran health. The society and the military has a long tradition in stigmatizing mental health disorders, creating barriers for help-seeking activities and heightening the risks for self-harming behaviors (Greene-Shortridge et al., 2007). A review of 144 studies found that (a) stigma has a small- to moderate-sized negative effect on help-seeking and (b) military service members are disproportionally deterred by stigma concerns (Clement et al., 2015). A review of the literature suggests that between 54–72.9% of military and veterans in need of mental

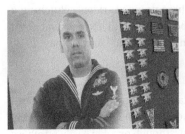

Figure 8.5 Ryan Larkin. In his parents' home, a photo of Ryan Larkin, a decorated Navy SEAL who committed suicide after suffering from undiagnosed Traumatic Brain Injury, is displayed next to the SEAL Tridents left by comrades on his casket. *Source:* AP photos

health care failed to seek care (Acosta et al., 2014). Despite increased intervention efforts, more than 6,100 veterans died by suicide in 2017 (i.e., about 17 individuals per day), reflecting a 2% increase since 2016 and a 6% increase over the last 12 years (Shane, 2019). Among military service members who participated in combat duty in Iraq and Afghanistan, concerns about stigma were greatest among those most in need of mental health services: individuals who scored positive on mental disorders were twice as likely as those who scored negative to show concerns about being stigmatized (Hoge et al., 2004). Compared to women, men are more likely to internalize stigma (Vogel et al., 2007).

Stigmatization of mental health issues must be understood within the military culture, which has little tolerance for (physical or psychological) weakness (Nash et al., 2009). Some of the top concerns that affect decisions to seek mental health care include: harm to career trajectory, loss of confidence in unit members, disparate treatment from unit leadership, loss of current/future security status, and concerns of record confidentiality (Acosta et al., 2014). A Perspectival Thinking approach to service members' concerns is to develop better mechanisms and procedures to safeguard personal information and records, avoid bias, and assure career trajectory.

However, Blocker and Miller (2013) warned that the recent procedures that aim to increase vigilance and preventive actions can result in a chilling effect causing soldiers to self-sensor and avoid seeking care. This is because a Perspectival Thinking approach cannot address concerns rooted in Magic Consciousness and Mythic Connection, which often define a military service member's identity and worldview. A soldier is expected to be a reliable and capable body that is ready to execute orders. As such, mental health concerns pose uncertainty to the reliability and trustworthiness of the body, resulting in a fundamental, disabling effect to a soldier's (or Marine's) identity (and thus, group membership). Recognizing that one has a failing, untrustworthy body that poses risks to his or her peers and uncertainties to complete orders from unit leaders is likely to generate shame.

Shame is an intense negative emotion having to do with the self in relation to standards/responsibilities. It is experienced as a global self-failure in one's community (Lewis, 1998). Unlike social stigma, which takes place in public, shame (and self-stigmatization) can be both public and private (Lewis, 1998). Shame is collective and community-oriented, reflecting the knowledge that one does not belong to the community. In contrast, **guilt** is the negative emotions one holds toward the failure of specific behaviors, not self, and thus, more likely to be experienced by people with Perspectival Thinking (which is more individualistic). Shame is an affective response to and a result of self-stigmatization. Hasson-Ohayon et al. (2012) found that shame, but not guilt, mediates one's insight and self-stigma. **Insight** is defined as individuals' awareness of their illness-condition and willingness to take action, ranging from complete denial of illness (i.e., lack of insight) to actively seeking treatment for an illness condition (Reddy, 2016). When a patient has high insight, they are "better" patients because they recognize that they are ill and thus, are more likely to seek healthcare services and adhere to treatment plans (Tessier et al., 2017). However, studies also suggest that the more one is aware of the illness label, the need for treatment, the illness implication, the more she is likely to experience shame, which in turn, leads to an increase in self-stigma. In addition, although the perception of public stigma has a significant impact on whether a person seeks mental health care, the relationship is fully mediated by self-stigma (Vogel et al., 2007). In other words, compared to perceived public stigma, self-stigma is a better and more direct predictor of whether a person would seek mental health care.

When individuals with predominantly Magic Consciousness or Mythic Connection believe that they fail to meet group standards, they are likely to feel shame (i.e., failure of self); in contrast, a person inhabiting Perspectival Thinking is likely to feel guilt (i.e., failure of specific behavior). Traditionally, the literature views the experience of guilt to be more adaptive because it focuses the person on the specific action taken or not taken (e.g., "Why did I do *that*?"), implying opportunities to change; in contrast, shame is considered maladaptive because it focuses the person toward the Self (e.g., "Why did *I* do that?"), paralyzing remedial actions that could have been taken (Dempsey, 2017). However, such categorization assumes that the person adopts Perspectival Thinking, and thus, is capable of fragmenting and distinguishing their actions from their identity. Recent literature has recognized that both shame and guilt can be both adaptive and maladaptive, depending on the contexts, including situational nuances and cultural variations (Dempsey, 2017).

If a veteran inhabits and exhibits Magic Consciousness or Mythic Connection about their identity as a group member, then their fear about career trajectory, confidence and trust from peers, and disparate treatment from leaders should be understood as the fear of losing group membership, rather than individual success. As they become more aware of their (hidden) mental illness, they recognize that they do not belong to the group that they identify with. In addition, they realize that insisting on staying in the group puts everything they love (their peers and the community) at risk – they are a potential danger to their community – the proverbial weak link in the chain. Self-stigmatization becomes inevitable. To avoid being ostracized by the community, label avoidance becomes necessary.

Label avoidance is defined as situations when people purposefully do not acknowledge symptoms or participate in mental health services in order to avoid the stigma and negative consequences resulting from a formal diagnostic label being applied to them (Ben-Zeev et al., 2012). The harmful effect of label avoidance is self-evident when individuals who are ill, purposefully work to avoid the stigmatizing label by concealing their symptoms and avoiding necessary diagnosis and treatment (i.e., staying "closeted;" Corrigan, 2018). However, label avoidance is not new to U.S. military service members. After all, label avoidance was the encouraged behavior of the 17-year policy of "Don't ask; Don't tell" that required LGBTQ military members to keep their sexuality a secret if they wanted to continue to serve in the military (Ben-Zeev et al., 2012). A Perspectival Thinking approach may consider providing a better safeguard for privacy (e.g., discrete location and entrance for a mental health clinic or providing anonymous counseling hotline) as solutions to address service members' label avoidance behaviors; in contrast, a Magic Consciousness or Mythic Connection approach recognizes that label avoidance is not about the "label" per se but about identity and belonging. Under Perspectival Thinking, a label is just a way to call things and can be changed arbitrarily; in contrast, under Magic Consciousness, as one is named, realities are invoked (i.e., one comes into existence); and under Mythic Connection, labels call forth the qualities and characteristics essential to the identity of the person. To truly address label avoidance for service members with magic or mythic identities, a new culture of the military community – redefining the meanings of reliable, trustworthy bodies that are ready and able for military duties – is necessary.

At this point, readers may wonder: Are there things that individual service members can do? For individuals with Magic Consciousness or Mythic Connection, their identities, moral codes, and ethics are tied to their communities. They are not (and cannot be) separated from the community. Not being part of the community means symbolic death as their existence becomes meaningless (and purposeless in the sense of Perspectival Thinking as magic people probably do not care about "purpose"). So, a short answer to the question would be: "No."

However, a more sophisticated answer would be: "Yes, if the service members develop an amenable Integral Fusion worldview." By *amenable*, we mean that the service members engage in interactive and continuing dialogues/conversations within their community to achieve mutually agreeable (and beneficial) objectives. For example, rather than completely surrendering and assimilate oneself into the Magic Consciousness or Mythic Connection of a military identity, a service member may reframe their mental illness with new meanings that are consistent with their valued identities in the community.

3. Reframing Veterans' Mental Health Issues

An example of an Integral Fusion worldview is to reframe the stigmatizing mental health disorders as physical injuries. For example, Nash et al. (2009) proposed the *stress injury* model, arguing that mental health disorders are a result of *physical* injury: "Ongoing preclinical and clinical studies of neurobiology are filling in the details in a coherent picture of the damage extreme stress can inflict on the brain" (p. 793). More recently, researchers and clinicians have argued that psychological trauma, depression, and mental resilience should be considered as part of *brain* health for military members and veterans (Friedl, 2014). Conceptualizing mental illness as physical injuries may first appear to adopt a Perspectival Thinking approach, particularly in the ways researchers and clinicians rely on scientific language (e.g., "brain injury" or advances in "neurobiology") to objectify individuals' suffering. However, reframing mental health issues as part of physical health is a strategy for short-circuiting **Cartesian dualism** (i.e., mind-body dualism: mind and body exist as separate entities; Switankowsky, 2000) that are foundational to the existing framework in western biomedicine.

A closer look suggests that such an approach reflects an Integral Fusion worldview, evoking Magic Consciousness and Mythic Connection that are particularly salient and powerful in addressing mental health concerns in military contexts.

Although service members can experience both physical and psychological wounds, service members' physical injuries do not carry the stigmatizing connotations of mental illness but are transformed into symbols of heroism. For example, when the U.S. Paralympics created the Paralympic Military Program in 2004, the goals were to emphasize "the rehabilitative benefits of sport," and to discover "potential elite athletes capable of representing the USA in international competitions"(Batts & Andrews, 2011). As "elite sports men and women with prosthetic limbs, wheelchairs and national flags draped around their shoulders," the display of "cyborg" bodies becomes a sense of pride and patriotism (Cree & Caddick, 2020, p. 266; see Figure 8.6). A physically "disabled" soldier is transformed into a survivor, a role model, and a top athlete, enjoying redemption and triumph through a "rehabilitated" body that is not just as good but *better* than most (Stassi, 2017).

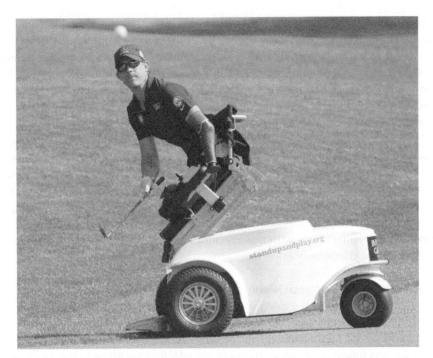

Figure 8.6 Invictus Games. A U.S. Marine Corps veteran competes in a golf tournament at the Invictus Games, an international Paralympic-style event for injured or sick military personnel and veterans. *Source:* DOD Photo / Alamy Stock Photo

Thus, by reframing mental illness as "physical injuries" to the "brain," and recasting mental health disorders as "invisible wounds" carried by soldiers, the emerging narratives create a new Mythic Connection for the *scars* they carry in their brains. Just like the lost limbs, these invisible wounds, though disruptive to the soldier's biography (e.g., career trajectory), also *reinforce* the soldier's identity as a member of the military community (i.e., **biographical reinforcement**) and provide a new resource to enrich their understanding of self (i.e., **biographical illumination**; e.g., finding strengths and resilience through mental health struggles; for a detailed discussion of biographical disruption, reinforcement, and illumination, see Chapter 3).

Through the narratives of mental illness as physical (brain) injuries, military and veterans' magic and/or mythic identities are secured because when seen as physical injuries, mental injuries are perceived as being much more amendable of rehabilitation. Consequently, the journey of recovery is more tangible/associatively relatable and understandable. It also becomes redemptive and even heroic. But more than this, these injuries are not mere residual "scars;" rather, under Magic Consciousness and Mythic Connection, they become a part of this person's identity *and* the group's identity. The disability is a continuation of the event that is not past but present and transformative of those who behold it. The injuries become stories that are memorialized through the common blood of the tribal "we."

In short, the Integral Fusion approach allows military and veterans to actively display their mental health scars as *evidence* of their group membership. The group membership is not dependent on the successful elimination of their mental illness, nor is it threatened when they show signs of "injury." If anything, their mental illness now understood as "physical injury" strengthened their group identity. For people with Mythic Connection, these scars are the symbols of a valued identity ready for storytelling. Joseph Campbell (1949/2008) argues that the most common mythic form recognized the world over is that of the hero: the one who sacrifices for the tribe. For people with Magic Consciousness, these scars are part of being who they are – disciplined bodies. Integral Fusion worldviews provide military service members and veterans the flexibility to identify the paths that best facilitate their healing and well-being, allowing them to connect their past with their future.

It is important to point out that an Integral Fusion worldview is not inherently better than other cultural perspectives. As we noted earlier in Chapter 5, cultural encounters add to the dimensions of our cultural understanding. As soldiers and Marines adopt the Magic Consciousness of military membership through socialization and training, they may continue to hold worldviews that they obtained prior to entering the military group. In recent years, researchers have raised the issue of moral injuries as a form of psychological trauma experienced by military and veterans. Litz et al. (2009) proposed the term **moral injury** as "the lasting psychological, biological, spiritual, behavioral, and social impact of perpetrating, failing to prevent, or bearing witness to acts that transgress deeply held moral beliefs and expectations" (p. 697). Researchers have found that perpetrating, failing to prevent, or witnessing **transgressive acts** (i.e., atrocities and killing that are "inhumane, cruel, depraved, or violent, bringing about pain, suffering, or death of others;" Drescher et al., 2011, p. 9) can have devastating impacts on a person's well-being (e.g., increased risks for depression, psychiatric distress, and suicide behaviors) and identities (e.g., existential despair and meaninglessness; Frankfurt & Frazier, 2016; Litz et al., 2009). Combat veterans are most at risk of moral injuries (Frankfurt & Frazier, 2016). However, although some claimed that drone operators are morally disengaged because of the "video game" like remote killing, recent evidence suggested that witnessing and executing remote killing in real-time can experience moral injuries because killing deemed permissible by others may not be consistent with their own moral principles (Enemark, 2019).

If a military service member is truly assimilated into the Magic Consciousness/ Mythic Connection of a military body/identity, they would not have experienced moral injuries because whatever atrocities and killings that took place were what was meant to be. A soldier or Marine holding a pure Perspectival Thinking perspective is also unlikely to experience moral injuries because they are not emotional nor concerned about morality or their actions. The mission is the goal and the rest are mere means to pursuing the linear objective. As the saying goes, in total war, all is fair. However, they may be frustrated as the killing was not necessary for achieving their objectives (i.e., efficiency concerns).

An Integral Fusion worldview requires integration between the military Magic Consciousness with other worldviews held by veterans. Moral injuries occur when these worldviews conflict with one another. A military service member or a veteran may obtain moral/religious beliefs of viewing human life as sacred prior to joining the military or after returning to civilian life. Litz et al. (2009) explained,

> [I]ndividual service members and units face unanticipated moral choices and demands and even prescribed acts of killing or violence may have a *delayed* but

lasting psychosocial–spiritual impact (e.g., guilt and shame). For example, it makes sense that most service members are able to assimilate most of what they do and see in war because of training and preparation, the warrior culture, their role, the exigencies of various missions, rules of engagement and other context demands, the messages and behavior of peers and leaders, and the acceptance (and recognition of sacrifices) by families and the culture at large. However, once redeployed and separated from the military culture and context (e.g., with family or after retirement), some service members may have difficulty accommodating various morally conflicting experiences. [emphasis added] (p. 697)

In other words, experiences of moral injury do not necessarily take place during combat duty. A veteran can experience moral injuries years later, at an unanticipated time in an unexpected manner. It is only natural that the veteran would feel overwhelmed, startled, and even devastated by the "new revelation" through their Integral Fusion worldviews.

Finally, conceptualizing veterans as a social group does not mean to simplify veterans' identities or cultural perspectives. Although we begin the section by noting that militaries purposefully assimilate individuals into a specific identity of Magic Consciousness to serve military missions, individual service members may develop different cultural understandings of their identities. We believe that many of the current mental health interventions are effective for service members and veterans with Perspectival Thinking. However, for individuals with Magic Consciousness or Mythic Connection, a perspectival approach, regardless of its efficiency or effectiveness, is not able to fully appreciate and respond to their barriers to care. Because Integral Fusion worldviews integrate and accommodate diverging cultural perspectives, they also provide opportunities for innovative solutions for individuals who are "stuck" in a particular cultural perspective. More importantly, because Integral Fusion worldviews are also fluid and amenable, the dynamics and interplay between different cultural worldviews can create tensions at a time and place that are unanticipated.

4. Innovative Solutions through Integral Fusion Approaches

Theory of Message Design Logic (O'Keefe, 1988, 1991) proposed three communicative approaches when individuals confront *multiple* and potentially conflicting goals: ***expressive* message design logic** (e.g., viewing communication as a process to express and receive thoughts and feelings); ***conventional* message design logic** (e.g., viewing communication as a cooperative game that is governed by social norms and rules); and ***rhetorical* message design logic** (e.g., viewing communication as the creation and negotiation of social selves and situations). For example, if a physician were to give criticism to improve a patient's treatment adherence, an expressive message user would say, "This is getting ridiculous. If you do not take your medication as prescribed, I will quit because you are wasting my time;" a conventional message user would say, "I've been your doctor for years and I care about you. If you want to be healthy, you need to take the prescribed medication;" in contrast, a rhetorical message user may say, "I need your advice. I notice that you are not taking the medication regularly, what can I do to help?" A rhetorical message user can not only transform a face-threatening criticism to face-enhancing advice-seeking and consensus-building but also achieve her goal of finding solutions to poor treatment adherence. Similar to our observation of the accrual of cultural dimensions, the three message design logic forms a "natural developmental progression": "Expressive Premise is a logical prerequisite to Conventional functioning, and the Conventional Premise is a logical prerequisite to Rhetorical functioning" (O'Keefe, 1988, pp. 97, 89).

Rhetorical message users must accumulate skills for expressive and conventional messaging (i.e., having the ability to express feelings and thoughts to perform conventionally defined actions), but they also have "the ability to reorder social situations through language," meaning that they "have an abstract sense of communication as a process in which ways of speaking and acting are not merely responses to the situation but constitutive of the situation" (O'Keefe, 1988, p. 89). In other words, rhetorical message users strategically reframe their situations to resolve potential tensions or conflicts through "integration": By altering "the situation to fit the action they want to perform," they reorganized conventionalized action to achieve their desired effects (O'Keefe, 1991, p. 140). O'Keefe (1988) explained,

> Rhetorical messages show a characteristic kind of connection to their context, for rather than being a reaction to some prior condition or taken-for-granted feature of the world, and rather than being a conventional response to some prior state of affairs, instead they are forward-looking and are connected to goals. (p. 88)

From this perspective, a rhetorical message user is a person with an Integral Fusion worldview. Their understanding of others' perspectives and needs, the situational demands, and their own objectives are valuable resources in helping them to find a creative solution that may not be transparent to others.

The strength of an Integral Fusion worldview does not lie in its "final," "ultimate," or "best" solution to a problem. Rather, its strengths lie in individuals' ability and willingness to *continuously* (re)connect and (re)engage with others in dialogues that preserve individual agency, address core values, and respond to tensions (see also Litz et al., 2009). Integral Fusion worldviews allow people to find creative solutions that may appear "outside of the box," including reframing the cause of tensions (e.g., conceptualizing mental health as physical injuries). As cultural participants of Integral Fusion worldviews "test" the strength of their solutions, the flexibility and richness of their worldviews provide the best chance of success.

B. LGBTQ as a Social Group

1. Two Puzzles regarding Stigmatized Identities

The literature on social stigma suggests two puzzles for minorities and marginalized populations: (a) they are encouraged and rewarded for accepting community standards and self-stigmatization; yet, self-stigma are often associated with negative consequences (e.g., shame, delayed diagnosis and treatment, and depression); and (b) individuals who strongly identify with their stigmatizing minority and marginalized status have more positive attitudes and adaptive behaviors than those who don't.

When a community relies on social stigma as a form of social control, cultural participants of the community are motivated to conform to the community rules. For

example, Kaiser and Wilkins (2010) found that the dominant group reacts more negatively toward individuals who strongly identify with a minority identity (e.g., proud to
be an ethnic minority or an LGBTQ individual) than individuals who weakly identify
with a minority identity. A community is motivated to punish people who do not
"know their place" (Herek et al., 2009). We reward weakly identified minorities with
"more opportunities for professional and social advancement than strongly identified
minorities" (Kaiser & Wilkins, 2010, p. 473). The carrot-and-stick approach allows the
community to maintain its social order. In fact, weakly identified minorities have been
found to focus on individual (rather than minority group-oriented) advancement and
exhibit dominant group favoritism (Ellemers et al., 2004; Kaiser & Wilkins, 2010). In
other words, stigmatized individuals are rewarded because they uphold community
standards by distancing their identification with their minority/marginalized group
and favoring the dominant out-group over their own minority in-group.

Management of social stigma is the management of information. As a result, peoples
with stigmatizing and stigmatized traits may actively conceal stigma-inducing information, cues, and traits to avoid discrimination (Goffman, 1963/2009). However, concealment also increases stigma-related stress (e.g., fear of discovery) and implies
self-stigmatization (e.g., accepting community standards; Frost, 2011). **Self-label**
involves adopting and agreeing with the assigned stigmatizing label and negative stereotype given by the community. A study found that the majority of young people with
psychiatric disorders do not passively accept the diagnostic labels that they were given,
but actively incorporate ambiguity and uncertainty when discussing their problems,
adopting a non-pathological depiction (e.g., "family problems" or "teenage problems")
of their struggles (Moses, 2009). In fact, compared to young people who resisted or
avoided the diagnostic label, the ones who self-labeled (i.e., referring to their problem
using psychiatric terms) also reported *higher* levels of self-stigma and depression
(Moses, 2009). Moses (2009) concluded that "self-labeling maybe demoralizing, stigmatizing, and disempowering" for adolescents with psychiatric disorders (p. 576).
Thus, the literature suggests a double bind and the picture that emerged is bleak. To
succeed in a community controlled by outgroup members, individuals of minority and
marginalized populations must learn to accept their assigned label of negative stereotypes, including self-stigma. You will be rewarded for "knowing your place" only when
you accept your inferior status. In short, label avoidance is bad; yet, self-label also leads
to self-stigma, which is also bad.

Recent studies have suggested that minorities and marginalized populations (e.g.,
African American, Latino, and LGBTQ groups) who identify with their stigmatized
groups may report higher self-esteem, less stress arising prejudice, and less self-harm-
ing/compromising behaviors. For example, **identity affirmation** (i.e., positive identity appraisal) with one's LGBTQ status is associated with greater well-being, life
satisfaction, and social connectedness, and less negative affect (Fredriksen-Goldsen et
al., 2017; Kertzner et al., 2009). Stronger identification of ethnic pride reduces Native
Americans students' chance of using illegal drugs and Latino students' cigarette smoking and alcohol use (Kulis et al., 2002). When Mexican-American students have a
strong identification with their cultural identity, they are less likely to engage in risky
health behaviors, including mixed-use of alcohol and drugs, heavy drinking, and regular marijuana use (Love et al., 2006). A meta-analysis of 102 studies found that when
parents instill pride for cultural heritage and ethnic identity in their children, such

messages can lead to children's positive self-perception, increased quality of interpersonal relationships, and buffer against maladaptive behaviors (Wang et al., 2020).

Is it possible for stigmatized groups to reap the benefit of identity affirmation of their stigmatized group without the downfall of accepting community standards, which expects one to also accept an inferior status (i.e., self-stigmatization)? LGBTQ populations' experiences of and success over social stigma can provide insight into potential solutions. LGBTQ populations have experienced stigma in our society and in law, subjecting them to violence, harassment, discrimination, and even criminal status (Leslie, 2000). From the historical oppression of policing and criminalizing sexual and gender "deviants" to the 2015 landmark case, *Obergefell v. Hodges*, when the U.S. Supreme Court held that bans on same-sex marriage are unconstitutional (Mogul et al., 2011; *Obergefell v. Hodges*, 2015), few stigmatized groups have made such success in transforming the larger society (see Figure 8.7). Although many LGBTQ individuals continue to report self-stigmatization and self-injury behaviors (House et al. 2011), others have developed strategies to resist discrimination and strengthen resilience.

2. Inclusive Strategies for Group Membership

Alternative support networks are critical in providing a buffer and creating resilience for LGBTQ populations. We define alternative support networks as individuals who serve as buffers and advocates for marginalized groups against community standards. For example, although family support may be unlikely or unreliable, LGBTQ individuals learn to seek advice, emotional support, socialization, and resources through partners and close friends (Hash & Rogers 2013). Among LGBTQ populations, these networks were found to mitigate mental health problems, reducing

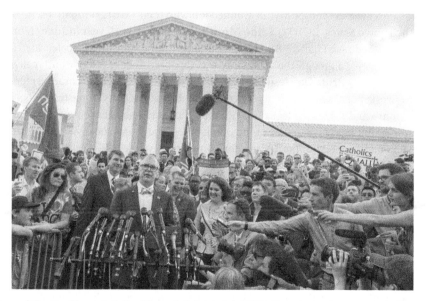

Figure 8.7   Jim Obergefell, Jim Obergefell, lead plaintiff, in the sex marriage case, speaks to the media in front of the United States Supreme Court in Washington, D.C., on June 26, 2015, after the Court's 5–4 ruling was announced that legalizes the ability for same-sex couples to marry nationwide. *Source:* UPI / Alamy Stock Photo

depression and self-stigma (Hash & Rogers, 2013). For transgender individuals, family and peer support were found to have a protective effect, creating resilience and reducing psychological distress (Bockting et al., 2013). In addition, individuals with high levels of peer support reported few negative impacts of actual experiences of discrimination (Bockting et al., 2013). However, because of the pervasiveness of stigma, Bockting et al. (2013) concluded that frequent contact with peers is necessary to reduce the negative impact of actual experiences of discrimination.

An alternative support network can include LGBTQ individuals as well as heterosexual allies. An **ally** is someone who identifies as a non-stigmatized group member, yet actively works to develop an understanding of the needs and experiences of the stigmatized groups and chooses to align with the social and political causes of the stigmatized groups. Jones et al. (2014) proposed that an LGBTQ ally is a heterosexual person who has "(a) knowledge about the experiences and history of LGBT groups, (b) awareness of the experiences of LGBT groups, (c) skills and confidence to assist LGBT persons if they are in need," and engages "(d) in social action efforts to promote change" (p. 182). In other words, social justice activism and advocacy is a salient component of an ally identity – having supportive attitudes are not enough to classify a person as an ally (Jones et al., 2014). LGBTQ allies are primarily motivated by fundamental principles (e.g., justice, civil rights, patriotism, religious beliefs, moral principles, and using privilege to positive ends) or by personal relationships/associations with an LGBTQ individual (Russell, 2011). A study of college athletes found that they are more likely to be engaged LGBTQ issues but not act as visible LGBTQ allies when they perceived that their coaches hold supportive attitudes toward LGBTQ groups; in contrast, athletes who adopt highly engaged and visible LGBTQ ally status are usually driven by a strong sense of social justice (Toomey & McGeorge, 2018). Because their decision to be an ally is value-driven, community-oriented, and closely tied to their sense of identity, they are likely to hold Magic Consciousness and/or Mythic Connection with their LGBTQ affiliations.

In the United States, **LGBTQ Pride Month** is celebrated each year in June (Library of Congress, n.d.; see Figure 8.8). The last Sunday in June was initially celebrated as a "Gay Pride Day" (although the actual day was flexible). Today, Pride Month celebrations and LGBTQ **Pride Day** festivals around the world include pride parades, picnics, parties, workshops, symposia and concerts that attract millions of participants. The Pride Month and Pride Day festival is not only the largest social event of the LGBTQ community but has become part of the public life of the larger society, creating ritual behaviors and business opportunities for commercial venders (Kates & Belk, 2001). **National Coming Out Day,** celebrated on October 11 every year in the United States, marks the anniversary of the National March on Washington for Lesbian and Gay Rights in 1987. Many people use the day to "share their personal coming out stories and support those who choose to keep their identities a secret or come out themselves" (Asmelash, 2019, para. 2).

As Pride Month celebrations and National Coming Out Day have become part of the public life and rituals of global communities, some researchers have raised concerns about how such practices commercialize LGBTQ identity to promote consumerism and implicitly suggest that an LGBTQ identity is so aberrant that it must be proclaimed (Birkhold, 2017; Kates & Belk, 2001). Nevertheless, the "display and show of market power may actually result in social legitimization of the gay and lesbian community" in the larger society (Kates & Belk, 2001, p. 415). A report by the Williams

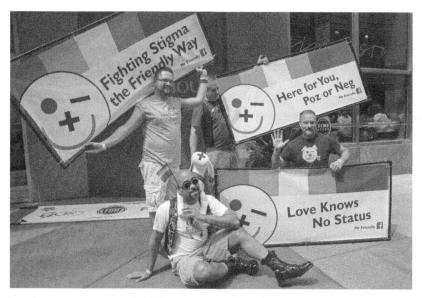

Figure 8.8 Pride parade in Detroit, Michigan. *Source:* Jim West / Alamy Stock Photo

Institute at the UCLA School of Law found that within five years of the Supreme Court's decision to extend marriage equality nationwide (*Obergefell v. Hodges,* 2015), an estimated 293,000 same-sex couples have married since *Obergefell,* boosting state and local economies by an estimated $3.8 billion and generated an estimated $244.1 million in state and local sales tax revenue (Mallory & Sears, 2020).

3. Facilitating Pan-Evolution through Integral Fusion Approaches

The history of the LGBTQ rights movement provides important insights into the management of social stigma for minority and marginalized populations. First, LGBTQ groups embrace differences and diversity when generating an Integral Fusion worldview of a cohesive identity. As a stigmatized group, LGBTQ populations have adopted *inclusive* strategies for group membership and actively built a community, celebrating positive identities for diverse members (Gold, 2018). "Gay" became popular in the 1960s. By the 1990s, the term has come to be used as a shorthand for an entire cluster of sexual and gender minorities (Invannone, 2018). Lesbian, bisexual, and queer (or questioning) were later included to highlight the diversity of the community. Members of sexual and gender minorities have formed alliances through broadening their membership. Invannone (2018) explained,

> Since the 1990s, different versions of the initialism have proliferated as increasingly nuanced ways to understand and define people's lived experience of gender and sexuality are articulated. One expanded version of the initialism in use is LGBTQQIP2SAA, which stands for: lesbian, gay, bisexual, transgender, queer, questioning, intersex, pansexual, two spirit, asexual, and ally. (para. 9)

Eventually, the LGBTQ community converged on the LGBTQ or LGBT+ initialism to balance efficiency and public awareness. Such an approach to LGBTQ group identity injects new meanings to their identities that are inclusive, non-judgmental, and positive, which are particularly effective in reducing self-stigma (Livingston et al., 2012). Through concerted efforts of youth outreach, public education, and leadership development, the LGBTQ movement minimizes the impact of self-stigma for LGBTQ youths and anchors itself to be part of the infrastructure of the larger community. The *evolving* inclusivity of the LGBTQ membership highlights the group's ability to reconcile and build Integral Fusion worldviews to facilitate group members' positive identities and successful coping.

Second, LGBTQ groups are not passive recipients of stigmatizing labels but actively redefine in-group and out-group boundaries that challenge the existing framework imposed by the larger society. Rather than accepting the community standards of an "us versus them" dualism based on sexual orientation, the LGBTQ group actively connected and engaged with heterosexual allies, conferring onto them membership status within the LGBTQ community. Such a strategy not only gave voice to the stigmatized groups but also effectively challenged the boundaries set by the dominant group, creating instability in the dominant groups' control over its community members. In other words, rather than focusing on one's stigmatized status, the LGBTQ community focused on efforts to facilitate the *pan-evolution* of the larger society (for discussion of pan-evolution, see Chapter 5). By embracing opportunities for cultural fusion and securing allies, LGBTQ groups transformed the larger community to support and even celebrate their uniqueness.

Third, LGBTQ groups' approaches to cultural fusion and Integral Fusion worldviews are not limited to that of its members' cultural perspectives, but also those of the members of the larger society. Commercial venders are likely to adopt Perspectival Thinking when contemplating cost-benefit analysis and strategizing its actions to maximize financial gains. Rather than resisting commercialization of the LGBTQ identities and activities, the LGBTQ community *leverages* its new-found commercial powers to legitimize and transform its status: LGBTQ identity is no longer stigmatized, but an identity worthy of (commercialized) ritual celebration. As a result, the LGBTQ community gains support from not just heterosexual allies who share Magic Consciousness or Mythic Connection with the community but also the dominant group "others" who find its commercial interests compatible with LGBTQ activities (i.e., Perspectival Thinking "others"). An LGBTQ individual with Magic Consciousness or Mythic Connection may be disgusted by the commercialization because of its perceived threat to the "authenticity" of LGBTQ identity, the "sacred, real, human, or historical meanings" of being a member of the LGBTQ community (Kates & Belk, 2001, p. 418). In contrast, an Integral Fusion worldview recognizes that "strong emotional and personal meanings attached to the [Pride Day] are not necessarily incompatible with its commercialization" (Kates & Belk, 2001, p. 422), which enhances the experiences of all in-group and out-group participants and ensures the visibility of LGBTQ issues in public discourse.

C. Conclusion

Social stigma has important implications for individuals' illness management and system-level health interventions. At an individual level, minority and marginalized populations are rewarded when they accept their stigmatized status. However, self-stigma can lead to label avoidance, including poor awareness of illness symptoms, delayed diagnosis and treatment, and poor treatment adherence. At an interpersonal level, courtesy stigma can lead to increased stress and pressure for family and friends who are associated with the stigmatized person. In addition, courtesy stigma can pressure members of a community to enforce community standards by distancing from and withdrawing support for stigmatized individuals. At a system-level, structural stigma and discrimination can result in silencing stigmatized groups' suffering and perpetuating inequity and injustice faced by minority and marginalized populations.

Although stigmatized groups are victims of communal violence, the dominant group justifies its use of social stigma to maintain its place with the power hierarchy and to exercise social control, ensuring the stability and viability of the community. Because the meanings and functions of social stigma differ for individuals with Magic Consciousness, Mythic Connection, and Perspectival Thinking, the effectiveness of interventions is dependent on its ability to address individuals' culture-specific concerns and perspectives.

Finally, Integral Fusion worldviews provide the best chance to break the stronghold of in-group and out-group boundaries set by community standards. Integration avoids dualistic ways of understanding relationships (e.g., us versus them or mainstream versus minority). Integration is not a zero-sum game. I can build my repertoire of cultural values. Because Integral Fusion worldviews are inclusive, diverse, and dynamic, individuals with Integral Fusion worldviews have more tools to respond to the challenges in their life journey and to appreciate the differences they encounter. More importantly, because Integral Fusion worldviews encourage its holders to view their relationships with larger communities to be collaborative and evolving, they are not "stuck" in a restrictive cultural perspective or ideology. By focusing on engaging others to achieve mutually agreeable objectives, people with Integral Fusion worldviews find innovative solutions (e.g., reframing the issue) to seemingly unfixable problems. More importantly, because an Integral Fusion worldview emphasizes individual agency and, at the same time, recognizes others' perspectives, it *integrates* differences and *transforms* the larger community. Whereas people of Magic Consciousness, Mythic Connection, or Perspectival Thinking are passive actors within a structure of fixed cultural rules and norms, people with Integral Fusion worldviews actively negotiate their roles and meanings with the larger community. An Integral Fusion approach provides minority and marginalized populations the opportunity to reap the benefit of identity pride without the downfall of social stigma.

III. Additional Resources

A. Key Terms and Theories

social stigma
prejudice
public stigma
self-stigma
structural stigma
courtesy stigma
xenophobia
shame

guilt
insight
label avoidance
Cartesian dualism
biographical disruption (see Chapter 3)
biographical reinforcement (see Chapter 3)
biographical illumination (see Chapter 3)
moral injury
transgressive acts
Theory of Message Design Logic
    expressive message design logic
    conventional message design logic
    rhetorical message design logic
self-label
identity affirmation
alternative support networks
ally
LGBTQ Pride Month
Pride Day
National Coming Out Day

B. Discussion Questions

1. Reflecting on your own, or your family member's experiences of illness, do you have any examples of experiences of the following types of stigma. What are they? Do they influence how you or your family member managed health information or health behaviors? In what ways?
   a. social stigma or prejudice
   b. self-stigmatization
   c. courtesy stigma
2. Reflecting on the public discourse about, and media representation of immigrants in the United States, can you identify and give examples of narratives that perpetuate social stigma to:
   a. keep immigrants down? Suggesting that immigrants are inferior?
   b. keep people in? Enforcing the norms and values of our communities?
   c. keep immigrants away? Suggesting that immigrants pose risks that threaten our communities?
3. The homelessness crises in several cities in California have led to public health concerns in recent years. In particular, the growing homeless population was blamed for a hepatitis A virus outbreak in San Diego in 2019, and an increased amount of fecal matter in California's waterways (Wooten 2019). By adopting Magic Consciousness, Mythic Connection, or Perspectival Thinking,
   a. Can you anticipate how each cultural perspective may frame the suffering and stigma experienced by the homeless population? How and why?
   b. Do you think they would propose different solutions? How and why?
4. Do you know anyone who is a veteran or a military service member?

    a. What type of cultural perspective do they hold with their military identity? Give an example and explain your observation.

    b. If you are planning a health intervention, which type of cultural perspective can lead to better outcomes? In other words, would it be easier to change behaviors if people have Magic Consciousness, Mythic Connection, or Perspectival Thinking? Why?

5. One of the reasons that the LGBTQ rights movement is successful is their ability to transform the larger community.

    a. Can you identify the different ways that society has changed in response to the LGBTQ rights movement?

    b. When some LGBTQ individuals argue that "strong emotional and personal meanings attached to the [Pride Day] are not necessarily incompatible with its commercialization" (Kates & Belk, 2001, p. 422), what kind of worldview do they hold? Why?

    c. Do you think it is appropriate or effective to allow "commercialization" of LGBTQ issues?

6. In recent years, "racist mascots" have been generating emotional and contested conversations among sports fans and local communities. Many of the mascots have names or appearances that reference or resemble Native Americans (see Not Your Mascots, 2020; Randle, 2020).

    a. Do you think Native Americans can or should follow similar strategies adopted by the LGBTQ populations?

    b. Do you think that the history and Magic Consciousness of Native American tribes may shape their willingness to adopt these strategies? Why or why not?

    c. Do you think adopting an Integral Fusion worldview to accept commercialization of their ethnic identity would make a person "lose" their Magic Consciousness or Mythic Connection as Native Americans? Why or why not?

C. References

Acosta, J. D., Becker, A., Cerully, J. L., Fisher, M. P., Martin, L. T., Vardavas, R., Slaughter, M. E., & Schell, T. L. (2014). *Mental health stigma in the military*. RAND. https://apps.dtic.mil/dtic/tr/fulltext/u2/a610275.pdf

Ali, A., Hassiotis, A., Strydom, A., & King, M. (2012). Self stigma in people with intellectual disabilities and courtesy stigma in family carers: A systematic review. *Research in Developmental Disabilities, 33*(6), 2122–2140.

Allport, G. W. (1958). *The nature of prejudice*. Doubleday.

Angermeyer, M. C., Schulze, B., & Dietrich, S. (2003). Courtesy stigma: A focus group study of relatives of schizophrenia patients. *Social Psychiatry and Psychiatric Epidemiology, 38*(10), 593–602.

Asmelash, L. (2019, October 11). *National Coming Out Day: What it is, and what people are saying about it*. CNN. https://www.cnn.com/2019/10/11/us/national-coming-out-day-trnd/index.html

Batts, C., & Andrews, D. L. (2011). 'Tactical athletes': The United States Paralympic Military Program and the mobilization of the disabled soldier/athlete. *Sport in Society, 14*(5), 553–568.

Bayer, R. (2008). Stigma and the ethics of public health: Not can we but should we. *Social Science & Medicine, 67*(3), 463–472.

Ben-Zeev, D., Corrigan, P. W., Britt, T. W., & Langford, L. (2012). Stigma of mental illness and service use in the military. *Journal of Mental Health, 21*(3), 264–273.

Berridge, K. C. (2017). Is addiction a brain disease? *Neuroethics, 10*(1), 29–33.

Bialik, K. (2017, November 10). *The changing face of America's veteran population.* Pew Research Center. https://www.pewresearch.org/fact-tank/2017/11/10/the-changing-face-of-americas-veteran-population

Birkhold, M. H. (2017, October 10). *It's time to end National Coming Out Day.* The Washington Post. https://www.washingtonpost.com/opinions/its-time-to-end-national-coming-out-day/2017/10/10/a9db94ec-ad2b-11e7-9e58-e6288544af98_story.html

Black, E. (2012). *War against the weak: Eugenics and America's campaign to create a master race.* Dialog Press.

Blocker, G.M., & Miller, J. A. (2013). Unintended consequences: Stigma and suicide prevention efforts. *Military Medicine, 178*(5), 473–473.

Bockting, W. O., Miner, M. H., Romine, R. E. S., Hamilton, A., & Coleman, E. (2013). Stigma, mental health, and resilience in an online sample of the US transgender population. *American Journal of Public Health, 103*(5), 943–951.

Buck v. Bell, 274 U.S. 200 (1927). https://www.oyez.org/cases/1900-1940/274us200

Burwell v. Hobby Lobby Stores, Inc., 573 U.S. 682 (2014). https://www.oyez.org/cases/2013/13-354

Campbell, J. (2008). *The hero with a thousand faces.* New World Library. (Original work published 1949)

City of Cleburne v. Cleburne Living Ctr., 473 U.S. 432 (1985). https://www.oyez.org/cases/1984/84-468

Clarke, A. (2016). Anticipated stigma and blameless guilt: Mothers' evaluation of life with the sex-linked disorder, hypohidrotic ectodermal dysplasia (XHED). *Social Science & Medicine, 158*, 141–148.

Clement, S., Schauman, O., Graham, T., Maggioni, F., Evans-Lacko, S., Bezborodovs, N., Morgan, C., Rüsch, N., Brown, J. S. L., & Thornicroft, G. (2015). What is the impact of mental health-related stigma on help-seeking? A systematic review of quantitative and qualitative studies. *Psychological Medicine, 45*(1), 11–27.

Cohen, A. (2016). *Imbeciles: The Supreme Court, American eugenics, and the sterilization of Carrie Buck.* Penguin.

Cooper, L., Caddick, N., Godier, L., Cooper, A., & Fossey, M. (2018). Transition from the military into civilian life: An exploration of cultural competence. *Armed Forces & Society, 44*(1), 156–177.

Corrigan, P. W. (2018). *The stigma effect: Unintended consequences of mental health campaigns.* Columbia University Press.

Cree, A., & Caddick, N. (2020). Unconquerable heroes: Invictus, redemption, and the cultural politics of narrative. *Journal of War & Culture Studies, 13*(3), 258–278.

Dempsey, H. L. (2017). A comparison of the social-adaptive perspective and functionalist perspective on guilt and shame. *Behavioral Sciences, 7*(4), Article 83. https://doi.org/10.3390/bs7040083

Drescher, K. D., Foy, D. W., Kelly, C., Leshner, A., Schutz, K., & Litz, B. (2011). An exploration of the viability and usefulness of the construct of moral injury in war veterans. *Traumatology, 17*(1), 8–13.

Ellemers, N., Van den Heuvel, H., de Gilder, D., Maass, A., & Bonvini, A. (2004). The underrepresentation of women in science: Differential commitment or the queen bee syndrome? *British Journal of Social Psychology, 43*(3), 315–338.

Enemark, C. (2019). Drones, risk, and moral injury. *Critical Military Studies, 5*(2), 150–167.

Foucault, M. (2005). *The order of things: An archaeology of the human sciences.* Routledge. (Original work published 1966)

Frankfurt, S., & Frazier, P. (2016). A review of research on moral injury in combat veterans. *Military Psychology, 28*(5), 318–330.

Fredriksen-Goldsen, K. I., Kim, H.-J., Bryan, A. E. B., Shiu, C., & Emlet, C. A. (2017). The cascading effects of marginalization and pathways of resilience in attaining good health among LGBT older adults. *The Gerontologist, 57*(Suppl. 1), S72–S83.

Friedl, K. E. (2014). Introduction: Evolution of military and veterans brain health research. *Alzheimer's & Dementia: The Journal of the Alzheimer's Association, 10*(3), S94–S96.

Frost, D. M. (2011). Social stigma and its consequences for the socially stigmatized. *Social and Personality Psychology Compass, 5*(11), 824–839.

Gallo, K. M. (1994). First person account: Self-stigmatization. *Schizophrenia Bulletin, 20*(2), 407–410.

Galton, F. (1883). *Inquiries into human faculty and its development.* Macmillan.

Gasper, T. (2015). A religious right to discriminate: *Hobby Lobby* and "religious freedom" as a threat to the LGBT community. *Texas A&M Law Review, 3*(2), 395–416.

Gill, J., & Liamputtong, P. (2011). Being the mother of a child with Asperger's syndrome: Women's experiences of stigma. *Health Care for Women International, 32*(8), 708–722.

Goffman, E. (2009). *Stigma: Notes on the management of spoiled identity.* Touchstone. (Original work published 1963)

Gold, M. (2018, June 21). *The ABCs of L.G.B.T.Q.I.A.+.* The New York Times. https://nyti.ms/2MICXY5

Gray, D. E. (2002). 'Everybody just freezes. Everybody is just embarrassed': Felt and enacted stigma among parents of children with high functioning autism. *Sociology of Health & Illness, 24*(6), 734–749.

Greene-Shortridge, T. M., Britt, T. W., & Castro, C. A. (2007). The stigma of mental health problems in the military. *Military Medicine, 172*(2), 157–161.

Guelzo, A. C. (2010). *Lincoln and Douglas: The debates that defined America.* Simon & Schuster.

Hash, K. M., & Rogers, A. (2013). Clinical practice with older LGBT clients: Overcoming lifelong stigma through strength and resilience. *Clinical Social Work Journal, 41*(3), 249–257.

Hassenstab, C. M. (2014). *Body law and the body of law: A comparative study of social norm inclusion in Norwegian and American laws.* De Gruyter Open.

Hasson-Ohayon, I., Ehrlich-Ben Or, S., Vahab, K., Amiaz, R., Weiser, M., & Roe, D. (2012). Insight into mental illness and self-stigma: The mediating role of shame proneness. *Psychiatry Research, 200*(2), 802–806.

Hatzenbuehler, M. L., Phelan, J. C., & Link, B. G. (2013). Stigma as a fundamental cause of population health inequalities. *American Journal of Public Health, 103*(5), 813–821.

Herek, G. M., Gillis, J. R., & Cogan, J. C. (2009). Internalized stigma among sexual minority adults: Insights from a social psychological perspective. *Journal of Counseling Psychology, 56*(1), 32–43.

Hoge, C. W., Castro, C. A., Messer, S. C., McGurk, D., Cotting, D. I., & Koffman, R. L. (2004). Combat duty in Iraq and Afghanistan, mental health problems, and barriers to care. *New England Journal of Medicine, 351*(1), 13–22.

House, A. S., Van Horn, E., Coppeans, C., & Stepleman, L. M. (2011). Interpersonal trauma and discriminatory events as predictors of suicidal and nonsuicidal self-injury in gay, lesbian, bisexual, and transgender persons. *Traumatology, 17*(2), 75–85.

Hurst, C. E., & McConnell, D. L. (2010). *An Amish paradox: Diversity and change in the world's largest Amish community.* Johns Hopkins University Press.

Invannone, J. J. (2018, June 9). *A brief history of the LGBTQ initialism.* Medium. https://medium.com/queer-history-for-the-people/a-brief-history-of-the-lgbtq-initialism-e89db1cf06e3

Isaac, J. (1964). *The teaching of contempt: The Christian roots of anti-semitism.* Holt, Rinehart and Winston.

Ismay, J. (2019, November 21). *Edward Gallagher, the SEALs and why the Trident Pin matters.* The New York Times. https://nyti.ms/2D9hROQ

Jones, K. N., Brewster, M. E., & Jones, J. A. (2014). The creation and validation of the LGBT Ally Identity Measure. *Psychology of Sexual Orientation and Gender Diversity, 1*(2), 181–195.

Kaiser, C. R., & Wilkins, C. L. (2010). Group identification and prejudice: Theoretical and empirical advances and implications. *Journal of Social Issues, 66*(3), 461–476.

Kates, S. M., & Belk, R. W. (2001). The meanings of Lesbian and Gay Pride Day: Resistance through consumption and resistance to consumption. *Journal of Contemporary Ethnography, 30*(4), 392–429.

Kertzner, R. M., Meyer, I. H., Frost, D. M., & Stirratt, M. J. (2009). Social and psychological well-being in lesbians, gay men, and bisexuals: The effects of race, gender, age, and sexual identity. *American Journal of Orthopsychiatry, 79*(4), 500–510.

Kim, N. (2018). *The gendered politics of the Korean Protestant Right: Hegemonic masculinity.* Springer.

Ko, L. (2016, January 29). *Unwanted sterilization and eugenics programs in the United States.* PBS. http://www.pbs.org/independentlens/blog/unwanted-sterilization-and-eugenics-programs-in-the-united-states

Kopelman, L. M. (2002). If HIV/AIDS is punishment, who is bad? *Journal of Medicine and Philosophy, 27*(2), 231–243.

Kramer, E. M., & Hsieh, E. (2019). Gaze as embodied ethics: Homelessness, the Other, and humanity. In M. J. Dutta & D. B. Zapata (Eds.), *Communicating for social change* (pp. 33–62). Palgrave Macmillan.

Kraybill, D. B. (2003). *The riddle of Amish culture.* Johns Hopkins University Press.

Kühl, S. (2002). *The Nazi connection: Eugenics, American racism, and German national socialism.* Oxford University Press.

Kulis, S., Napoli, M., & Marsiglia, F. F. (2002). Ethnic pride, biculturalism, and drug use norms of urban American Indian adolescents. *Social Work Research, 26*(2), 101–112.

Leshner, A. I. (1997). Addiction Is a brain disease, and it matters. *Science, 278*(5335), 45–47.

Leslie, C. R. (2000). Creating criminals: The injuries inflicted by unenforced sodomy laws. *Harvard Civil Rights-Civil Liberties Law Review, 35*(1), 103–182.

Lewis, M. (1998). Shame and stigma. In P. Gilbert & B. Andrews (Eds.), *Shame: Interpersonal behavior, psychopathology, and culture* (pp. 126–140). Oxford University Press.

Library of Congress. (n.d.). *Lesbian, gay, bisexual, transgender and queer pride month: About.* Retrieved August 8, 2020, from https://www.loc.gov/lgbt-pride-month/about

Lincoln, A., & Douglas, S. A. (1860). *Political debates between Hon. Abraham Lincoln and Hon. Stephen A. Douglas, in the celebrated campaign of 1858 in Illinois: Including the preceding speeches of each at Chicago, Springfield, etc., Also the two great speeches of Mr. Lincoln in Ohio, in 1859, as carefully prepared by the reporter of each party and published at the times of their delivery.* Follett, Foster and Co. https://books.google.com/books?id=6TgzAQAAMAAJ

Link, B. G., & Phelan, J. C. (2001). Conceptualizing stigma. *Annual Review of Sociology, 27*, 363–385.

Litz, B. T., Stein, N., Delaney, E., Lebowitz, L., Nash, W. P., Silva, C., & Maguen, S. (2009). Moral injury and moral repair in war veterans: A preliminary model and intervention strategy. *Clinical Psychology Review, 29*(8), 695–706.

Livingston, J. D., Milne, T., Fang, M. L., & Amari, E. (2012). The effectiveness of interventions for reducing stigma related to substance use disorders: A systematic review. *Addiction, 107*(1), 39–50.

Love, A. S., Yin, Z., Codina, E., & Zapata, J. T. (2006). Ethnic identity and risky health behaviors in school-age Mexican-American children. *Psychological Reports, 98*(3), 735–744.

Mallory, C., & Sears, B. (2020, May). *The economic impact of marriage equality five years after Obergefell v. Hodges.* The Williams Institute. https://williamsinstitute.law.ucla.edu/publications/econ-impact-obergefell-Five-years

Matthews, S., Dwyer, R., & Snoek, A. (2017). Stigma and self-stigma in addiction. *Journal of Bioethical Inquiry, 14*(2), 275–286.

Medical Humanities-Health Studies Program. (n.d.). *Indiana eugenics: History and legacy 1907–2007.* Indiana University-Purdue University, Indianapolis. Retrieved August 8, 2020, from https://www.iupui.edu/~eugenics

Mogul, J. L., Ritchie, A. J., & Whitlock, K. (2011). *Queer (in)justice: The criminalization of LGBT people in the United States.* Beacon Press.

Moses, T. (2009). Self-labeling and its effects among adolescents diagnosed with mental disorders. *Social Science & Medicine, 68*(3), 570–578.

Mukherjee, S. (2016). *The gene: An intimate history.* Scribner.

Nash, W. P., Silva, C., & Litz, B. (2009). The historic origins of military and veteran mental health stigma and the stress injury model as a means to reduce it. *Psychiatric Annals, 39*(8), 789–794.

National Center for Veterans Analysis and Statistics. (2020). *Quick facts.* https://www.va.gov/vetdata/Quick_Facts.asp

New International Version. (2011). Biblica. https://www.biblica.com/bible/(Original work published 1978)

Not Your Mascots. (2020). Facebook. https://www.facebook.com/notyourmascots

O'Keefe, B. J. (1988). The logic of message design: Individual differences in reasoning about communication. *Communication Monographs, 55*(1), 80–103.

O'Keefe, B. J. (1991). Message design logic and the management of multiple goals. In K. Tracy (Ed.), *Understanding face-to-face interaction: Issues linking goals and discourse* (pp. 131–150). Erlbaum.

Obergefell v. Hodges, 376 U.S. ____ (2015). https://www.oyez.org/cases/2014/14-556

Olson, L. R., Cadge, W., & Harrison, J. T. (2006). Religion and public opinion about same-sex marriage. *Social Science Quarterly, 87*(2), 340–360.

Parsons, T. (1951). *The social system.* Quid Pro Books.

Phelan, J. C., Link, B. G., & Dovidio, J. F. (2008). Stigma and prejudice: One animal or two? *Social Science & Medicine, 67*(3), 358–367.

Phillipps, D. (2019, November 19). *Navy wants to eject from SEALs a sailor cleared by Trump, officials say.* The New York Times. https://www.nytimes.com/2019/11/19/us/ navy-seals-edward-gallagher-trident.html

Randle, A. (2020, January 11). *Officials called 'Redmen' a racist mascot. Then voters weighed in.* The New York Times. https://www.nytimes.com/2020/01/11/nyregion/ killingly-redmen-mascot.html

Reddy, M. S. (2016). Lack of insight in psychiatric illness: A critical appraisal. *Indian Journal of Psychological Medicine, 38*(3), 169–171.

Reilly, P. (1991). *The surgical solution: A history of involuntary sterilization in the United States.* Johns Hopkins University Press.

Reilly, P. R. (2015). Eugenics and involuntary sterilization: 1907–2015. *Annual Review of Genomics and Human Genetics, 16*(1), 351–368.

Russell, G. M. (2011). Motives of heterosexual allies in collective action for equality. *Journal of Social Issues, 67*(2), 376–393.

Schüklenk, U., Stein, E., Kerin, J., & Byne, W. (1997). The ethics of genetic research on sexual orientation. *Hastings Center Report, 27*(4), 6–13.

Shane, L., III. (2019, September 20). *Veteran suicides increase despite host of prevention, mental health efforts.* MilitaryTimes. https://www.militarytimes.com/news/pentagon- congress/2019/09/20/veteran-suicides-increase-despite-host-of-prevention-mental- health-efforts

Silver, M. G. (2004). Eugenics and compulsory sterilization laws: Providing redress for the victims of a shameful era in United States history. *George Washington Law Review, 72*(4), 862–891.

Skinner v. Oklahoma, 316 U.S. 535 (1942). https://www.oyez.org/cases/1940-1955/316us535

Smith, R. A. (2007). Language of the lost: An explication of stigma communication. *Communication Theory, 17*(4), 462–485.

Stassi, L. (2017). After injury, soldier aims for new way to serve. *Army Magazine, 67*(2), 71.

Stuber, J., Meyer, I., & Link, B. (2008). Stigma, prejudice, discrimination and health. *Social Science & Medicine, 67*(3), 351–357.

The Supreme Court ruling that led to 70,000 forced sterilizations. (2016, March 7). NPR. https://www.npr.org/sections/health-shots/2016/03/07/469478098/the-supreme-court- ruling-that-led-to-70-000-forced-sterilizations

Switankowsky, I. (2000). Dualism and its Importance for medicine. *Theoretical Medicine and Bioethics, 21*(6), 567–580.

Tessier, A., Boyer, L., Husky, M., Baylé, F., Llorca, P.-M., & Misdrahi, D. (2017). Medication adherence in schizophrenia: The role of insight, therapeutic alliance and perceived trauma associated with psychiatric care. *Psychiatry Research, 257*, 315–321.

Thornicroft, G., Rose, D., Kassam, A., & Sartorius, N. (2007). Stigma: Ignorance, prejudice or discrimination? *The British Journal of Psychiatry, 190*(3), 192–193.

Toomey, R. B., & McGeorge, C. R. (2018). Profiles of LGBTQ ally engagement in college athletics. *Journal of LGBT Youth, 15*(3), 162–178.

Ungar, M. (2000). State violence and lesbian, gay, bisexual and transgender (LGBT) rights. *New Political Science, 22*(1), 61–75.

Vogel, D. L., Wade, N. G., & Hackler, A. H. (2007). Perceived public stigma and the willingness to seek counseling: The mediating roles of self-stigma and attitudes toward counseling. *Journal of Counseling Psychology, 54*(1), 40–50.

Wang, M.-T., Henry, D. A., Smith, L. V., Huguley, J. P., & Guo, J. (2020). Parental ethnic-racial socialization practices and children of color's psychosocial and behavioral adjustment: A systematic review and meta-analysis. *American Psychologist, 75*(1), 1–22.

Weiner, B., Perry, R. P., & Magnusson, J. (1988). An attributional analysis of reactions to stigmas. *Journal of Personality and Social Psychology, 55*(5), 738–748.

Wiser, C. T. (Director). (2014). *The Amish: Shunned*. [Film]. American Experience. https://www.pbs.org/wgbh/americanexperience/films/amish-shunned

Wooten, D. A. (2019). Forgotten but not gone: Learning from the hepatitis A outbreak and public health response in San Diego. *Topics in Antiviral Medicine, 26*(4), 117–121.

9

Uncertainty in Health and Illness

From Perspectival Thinking to Integral Fusion

In Chapter 9, we will explore how different cultural perspectives shape individuals' and societies' understanding and management of uncertainty in health contexts. We first survey major theories on the management of uncertainties in health contexts, examining their corresponding assumptions and cultural perspectives. By questioning the emphasis of information management in the literature of uncertainty management, we will investigate the different ways uncertainties are negotiated. In particular, we examine how storytelling and humor allow individuals to manage uncertainty by transforming the meanings of uncertainty. We conclude the Chapter by examining the interactive nature of uncertainty management and the functions of ambiguity in achieving an Integral Fusion worldview.

I. Uncertainty in Health and Illness

A. Uncertainties in Medicine

The rapid development of science and medicine can encourage confidence that we have the knowledge of, and control over, illness, disease, and treatment outcomes. But such confidence may be unwarranted. Medicine is inherently filled with uncertainties. According to Brashers (2001), "Uncertainty exists when details of situations are ambiguous, complex, unpredictable, or probabilistic; information is unavailable or inconsistent; and when people feel insecure in their own state of knowledge or the state of knowledge in general" (p. 478). Communicating uncertainty can be particularly problematic in health contexts. Medicine is not just about new technology or medical jargon. To understand medical language, individuals need to understand medical worldviews (e.g., anatomy and probabilities), interpret their corresponding meanings (e.g., what does it mean when ovaries produce different types of hormone after menopause), and apply their understanding to their personal preferences and life goals (for discussions on *health literacy*, see Chapter 7). Medical language is situated in the natural world and patients' illness experience is situated in their everyday life.

Beresford (1991) proposed three *sources* of uncertainty in medicine: technical, personal, and conceptual. **Technical uncertainty** arises when there is inadequate scientific data to predict the effects of certain factors in the progress of a disease or the outcome of certain interventions. **Personal uncertainty** is rooted in physician-patient relationships when physicians were unable to discern a patient's preferences or when they feel that they are too attached to patients. **Conceptual uncertainty** is caused by difficulties in applying abstract criteria or values to concrete situations (e.g., how to distribute scarce medical resources between two patients). Medical sociologist Renée Fox (2002) explained that the changing nature of medicine (e.g., emergence and re-emergence of infectious disease and advances in genetic medicine) and increased effects of **iatrogenesis** in modern medicine (i.e., side-effects caused by medical treatment) can also heighten physicians' uncertainty in clinical decision-making. Finally, evidence-based medicine, the gold standard of modern medicine, confronts a unique form of uncertainty – **epistemological uncertainty** (i.e., uncertainty related to applying "evidence-based," universal knowledge gained through standardized clinical trials and experiments to the specific patient or case at hand) because clinical decision-making and situations are often far more complicated and nuanced than the narrowly defined scientific questions posed in clinical studies (Fox, 2002; Griffiths et al., 2006).

These sources of uncertainty can lead to significant challenges in physicians' clinical practices. For example, physicians can experience **diagnostic uncertainty**, which is defined as "subjective perception of an inability to provide an accurate explanation of the patient's health problem" (Bhise et al., 2018, p. 111). Diagnostic uncertainty can be caused by any of the three basic sources of uncertainty. For example, the time-constraint in a medical encounter, patients' lack of communicative competence, and the limitations of diagnostic tests can lead to both technical and personal uncertainties. The complexity of medical options, the balancing act between treatment efficacy and complications, and the lack of evidence-based best practices can lead to conceptual uncertainty. Inappropriate management of diagnostic uncertainty has been linked to diagnostic errors as well as excessive healthcare utilization, including over-testing, over-prescribing, unnecessary surgeries, more hospitalizations and referrals, and increased health costs (Bhise et al., 2018). Due to the potentially significant and damaging consequences to patients' process and quality of care, researchers and medical educators have proposed interventions to *reduce* diagnostic uncertainty. Such an approach highlights Perspectival Thinking within medicine, which has little tolerance for ambiguity and uncertainty. As a result, interventions often focus on reducing uncertainty by providing physicians best practices, training, or tools for better clinical decision-making (e.g., Cohen et al., 1987; Kim & Lee, 2018).

However, medical educators are increasingly urging a shift in conceptualizing uncertainty in medicine. Rather than viewing medical uncertainty as something to be eliminated, they propose that physicians should develop better skills to *tolerate* and communicate uncertainty in clinical settings. (Luther & Crandall, 2011; Simpkin & Schwartzstein, 2016). For example, Simpkin and Schwartzstein (2016) explained,

> [M]any current medical students, the digital natives, seek structure, efficiency, and predictability; they insist on knowing "the right answer" and are frustrated when one cannot be supplied. This attitude no doubt increases the likelihood that they will perceive uncertainty as a threat. ... Our curricula should recognize diagnosis as dynamic and evolving – an iterative process that accounts for multiple, changing perspectives. We can speak about "hypotheses" rather than "diagnoses," thereby changing the expectations of both patients and physicians and facilitating a shift in culture. (p. 1714)

"Structure, efficiency, and predictability" are hallmarks of Perspectival Thinking as its cultural participants aim to control the "chaos" by imposing ever-increasingly precision, structural units to ensure efficiency and predictability. By replacing "diagnosis," which implies a singular, definitive, and positivistic answer to a patient's unstructured symptoms in her Lifeworld, with "hypothesis," which accommodates probabilities and uncertainties in a provider's Voice of Medicine, providers and patients' are oriented to an Integral Fusion worldview that emphasizes the temporal aspect of medicine as a process with a dynamic and interactive nature, which includes uncertainty.

Physicians' uncertainty is not limited to their control of an objective, external reality. Medical sociologist Rene Fox (2002) emphasized that physicians' experiences of uncertainty in medicine are both *cognitive* and *existential* in nature as they constantly struggle with (a) the impossibility of mastering the entire corpus of medical knowledge and skills, (b) the gaps and limitations in medical knowledge and effectiveness that exists despite medicine's continuous advances, and (c) the "difficulties associated with distinguishing between personal ignorance and ineptitude; and the lacunae and incapacities of medicine itself" (p. 237). In other words, physicians' management of uncertainty involves not only their abilities to navigate the medical terrains of scientific knowledge and clinical realities but also their identities as health professionals. When reflecting on his life as a brain surgeon, Marsh (2017) explained, "We need, of course, self-confidence to cope with the fact that surgery is dangerous and we sometimes fail. We also need to radiate confidence to our frightened patients, but deep down most of us know that we might not be as good as we make out" (p. 68). Marsh (2017) concluded:

> There's nothing more frightening for a patient than a doctor, especially a young one, who is lacking in confidence. Furthermore, patients want hope, as well as treatment.
>
> So we quickly learn to deceive, to pretend to a greater level of competence and knowledge than we know to be the case, and try to shield our patients a little from the frightening reality they often face. And the best way of deceiving others, of course, is to deceive yourself. You will not then give yourself away with all the subtle signs which we are so good at identifying when people lie to us. [Self-deception ...] is an important and necessary clinical skill we must all acquire at an early stage in our career. (p. 244)

Physicians' cognitive and existential concerns stemming from clinical uncertainty, thus, take on a communicative dimension with direct consequences for on patient's quality of care. Communicating uncertainty becomes a coordinated activity between providers and patients to set expectations for, including their identities, relationships, and tasks (Politi et al., 2011a; Portnoy et al., 2013; Scott et al., 2020). We will revisit the interactive nature of uncertainty management later in the Chapter.

Physicians' "confidence" also comes at a price. In a study that examines established practices, Prasad et al. (2013) noted that 40.2% of the 363 studies published in high-impact journals between 2001–2010 found the existing standards of care ineffective, resulting in **medical reversals** (i.e., when a medical practice is found to be inferior to some lessor or prior standards of care). The high rate of medical reversal may be a result of overconfidence because many established practices became accepted through the advocacy of prominent figures rather than evidence-based studies (Hatch, 2017). The need for "self-deception" in order to support patients' desire for hope may encourage physicians to move away from Perspectival Thinking, which defines and grounds medical science, and to embrace other cultural perspectives.

This brings us back to Talcott Parsons (1951), one of the earliest sociologists who investigated uncertainty in medical contexts. Parsons argued that both physicians and patients are likely to adopt Magic Consciousness to manage uncertainty in clinical contexts because the basic function of magic is "to bolster the self-confidence of actors in situations where energy and skill do make a difference but where because of uncertainty factors, outcomes cannot be guaranteed" (Parsons, 1951, p. 329). Parsons (1951) explained, "Magical beliefs and practices tend to cluster about situations where there is an important uncertainty factor and where there are strong emotional interests in the success of action. ... The health situation is a classic one of the combination [sic] of uncertainty and strong emotional interests which produce a situation of strain and is very frequently a prominent focus of magic" (pp. 328–329). Although the scientific tradition of modern medicine may "preclude outright magic," physicians also adopt "rituals" that promote optimism, "bias in favor of active intervention," and "fashion change" in medical practices that are indicative of a Magic Consciousness perspective (Parsons, 1951, p. 329).

Despite their scientific training and Perspectival Thinking, physicians' ways of communicating uncertainty often reflect considerations for Magic Consciousness or Mythic Connection. By associating prognoses "with the limits of their diagnostic and therapeutic powers, and with the grave illnesses and impending deaths of patients," physicians developed "magic-infused clinical thinking" (Fox, 2002, p. 241). For example, when physicians reported that discussions about poor prognoses can "make people depressed" or "take away hope," their saying-it-make-it-so attitude highlights Magic Consciousness (Mack & Joffe, 2014; Mack & Smith, 2012). When President Trump was hospitalized after contracted COVID-19, his physician, Navy Cmdr Dr. Sean Conley, explained that he omitted information about "alarming drops in the President's oxygen levels" during the news conference the day before because he did not want to "to give any information that might *steer the course of illness* in another direction" [emphasis added] (Reston, 2020, para. 4). By emphasizing the lack of certainty for a definitive timeframe, providers shift into an Integral Fusion worldview by recognizing the perspectival limitations of modern medicine (Hancock et al., 2007). As a result, physicians often systematically downplay the negative aspect of a patient's condition when discussing uncertainties in a patient's illness event. For example, a study found that radiation oncologists' predicted survival was, on average, 12.3 weeks longer than their cancer patients' actual survival (Chow et al., 2005). In addition, among cancer patients whose actual survival was 12 weeks or less, their oncologists overestimated by 21.9 weeks (Chow et al., 2005). Another study found that compared to advanced cancer patients' actual survival, clinicians' predicted survival was overestimated by 19 weeks on average (Razvi et al. 2019). More importantly, among patients whose actual survival was 12 weeks or less, radiation oncologists overestimated by 24.9 weeks on average; in contrast, among patients whose actual survival was 52 weeks or more, clinicians' only overestimated by .1 week on average (Razvi et al. 2019). Rather than suggesting that physicians are less "accurate" when a patient is close to a

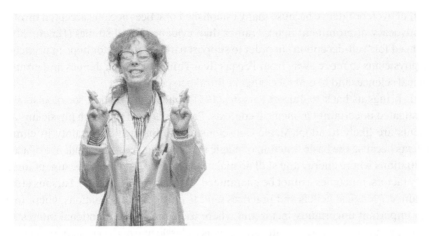

Figure 9.1 Ritualization of optimism. Should doctors share the whole truth with you, including their uncertainties, or should they "hope for the best" with you? *Source:* Aaron Amat / Alamy Stock Photo

looming death, we argue that the discrepancies highlight providers' willingness to incorporate other non-Perspectival considerations (e.g. maintaining hope for patient and themselves) when they face the limits of perspectival, modern medicine. Christakis (1998) proposed the term **"ritualization of optimism"** to describe physician's presentation of "the favorable outlook regarding a patient's outcome in spite of, and as a result of, the uncertainty inherent in the patient's predicament, and often in spite of evidence suggesting an unfavorable prognosis" (p. 82; see Figure 9.1).

In summary, uncertainty is inherent in medicine. It is inevitable in its Perspectival Thinking and its limitations of the tools we have for precision. Physicians face limitations in their knowledge as the field of medicine is expansive and fast-changing. Medicine continually finds new gaps in knowledge. Limitations can also be shaped by practitioners' technical skills and accompanying technologies. In addition, clinicians' uncertainty is intertwined with their identities as health professionals. Thus, communicating uncertainty involves not only an accurate assessment of the risks or probabilities involved but also entails coordination of other interpersonal, relational, and task goals with their patients. Uncertainty management becomes interpersonal, interactive, and evolving. Patients' and physicians' strong emotional interests for the outcome can shift the stronghold of Perspectival Thinking in medicine to other cultural perspectives, including Magic Consciousness and Mythic Connection.

B. From Uncertainty Reduction to the Management of Multiple Goals

1. The Evolution of Theoretical Approaches to Uncertainty

When researchers first conceptualized the role of uncertainty in shaping interpersonal communication, their approach highlights a Western attempt to control nature through its pursuit of certainty or predictability (Bradac 2001; Case et al., 2005). **Uncertainty Reduction Theory** (URT), proposed by Berger and Calabrese (1975), was one of the first communication theories to examine the role of uncertainty in interpersonal communication. URT assumes that individuals are driven to reduce their uncertainty, noting that "when strangers meet, their primary concern is one of uncertainty *reduction* or increasing *predictability* about the behavior of both themselves and others in the interaction" [emphasis added] (Berger & Calabrese, 1975, p. 100). In addition, information seeking is necessary to reduce uncertainty as individuals would "interrogate each other in order to gain information which might be instrumental in uncertainty reduction" (Berger & Calabrese, 1975, p. 103). Under URT, uncertainties are perceived to be undesirable and thus, individuals are driven to eliminate uncertainty through information-seeking. The Western understanding of information – information/knowledge is power – serves as the underlying foundation of URT (see also Cultural Functions and Meanings of Information in Chapter 6). Uncertainty reduction is attractive to western medicine because it is compatible with the biomedical paradigm of Perspectival Thinking, which is in constant pursuit of better tests for illnesses and greater certainty in their causal pathways (Babrow & Kline, 2000). In addition, uncertainty reduction is attractive in cultures that value personal control and individual agency (Babrow & Kline, 2000).

Extending URT, Gudykunst (1998) proposed **Anxiety/Uncertainty Management** (AUM) Theory to intercultural and intergroup interactions. Despite acknowledging that cultural sojourners may not wish to have complete predictability when interacting with the host society, Gudykunst equated uncertainty with anxiety and noted that when a cultural sojourner's "anxiety is high, they must cognitively manage their anxiety to communicate effectively and adjust to the host cultures" (p. 229). Whereas URT does not particularly emphasize the role of affect in uncertainty management (and thus, is highly consistent with the cultural perspectives of Perspectival Thinking), AUM connects the cognitive response of uncertainty with the affective response of anxiety, noting that effective communication is dependent on the "appropriate" level of uncertainty to motivate but not overwhelm individuals' information-seeking intentions and behaviors (Yoshitake, 2002). Although AUM emphasizes the importance of empathy, its conceptualization of empathy centers on the "functions" and "use" of empathy (Gudykunst, 2003b; Yoshitake, 2002). In other words, empathy becomes a tool, something that can be manipulated and performed to achieve a desired objective: "Individuals can *choose* to be empathic when they *want* to communicate effectively" [emphasis added] (Gudykunst, 2003b, p. 33). The emphasis on individuals' choice and the pursuit of effective and efficient communication (from the perspective of the communicator) makes AUM a theory with strong Western bias, rendering communication into a linear pursuit of goal-oriented, individualistic acts. However, AUM is not a theory of pure Perspectival Thinking because by noting that anxiety of the unknown is a major motivator for individuals to reduce uncertainty, AUM shifts the Perspectival Thinking in URT into Mythic Connection. Uncertainty becomes a drama that needs to be maintained, reconciled, and negotiated to achieve a desired outcome.

At first glance, connecting uncertainty with anxiety appears intuitive in health contexts because individuals' illnesses, which are presumed to be undesirable and perceived as threats, are likely to create negative affects that motivate information-seeking. However, a closer look at the spectrum of individuals' health issues and behaviors suggests that uncertainty does not always entail anxiety in health contexts. For example, when a person is diagnosed with a terminal illness that is near the end-of-life, the certainty of death is high, but a person may experience significant anxiety. Alternatively, an individual may actively seek multiple opinions and alternative treatments to *increase* (as opposed to reduce) uncertainty of the end-of-life prognosis. On the other hand, when a patient is confronted with health-related uncertainty (e.g., a lump in breast tissue or a suspicious skin tag), a person may intentionally ignore the warning signs to avoid anxiety rather than actively seeking a diagnosis to confirm or eliminate uncertainty. In short, starting from the 1990s, researchers began to recognize that uncertainty is not directly connected to anxiety. Rather, when individuals experience uncertainty, it is their *appraisal* of the uncertainty (rather than the uncertainty itself) that leads to specific coping behaviors (Babrow, Kasch, & Ford, 1998; Brashers et al., 1998; Mishel, 1990, 1997, 1999).

Mishel (1988) defined uncertainty as a cognitive state when a person lacks the ability to determine the *meanings* of illness-related events. In her **Reconceptualized Uncertainty in Illness Theory** (RUIT), Mishel (1990) proposed that uncertainty can be appraised to be a *danger* (i.e., negative appraisal) or an *opportunity* (i.e., positive appraisal). Negative appraisals likely lead to negative affects (e.g., anxiety, anger, and frustration). Positive appraisals are likely to be associated with positive affects (e.g., hope and excitement). Depending on whether illness-related uncertainty is perceived as a threat or a hope, individuals may have different coping strategies (e.g., information-seeking, information avoidance, or fatalistic attitudes) and health outcomes (e.g., mental health and quality of life; Mishel, 2013; see Figure 9.2).

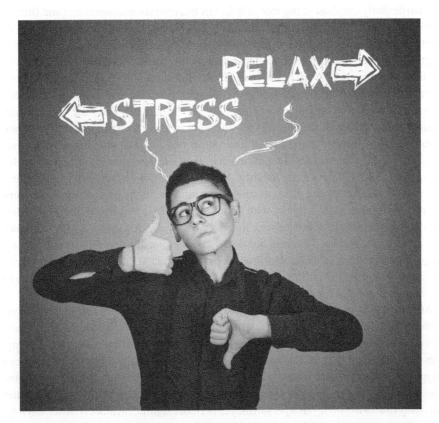

Figure 9.2 Uncertainty appraisal. Uncertainty is not inherently good or bad. Our responses to uncertainty are shaped by the meanings that we attribute to it. *Source:* Ion Chiosea/123RF

At first glance, Babrow's (2001) **Problematic Integration Theory** (PI) may appear to be highly perspectival as it argues that individuals' cognitive conflicts can trigger efforts to address underlying uncertainties when their *assessment of probabilities* of the event (i.e., **probabilistic orientation**) and the *evaluation of the event or outcome* (i.e., **evaluative orientation**) become *problematic* (see also Babrow, 1992). For example, a person may become uncertain about whether to take an important business trip to China when early reporting of coronavirus infections suggests an alarming trend (i.e., increasing probability of contracting a highly contagious and somewhat dangerous illness). Despite the seemingly mathematical and mechanical approach to one's cognitive process, PI, in fact, adopts an Integral Fusion approach to individuals' experiences of uncertainty. PI recognizes that individuals' assessments and evaluations are dynamic, interactive, and evolving, noting that probabilistic and evaluative orientations are "interdependent" with one another, "integrated in experiences," and integrated with "broader complexes of knowledge, feelings, and behavior intentions" (Babrow, 2001, pp. 554–555). In other words, an individual's appraisal of uncertainty is contextually situated and interactively negotiated. It incorporates a sense of temporal dimension, noting that past experiences provide individuals resources to interpret the meanings of current uncertainty. In addition, the integrative process is often problematic, requiring individuals to reconcile tensions between different values, emotions, ambiguity, ambivalence, probabilities, and possibilities (Babrow, 2001). As a result, PI does not project a linear or definitive answer to addressing uncertainty nor does it presume that certain outcomes are universally valuable. By embracing the "dynamic, contextual, and unpredictable nature" of problematic integration, cultural participants are free to create, negotiate, and coordinate the meanings of uncertainty that define and empower their agency and experiences.

Finally, **Uncertainty Management Theory** (UMT), proposed by Brashers (2001), focuses on individuals' information behaviors when faced with uncertainty. UMT argues that individuals' experiences of uncertainties are multilayered, interconnected, and temporal. **Multilayered** means that uncertainty of a single event is situated in layers of contexts, which may produce "complementary and contradictory forces" (Brashers & Babrow, 1996, p. 249). For example, learning about one's diagnosis of a terminal illness may lead to uncertainties about identities (e.g., disruption to life biography), relationships (e.g., whether the proposed treatment may make a person unable to have sex and thus, pose threats to a romantic relationship), and other concerns (e.g., finances) that are *specific to the diagnosis*. **Interconnected** means that one area of uncertainty can trigger uncertainties in *other areas*. For example, difficulties in finding effective treatments for medically unexplained symptoms can lead to uncertainty about self-concept, financial well-being, and career trajectories. **Temporal** means that the duration, evolving nature, and revolutionary changes of uncertainty must be understood through a temporal dimension. For example, a concussion involves short-term uncertainty for most people; in contrast, an NFL athlete may view concussion as a continuing trauma. As a professional football player, one subjects himself to compromised quality of life at an early age – thus, the meanings of concussion for an NFL player may evolve over his life career and may suddenly change due to a major incident. Although a concussion diagnosed on a football field may bring a certain level of uncertainty, a diagnosis of bleeding in the brain after the game may result in the early termination of a promising career.

Two aspects of UMT offers a particularly sophisticated understanding of information management. First, UMT recognizes that the "relationship between information and uncertainty is not straightforward" (Hogan & Brashers, 2009, p. 48). UMT recognizes that uncertainty is a *tool*, rather than a result, of some patients' illness management – they may intentionally seek or avoid information to increase, maintain, or reduce uncertainty as a coping strategy (Brashers et al., 2004). For example, a patient with an end-of-life prognosis may intentionally seek information about alternative treatment to create ambiguity toward imminent death. Alternatively, a terminal patient may actively avoid information to engage in denial behaviors to reduce uncertainty. In other words, UMT rejects the linear relationship between information seeking and uncertainty reduction. UMT argues that individuals actively cultivate, maintain, or reduce uncertainty in response to their communicative goals. Second, UMT proposes that uncertainty management is situated in and coordinated within individuals' social networks (Barbour et al., 2011; Brashers et al., 2002; Goldsmith & Brashers, 2008). Because individuals may prefer to *reduce* or *increase* uncertainty during different stages of an illness event, patients and their supportive others may engage in complex coordination of information to manage uncertainty. For example, when an elderly parent is diagnosed with pancreatic cancer, their adult children may coordinate tasks between themselves (e.g., the child who has a medical background may seek information from the latest medical journals; the child who accompanies the parent to appointments may prepare a list of questions to ask the physician) and selectively provide information to their parent (e.g., telling the ill parent to focus on the treatment, shielding the parent from unpleasant information, and providing necessary information to assist decision-making).

Both PI and UMT adopt heuristic approaches to uncertainty management, providing theoretical explanations to any situations in which individuals experience subjective uncertainty (Babrow & Striley, 2014; Bradac, 2001). By recognizing that the meanings of uncertainty are not fixed but rather appraised through social interactions, researchers have explored how individuals collaborate with others to manage information in order to achieve their desired level of uncertainty. Individuals' management of information includes their considerations for the types and sources of information as well as different communicative goals, including identity, relational, and task goals (Barbour et al., 2011; Brashers et al., 2006; Martin et al., 2010). In summary, by recognizing the co-existence of potentially competing and conflicting goals and incorporating the need to negotiate and coordinate one's communicative goals with others to achieve successful coping, UMT also adopts an Integral Fusion worldview for the management of uncertainties.

2. From Tolerating Uncertainty to Integrating Uncertainty

The literature of uncertainties in health contexts has gone through major changes. As we discussed earlier, modern medicine is rooted in Perspectival Thinking (see Chapter 4). Under Perspectival Thinking, uncertainty is not tolerated or tolerable. It is important to note that the very notion of "managing" uncertainty highlights Perspectival Thinking. It presumes a sense of agency and control. Under Magic Consciousness, people live in the here-and-now. Because everything is complete "as is," there is no need for individual agency or control. In contrast, under Perspectival Thinking, individuals exercise agency to parse their realities into "manageable" units for better "control." Thus, managing uncertainty becomes hypertrophic under Perspectival Thinking. The drive for greater precision and greater tools to increase fragmentation (and thus, precision) is inherent in all pursuits under Perspectival Thinking. Philosopher Nicolas Rescher (1998) argued uncertainty is the main obstacle to scientific prediction and that "successful prediction is one of the cardinal aims of science" (p. 159; see also Guillán, 2017). There may be scientific language that "tolerates" uncertainty, such as "margin of error" (i.e., the range of values above and below the sample statistic in a confidence interval; in other words, it is the variability of the result that may differ from the "actual" sample). However, uncertainty is not really tolerated because the scientific pursuit always aims to reduce the margin of error, which itself is a measure based on fragmentation. Elimination of uncertainty is the ultimate goal of Perspectival Thinking.

Because of the evolution of theories of uncertainty management and the strong Western bias in the early theories (e.g., URT and AUM), later theories often centered on the management of information as the main coping strategy for uncertainty management (Case et al., 2005). In addition, the relationship between uncertainty and information management has been conceptualized as a circular one, with individuals constantly balancing the equilibrium between their information needs and a tolerable level of uncertainty (Hogan & Brashers, 2009). However, conceptualizing uncertainty through its relationship with information management reflects a Perspectival Thinking approach. If we were to appreciate the complexity of uncertainty and individuals' coping strategies, we need to look beyond individuals' information behaviors and explore how other cultural approaches may understand uncertainty or frame its cultural participants' understanding, experiences, and coping with uncertainty.

In her pioneering work in the 1950s, Renée Fox (1980) has challenged the presumed certainty of medicine by demonstrating how medical education transforms physicians' perspectives by helping them "coming to terms with uncertainty" (p. 7). As students enhance their cognitive mastery of a situation (e.g., acquiring more medical knowledge and technical skills), they also learn to accept uncertainty, recognize their own limitations, and develop their coping strategies (e.g., medical humor and self-mockery). When cultural participants who are predominantly perspectival modern recognize its true limitations – that there will always be uncertainty due to the limits of medical science, their own ignorance, and the difficulties in distinguishing the two – they may be motivated to break the cultural frame of Perspectival Thinking because it is no longer functional or effective. In fact, faced with extraordinary and often tragic uncertainty, physicians have been found to take "laughter-accompanied bets on such serious matters as the diagnosis of a patient's illness, the impact of their therapy, its prognosis, the outcome of a particularly important or risky experiment that they conducted on a patient-subject and, most audacious of all, whether one of their patients would live or die" (Fox, 1980, p. 8). *House M.D.*, a television series, often featured bets between physicians as a recurring theme ("What Would *House M.D.* be Without Bets??", 2012). Although such reactions may appear inappropriate or offensive to patients, "insider" humor and stories highlight physicians' attempts to shift into an Integral Fusion approach to uncertainty.

Without abandoning their role in biomedicine, providers utilize humor and institutional stories as a vehicle for Magic Consciousness (e.g., identity claim) and Mythic Connection (e.g., storytelling) and for the eventual development of an Integral Fusion worldview. Medical students do not just learn the mechanical, perspectival aspect of becoming a physician but are also socialized with the coping strategies that recognize their human frailty. For example, during clinical clerkships, medical students often observed residents and physicians' use of humor and slang in hospitals. Medical students noted that humor helped residents build team cohesion, cope with frustrations of their jobs (e.g., difficult or unappreciative patients, demanding workload, and medical efforts that often do not improve patients' outcomes), cope with negative emotions or events (e.g., sadness and death), and reconcile cognitive dissonance (e.g., having to hurt people), and build team cohesion (Parsons et al., 2001). Though certain kinds of humor may be inappropriate or offensive to outsiders, they serve the valuable function of creating a sense of community and, thus, solidarity. "We get it." Stories bind communities.

A common genre among medical students is called *cadaver stories*, an oral culture of medical training (see Figure 9.3). Hafferty (1988) explained,

> Cadaver stories are narratives describing "jokes" played by medical student protagonists on unsuspecting and emotionally vulnerable victims. In these stories, medical students physically (and thus symbolically) manipulate whole cadavers or certain cadaver parts-often extremities or sexual organs-for the dual purpose of shocking their intended victims and deriving humor from their victim's distress. The victims in cadaver stories are either lay people or what the narratives portray as emotionally vulnerable medical students. (p. 344)

The telling of cadaver stories is "particularly endemic in that period directly before and during the first few weeks of lab. ... Once lab ends, cadaver stories disappear, but they are not forgotten" (Hafferty, 1988, p. 349). Hafferty (1988) concluded, "The act of telling cadaver stories (as well as their content) marks the anxious anticipation of anatomy lab, the initial adjustment to lab, and those periods in lab when the cadaver is most likely to appear as a human referent" (p. 349).

On the other hand, the actual manipulation of cadavers can entail the magic impact of immediate shock before language and rationalization engage. Actual manipulation is not storytelling but evocative and invocative performance at the magic level of existence. It involves the transformation of a person's body into an object for fun, and in the process, it creates magic dissonance involving the identity of the corpse as a real

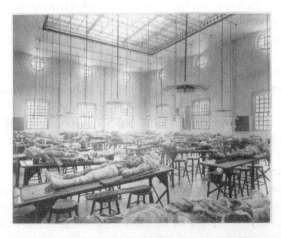

Figure 9.3 Dissecting room, Jefferson Medical College in 1902. When we see a body treated as an object to be dissected and analyzed, the Magic Consciousness of our embodied experiences as a human being starts to crack. *Source:* The Library of Congress

person and a prop for emotional impact. The dissonance may be resolvable once mythic and perspectival rendering occurs. But prior to "thinking about" what happened, and making sense of it (e.g., retelling it), it has already happened to the student. Its impact is immediate, and it serves to transform the naïve student into a doctor who must come to see human bodies in a somewhat objective, disinterested way. Such desensitization is regarded as part of the process of becoming professional (i.e., a new identity), and of becoming more able to bracket emotions that might otherwise hinder physical assessment and treatment.

Cadaver stories allow students to cope with some of the most anxiety-producing activities (e.g., dissecting sexual organs and the face) by encouraging students to see the event from the perspective of an outsider *and* an insider: cadaver stories would not be funny without the student empathizing with the "emotionally vulnerable" layperson and recognizing that this is a "joke" meant for medical professionals. As one listens and laughs, the medical student becomes one of "us," the in-group. More importantly, in these high uncertainty events, the medical students learn to reduce uncertainty not through information-seeking or information avoiding, but through transforming the meanings of their uncertainty. In other words, rather than manipulating the amount of information as a strategy for uncertainty management, medical students manage their uncertainty by changing the *quality* of the event/uncertainty (see also Theory of Message Design Logic in Chapter 8): They come to see differently (i.e., a new reality) because they are transformed (i.e., a new cultural perspective).

Humor as a speech activity highlights the interactive and collaborative display of shared knowledge and agreed-upon norms (Kotthoff, 2007) – a joke is not successful if only the speaker thinks it is funny. At the same time, humor allows individuals to make sense of "modifications and transgressions in communicative processes" (Kotthoff 2007, p. 263). Humor, in such contexts, becomes the vehicle for cultural values and social norms – elements essential for Mythic Connection. When examining individuals' use of humor in palliative care, Dean and Gregory (2004) argued, "The value of humor resides not in its capacity to alter physical reality, but in its capacity for affective or psychological change that enhances the humanity of the experience" (p. 146). The transformative, interactive, and collaborative nature of humor allows healthcare providers, patients, and families to build therapeutic relationships, contend with circumstances (e.g., relieve tension), and express sensibility (e.g., protect dignity and a sense of worth). In other words, humor allows participants to maintain and manage multiple competing (if not conflicting) goals by providing multiple frames to interpret the meanings of uncertainty (Dean & Gregory, 2004; Kotthoff, 2007).

3. Comparisons of Cultural Perspectives toward Uncertainty

Uncertainty is a salient topic, a sore thumb, under Perspectival Thinking. It creates a glaring weakness of the system that cultural participants must learn to "tolerate." In contrast, uncertainty under Mythic Connection and Magic Consciousness is qualitatively different – it is not a weakness, but part of reality and an essential part of the story. It is integrated into the meanings of reality. However, these two cultural perspectives entail distinctive approaches to uncertainty.

Under Magic Consciousness, people do not experience (un)certainty nor ambiguity. Magic is a performance that is not symbolic. Thus, it does not point beyond the act or talk itself. Magic is spaceless and timeless and, thus, without perspective/position. Under Magic Consciousness, people live in the here and now. For them, (un)certainty is a non-issue because their reality/world is not fragmented (i.e., it's taken-for-granted). It (identity) is tautological. It is what it is. I am what I am. Interpretation is nonexistent. Doubt and certainty are not involved in Magic Consciousness. As a result, when people hold Magic Consciousness, they do not experience uncertainty. The translation of the ancient Jewish mythologeme harkens back to the magic origin. In Exodus 3: 13–14: (*New International Version,* 1978/2011)

> Moses said to God, "Suppose I go to the Israelites and say to them, 'The God of your fathers has sent me to you,' and they ask me, 'What is his name?' Then what shall I tell them?"
>
> God said to Moses, "I AM WHO I AM. This is what you are to say to the Israelites: 'I AM has sent me to you.'"

God's name is *Yahweh,* "I am." The sentence, "God is" is a simple acknowledgment of truth (verition) of being (Gebser, 1949–1953/1985; Kramer, 1997). It is not an explanation, or a description, or a story, or an argument, or a justification. In that sense, it has no meaning. It is what is – a taken-for-granted reality.

In contrast, uncertainty is essential for Mythic Connection. Inherent in uncertainty is the ambiguity of meanings, which demands interpretation. Because we need interpretation to decipher the meanings, we rely on symbolic communication (e.g., imagination and creativity through storytelling) to reconcile ambiguity inherent in realities. Through stories and storytelling, Mythic Connection finds its points of reference, be it found in religion or science, that enable people to make sense of (orient toward) novel situations. In short, the presence of uncertainty gives meaning to one's reality. For example, if the existence of God is certain, the value of religious devotion becomes less meaningful. If God is a certainty for a person, doubt, interpretation, or explanation is not necessary or provoked. God does not need devotion, as such because its existence simply is the case. The "leap of faith," an awareness of uncertainty but also a commitment to the unknown, empowers individuals with Mythic Connection.

Studies found that when individuals experience high uncertainty, they increase their belief in a God that is in control of chaos (Kay et al., 2010; see also religious coping in Chapter 13). When people are primed to think about God, they are more likely to take risks (Chan et al., 2014). Such findings may entail different processes under different cultural perspectives. By shifting into Magic Consciousness, one eliminates all uncertainty (i.e., "It's God's will."). In an interesting way, by relinquishing the agency and control that one is presumed to have under Perspectival Thinking, the person is free from their anxiety due to lack of control. In our studies about Indonesian women with diabetes, they explained how recognizing their illness as God's will can be an empowering experience:

> Marni explained, "I don't want people to visit me in the hospital and cry. I'm so prepared for this, and I feel I'm strong! I resign my fate to God." Surti also explained, "[My diabetes] doesn't make me depressed at all. Rather, it makes me grateful that God still looks after me. Thus, although I get sick, I can still do my daily activities." (Pitaloka & Hsieh, 2015, p. 1161)

In a study of women with end-stage renal disease, a participant reported, "You have to be *a believer first*. If you say, 'I don't believe that this can happen or this and that,' then you will not be healed" [emphasis added] (Tanyi & Werner, 2008, p. 40). Another patient noted, "[spirituality] doesn't allow me to give up so easily whatever my fight is" (Tanyi & Werner, 2008, p. 40). In short, by assuming Magic Consciousness, these patients are empowered to accept their suffering (without pitying themselves) and fight their hardest struggles (without worrying about the outcomes). It is what it is. Uncertainty is a non-issue.

In contrast, by shifting into Mythic Connection, one can find meanings even in the face of great adversities (e.g., "This is a test from God for me to show grace in adversities."). For example, Fitri, another Indonesian patient with diabetes, explained:

> God has a beautiful plan for us. Whatever that is, I will accept it with patience. This illness means that God still loves me. He wants me to remember that there are many people out there that live a more unfortunate life than I do.... It is part of His blessings. (Pitaloka & Hsieh, 2015, p. 1161)

By reframing their illness experiences as a blessing, these patients were able to find the silver lining in God's plan, maintaining hope and strength as they cope with daily struggles (Sadati et al., 2015). When discussing her experience with end-stage renal disease, a patient concluded, "You just come to understand there is a bigger meaning in the universe than you" (Tanyi & Werner, 2008, p. 46). Thus, under Mythic Connection, a person may experience uncertainty, but they also come to appreciate that their life/fate is not their own (i.e., connection to a larger community). As a result, their uncertainty is not within their control. By surrendering themselves to the greater meaning/purpose (that they may not comprehend), they are empowered in their illness management. One study found that women with lower socioeconomic status, minorities, and those with more severe disease are more likely to see the "benefits" when first diagnosed with breast cancer (Tomich & Helgeson, 2004). From this perspective, a patient may shift from Perspectival Thinking to Magic Consciousness and Mythic Connection as a coping strategy for uncertainty management when they have limited control over the illness (e.g., aggressive or advanced cancer) or limited resources to cope with the illness.

Many scholars have argued that from this perspective, what appears as fatalistic strategies under Perspectival Thinking are, in fact, active and adaptive behaviors under Magic Consciousness and Mythic Connection that empower cultural participants to exercise agency and maintain hope in their illness experiences (Pitaloka & Hsieh, 2015; Sadati et al., 2015). We have relied primarily on faith/spirituality to discuss Magic Consciousness and Mythic Connection because religion is a common coping mechanism when one shifts cultural perspectives. However, it is important to note that Magic Consciousness and Mythic Connection need not derive from religion. For example, mothers with mental illness may rely on their relationships with their children to maintain hope (e.g., "My children give me strength, they give me hope, they give me the will to survive...;" Nicholson, 2010, p. 376). By emphasizing their identity as a mother (i.e., a parent-child bond under Magic Consciousness) rather than as a patient, mothers who are coping with a severe illness often reported a sense of empowerment in great adversities. By changing the *quality* (as opposed to the quantity) of uncertainty, one can (re)gain control over their experiences of uncertainty. Uncertainty management becomes a resource to claim agency and control. Uncertainty is integrated into one's worldview and, thus, is always meaningful and valuable.

For example, whereas the linear life narratives dominant in Western culture construct uncertainty as a cause of biographical disruption (for a detailed discussion about biographical disruption, biographical reinforcement, and biographical illumination, see Chapter 3), researchers have found that patients develop alternative narratives to regain control of their life stories. Parents of babies with disabilities actively engage in storytelling with "overlaid and interwoven values that are applied to interpret uncertainty as an opportunity to focus on the quality of life in the present" (Fisher & Goodley, 2007, p. 74). Rather than feeling powerless toward an uncertain future, these parents construct their life stories as "open-ended uncertainty" (Fisher & Goodley, 2007, p. 75). They portray the present as ongoing, evolving, and always intertwined with others' lives. A mother explained how her child with disability had "enriched her life and the lives of many people he had come into contact with. She felt he was special and was blessed with the ability to reach out and touch people and bring people together in new ways" (Fisher & Goodley, 2007, p. 75). Another mother said that she would be happy to have another child with autism, "They are lovely kids. They've really taught me something. They've taught me to look at people in different ways" (Fisher & Goodley, 2007, p. 75). Rather than focusing on a hope that targets a concrete goal, such parents develop "transcendent" hope that allows them to connect and empathize with others and embrace future possibilities, meanings, and values. In other words, by moving away from a singular focus under Perspectival Thinking, people may incorporate other cultural perspectives and develop an Integral Fusion worldview that create desired meanings for their uncertainty (and everyday life).

From this perspective, time (or *temporal* dimension) plays a vital role as individuals develop an Integral Fusion worldview (Heidegger, 1927/1962; Husserl, 1964/2019), a point also echoed by Problematic Integration Theory and Uncertainty Management Theory. How we react to situations is often layered with previous experiences. Our phobias and anxieties are rooted in our pasts. Our coping in the present often involves projecting future outcomes to moderate those anxieties. The layering of temporal scenes is the process of integration. Experience is blended with current conditions and projected future actions. This is the four-dimensional process and mode of experience, borrowing from Gebser (1949–1953/1985), we call the Integral Fusion. The Integral Fusion is not limited to dominant emotional states or linear thinking. It enables a multiplicity of coping mechanisms drawing on all temporal vectors (past, present, future, and the integration of them). Memory of the "past" occurs now as does projection for the future, and all the while the now is moving/changing, requiring constant integration of new recollections and new potentials. Some cultures call this wisdom. It is the fundamental hermeneutic aspect of human experience (Derrida, 1975–1976/2020; Gebser, 1949–1953/1985; Kramer, 1997). Thus, the future becomes an open horizon. Even the certainty of adversities (e.g., looming death in end-of-life care) can take on a multiplicity of meanings forming a complex process. This Integral Fusion worldview encompasses the perspectival precision of calling the time of death (as a single event) and all the other channels of flowing information that lead up to, through, and continue beyond the event so that the event becomes part of an ongoing temporal process that is not only personal but also collective understanding of realities (Whitehead, 1929/2010).

In conclusion, the early development of theories of uncertainty highlighted the inherent bias of Perspectival Thinking by assuming uncertainty to be undesirable, and people as predisposed to eliminate uncertainty – almost as by instinct. In addition, information-seeking was conceptualized as the primary method for uncertainty management. However, when we assume other cultural perspectives on uncertainty, it becomes apparent that personal information-seeking behavior is only one of the many ways people deal with uncertainty. Magic Consciousness and Mythic Connection transform the nature of uncertainty to something qualitatively different from the uncertainty experienced by Perspectival Thinking. Physicians use humor, which may be perceived to be inappropriate or offensive to outsiders, to maintain a sense of community (i.e., an essential element for mythic and magic cultural perspectives). Through humor, they empathize with others and socialize emotional coping strategies in particularly high stress and tragic situations. Patients and family members embrace uncertainty as a resource that is empowering, relationship-strengthening, and life-affirming. They are not passive recipients (or victims) of uncertainty. Rather, through reframing uncertainty, they regain agency (i.e., a sense of control). Uncertainty is not merely tolerated but actively *integrated* into their life stories, shaping meanings beyond their experiences of uncertainty. By doing so, these people develop an Integral Fusion worldview that accommodates competing perspectives, including communicative goals and conflicting tensions of uncertainty.

II. Cultural Approaches to Uncertainty Management

A. The Interactive Nature of Uncertainty Management

The research community across diverging disciplines has now come to the consensus that reducing uncertainty is not always desirable. In the fields of intercultural communication and cross-cultural psychology, researchers have noted cultures have different levels of **uncertainty avoidance**. Uncertainty avoidance is the level of tolerance one has for unpredictability. Having high uncertainty avoidance means that one has a strong desire to avoid uncertainty. As a result, such cultures are likely to prefer highly formalized and structured forms of communication and procedures, often reflected in their extensive collections of laws, libraries, and policies. Perspectival Thinking is the embodiment of high uncertainty avoidance. In contrast, cultures with low uncertainty avoidance mean that they are not obsessed with predictability. As a result, they are not driven to eliminate uncertainty: they "accept dissent" and have "lower stress and weaker superegos" (Gudykunst, 2003a, p. 19). Hofstede (2001) noted that members of high uncertainty avoidance find "what is different is dangerous;" in contrast, members of low uncertainty avoidance find "what is different is curious" (p. 161). Generally speaking, Perspectival Thinking is higher in uncertainty avoidance than Mythic Connection and Magic Consciousness.

At an individual level, researchers have noted the concept of **ambiguity aversion**, a psychological trait studied extensively in behavioral economics and risk psychology. Ambiguity aversion refers to individuals' preference for taking risks of *known* probabilities over risks of *unknown* probabilities. Although the majority of people are ambiguity averse, some people (e.g., individuals with highly optimistic personalities) are less ambiguity averse than the rest (Pulford, 2009). In the medical literature, however, some researchers have used ambiguity aversion as a general description as preferences to avoid uncertainty (e.g., Portnoy et al., 2013).

In this sense, ambiguity can be used interchangeably as uncertainty. Because ambiguity aversion is conceptualized as a psychological trait, it is viewed as a fixed, stable personality trait, rather than an attitude that can be interactively negotiated. Because multiple studies have identified negative impacts when health professionals have low tolerance for ambiguity (e.g., increased test-ordering, failure to comply with evidence-based guidelines, fear of malpractice litigation, defensive practice, and discomfort in the contexts of death and grief), some have proposed using a measure of tolerance for ambiguity as a criterion for selecting applicants for medical school (Geller, 2013).

Although the discipline of psychology tends to view social groups or individuals' preferences as stable, innate personality characteristics, recent studies in communication have highlighted individuals' understandings of uncertainty as being socially constructed and interactively negotiated with their supportive others. The interdependent and interpersonal nature of uncertainty management is especially important in health-care contexts given the unpredictable, complex, and ambiguous nature of physician-patient interactions and medical procedures (Brashers, 2001). Patients frequently seek or avoid information as a means of maintaining illness-related uncertainty in order to sustain hope or deniability, continue with life, manage overwhelming or flawed information, and/or maintain boundaries (Barbour et al., 2011; Beach & Dozier, 2015). Providers' responses to patient uncertainty influence their ability to diagnose and connect with patients, their referral and disclosure patterns (Prochniak et al., 2012), and patient satisfaction (Politi et al., 2011b), all of which also shape patients' experiences of illness-related uncertainty. Brashers et al. (2000) explained, "One of the ways individuals can manage uncertainty (and thus manage emotional responses to it) is by managing interaction" (p.66).

Uncertainty management is situated in and coordinated within individuals' social networks. Uncertainty can be created, challenged, and successfully negotiated within a single conversation (Beach & Dozier, 2015; Gutzmer & Beach, 2015). A person's choice of withholding or disclosing specific information may influence another's uncertainty about self, the other, and the relationship (Goldsmith, 2009; Knobloch & Satterlee, 2009). Individuals do not have total control over their uncertainty or its corresponding meanings. The meanings of uncertainty are socially constructed and interactively negotiated. For example, a person may recognize the possibility of increasing conversational partners' uncertainty or even violating their uncertainty preferences, but feel obligated or compelled to share certain information, such as sexual disclosure or cancer risk estimates (Han et al., 2011; Lo et al., 2009). Providers' perceptions of patient attitudes toward uncertainty may influence their disclosure patterns. In particular, when physicians believe that patients may have negative reactions to a discussion about the scientific uncertainties or disagreements surrounding a controversial medical test or treatment, they are likely to adopt a paternalistic approach, avoiding discussions about scientific uncertainty or involving them in decision-making (Portnoy et al., 2013).

In addition, *how* physicians communicate risk-estimates (e.g., textual and/or visual formats) can influence whether a patient experiences heightening worries or negative affect (Han et al., 2011). For example, an interpreter recalled two incidents in which physicians' responses to patient uncertainty led to different outcomes:

> [The patient could not decide whether to receive an amniocentesis, and the doctor said], "I cannot make this decision for you. You have to make it for yourself." And the patient went home confused. And that's where it stood. ... And a week later, I had the very same situation with another doctor and the doctor simply said, "You know what, this is what I tell my patients. My wife never had the amnio, because she said whatever the baby is, I'm still having it. So, she never had the amnio." So, the patient went home so happy. (Hsieh, 2006, p. 724)

By sharing a story about his wife, the second physician was able to effectively address the patient's uncertainty without violating patient autonomy. When discussing poor prognosis of a malignant disease, patients and doctors together used certain key terms ambiguously (e.g., "you are *stable* at the moment" or "everything is going *okay*"), in a manner which allowed doctors to feel that facts were not misrepresented and the patient to feel reassured (Skelton et al., 1999; see Figure 9.4).

Because uncertainty is multilayered and interconnected, individuals often need to coordinate and collaborate with others to manage different areas of uncertainty and different communicative goals (Knobloch & Satterlee, 2009; Martin et al., 2010; Tait et al., 2009). (For more discussions on social support, see Chapter 10.)

Relational others are critical in providing evaluative frameworks to assist individuals in interpreting uncertainty (Brashers et al., 2004). For example, parents' communicative behaviors and frames can influence children's understanding of reality. When parents experience higher levels of stress, report higher levels of uncertainty, or

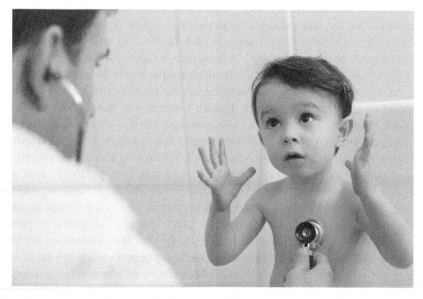

Figure 9.4 Uncertainty is interactively negotiated. How we talk about the "facts" makes a big difference in how we understand our realities and uncertainties. *Source:* Cultura Creative (RF) / Alamy Stock Photo

perceive their children to be more vulnerable, their children also experience higher levels of illness-related uncertainty, which heightens children's experiences of pain or depressive symptoms (Mullins et al., 2007; Page et al., 2012).

Physicians help patients to develop specific interpretive frames to manage their uncertainty. For example, providers may use specific contextualization cues in their conversation to "orient patients' understanding of their conditions and guide their interpretation of providers' intended meanings" (Hsieh et al., 2016, p. 1196). An analysis of conversations between patients with a serious malignant disease and a hematologist found that providers offer evaluative frames to offer assurance to patients' uncertainty (e.g., "I'm not too worried." "Don't worry too much." "It doesn't look rosy but how serious it is, I can't say."; Skelton et al., 1999). By referring to the surgical option for cancer treatment as an "incredibly morbid procedure" and "a big, big surgery," an oncologist discouraged the patient from the specific treatment (Hsieh et al., 2016). When a patient expressed concerns about an earlier CT scan that suggested that her cancer may have metastasized to her lungs, the provider contradicted the diagnostic CT scan by offering her personal observation as an expert, noting, "I'm doubtful that we'll see much just because you're sitting here looking fairly normal. You know, people with a belly full of tumors come in, and they don't feel good" (Hsieh et al., 2016, p. 1194). Thus, the provider encouraged the patient to rely on her observation, rather than the CT scan, as the interpretive frame. Providers may also offer assurance and control meaning by explaining that the treatment offered is standardized, best practices, for all patients and thus, preemptively block specific interpretive frames (e.g., a more aggressive option is not offered due to patients' advanced age; Hsieh et al., 2016).

A physician's choice of interpretive frame can have a significant impact on a patient's understanding. For example, a physician may choose to communicate illness-related uncertainty through *numbers* (e.g., probability, ranges, or distribution; "the mortality rate is 20–25%") or *evaluative labels* (e.g., high or low; good or bad; "the mortality rate is high"). Numerical uncertainty ranges (e.g., confidence intervals: the associated confidence level that the true parameter is in the proposed range) and evaluable labels highlight different aspects of uncertainty. Physicians often rely on statistical probabilities to communicate uncertainty (e.g., "Among patients who took the diagnostic test in our clinic, 95% were negative; but if the result is positive, one in five survive more than three years"). A patient's ability to understand the meanings of a risk-estimate is dependent on their health numeracy. **Health numeracy** is defined as "individual-level skills needed to understand and use *quantitative* health information, including basic computation skills, ability to use information in documents and non-text formats such as graphs, and ability to communicate orally" [emphasis added] (see also discussion on health literacy on Chapter 7; Ancker & Kaufman, 2007, p. 719). Patients with low health numeracy experience increased uncertainty due to difficulties in understanding risk estimates, follow complex health regimens, or make informed decisions (Manganello & Clayman, 2011; Peters et al., 2007). Peters et al. (2009) explained, "Decision makers need help in interpreting not only what the numbers are but what they mean" (p. 226). As a result, **evaluative labels** may be particularly helpful for situations involving unfamiliar, not easily evaluable numeric information or for individuals with low numeracy. Dieckmann et al. (2012) noted some advantages and disadvantages of using evaluative labels for decision-making purposes. On the one hand, laypeople have an easier time understanding the general concept of uncertainty when an evaluative label is provided. In particular, evaluative labels help individuals with low numeracy to better integrate relevant information for decision-making and minimize influences from irrelevant information (Dieckmann et al., 2012; Peters et al., 2009). However, some people may overemphasize evaluative labels, resulting in decisions that were inconsistent with their previously stated attitudes. Dieckmann et al. (2012) concluded, for people with low numeracy, "putting an evaluative label on a particular element of a display may signal to a layperson that this element is paramount to the decision at hand. … The simplicity and power of evaluative labels is a double-edged sword" (p.733).

In summary, as uncertainty is communicated, individuals inevitably have to decide how, and to what extent, they will disclose uncertainty. The meanings of uncertainty are socially constructed and interactively negotiated. The goals of communication, however, do not always aim to reduce or eliminate uncertainty. Instead, both patients and providers actively and strategically use different linguistic devices (e.g., evaluative labels, interpretive frames, and risk estimates) to manipulate the meanings of uncertainty in order to achieve specific communicative goals (e.g., discouraging certain options or facilitating informed decision-making).

B. Pragmatic Functions of Ambiguity

Depending on one's cultural perspectives, uncertainty can lead to different approaches for illness management. Under Perspectival Thinking, certainty is meaningful. Uncertainty should be eliminated because it frustrates the linear pursuit of Perspectival Thinking and is a barrier to an individual's ability to assess "reality." The literature on uncertainty management, health literacy, and medical decision-making has traditionally centered on achieving informed decision-making by eliminating uncertainty. By ensuring that individuals have an "accurate" understanding of reality (e.g., risk estimates), individuals are presumed to be capable of making decisions that are consistent with their values.

In contrast, because uncertainty is part of the taken-for-granted reality in Magic Consciousness and Mythic Connection, uncertainty is not perceived to be a void in need of interpretation or something to be eliminated. Uncertainty may be preferred over final solutions and such extended ambiguity is meaningful for many reasons. As long as the case is "open," discussion can continue, and everyone can feel engaged and respected. Many scholars have noted that magic and mythic people tend to leave conflicts unresolved and to argue in circles for three reasons (Greenhouse, 1989; Javidan, 2007; Zimbardo & Boyd, 2015). First, in an intimate community, it is best to leave things somewhat unresolved rather than totally defeating a fellow community member and leaving them with no face (i.e., relationship maintenance). Second, there is no sense of urgency to resolve things or to finish things "on schedule" (i.e., an absence of temporal urgency). Third, there is less concern to disambiguate identities and events (i.e., low ambiguity aversion).

The literature traditionally has used the term uncertainty and ambiguity interchangeably. So far, we also have used these two terms interchangeably in this Chapter. However, in recent years, some researchers have distinguished the two concepts. Some argued that **ambiguity** is a form of uncertainty, specific to the "lack of reliability, credibility, or adequacy of risk estimates" (Han et al., 2011, p. 833). Ellsberg (1961), an economist, noted that ambiguity exists when the probability of the risk is *unknown*, and uncertainty arises when the probability of the risk is *known*. Ambiguity is mathematically presented as "the confidence level around individual probability estimates," signaling "uncertainty about uncertainty" (Dhawale et al., 2017, p. 867). Grenier et al., (2005) proposed that ambiguity concerns the circumstances of the *present*; in contrast, **uncertainty** concerns unpredictable circumstances of the *future*. It is beyond the scope of the current Chapter to delineate the differences or similarities between uncertainty and ambiguity, as the literature involves diverse disciplines, diverging approaches, and conflicting claims. Nevertheless, we have decided to choose the term ambiguity to highlight our interests and focus for the current section: the pragmatic functions of maintaining uncertainty in difficult, complex situations in health contexts. By changing our use of the term from uncertainty to ambiguity, we aim to connect to the larger literature on strategic ambiguity, intentional ambiguity, and equivocal communication. Our focus is on the purposeful maintenance of ambiguity in medical encounters.

Researchers have observed that when discussing serious illness, providers' talk often involves ambiguity resulting from structurally and pragmatically inconsistent information (Batten et al., 2019; Hsieh & Terui, 2015). For example, it is not uncommon for providers to provide both optimistic and pessimistic statements in a single medical encounter (Robinson et al., 2008). When observing oncologist-patient interactions, Hsieh and Terui (2015) noted that oncologists often adopt conversational tactics that create ambiguity. For example, one oncologist explained to a patient, "The report doesn't see anything big, spread, *which is good. They don't even see that cancer that's there.* ... CAT scans are a little bit- I mean *they're helpful, and then they're not helpful* because we know you have a cancer and they don't even comment on it" (Hsieh & Terui, 2015, p. 147). Another oncologist stated to a different patient, "So I think what my examination says is that you're better than average in terms of the way, you know, your exam is. And *I'm not seeing anything scary.* Okay? *So the only thing scary is the biopsy result*, not anything about your physical exam at all, so *that's awesome*, okay?" (Hsieh & Terui, 2015, p. 147). What does it mean to say something is "helpful but not helpful?" How about "Not seeing anything scary, except one scary thing. So that's awesome!" It is important to note that these self-conflicting remarks may not be the speakers' failure or mistake in providing a coherent meaning. These structural and pragmatic inconsistencies may be intended structure to "cover all grounds" (Hsieh & Terui, 2015, p. 148). Ambiguity should not be viewed exclusively as inefficiencies in the discursive process or a result of miscommunication (Xafis & Wilkinson, 2019). Rather, they serve specific functions.

First, ambiguity is **multivocal** (or polyvocal). Multivocality means the co-existence of multiple voices, meanings, and interpretations (Bakhtin, 1981; Baxter & Montgomery, 1996). Ambiguity destabilizes a unitary understanding of reality. As such, ambiguity becomes a tool and a resource for use by participants within a communicative activity to negotiate tensions, meanings, and identities. For example, patients may use a rhetorical question to mitigate their true questions or other face-threatening acts (e.g., challenging the physician's competence; Ainsworth-Vaughn, 1994). During a clinical appointment, a patient may reference conversations with another physician who suggests that a "cure" to his cancer was possible as an indirect strategy to solicit the current physician's opinion (Skelton et al., 1999). **Indirect information-seeking** (e.g., talking around the issue, disclosing information in hopes of receiving reciprocal disclosure) is common in health contexts (Brashers et al., 2002). It allows individuals to search for information "without the potential costs associated with direct discussions of the issue(s)" and "may improve the chances of being pleasantly surprised by the information received" (Afifi et al., 2004, pp. 433, 446). The success of indirect information-seeking lies in its ability to be ambiguous. Because multiple meanings co-exist, information seekers may minimize face threats to others and to themselves and their communicative goals (Davis, 2007).

Second, ambiguity allows participants to manage competing goals. Indirect information-seeking provides patients the opportunities to achieve competing communicative goals (e.g., challenging physicians' authority and minimizing potential face threats or identifying the status of illness without eliminating hope). "Certainty is not necessarily a goal of the consultation," particularly when patients are confronted with bad news (Skelton et al., 1999, p. 623). A patient may have a fairly certain course of treatment for the immediate future, but the long-term prognosis is poor. As a result, physicians have been observed to provide detailed discussions about treatments to facilitate informed decision-making and offer "less, and vaguer information about prognosis [sic], citing its uncertainty and lesser relevance to future actions as reasons" (Miyaji, 1993, p. 249). A hematologist explained, "I am vague about what the timescale is because I don't know what the timescale is usually" (Skelton et al., 1999, p. 623). Miyaji (1993) argued that by being specific about treatment plans but vague about illness trajectory, physicians aimed to manage the competing goals of honoring patient autonomy, protecting patients' hope, and preserving possibilities for medical advances.

Third, ambiguity allows participants to negotiate meanings, providing the flexibility needed to "agree to disagree." For example, Batten et al. (2019) demonstrated that patients and physicians often have significantly different understandings of *treatability statements* (e.g., "this is a treatability condition;" "we have treatments for your loved one") in the contexts of serious illness. Whereas physicians may not intend for a statement to suggest that there will be an improvement of prognosis or quality of life, patients often understand statements to be forms of encouragement to evoke hope and encourage the pursuit of further treatment. Strategic ambiguity has been identified as a communicative behavior utilized by many to manage conflicting goals (Bavelas et al., 1990). Xafis and Wilkinson (2019) argued when patients and providers have diverging understandings of the meanings conveyed in a treatability statement, it may not necessarily be a result of miscommunication. Rather, Xafis and Wilkinson (2019) proposed that physicians may rely on **intentional ambiguity** to manage competing communicative goals: (a) maintaining hope for the patient with terminal cancer, (b) fulfilling obligations as a health professional (e.g., telling the truth and providing health interventions), and (c) deferring decision-making regarding how best manage uncertainty (e.g., ambiguity allows clinicians to defer their responses toward stress or negative reactions from the patients, families, and even themselves to a later time). In other words, physicians may narrow their meanings of treatment to the immediate present and allow patients to maintain alternative meanings of treatment for the broader illness trajectory. The flexibility (and ambiguity) of meanings intended for the local context (e.g., the specific conversations for immediate decision-making) or the global/broader context (e.g., illness trajectory as a whole) allow physicians and patients to negotiate meanings and satisfy competing goals.

Finally, ambiguity provides agency to the recipient of the message to determine their course of action. Previous studies have suggested that patients are often at the mercy of providers' information disclosure (Miyaji, 1993). Once explicit information is given through direct communication, the information cannot be unheard. However, when a message is ambiguous, the recipient of the message has an opportunity to shape the meaning and trajectory of the disclosure. For example, if a provider says, "I'm glad that the tumor is now under control," a patient can say, "That's great." Such a response accepts the multivocality of the term "control," allowing "the doctor to feel that facts were not misrepresented while perhaps permitting the patient to feel reassured" (Skelton et al., 1999, p. 620). Alternatively, a patient may use the follow-up question to ask for an evaluative label (e.g., "Is that good news?"), seek clarification (e.g., "What do you mean by control?"), or address specific concerns (e.g., "Am I going to be cured? How long will I live?"). From this perspective, providers' intentional ambiguity provides patients the power to control their preference for information, desired level of uncertainty, and how and what information they wish to receive. In other words, ambiguity may not be the result of ineffective communication or a product of providers' hegemonic control of information. Instead, ambiguity can be a collaborative accomplishment between providers and patients to achieve mutually agreeable goals for optimal quality of care.

In summary, ambiguity in medical encounters is not necessarily a failure of effective communication (as perceived by Perspectival Thinking). The worldviews of Magic Consciousness and Mythic Connection embrace ambiguity. When ambiguity accommodates different meanings and empowers participants to reconcile and accommodate competing meanings, an Integral Fusion worldview that is shared by all participants emerges.

III. Additional Resources

A. Key Terms and Theories

sources of uncertainty
technical uncertainty
personal uncertainty
conceptual uncertainty
iatrogenesis
epistemological uncertainty
diagnostic uncertainty
medical reversal
ritualization of optimism
Uncertainty Reduction Theory (URT)
Anxiety/Uncertainty Management (AUM)
Reconceptualized Uncertainty in Illness Theory
Problematic Integration Theory
    Probabilistic orientation
    Evaluative orientation
Uncertainty Management Theory
    multilayered (uncertainty)
    interconnected (uncertainty)
    temporal (uncertainty)

uncertainty avoidance
ambiguity aversion
health numeracy
evaluative label
ambiguity (versus uncertainty)
multivocality
indirect information-seeking
intentional ambiguity

B. Discussion Questions

1. When there is an emerging pandemic crisis of a highly infectious and potentially deadly virus (e.g., COVID-19), there are many different sources and layers of uncertainty. Please review the sources and types of uncertainty discussed in the Chapter and answer the following questions?
   a. Can you give examples of the following sources of uncertainty:
      i. technical uncertainty
      ii. personal uncertainty
      iii. conceptual uncertainty
      iv. epistemological uncertainty
      v. diagnostic uncertainty
   b. Do you think different people may face different uncertainties in the same event? What kinds of uncertainties would the following persons have:
      i. physicians
      ii. policymakers
      iii. the general public
      iv. a person who is experiencing minor fever
   c. Can you give examples showing how their uncertainties can be multilayered and interconnected?
   d. How does the temporal dimension influence
      i. the sources of uncertainty in (a)(i)-(v)?
      ii. the kinds of uncertainties in (b)(i)-(iv)?
   e. How can we best resolve these uncertainties?
      i. Do you think different people (e.g., policymakers v. a potential patient) would resolve their uncertainty differently? Why?
      ii. Do you think different sources of uncertainties require different solutions? Why?
2. Do you agree that the meanings of uncertainties need to be appraised before people can choose their coping strategies?
   a. How would a person with Magic Consciousness answer this question?
   b. How about a person with Mythic Connection?
   c. How about a person with Perspectival Thinking?
3. Think of a time or an event in your life that you experienced high uncertainty (e.g., your mother was in ICU after a car accident; your cancer is in remission after intensive chemotherapy).
   a. How did you feel about the uncertainty? Did you feel excited or anxious?
      i. Did you try to reduce your uncertainty? How?
      ii. Did you try to increase your uncertainty? How?

     iii. Did you seek spiritual or religious coping? Was it helpful? Why?

     iv. Did you talk to friends? In what ways were they helpful? If you were to categorize their support, which cultural perspectives (i.e., Magic Consciousness, Mythic Connection, Perspective Thinking, or Integral Fusion) best explain their responses?

  b. Looking at your strategies/solutions for uncertainty management, which cultural perspective(s) (i.e., Magic Consciousness, Mythic Connection, Perspective Thinking, or Integral Fusion) best explain your responses? Why?

     i. Now looking back, do you think you could have tried different cultural perspectives? What would they look like?

  c. Do you think a particular cultural perspective is better or more efficient in managing uncertainties? Why or why not?

  d. Do you prefer one cultural perspective over another when managing uncertainties? Why?

4. Let's try a hypothetical. Your best friend's dad just received a diagnosis of pancreatic cancer. Your friend is extremely upset and distressed by the news. You want to help them manage their uncertainties.

  a. If your friend holds Magic Consciousness about her father's diagnosis, what would they believe and/or say? Do you think they experience uncertainty? How would you help?

  b. If your friend holds Mythic Connection about her father's diagnosis, what would they believe and/or say? Do you think they experience uncertainty? How would you help?

  c. If your friend holds Perspectival Thinking about her father's diagnosis, what would they believe and/or say? Do you think they experience uncertainty? How would you help?

5. Why do you think physicians adopt the ritualization of optimism if they, at the same time, also believe the importance of informed decision-making? Are they contradictory in their beliefs and/or practices?

6. Think of an example that you intentionally tried to maintain ambiguity when talking to another person. Explain the event/example.

  a. How did you maintain ambiguity? (e.g., did you adopt any specific behavioral, verbal, or nonverbal strategies?)

  b. Why did you maintain ambiguity?

  c. Do you think maintaining ambiguity in those situations is good or bad?

  d. Are there good reasons to maintain ambiguity?

  e. Do you think physicians' ritualization of optimism conflicts with the principles of informed decision-making, patient-centered care, and/or patient autonomy?

C. References

Afifi, W. A., Dillow, M. R., & Morse, C. (2004). Examining predictors and consequences of information seeking in close relationships. *Personal Relationships*, *11*(4), 429–449.

Ainsworth-Vaughn, N. (1994). Is that a rhetorical question? Ambiguity and power in medical discourse. *Journal of Linguistic Anthropology*, *4*(2), 194–214.

Ancker, J. S., & Kaufman, D. (2007). Rethinking health numeracy: A multidisciplinary literature review. *Journal of the American Medical Informatics Association*, *14*(6), 713–721.

Babrow, A. S. (1992). Communication and problematic integration: Understanding diverging probability and value, ambiguity, ambivalence, and impossibility. *Communication Theory*, *2*(2), 95–130.

Babrow, A. S. (2001). Uncertainty, value, communication, and problematic integration. *Journal of Communication*, *51*(3), 553–573.

Babrow, A. S., Kasch, C. R., & Ford, L. A. (1998). The many meanings of uncertainty in illness: Toward a systematic accounting. *Health Communication*, *10*(1), 1–23.

Babrow, A. S., & Kline, K. N. (2000). From "reducing" to "coping with" uncertainty: Reconceptualizing the central challenge in breast self-exams. *Social Science & Medicine*, *51*(12), 1805–1816.

Babrow, A. S., & Striley, K. M. (2014). Problematic integration theory and uncertainty management theory: Learning to hear and speak to different forms of uncertainty. In D. O. Braithwaite & P. Schrodt (Eds.), *Engaging theories in interpersonal communication: Multiple perspectives* (2nd ed., pp. 103–114). Sage.

Bakhtin, M. M. (1981). *The dialogic imagination: Four essays by M. M. Bakhtin*. (M. Holquist & C. Emerson, Trans.). University of Texas Press.

Barbour, J. B., Rintamaki, L. S., Ramsey, J. A., & Brashers, D. E. (2011). Avoiding health information. *Journal of Health Communication*, *17*(2), 212–229.

Batten, J. N., Wong, B. O., Hanks, W. F., & Magnus, D. C. (2019). Treatability statements in serious illness: The gap between what is said and what is heard. *Cambridge Quarterly of Healthcare Ethics*, *28*(3), 394–404.

Bavelas, J. B., Black, A., Chovil, N., & Mullett, J. (1990). *Equivocal communication*. Sage.

Baxter, L. A., & Montgomery, B. M. (1996). *Relating: Dialogues and dialectics*. Guilford Press.

Beach, W. A., & Dozier, D. M. (2015). Fears, uncertainties, and hopes: Patient-initiated actions and doctors' responses during oncology interviews. *Journal of Health Communication*, *20*(11), 1243–1254.

Beresford, E. B. (1991). Uncertainty and the shaping of medical decisions. *Hastings Center Report*, *21*(4), 6–11.

Berger, C. R., & Calabrese, R. J. (1975). Some explorations in initial interaction and beyond: Toward a developmental theory of interpersonal communication. *Human Communication Research*, *1*(2), 99–112.

Bhise, V., Rajan, S. S., Sittig, D. F., Morgan, R. O., Chaudhary, P., & Singh, H. (2018). Defining and measuring diagnostic uncertainty in medicine: A systematic review. *Journal of General Internal Medicine*, *33*(1), 103–115.

Bradac, J. J. (2001). Theory comparison: Uncertainty reduction, problematic integration, uncertainty management, and other curious constructs. *Journal of Communication*, *51*(3), 456–476.

Brashers, D. E. (2001). Communication and uncertainty management. *Journal of Communication*, *51*(3), 477–497.

Brashers, D. E., & Babrow, A. S. (1996). Theorizing communication and health. *Communication Studies*, *47*, 243–251.

Brashers, D. E., Goldsmith, D. J., & Hsieh, E. (2002). Information seeking and avoiding in health contexts. *Human Communication Research*, *28*(2), 258–271.

Brashers, D. E., Hsieh, E., Neidig, J. L., & Reynolds, N. R. (2006). Managing uncertainty about illness: Health care providers as credible authorities. In R. M. Dailey & B. A. Le Poire (Eds.), *Applied interpersonal communication matters: Family, health, and community relations* (pp. 219–240). Peter Lang.

Brashers, D. E., Neidig, J. L., & Goldsmith, D. J. (2004). Social support and the management of uncertainty for people living with HIV or AIDS. *Health Communication*, *16*(3), 305–331.

Brashers, D. E., Neidig, J. L., Haas, S. M., Dobbs, L. K., Cardillo, L. W., & Russell, J. A. (2000). Communication in the management of uncertainty: The case of persons living with HIV or AIDS. *Communication Monographs*, *67*(1), 63–84.

Brashers, D. E., Neidig, J. L., Reynolds, N. R., & Haas, S. M. (1998). Uncertainty in illness across the HIV/AIDS trajectory. *Journal of the Association of Nurses in AIDS Care*, *9*(1), 66–77.

Case, D. O., Andrews, J. E., Johnson, J. D., & Allard, S. L. (2005). Avoiding versus seeking: The relationship of information seeking to avoidance, blunting, coping, dissonance, and related concepts. *Journal of the Medical Library Association*, *93*(3), 353–362.

Chan, K. Q., Tong, E. M. W., & Tan, Y. L. (2014). Taking a leap of faith: Reminders of God lead to greater risk taking. *Social Psychological and Personality Science*, *5*(8), 901–909.

Chow, E., Davis, L., Panzarella, T., Hayter, C., Szumacher, E., Loblaw, A., Wong, R., & Danjoux, C. (2005). Accuracy of survival prediction by palliative radiation oncologists. *International Journal of Radiation Oncology Biology Physics*, *61*(3), 870–873.

Christakis, N. A. (1998). Predicting patient survival before and after hospice enrollment. *The Hospice Journal*, *13*(1-2), 71–87.

Cohen, P. R., Day, D., De Lisio, J., Greenberg, M., Kjeldsen, R., Suthers, D., & Berman, P. (1987). Management of uncertainty in medicine. *International Journal of Approximate Reasoning*, *1*(1), 103–116.

Davis, W. A. (2007). *Implicature: Intention, convention, and principle in the failure of Gricean theory*. Cambridge University Press.

Dean, R. A. K., & Gregory, D. M. (2004). Humor and laughter in palliative care: An ethnographic investigation. *Palliative and Supportive Care*, *2*(2), 139–148.

Derrida, J. (2020). *Life death*. (P.-A. Brault & M. Naas, Trans.; P.-A. Brault & P. Kamuf, Eds.). University of Chicago Press. (Original work published 1975–1976)

Dhawale, T., Steuten, L. M., & Deeg, H. J. (2017). Uncertainty of physicians and patients in medical decision making. *Biology of Blood and Marrow Transplantation*, *23*(6), 865–869.

Dieckmann, N. F., Peters, E., Gregory, R., & Tusler, M. (2012). Making sense of uncertainty: Advantages and disadvantages of providing an evaluative structure. *Journal of Risk Research*, *15*(7), 717–735.

Ellsberg, D. (1961). Risk, ambiguity, and the Savage axioms. *The Quarterly Journal of Economics*, *75*(4), 643–669.

Fisher, P., & Goodley, D. (2007). The linear medical model of disability: Mothers of disabled babies resist with counter-narratives. *Sociology of Health & Illness*, *29*(1), 66–81.

Fox, R. C. (1980). The evolution of medical uncertainty. *The Milbank Memorial Fund Quarterly. Health and Society*, *58*(1), 1–49.

Fox, R. C. (2002). Medical uncertainty revisited. In G. Bendelow, M. Carpenter, C. Vautier, & S. Williams (Eds.), *Gender, health and healing: The public/private divide* (pp. 236–253). Routledge.

Gebser, J. (1985). *The ever-present origin*. (N. Barstad & A. Mickunas, Trans.). Ohio University Press. (Original work published 1949–1953)

Geller, G. (2013). Tolerance for ambiguity: An ethics-based criterion for medical student selection. *Academic Medicine*, *88*(5), 581–584.

Goldsmith, D. J. (2009). Uncertainty and communication in couples coping with serious illness. In T. D. Afifi & W. A. Afifi (Eds.), *Uncertainty, information management, and disclosure decisions: Theories and applications* (pp. 203–225). Routledge.

Goldsmith, D. J., & Brashers, D. E. (2008). Communication matters: Developing and testing social support interventions. *Communication Monographs*, *75*(4), 320–329.

Greenhouse, C. J. (1989). Just in time: Temporality and the cultural legitimation of law. *The Yale Law Journal*, *98*(8), 1631–1651.

Grenier, S., Barrette, A.-M., & Ladouceur, R. (2005). Intolerance of uncertainty and intolerance of ambiguity: Similarities and differences. *Personality and Individual Differences*, *39*(3), 593–600.

Griffiths, F., Green, E., & Bendelow, G. (2006). Health professionals, their medical interventions and uncertainty: A study focusing on women at midlife. *Social Science & Medicine*, *62*(5), 1078–1090.

Gudykunst, W. B. (1998). Applying anxiety\uncertainty management (AUM) Theory to intercultural adjustment training. *International Journal of Intercultural Relations*, *22*(2), 227–250.

Gudykunst, W. B. (Ed.). (2003a). *Cross-cultural and intercultural communication*. Sage.

Gudykunst, W. B. (2003b). Understanding must precede criticism: A response to Yoshitake's critique of Anxiety/Uncertainty Management Theory. *Intercultural Communication Studies*, *12*(1), 25–40.

Guillán, A. (2017). *Pragmatic idealism and scientific prediction: A philosophical system and its approach to prediction in science*. Springer.

Gutzmer, K., & Beach, W. A. (2015). "Having an ovary this big is not normal": Physicians' use of normal to assess wellness and sickness during oncology interviews. *Health Communication*, *30*(1), 8–18.

Hafferty, F. W. (1988). Cadaver stories and the emotional socialization of medical students. *Journal of Health and Social Behavior*, *29*(4), 344–356.

Han, P. K. J., Klein, W. M. P., & Arora, N. K. (2011). Varieties of uncertainty in health care: A conceptual taxonomy. *Medical Decision Making*, *31*(6), 828–838.

Han, P. K. J., Klein, W. M. P., Lehman, T., Killam, B., Massett, H., & Freedman, A. N. (2011). Communication of uncertainty regarding individualized cancer risk estimates: Effects and influential factors. *Medical Decision Making*, *31*(2), 354–366.

Hancock, K., Clayton, J. M., Parker, S. M., Wal der, S., Butow, P. N., Carrick, S., Currow, D., Ghersi, D., Glare, P., Hagerty, R., & Tattersall, M. H. (2007). Truth-telling in discussing prognosis in advanced life-limiting illnesses: A systematic review. *Palliative Medicine*, *21*(6), 507–517.

Hatch, S. (2017). Uncertainty in medicine. *BMJ*, 357, Article j2180. https://doi.org/10.1136/bmj.j2180 .

Heidegger, M. (1962). *Being and time*. (J. Macquarrie & E. Robinson, Trans.). Harper. (Original work published 1927)

Hofstede, G. (2001). *Culture's consequences: Comparing values, behaviors, institutions and organizations across nations*. Sage.

Hogan, T. P., & Brashers, D. E. (2009). The theory of communication and uncertainty management: Implications from the wider realm of information behavior. In T. D. Afifi & W. A. Afifi (Eds.), *Uncertainty, information management, and disclosure decisions: Theories and application* (pp. 45–66). Routledge.

Hsieh, E. (2006). Conflicts in how interpreters manage their roles in provider-patient interactions. *Social Science & Medicine, 62*(3), 721–730.

Hsieh, E., Bruscella, J., Zanin, A., & Kramer, E. M. (2016). "It's not like you need to live 10 or 20 years": Challenges to patient-centered care in gynecologic oncologist-patient interactions. *Qualitative Health Research, 26*(9), 1191–1202.

Hsieh, E., & Terui, S. (2015). Inherent tensions and challenges of oncologist–patient communication: Implications for interpreter training in health-care settings. *Journal of Applied Communication Research, 43*(2), 141–162.

Husserl, E. (2019). *The phenomenology of internal time-consciousness.* (J. S. Churchill & M. Heidegger, Eds.). Indiana University Press. (Original work published 1964)

Javidan, M. (2007). Forward-thinking cultures. *Harvard Business Review, 85*(7–8), 20.

Kay, A. C., Gaucher, D., McGregor, I., & Nash, K. (2010). Religious belief as compensatory control. *Personality and Social Psychology Review, 14*(1), 37–48.

Kim, K., & Lee, Y.-M. (2018). Understanding uncertainty in medicine: Concepts and implications in medical education. *Korean Society of Medical Education, 30*(3), 181–188.

Knobloch, L. K., & Satterlee, K. (2009). Relational uncertainty: Theory and application. In T. D. Afifi & W. A. Afifi (Eds.), *Uncertainty, information management, and disclosure decisions: Theories and applications* (pp. 106–127). Routledge.

Kotthoff, H. (2007). Oral genres of humor: On the dialectic of genre knowledge and creative authoring. *Pragmatics: Quarterly Publication of the International Pragmatics Association, 17*(2), 263–296.

Kramer, E. M. (1997). *Modern/postmodern: Off the beaten path of antimodernism.* Praeger.

Lo, S. C., Zea, M. C., & Poppen, P. J. (2009). Information, uncertainty, and sexual disclosures in the era of HIV/AIDS. In T. D. Afifi & W. A. Afifi (Eds.), *Uncertainty, information management, and disclosure decisions: Theories and applications* (pp. 254–276). Routledge.

Luther, V. P., & Crandall, S. J. (2011). Commentary: Ambiguity and uncertainty: Neglected elements of medical education curricula? *Academic Medicine, 86*(7), 799–800.

Mack, J. W., & Joffe, S. (2014). Communicating about prognosis: Ethical responsibilities of pediatricians and parents. *Pediatrics, 133*(Suppl. 1), S24-S30.

Mack, J. W., & Smith, T. J. (2012). Reasons why physicians do not have discussions about poor prognosis, why it matters, and what can be improved. *Journal of Clinical Oncology, 30*(22), 2715–2717.

Manganello, J. A., & Clayman, M. L. (2011). The association of understanding of medical statistics with health information seeking and health provider interaction in a national sample of young adults. *Journal of Health Communication, 16*(Suppl. 3), 163–176.

Marsh, H. (2017). *Admissions: Life as a brain surgeon.* St. Martin's Press.

Martin, S. C., Stone, A. M., Scott, A. M., & Brashers, D. E. (2010). Medical, personal, and social forms of uncertainty across the transplantation trajectory. *Qualitative Health Research, 20*(2), 182–196.

Mishel, M. H. (1988). Uncertainty in illness. *Image: The Journal of Nursing Scholarship, 20*(4), 225–232.

Mishel, M. H. (1990). Reconceptualization of the uncertainty in illness theory. *Image: The Journal of Nursing Scholarship, 22*(4), 256–262.

Mishel, M. H. (1997). Uncertainty in acute illness. *Annual Review of Nursing Research, 15*(1), 57–80.

Mishel, M. H. (1999). Uncertainty in chronic illness. *Annual Review of Nursing Research*, *17*(1), 269–294.

Mishel, M. H. (2013). Theories of uncertainty in illness. In M. J. Smith & P. R. Liehr (Eds.), *Middle range theory for nursing* (3rd. ed., pp. 53–86). Springer.

Miyaji, N. T. (1993). The power of compassion: Truth-telling among American doctors in the care of dying patients. *Social Science & Medicine*, *36*(3), 249–264.

Mullins, L. L., Wolfe-Christensen, C., Hoff Pai, A. L., Carpentier, M. Y., Gillaspy, S., Cheek, J., & Page, M. (2007). The relationship of parental overprotection, perceived child vulnerability, and parenting stress to uncertainty in youth with chronic illness. *Journal of Pediatric Psychology*, *32*(8), 973–982.

New International Version. (2011). Biblica. https://www.biblica.com/bible/ (Original work published 1978)

Nicholson, J. (2010). Parenting and recovery for mothers with mental disorders. In B. L. Levin & M. A. Becker (Eds.), *A public health perspective of women's mental health* (pp. 359–372). Springer.

Page, M. C., Fedele, D. A., Pai, A. L., Anderson, J., Wolfe-Christensen, C., Ryan, J. L., & Mullins, L. L. (2012). The relationship of maternal and child illness uncertainty to child depressive symptomotology: A mediational model. *Journal of Pediatric Psychology*, *37*(1), 97–105.

Parsons, G. N., Kinsman, S. B., Bosk, C. L., Sankar, P., & Ubel, P. A. (2001). Between two worlds: Medical student perceptions of humor and slang in the hospital setting. *Journal of General Internal Medicine*, *16*(8), 544–549.

Parsons, T. (1951). *The social system.* Quid Pro Books.

Peters, E., Dieckmann, N. F., Västfjäll, D., Mertz, C. K., Slovic, P., & Hibbard, J. H. (2009). Bringing meaning to numbers: The impact of evaluative categories on decisions. *Journal of Experimental Psychology: Applied*, *15*(3), 213–227.

Peters, E., Hibbard, J., Slovic, P., & Dieckmann, N. (2007). Numeracy skill and the communication, comprehension, and use of risk-benefit information. *Health Affairs*, *26*(3), 741–748.

Pitaloka, D., & Hsieh, E. (2015). Health as submission and social responsibilities: Embodied experiences of Javanese women with type II diabetes. *Qualitative Health Research*, *25*(8), 1155–1165.

Politi, M. C., Clark, M. A., Ombao, H., Dizon, D., & Elwyn, G. (2011a). Communicating uncertainty can lead to less decision satisfaction: A necessary cost of involving patients in shared decision making? *Health Expectations*, *14*(1), 84–91.

Politi, M. C., Clark, M. A., Ombao, H., & Legare, F. (2011b). The impact of physicians' reactions to uncertainty on patients' decision satisfaction. *Journal of Evaluation in Clinical Practice*, *17*(4), 575–578.

Portnoy, D. B., Han, P. K. J., Ferrer, R. A., Klein, W. M. P., & Clauser, S. B. (2013). Physicians' attitudes about communicating and managing scientific uncertainty differ by perceived ambiguity aversion of their patients. *Health Expectations*, *16*(4), 362–372.

Prasad, V., Vandross, A., Toomey, C., Cheung, M., Rho, J., Quinn, S., Chacko, S. J., Borkar, D., Gall, V., Selvaraj, S., Ho, N., & Cifu, A. (2013). A decade of reversal: An analysis of 146 contradicted medical practices. *Mayo Clinic Proceedings*, *88*(8), 790–798.

Prochniak, C., Martin, L., Miller, E., & Knapke, S. (2012). Barriers to and motivations for physician referral of patients to cancer genetics clinics. *Journal of Genetic Counseling*, *21*(2), 305–325.

Pulford, B. D. (2009). Is luck on my side? Optimism, pessimism, and ambiguity aversion. *Quarterly Journal of Experimental Psychology, 62*(6), 1079–1087.

Razvi, Y., Chan, S., Zhang, L., Tsao, M., Barnes, E., Danjoux, C., Sousa, P., Zaki, P., McKenzie, E., Lam, H., Deangelis, C., & Chow, E. (2019). Are we better a decade later in the accuracy of survival prediction by palliative radiation oncologists? *Annals of Palliative Medicine, 8*(2), 150–158.

Rescher, N. (1998). *Predicting the future: An introduction to the theory of forecasting*. State University of New York Press.

Reston, M. (2020, October 4). *Trump update spurs more questions than answers, again*. CNN. https://www.cnn.com/2020/10/04/politics/donald-trump-coronavirus-alternate-reality/index.html

Robinson, T. M., Alexander, S. C., Hays, M., Jeffreys, A. S., Olsen, M. K., Rodriguez, K. L., Pollak, K., Abernethy, A. P., Arnold, R., & Tulsky, J. A. (2008). Patient–oncologist communication in advanced cancer: Predictors of patient perception of prognosis. *Supportive Care in Cancer, 16*(9), 1049–1057.

Sadati, A. K., Lankarani, K. B., Gharibi, V., Fard, M. E., Ebrahimzadeh, N., & Tahmasebi, S. (2015). Religion as an empowerment context in the narrative of women with breast cancer. *Journal of Religion and Health, 54*(3), 1068–1079.

Scott, A. M., Harrington, N. G., & Spencer, E. (2020). Primary care physicians' strategic pursuit of multiple goals in cost-of-care conversations with patients. *Health Communication*, 1–13. Advance online publication. https://doi.org/10.1080/10410236.2020.1723051

Simpkin, A. L., & Schwartzstein, R. M. (2016). Tolerating uncertainty – the next medical revolution? *New England Journal of Medicine, 375*(18), 1713–1715.

Skelton, J. R., Murray, J., & Hobbs, F. D. (1999). Imprecision in medical communication: Study of a doctor talking to patients with serious illness. *Journal of the Royal Society of Medicine, 92*(12), 620–625.

Tait, R. C., Chibnall, J. T., & Kalauokalani, D. (2009). Provider judgments of patients in pain: Seeking symptom certainty. *Pain Medicine, 10*(1), 11–34.

Tanyi, R. A., & Werner, J. S. (2008). Women's experience of spirituality within end-stage renal disease and hemodialysis. *Clinical Nursing Research, 17*(1), 32–49.

Tomich, P. L., & Helgeson, V. S. (2004). Is finding something good in the bad always good? Benefit finding among women with breast cancer. *Health Psychology, 23*(1), 16–23.

What would House M.D. *be without bets??* (2012, May 19). houseunited. http://houseunited.wikidot.com/wiki:bets

Whitehead, A. N. (2010). *Process and reality*. (D. R. Griffin & D. W. Sherburne, Eds.; Corrected ed.). Free Press. (Original work published 1929)

Xafis, V., & Wilkinson, D. (2019). Commentary: Treating ambiguity in the clinical context: Is what you hear the doctor say what the doctor means? *Cambridge Quarterly of Healthcare Ethics, 28*(3), 422–432.

Yoshitake, M. (2002). Anxiety/uncertainty management (AUM) theory: A critical examination of an intercultural communication theory. *Intercultural Communication Studies, 11*(2), 177–193.

Zimbardo, P. G., & Boyd, J. N. (2015). Putting time in perspective: A valid, reliable individual-differences metric. In M. Stolarski, N. Fieulaine, & W. van Beek (Eds.), *Time perspective theory; Review, research and application: Essays in honor of Philip G. Zimbardo* (pp. 17–55). Springer.

10

Social Support

Understanding Supportive Relationships Through
Cultural Perspectives

Chapter 10 provides an overview of the literature on social support, highlighting its multi-dimensional meanings as situated in interpersonal and social contexts. By situating the meanings of social support in cultural contexts, we acknowledge that social support is a cultural phenomenon that needs to be understood, interpreted, and enacted through its cultural norms. By adopting a normative approach to individuals' interpretation and evaluation of social support, we will explore the challenges to identity management and illness management faced by patients and their supportive others in offering different forms of social support.

I. Social Relationships in Health Contexts

As social beings, we inherently recognize that social relationships are essential if we want to survive and thrive in our environments and communities. Economists found that people who face extreme poverty and food insecurity – people who have almost nothing to lose – are often reluctant to leave their communities to pursue better economic opportunities due to concerns about losing family ties and social support at home (Banerjee & Duflo, 2019). Despite the significant financial incentives for emigration, people believe that moving away from their hometown and families can entail significant financial costs (e.g., no more free babysitting from grandma), reputational downsides (e.g., no one can vouch for your reliability and trustworthiness as a business owner), and psychological suffering (e.g., loneliness and feeling homesick; Banerjee & Duflo, 2019).

Social support has been a central topic in various disciplines, including psychology, economics, communication, and medicine, among others. **Social support** is defined as supportive others' provision of "psychological and material resources intended to benefit an individual's ability to cope with stress" (Cohen, 2004, p. 676). Through interdisciplinary approaches, researchers have agreed that social support is a multidimensional construct, involving emotional (e.g., feeling assured or anxious), cognitive (e.g., assessing whether and what type of support is available), behavioral (e.g., soliciting and offering support), and normative (e.g., what is considered supportive based on social norms) components. Social support has been found to have significant impacts on *both* support

Rethinking Culture in Health Communication: Social Interactions as Intercultural Encounters,
First Edition. Elaine Hsieh and Eric M Kramer.
© 2021 John Wiley & Sons, Inc. Published 2021 by John Wiley & Sons, Inc.

providers' and support recipients' coping strategies, identities, relationships, and even health statuses, including psychological and physiological outcomes.

Social support can involve different forms of support. Some of the commonly identified types of support include: **instrumental support** (i.e., provision of material resources, such as offering financial assistance or assisting daily tasks; also referred to as **tangible support**), **informational support** (i.e., provision of relevant information to promote successful coping, such as giving advice about preparing for exams), **emotional support** (e.g., provision of social connection that acknowledges, elaborates, and legitimizes a person's identity and emotions that make them feel heard; sometimes also referred to as **esteem support**, which often focuses on giving reassurance of self-worth), **appraisal support** (e.g., provision of perspectives that assists individuals to evaluate the issues at stake, such as constructive feedback), and **network support** (i.e., opportunities for socializing or belonging to a group; Cohen, 2004; Goldsmith, 2004; Heaney & Israel, 2008).

A. The Protective Functions of Social Support

Researchers have long noted that strong social support is essential to individuals' *psychological* and *physical* wellbeing in both *good* times and *bad* times (Feeney & Collins, 2015; Roy, 2011). Social support helps people to thrive when coping with stressful life adversities as well as pursuing life opportunities for growth and development. In particular, social support functions as (a) a source of strength that promotes thriving through adversity and (b) as a relational catalyst that promotes thriving through "full participation in life opportunities for exploration, growth, and development in the absence of adversity" (Feeney & Collins, 2015, p. 118).

1.   Buffering Effects in Life Adversities

A plethora of research in the 1980s investigated **buffering effects** of social support for stressful life events (Dean & Lin, 1977; Roy, 2011; Thoits, 1982). By acting as "buffers" against life adversities, social support is triggered under stressful life circumstances as it promotes individuals' resilience. In Western societies, spousal or partner relationship is one of the most powerful buffers in assisting individuals in mitigating the negative impacts of stressful life events (Roy, 2011). **Stressful life events** are typically conceptualized as major life events (e.g., death of spouse/parent/child, leaving home for an out-of-state education/job, getting married/divorced, or becoming new parents) that are expected to result in "psychological and physiological stress responses for the average person"(Cohen et al., 2019, p. 579). Stressful life events have been linked to a wide range of illnesses that involve affect regulation (e.g., depression and anxiety), health behaviors (e.g., poor sleep and smoking), hormones, and/or the autonomic nervous system (Cohen et al., 2019). Experiencing stressful life events is associated with increased risks of depression, cardiovascular disease, infectious disease, and cancer-related mortality (Cohen et al., 2019). Three types of stressful life events have been found to be particularly damaging to individuals' health: interpersonal problems (e.g., workplace conflict or death of a oved one), loss of social status (e.g., divorce or being bullied), and employment (e.g., unemployment or underemployment; Cohen et al., 2019).

Emotional support and informational support have consistently demonstrated to have buffering effects because they enhance a wide range of coping strategies for the support recipient (Burleson & MacGeorge, 2002; Cohen & Wills, 1985). Feeney and Collins (2015) noted that when individuals are faced with adversities, they rely on social support to provide a safe haven (e.g., a place that offers emotional and physical comfort free of negative judgments), develop fortification (e.g., nurture and embrace hidden talents and abilities), assist reconstruction process (e.g., coping with adversities in a positive manner), and reframe/redefine adversities for positive change.

In their extensive review of the literature, Cohen and Wills (1985) suggested that social support has buffering effects when interpersonal resources are responsive to the needs elicited by stressful life events. The **matching model** proposes that "social support is effective in reducing the effects of stressful events only in so far as the form of assistance matches the demands of the event" (Cohen, 2004, p. 677). For example, lending someone money may be helpful when the support recipient has lost a job, but it may be useless if the support recipient is grieving over the death of a loved one. The matching model of social support, however, has *failed* to find clear evidence to support buffering effects (Burleson & MacGeorge, 2002; Goldsmith, 2004). This is partly due to the complex interrelationships between different types of support and the wide range of factors moderating individuals' experiences of social support. For example, a single stressful event can result in needs for different types of support. When a person experiences the death of a spouse, they may concurrently face financial uncertainty, loss of social status, and anxiety related to self-worth. Thus, offering money to a person who is grieving over the death of a spouse can be helpful not only in addressing financial uncertainty but also communicating care and love for the person. In other words, support recipients may attribute meanings (e.g., esteem support) to the act of instrumental support (e.g., giving money).

Second, individuals' appraisal of the support received may be moderated by other factors. For example, by recognizing a friend who has little money but offers a shoulder to cry on is doing her best to help, a support recipient may find the strength to develop a wide range of coping strategies that she otherwise would not have had. Similarly, a person is unlikely to appraise emotional support to be sincere and genuine if the person who offers it repeatedly snubs extending instrumental or appraisal support when they can easily afford to do so. Goldsmith (2004) explained, "The matching metaphor fails to adequately acknowledge the ways in which situations may be represented and constructed in communication" (p. 84). A support provider may view giving a ride to an alcoholic friend to an AA meeting versus a liquor store means very different things; in contrast, a support recipient may not differentiate the meanings of the rides. Although support typologies can be distinguished conceptually, it is likely that peoples' understanding of social support offered and received are dynamically negotiated and contextually situated (Goldsmith, 2004). In short, the matching model, despite its intuitive appeal, oversimplifies complex relationships and processes of social support in real life (Burleson & MacGeorge, 2002).

Interestingly, Cohen and Wills (1985) found buffering effects with perceived social support, but not with received social support or support structure. Similarly, Roy (2011) found that intimacy of close relationships, rather than the size of a person's support network, is a stronger predictor of buffering effects. Even one single, reliable source of social support (e.g., a confidant) is sufficient and effective as a stress buffer to provide appropriate aide (Cohen, 2004). **Perceived social support** is defined as individuals' perception concerning the *general* availability of support and/or *global* satisfaction with support provided (Haber et al., 2007). It represents a global understanding of one's perception and satisfaction with the availability of social support. In contrast, **received social support** is defined as the *specific* supportive behaviors received in the past; **support structure** is assessed through objective measures of an individuals' support network (e.g., number of friends or frequency of contacts).

Researchers were intrigued by the consistent findings of perceived social support as a predictor of health, but not received social support (Haber et al., 2007). After all, the received social support is a more accurate, objective measure of the extent of supportive behaviors received by a recipient. In contrast, perceived social support may not be representative of the actual support received in reality, and can be influenced by support recipients' bias, judgment, and memory. Nevertheless, researchers have noted that compared to perceived social support, receiving actual support can entail significant risks (e.g., disclosing one's illness status may result in potential stigmatization) or future obligations (e.g., expectations of paying back the favors in the future) that may dampen the benefits of social support – making received social support a less powerful predictor of health than perceived social support. In addition, maintaining an extensive support network may demand a significant investment of one's time and resources – mitigating the positive effects of social support. On the other hand, the belief that others will provide necessary resources if asked (i.e., perceived social support) can bolster one's ability to cope with stress and mitigate maladaptive behaviors (e.g., avoidance) without the risks and ensuing obligations of received social support (Cohen, 2004). As a result, "although the perception that support is available is associated with better adjustment, the perception that one has been the recipient of specific supportive act is not" (Bolger et al., 2000, p. 958).

2. Direct Effect in Everyday Life

Although early studies focused on the buffering effects of social support against stress, researchers have increasingly recognized that social support can constitute valuable resources in everyday life, not just in stressful moments. According to the **direct effect** model (also called the **main effect** model), Researchers argued that social support is beneficial "irrespective of whether one is under stress" (Cohen, 2004, p. 678). Feeney and Collins (2015) explained that in the absence of adversity, social support continues its influence by providing a *secure base* to encourage ones' exploration behaviors (e.g., desires to learn, grow, discover, and accomplish goals). In the absence of adversities, social support encourages individuals to create, reframe, recognize, embrace, and prepare for life opportunities (e.g., challenge oneself to reach outside of one's comfort zone).

From this perspective, social support exerts its impact when individuals engage in **social integration** (i.e., participation in a broad range of social relationships), providing a sense of normative rules that enhance their sense of identity, relationship, life-meaning, belonging, self-worth, security, and stability (Cohen, 2004). Researchers have argued that social support in intimate relationships has not only buffering effects in times of stress but also direct effects in everyday life (Roy, 2011).

Social integration involves a *behavioral* component (e.g., active engagement in a wide range of social activities or relationships) and a *cognitive* component (e.g., a sense of community and identification with one's social roles; Brissette et al., 2000). People who demonstrate a strong level of social integration with their communities or relationships (e.g., married, have close family and friends, belong to social and religious groups) have been found to have a better chance of survival after heart attacks, less risk for cancer recurrence, less depression and anxiety, less severe cognitive decline with aging, and better resistance against infectious disease (Cohen, 2004).

More importantly, social integration suggests that both receiving social support *and* providing social support can lead to positive outcomes. A study of churchgoers found that the negative impacts of financial strain on mortality were reduced for elderly churchgoers who provided more emotional support to fellow church members (Krause, 2006). "**Paying it forward** (PIF)" has now become a social movement, encouraging individuals to provide random acts of kindness to others (Cobb, 2015; see Figure 10.1). A recent study found that both receivers and givers of random acts of kindness experience positive benefits to their well-being, noting that "PIF givers reported increased overall PA [positive affect], optimism, gratitude, life satisfaction, and joviality, with the largest changes found in PA and joviality" (Pressman et al., 2014, p. 6). In addition to experiences of positive mood, receivers of acts of kindness often demonstrate desire and behaviors of paying the kindness forward (Pressman et al., 2014). This is a proliferating, upward-and-forward effect of goodwill that has also been observed by other studies on PIF, altruism, and generosity (Chang et al., 2012; Dass-Brailsford et al., 2011; Tsvetkova & Macy, 2014).

Acts of kindness can spread through a social network, creating a compounding impact with an increasing number of people choosing to "pay it forward" as they become inspired and revitalized by others' acts of kindness. In short, acts of kindness energize the givers; at the same time, they inspire and revitalize recipients to pass on the goodwill. It catches on. Researchers argued that groups with altruistic members would become more altruistic as a whole, resulting in a higher likelihood of survival than selfish groups (Fowler & Christakis, 2010; Klein, 2014; van Doorn & Taborsky, 2012). Being mindful of others' acts of kindness may just be the key to providing the needed energy for us to create, support, and maintain the community that we love. It creates a community in which everyone can be seen, heard, and thrive.

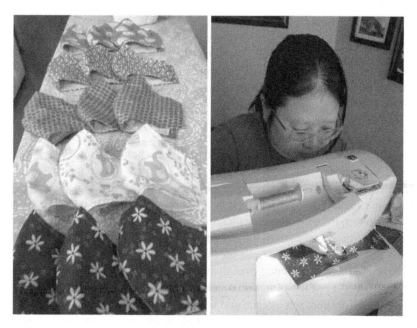

Figure 10.1 Pay it forward. During the COVID-19 pandemic, many citizens volunteered to sew facemasks for frontline health professionals and whoever need them. *Source:* Elaine Hsieh

B. Potentially Negative Impacts of Social Support

Recent studies have highlighted the complex relationships of social support and its corresponding impacts. Although social support is given with the intent to be beneficial to the recipients, researchers have noted that support offered may be unwanted, undesirable, or negative to support recipients (Goldsmith, 2004; Roy, 2011). Successful provision of social support requires the participants to "construct together a vision of the situation and coping options that is coherent – internally, externally, and between partners" (Goldsmith, 2004, p. 150). In other words, the participants of supportive communication need to develop a mutually agreeable understanding of the event and coordinate their efforts to meet the demands of the situation.

How people evaluate the helpfulness of social support may be moderated by a wide range of factors. For example, relationships between support providers and support recipients and the timing of the support (e.g., whether support was solicited) have been found to influence the helpfulness of emotional support; similarly, source credibility and the co-existence of other forms of support may influence support recipients' assessments of the helpfulness of informational support (Brashers et al., 2006; Burleson & MacGeorge, 2002). How support is delivered may also shape individuals' evaluations of the helpfulness of the support. For example, receiving social support can implicate costs or risks to one's identity, relationship, or future obligations (e.g., accepting money from a friend may suggest that a person is unable to financially support oneself imposes additional burdens to a friend, or requires one to pay back or offer money in the future). As a result, a relational partner may intentionally offer assistance in indirect or tactful ways (e.g., concealing the assistance provided, completing tasks without mentioning it, and shielding a support recipient from concerns or problems) so that the support recipients does not experience threats to self-esteem or feelings of obligation and dependence (Goldsmith, 2004). For example, a sibling may offer significant cash to celebrate his elderly sister's birthday, labeling the cash gift as a birthday present for a life milestone (e.g., a normative practice) rather than instrumental support to assist her dire financial situation. In a study of 68 couples in which one partner was preparing for the New York State Bar Examination, Bolger et al. (2000) found that partners' report of support provision was related to an examinee's feeling less depressed the next day; however, when examinees reported receiving support, their levels of anxiety and depression tended to be greater the following day. As a result, during the most stressful time (i.e., the final week before the bar exam), **invisible support** (i.e., when a support provider reported offering support, but the support recipient did not report receiving it) demonstrated the best outcome. From this perspective, "the most effective support may be that which goes unrecognized as support" (Goldsmith, 2004, p. 117).

In certain situations, the provision of social support does not always guarantee positive influences on the support recipients. And social support can even lead to negative outcomes (e.g., increased anxiety and stress) for the support provider (Burg & Seeman, 1994; Roy, 2011). For example, despite the benefits of social integration, staying unhappily married is more detrimental than divorcing because people in low-quality marriages are (a) less happy than individuals who divorce and remarry and (b) have lower levels of life satisfaction, self-esteem, and overall health than people who divorce and remained unmarried (Hawkins & Booth, 2005). Negative interactions with support networks may increase stress, resulting in maladaptive behaviors and physiological responses that compromise health status (Cohen, 2004). Supportive behaviors that aim to offer support to a spouse who suffered a heart attack may be viewed as nagging or controlling, resulting in threats to identity and the relationship (Goldsmith et al., 2006).

Offering support can also be draining for the support giver. A supportive other who offered emotional support by listening to a friend in distress may feel more sadness afterward, particularly when they feel that they are responsible for the circumstances or fail to improve the support recipients' distress (Perrine, 1993). When faced with increasing demands to offer social support to their online communities, participants of social networking sites may feel exhausted, reduce usage intensity, or even stop visiting these sites (Maier et al., 2015). Interestingly, a study of female breast cancer patients and their male partners' relational satisfaction and illness-related distress found that the male partners' unsupportive behaviors resulted in negative consequences *only when* the patients perceived their behaviors as unsupportive (Manne et al., 2006). In other words, the impacts of enacted social support may be determined not by the exact forms it takes in reality but in how the support is negotiated, interpreted, and coordinated in a support network (Goldsmith et al., 2012; Goldsmith & Miller, 2013).

II.   Cultural Approaches to Social Support

Although the literature on social support has been extensive and researchers have been cognizant of the cultural or normative variations of social support (e.g., Goldsmith, 2004), there are limited studies that examine the cultural perspectives of social support. The literature of social support and its impacts on health and illness is predominately Western and often entails a Judeo-Christian bias (Roy, 2011). Nevertheless, in the following section, our goal is to reframe the existing literature through the cultural perspectives that set the foundations of this book.

A.   Social Support through Magic Consciousness: This Is Who We Are

For people with Magic Consciousness, social support is not something to be given or received, nor is it communicated to signal love, assistance, or "support." Supportive behaviors and communication are not something external to the we-identity, relationships, and social norms that form the group. More importantly, by the qualities of Magic Consciousness, "supportive acts" are not categorized as such. Rather, they enact such behaviors and communicative acts because that is what they (i.e., members of the Magic Consciousness community) do. Your needs are my needs. We are one. Support is presumed and nondirectional (i.e., the concepts of support "giver" versus "recipients" are nonexistent as Magic Consciousness is nonspatial). We live within a supportive environment that nurtures us as a whole. It is inherent in life itself.

1.   Support Is Unreflective, Taken-for-Granted

One of the best examples for social support through Magic Consciousness often takes place within a family unit – one of the most ancient, primal community of Magic Consciousness bound by blood. When we offer support to our children or parents, we do not think about whether we have the capacity, ability, or resources to offer support. When a child being held by its mother reaches for something it cannot grasp, the mother extends the child, and reaches for them to grasp for them as a single motion-identity (Merleau-Ponty, 1945/2002). Anthropologists have called this "sympathetic magic" (Lévy-Bruhl, 1926/2018) or "participation mystique" (Jung et al., 2012). We just do it. The newspapers are full of stories of **hysterical strength** (i.e., a display of extreme strength by humans beyond what is normal). For example, a BBC report noted:

> In 2012, Lauren Kornacki, a 22-year-old woman in Glen Allen, Virginia, raised a BMW 525i off her father when the car toppled from a jack. Seven years earlier, a man named Tom Boyle hoisted a Chevy Camaro, freeing a trapped cyclist in Tucson, Arizona. The events don't always involve vehicles, like when Lydia Angyiou went toe-to-toe with a polar bear in northern Quebec to protect her son and his friends while they played hockey. (Hadhazy, 2016, para. 2)

In these moments of profound identification, support providers do not hesitate. They do not calculate what support is necessary or whether they are capable of offering such support. The support was offered immediately, without requests from the support recipient *and* without any analysis of the costs to the support provider. What they are attempting to do may seem illogical – unrealistic. In such moments, it is said that individuals who exhibit hysterical strength (i.e., the support providers) ignore pain and fatigue, and push their performance to the extreme. In hindsight, observers may suggest that they experienced an "adrenaline rush," but that is a reductionist and perspectival explanation after the fact. The person performing the feat of hysterical strength experiences nothing but a profound sense of urgency that slows time to a point and restricts spatialized emotional "distance." For example, "only upon returning home from having lifted a car off of a teenager, Boyle – the Arizonian man – felt pain in his mouth. It turned out he had unknowingly cracked eight of his teeth, apparently from clenching his jaw during the intense lift" (Hadhazy, 2016, "Adrenaline rush" section). There were no calculations of cost-benefit analysis nor appeal to morality or cultural values. The supportive acts were enacted with little internal reflection or external appeal – it's simply what we do for one another.

The **clan culture** within the Chinese family system reflects social support through Magic Consciousness. In a study of Chinese working mothers, a participant explained, "The clan is most important to us. During the most critical moments, we can always rely on our clan members. Friends are helpful, but they can only give short-term help. If we need long-term help, we will always rely on our clansmen" (Yuen-Tsang, 2018, p. 140). Support was given and received simply because they shared common blood ties, "the only criteria for making the decision on whether support should be given or withheld" (Yuen-Tsang, 2018, p. 140). Clan members utilize a wide range of resources to help each other to find jobs and resources.

Social support among clan members involves a "common strength." By "pooling their resources together for use by network members as and when the need arose," they view the success of a single clan member not as an achievement of the individual but as an achievement of "the entire family network" – because the individual's success could bring financial and material support to the whole clan in the long-run (Yuen-Tsang, 2018, pp. 150–151). Social support to other clan members is often spontaneous, extremely generous, and entirely selfless, reflecting a Magic Consciousness orientation; in contrast, support to "secondary support network" is often transactional and calculative, a Perspectival Thinking approach (Yuen-Tsang, 2018). The family is the most important source of social support for aging parents, who received relatively little support from friends, neighbors, or any social or governmental organizations (Chen et al., 2014).

Within the clan culture, Chinese parents and their children's success are intertwined as one (Zhang, 2019). One study found that one-third of Chinese parents in China relied on their adult children for income at old age (Logan & Bian, 2003). It is not an economic exchange but rather a holistic effort for the success of the clan. Only in modern times have economists compared this familial process with dissociated governmental support, which is impersonal and bureaucratic. In traditional clans, the elderly parents view their son's success as theirs. Chinese parents still often offer financial support, assist housework, provide free housing and childcare, and live with their adult children. As a result, there is a significant pooling of resources, including finances and labor, to ensure "individual" success within the clan – after all, success of one is success of all – they are nearly identical. For example, it is not uncommon for Chinese grandparents to live with their grandchildren and be their primary caregivers for years, allowing their adult children to pursue financial/career opportunities out-of-town (Chen et al., 2011). Providing instrumental support to adult children (e.g., assisting housework and babysitting grandchildren) are particularly beneficial to Chinese parents who subscribe to traditional cultural norms, *enhancing* their morale and overall well-being (Chen & Silverstein, 2000). Under Magic Consciousness, offering social support is not draining but empowering and *reenergizing* – as the social act reinforces one's identity as an in-group member. In short, in a community of Magic Consciousness, social support is not a resource to be mined or parsed. The community (e.g., a family clan) acts as one, pooling resources together and treating individual success as collective success. The support provider is energized and empowered through community success. Although a person of Perspectival Thinking may consider such supportive acts to be "selfless," "generous," or "altruistic," it is important to remember that for a person with Magic Consciousness – there is no "self" and thus, as support providers, they are not "selfless" per se but simply act the way they assume to be the only way to act – as part of the clan. Similarly, they do not consider themselves generous or altruistic either because their actions are not meant to benefit "others" at the expense of "self," but rather to assure the survival of the communal system.

2. Community Norms Dictates Behavioral Patterns

Under Magic Consciousness, community norms govern individual behaviors. At times, social support among community members of Magic Consciousness can appear problematic, if not risky, to outsiders. In the sitcom *Friends*, Rachel, a nonsmoker, decided to take up smoking in her new workplace because she felt that she was not part of the group when her co-workers and supervisors went for smoking breaks without her (Curtis & Holland, 1999). In fact, when group norms reinforce smoking behaviors as a social habit (e.g., colleagues engage relationship-building chats when taking a smoke break), smokers are less likely to quit smoking (Caplan et al., 1975). When examining the impact of job-related stress on individuals' smoking behaviors, Westman et al. (1985) concluded that supportive others who smoke can reinforce a stressed smokers' intention to smoke, counteracting any tendency to quit smoking.

Group norms reinforce individuals' behaviors (see also the Theory of Reasoned Action and Theory of Planned Behaviors in Chapter 6). **Norms** are socially-enforced rules that embody community values and worldviews (Horne, 2009). Community members are motivated to enforce norms by rewarding members who abide by these social rules and punishing those who do not. The more a person identifies with a community, the more likely they follow group norms. For example, students who believe that it is normal for students to have unhealthy eating habits *and* hold strong identification for their identity as students, are more likely to adopt poor diet practices (Louis et al., 2007). College students are more likely to intend to binge drink when they perceive normative support from their friends and peers at university to engage in binge drinking and perceive more pressure from significant others to binge drink (Johnston & White, 2003). Researchers have argued social integration into the military's fatalistic masculinity (e.g., soldiers sacrifice for others and do not bring attention to their pain) is a major contributor to the high rate of military suicide (Braswell & Kushner, 2012). Horne (2009) explained, "Social relationships ... can lead to enforcement efforts that are counterproductive. People might enforce norms that they would rather not enforce because of their connections to others. This means that even rational people can enforce norms in ways that are damaging" (p. 64).

Our history is full of extreme brutality and horrifying acts that ordinary people participate in the most uneventful, routine manners as part of their everyday life in their communities (Baron-Cohen, 2012). Nazi concentration/extermination camps and China's Cultural Revolution had created death tolls in the millions yet received strong support from their citizens at the time. Human slavery/trafficking, honor killings, and forced sterilization continue plague in many parts of the world today (Bales & Soodalter, 2010; Kulczycki & Windle, 2011; World Health Organization, 2014). It is important to point out that individuals within a community of Magic Consciousness are not calculating the benefits to be gained nor the horror to be invoked through their acts. People with Magic Consciousness engage in group norms because that's what they do. They do not question the behaviors, nor do they attach ethical or moral standards to the act. Consequently, for people of Magic Consciousness, when problematic health behaviors are part of the groups' normative behaviors, they can be particularly detrimental to individual members' health.

B. Social Support through Mythic Connection: This Is What Is Right

Under Mythic Connection, social support is attached with values that community members aspire to, acting as the embodiment of community values. Whereas social support under Magic Consciousness is primal and unreflective (i.e., presumed and taken-for-granted), social support under Mythic Connection reflects what we think "good" people should do.

1. Shared Identities Encourages Support Provision

Social support through Mythic Connection highlights community aspirations. For example, during 2019–2020, COVID-19, a novel coronavirus, was the cause of a global pandemic. By May 2020, 185+ countries/regions around the world faced dire situations requiring many local communities to impose travel bans, shelter-in-place, or stay-at-home orders to ensure public health safety and conserve medical resources

(Johns Hopkins Coronavirus Resource Center, 2020). Along with many governmental responses, many grassroots activities reflected some of the best social support offered between strangers in our society. For example, in early February in Taiwan, as face-mask inventories became depleted and the government imposed individual quotas, "我 OK, 你先領 (I'm okay, you get it first)" became a trending slogan, framing many Taiwanese people's profile picture on social media, encouraging people to save the facemasks to the people who need them most. The social movement of saving face-masks for those who need them the most allowed people who "sacrificed" their rights, to feel good about their good deeds. Simultaneously, the messaging created social pres-sure to make others who were ambivalent or unwilling to follow the movement to feel ashamed of their selfishness (Chu, 2020). Likewise, in late March, when New York and California had imposed shelter-in-place and/or stay-at-home orders, hospital workers posed pictures of their bruised faces after wearing N95 facemasks for long hours, and with them holding signs that said, "I stayed at work for you, you stay at home for us" (Williams, 2020; see Figure 10.2). College students who decided to enjoy their spring breaks in New Orleans, who went clubbing on St. Patrick's Day weekend, and who visited public beaches in Florida all faced a hostile backlash for being "selfish" or "ignorant," common labels used in the mass media and social media commentary (Flynn, 2020; Mounk, 2020). By praising healthcare professionals' sacrifice and assign-ing negative labels to norm violators, a society can assert its control over community members.

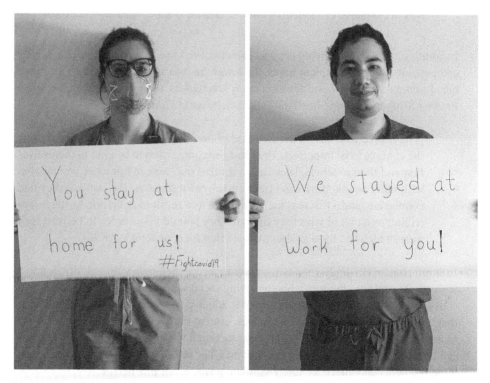

Figure 10.2 "I stayed at work for you; you stay at home for us." During the COVID-19 pandemic, healthcare providers have used their social media posts to show solidarity with the public at a time of great anxiety and fear. Photo by Dr. Preston E Kramer, MD, at Swedish Medical Center at Seattle, WA. *Source:* Elaine Hsieh

Social support through Mythic Connection, employing stories that portray moral standards, can be rewarding for individuals who act as "good" citizens in their communities. Crocker and Canevello (2008) investigated the different outcomes of people who offered social support motivated by compassionate goals versus self-image goals. **Compassionate goals** involve focusing on "supporting others, not to obtain something for the self, but out of consideration for the well-being of others;" in contrast, **self-image goals** involve the desire to "construct, maintain, and defend desired public and private images of the self to gain or obtain something for the self" (Crocker & Canevello, 2008, p. 557). Compassionate goals reflect a Mythic Connection approach to social support; in contrast, self-image goals echo a Perspectival Thinking approach. Crocker and Canevello (2008) concluded that "people with compassionate goals create a supportive environment for themselves and others, but only if they do not have self-image goals" (p. 555). In particular, they explained,

> Compassionate goals were associated with spiritual transcendence, specifically, the belief that all life is interconnected. People with compassionate goals do not view relationships as non–zero sum, with positive outcomes for the self being achieved at the expense of others. These people have compassion for themselves, as well as others. ... [People] with compassionate relationship goals do not give support strategically to obtain support for themselves; ... compassionate goals ... reflect a non–zero-sum perspective. Indeed, students who strive to give support to others reap considerable benefits in social support received, increased trust, feelings of closeness, low loneliness, and decreased conflict. (p. 572)

In addition, although receiving support can entail risks (e.g., face threats), the higher compassion a support recipient holds, the lower the stressed responses are (e.g., lower blood pressure reactivity and lower cortisol reactivity; Cosley et al., 2010). As Brené Brown (2010) explained in her TED Talk, *The Power of Vulnerability*:

> [The people who have a strong sense of love and belonging had], very simply, the courage to be imperfect. They had the compassion to be kind to themselves first and then to others, because, as it turns out, we can't practice compassion with other people if we can't treat ourselves kindly. And the last was they had connection, and – this was the hard part – as a result of authenticity, they were willing to let go of who they thought they should be in order to be who they were, which you have to absolutely do that for connection. (08:36)

In short, people with high compassion goals embrace their own vulnerability, connect with others, and benefit more when receiving social support.

In contrast, people with self-image goals adopt a zero-sum perspective, believing that "people should take care of themselves, even at the expense of others" (Crocker & Canevello, 2008, p. 572). They adopt a transactional view of social support (i.e., what can I receive in return by offering the support). The self-image goals ultimately undermine the beneficial effects of compassionate goals. From this perspective, like social support under Magic Consciousness, social support under Mythic Connection creates a non-zero-sum relationship between support providers and support recipients. By framing social support as gains for one's community *and* assurance of one's community membership, social support substantiates its positive effects to both the giver and the recipient.

2. Support Prioritizes In-Group Members

Mythic Connection bridges supportive behaviors with cultural values that energize support providers. The Myth of a people links all members together through a common worldview. For example, although Chinese family caregivers of elderly persons face chronic stress, the stronger the caregivers identify with the cultural values of *filial piety* (i.e., Confusion ethics rooted in Chinese culture that instructs individuals to be respectful and obedient to their parents, placing family needs above individual interests), the more likely they will view their caregiving tasks as positive, beneficial, and less costly (Lai, 2009). Similarly, the more children subscribe to the cultural norms of filial piety, the more likely they are to increase their social support in response to the growing health needs of their parents (Silverstein et al., 2006). Support providers and recipients under Magic Consciousness enact their social support without recognizing those as supportive acts (because they do not differentiate self-versus-others and thus, the acts are not meant to be "supportive" of one another). In contrast, individuals of Mythic Connection recognize that it's their cultural values and social norms that obligate community members' supportive behaviors toward one another.

Under Mythic Connection, members of a community share stories with one another, from one generation to the next, reinforcing their cultural values and forming a cultural heritage. Storytelling has the form of drama – emotional identification. Myths explain the universe to us, our place within it, what are proper and improper behaviors. The identity of the members is conferred by the system as members affirm each other's membership and existence. This is what Niklas Luhmann (1997/2012) called "recursive communication." We come to embody our social structures and cultural beliefs. The structure gives identity and meaning to its members, and they, in turn, maintain the structure by enacting its patterned, normative formations. This is the fundamental dialectic of the whole of human reality. Structure is thus a verb, not a noun, and it is a process of continual maintenance through enactment – structuration (Whitehead, 1929/2010). The stories we tell help to socialize people to become members and to assume roles with the social construct. The stories give us a general guide for how to exist and behave, a syntagmatic structure, including the compulsion to retell them to the next generation.

Silverstein et al. (2012) proposed that **moral capital** can serve as "the stock of internalized social values that obligates children to care for and support their older parents" (p. 1252). In this case, children are socialized into the cultural values of filial piety. Moral capital is a normative form of social regulation, providing "the certainty with which one can anticipate that others hold particular values from which they anticipate a benefit" (p. 1252). Although Silverstein et al. (2012) adopted a perspectival understanding of the transactional economy of moral "capital," we argue that the foundational strength of the moral capital is the cohesiveness of the moral community, not the capital earned or owed. In other words, it is the moral values imposed through cultural norms that hold community members accountable for one another. As international communities struggled to respond to the rapidly growing COVID-19 pandemic, The Director-General of World Health Organization, Dr. Tedros Adhanom

Ghebreyesus, urged, "Washing your hands will help to reduce your risk of infection. But it's also *an act of solidarity* because it reduces the risk you will infect others in your community and around the world. Do it for yourself, *do it for others*" [emphasis added] (Tedros, 2020). This is an appeal to community values, a call for social support through Mythic Connection. From this perspective, social support under Mythic Connection can serve as a tool for social control, encouraging community members to act in a collaborative and collective manner that supports the public good.

Because community is central to Mythic Connection, social support under Mythic Connection is not universally granted. Joseph Campbell (1988/2011) explained that myths are bounded: The local culture has its landscape, flora and fauna, and myths. For example, Maner and Gailliot (2007) found that empathy-driven helping behaviors are dependent on relational contexts. For close personal relationships (e.g., kinship), social support can be motivated by empathic concerns and "a true desire to help the welfare of another person;" however, empathy is not a significant motivator for supportive behaviors offered to a distant relationship (e.g., a stranger). Similar attitudes are exhibited in Chinese families. Unquestioned support is limited to members of their primary support networks (e.g., clan members). A more transactional approach is taken toward their secondary support networks (e.g., friends and colleagues; Yuen-Tsang, 2018). Social support is prioritized for in-group members under Mythic Connection. As a result, if a person views only family members with "blood ties" as in-group, the person may even limit his or her support to in-laws or adopted children, even though they are considered family members by secular law. On the other hand, if a person views all human-beings (or all living creatures) as in-group members, then support is extended to all. One's definition of community sets the boundaries for acts of sympathetic support, and acts of denial, rejection, and repudiation.

Finally, because social support under Mythic Connection prioritizes in-group members but also focuses on public goods, it is likely that support-seeking behaviors may be suppressed through Mythic Connection to maximize group interests. For example, although the collectivist cultural orientation in East Asian cultures may suggest that social support is freely offered (under Magic Consciousness) or is obligated through social norms (under Mythic Connection), researchers were surprised to find individuals who are in need of support actively avoid support-seeking behaviors. Kong and Hsieh (2012) found that although many elderly Chinese immigrants believed that their adult children or relatives would not hesitate to offer help (e.g., taking them to clinics), they nevertheless felt guilty for being a burden to others. They actively silenced their suffering. For example, an elderly couple talked about how they managed minor illnesses with Chinese herbal medicine without going to the doctor. The husband concluded, "It's not right to always ask [our nieces] for help. You actually bring trouble to them" (Kong & Hsieh, 2012, p. 845). Another elderly participant echoed, "[Somebody says,] I am old; I have to depend on my children. They should do this and that for me. That's wrong" (Kong & Hsieh, 2012, p. 845). Kong and Hsieh (2012) explained,

> The reason that such behaviors are "wrong" is not because elderly Chinese should not ask for family support, but that such behaviors conflict with their desired social roles within the family structure (i.e., they should be the caregivers for the family and the primary caretakers for the grandchildren) in the United States. (p. 845)

Similarly, through a series of studies on Asians and Asian Americans' support-seeking behaviors, Taylor et al. (2004) concluded, "East Asian cultural norms appear to discourage the active engagement of one's social support network for help in solving problems or for coping with stress" (p. 360). Taylor et al. (2004) explained,

> In individual cultural contexts, relationships may be seen as means for promoting individual goals, and as such, one may recruit explicit help or aid from those in one's social networks in order to achieve one's personal goals. In collectivist cultural contexts, individual goals may be seen as a means for promoting relationships. Pursuing the goals of the self may risk straining relationships if one calls on his or her social support network for aid. Thus, a person from an interdependent country may feel that he or she has less to gain personally than he or she can lose socially by calling on others for help. That is, if pursuing the goals of relationships is primary, then a person may prefer not to burden the social network and to solve problems individually instead. (p. 360)

Under Mythic Connection, these individuals allied with the normative morals of the collective. It made them "good" members and gave them solace. As a result, even as they "deny" their own needs, they view such acts as their contribution to the system. They were happy to sacrifice, to do their part, to be involved not by taking but by actively declining resources.

In summary, social support under Mythic Connection can impose social pressure to encourage desirable behaviors. The definition of community highlights the availability and boundaries of social support. Being members of a mythic community has inherent value, which represents the shared moral dimension of identity and relationship in the mythic worldview. The parents need not "earn" the respect and support of the children and vice versa. Rather, through group identity, the inherent obligations, rights, and privileges are presumed by in-group members. By highlighting public goods of shared communities, support providers are energized through their "good deeds." At the same time, support recipients can reasonably anticipate that their in-group membership will entitle them to anticipated resources from other community members. Nevertheless, because Mythic Connection emphasizes public interests (rather than individual needs), individuals may also be encouraged to suppress their support-seeking behaviors to conserve community resources.

C. Social Support through Perspectival Thinking: This Is What Is Needed

Social support through Perspectival Thinking adopts a mechanical and/or transactional approach to social support. A Perspectival Thinking approach to social support can take on many different forms.

1. Social Support as a Mechanical and/or Transactional Process

One of the examples of Perspectival Thinking is reducing individual actions and supportive behaviors to biological processes, arguing that it's the hormonal production that motivates our social behaviors and shapes individuals' health status (Uchino,

2006). For example, some researchers argued that social support can reduce one's cortisol levels (i.e., a high level of cortisol indicates a stressed response that has immunosuppressive effects), allowing individuals to have a stronger immune system to fight infectious disease (Uchino, 2006). In a TED Talk, Psychologist McGonigal (2013) emphasized the importance of oxytocin, a neuro-hormone, in motivating individuals' support-seeking behaviors. By noting that oxytocin's nickname is "the cuddle hormone" because it is released when you hug someone, McGonigal (2013) explained,

> [Oxytocin] is a stress hormone. Your pituitary gland pumps this stuff out as part of the stress response. It's as much a part of your stress response as the adrenaline that makes your heart pound. And when oxytocin is released in the stress response, it is motivating you to seek support. [....] When life is difficult, your stress response wants you to be surrounded by people who care about you. (08:07)

Thus, a physiological approach biomedicalizes one's processes and experiences of social support, including their stress responses, supportive behaviors, and health outcomes.

Another example of a perspectival approach is the legalization of support obligations. When Magic Consciousness and/or Mythic Connection no longer bound community members to offer support, individuals and communities may resort to legal means to ensure the availability of social support. For example, as Chinese societies become more westernized and modernized, clan culture and filial piety may have less influence over individuals' supportive behaviors (Cheung & Kwan, 2009). As a result, Chinese parents have resorted to contractual agreements to ensure that adult children will provide support to them in their old age (Chou, 2011). In 2007, South Korea passed filial piety legislation to encourage "the practice of filial duties and responsibilities within the family unit, the community, and the wider society" (Park, 2015, p. 281). Relying on the legal system to ensure the provision of social support is a perspectival approach because it eliminates any sentimentalities or moral obligations that bond support providers with recipients. Dissociation creates an emotional "distance" between people and caring diminishes.

A transactional approach to social support entails **reciprocity**: providing support to others will result in the receipt of (future) support from others. Silverstein et al. (2012) explained, "Norms of reciprocity, backed up with punishment for defection, encourage people to respond to cooperation with cooperation and to give with giving in return. Thus, people can elicit support from others by giving it first, obligating the support recipient to reciprocate" (p. 556). For example, parents who provide financial assistance to their adult children are more likely to receive support from them in old age (Silverstein et al., 2012). A study of social support among coworkers found that reciprocity relationships are positively related to social support availability – the amount of social support received is dependent on whether they offered support in the past (Bowling et al., 2004). Because reciprocity operates through a sense of equity and fairness (i.e., social support should be somewhat equitable in the exchange), individuals are more likely to hold each other accountable for support reciprocity when they share equal status (Buunk et al., 1993). For example, we are more likely to demand support reciprocity from coworkers and siblings than from supervisors or parents. From this perspective, social support under Perspectival Thinking is sensitive to relational contexts, but not in the sense of community, but in terms of the power hierarchy.

Under Magic Consciousness, reciprocity is not calculated or expected. Aid is simply always part of life and if one person helps another more than they "get back," that is not a concern. Parenting among all animals is instinctive and the "altruism" shown is not toward individuals but the entire group (species, "We, the People"). You succeed, so we all succeed. The clan endures. The man who lifts a car off of a child does not think or ask for assurances of reciprocity before "expending" his energy. Whereas social support under Magic Consciousness can be considered "unconditional" by the standards of Perspectival Thinking, what is implied is that "conditions" are directional and part of the calculation. Under Perspectival Thinking, support without conditions is often viewed as "irrational" as it ignores the perspectives of cost/benefit and hedonic calculus.

Without reciprocity and the sense of "balance" (as in reason, ratio, and accounting), a perspectival person may feel justified by withholding resources. What is "fair" in the perspectival world, is a sense of balance/equality. That is not the case in magic or mythic worlds where power distance (i.e., the acceptance of inequality between those in power and the subordinates as natural and normal) prevails. Filial piety does not depend on the parents reciprocating the children's support. The parents must show deference to their parents; at the same time, they also expect it from their children. There is no person-to-person reciprocity or equality. Rather, all equally have inherent obligations and rights, but not to each other in the same ways. Equality in the perspectival world is spatial and therefore, it is based on "balance." Equality strips away Mythic Connection, which gives roles various inherent meanings and statuses. Social support can be presumed in a magic or mythic collective. It cannot be presumed by perspectival individuals.

2. Social Support as Exchanges of Individual Interests

Because social support under Perspectival Thinking is mechanical and transactional, support recipients can be cynical or critical of supportive behaviors. For example, support recipients' mood and well-being may be harmed if they believe that (a) a support provider was motivated by self-image goals (e.g., the support offered in the hope that it will result in a trade-off), or (b) that their self-image goals (e.g., desire to appear competent) may be compromised as a result of receiving support (Crocker & Canevello, 2008). As a result, a transactional view of social support minimizes the benefits of social support because social support is reduced to a cost-benefit analysis without a sense of interconnectedness or moral aspirations rooted in the sense of shared community.

Some researchers have coined the term **"social capital"** to conceptualize social support. The term "capital" is predominantly perspectival because it suggests a quantifiable set of reserve assets that can be accumulated, exchanged, and depleted by individuals. This is an economic approach to social relationships, which are conceptually anchored through individualistic and capitalistic approaches to identity and relationships (Schuller et al., 2000; see Figure 10.3). Social capital has been theorized in two primary ways: as resources and as social norms (Fulkerson & Thompson, 2008). As a *resource* grounded through interpersonal relationships and networks, social capital can be transacted and exchanged into other forms of resources (e.g., money or status; Fulkerson & Thompson, 2008). Viewing social capital as a resource fits squarely with Perspectival Thinking. In contrast, when viewed as a social norm, social capital entails debts and favors that one accumulates through *reciprocity transactions* (i.e., expectations of reciprocal, rational exchange of intangible goods) and *value introjection* (i.e., the moral expectations that underlies and precedes contractual relationships and economic behaviors; Fulkerson & Thompson, 2008; see also Silverstein et al., 2012). Depending on how one orients her obligations and relationships, such normative expectations can be driven by either Perspectival Thinking (e.g., an impersonal exchange with business-like expectations and obligations) or Mythic Connection (e.g., doing the "right" thing as a good member of the collective).

Many researchers have warned how a transactional approach to social support can become problematic. For example, researchers observed that "parents who worry about being abandoned in old age may strategically underinvest in the education of their children to make sure they do not have the option of moving to the city" (Banerjee & Duflo 2019, p. 36). In other words, to guarantee their future support, parents may strategically limit their support to their children. Because Perspectival Thinking is strategic and calculating, individuals are driven to maximize their *individual* interests. This approach dissociates, rather than associates, individuals from their community and support network. Others are regarded as mere resources to be exploited. In his book, *The Science of Evil: On Empathy and the Origins Of Cruelty*, Baron-Cohen (2012) cautioned,

> Treating other people as if they were just objects is one of the worst things you can do to another human being, to ignore their subjectivity, their thoughts and feelings. When people are solely focused on the pursuit of their own interests, they have all the potential to be unempathic. (pp. 7–8)

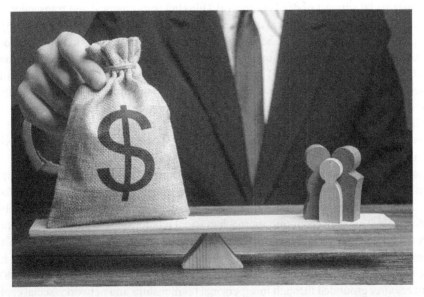

Figure 10.3 Social support as social capital. What can be more perspectival and transactional when we treat relationships as a resource, with values to be realized through exchanges? *Source:* Andrii Yalanskyi / Alamy Stock Photo

Zero degrees of empathy is ultimately a lonely kind of existence, a life at best misunderstood, at worst condemned as selfish. It means you have no brakes on your behavior, leaving you free to pursue any object of your desires, or to express any thought in your mind, without considering the impact of your actions or words on any other person. (p. 44)

In summary, support provision under Perspectival Thinking is strategic and transactional, focusing on a narrowed understanding of zero-sum analysis of costs and benefits. This is equated with rational choice and rational decision-making. Reciprocity demands through psychological processes, normative expectations, or even legal mechanisms serve to explain and guarantee the exchange of social support. Such an approach to social support, however, is driven by individuals' self-interests. As a result, even the closest of social ties do not warrant support provision if the support provision may lead to diminishing self-interests.

III. An Integral Fusion Approach to Social Support

Because there are many different ways to understand culture, we have worked to avoid limiting discussions of cultural variations through the lenses of national, ethnic, or racial cultures. Such an approach also overlooks the variations between cultural subgroups, individual differences, and contextual considerations (e.g., issues at stake, relationships, and support availability). When we referenced ethnic or group cultures, our focus was not on the ethnic or group differences, but on how specific cultural perspectives (e.g., Magic Consciousness, Mythic Connection, and Perspectival Thinking) are enacted. For example, we explored how social support within familial clans in Chinese societies can operate through Magic Consciousness, how filial piety, a Chinese cultural value, can create normative pressure for both support givers and support recipients, and how legal systems are utilized to ensure support between adult children and elderly parents in recent years. By recognizing the complexity of cultures (e.g., culture as ethnic/racial groups, speech communities, worldviews, and as a living process), our analytical focus centers on how support is appraised, negotiated, and coordinated among multiple parties.

A. Empathy and Support Enacted through Communication

An Integral Fusion approach requires individuals to have the ability to not only understand others' perspectives but also to respond to their perspectives in a way that accommodates (rather than patronizes) differences. If one recognizes others' perspectives but patronizes their concerns, his or her approach is Perspectival Thinking because such an approach centers on accomplishing one's own objectives *and* objectifying others' perspectives for strategic gain (see also "Exploitations" when Cultural Perspectives Collide in Chapter 13). Our understanding of an Integral Fusion approach is akin to the concept of **empathy** proposed by psychologist Baron-Cohen (2012):

Empathy is our ability to identify what someone else is thinking or feeling and to respond to their thoughts and feelings with an appropriate emotion. This suggests there are at least two stages in empathy: recognition and response. Both are needed, since if you have the former without the latter you haven't empathized at all. If I can see in your face that you are struggling to lift your suitcase onto the overhead rack on the train and I just sit there and watch, then I have failed to respond to your feelings (of frustration). Empathy therefore requires not only that you can identify another person's feelings and thoughts, but that you respond to these with an appropriate emotion. (pp. 16–17)

In this sense, empathy is not just an emotional state but involves both cognitive components (e.g., identifying another person's feelings and thoughts) and behavioral components (i.e., responding with actions that convey the appropriate emotions).

Goldsmith (2004) proposed that communication is how social support is enacted in interpersonal relationships. She explained, "**Enacted support** occurs in the context of conversation, which includes an exchange of messages as well as processes of interpretation and coordination between conversational partners" (p. 26). Goldsmith (2004) explained,

Rather than picturing enacted support as a resource that is handed over unproblematically from one person to another, we should see enacted social support as a *process* through which conversational partners construct together a view of the situation, including the nature of the problem, the options for coping, the implications for valued images of self, and the significance for the relationship. If and when social support facilitates coping, it is not only by virtue of having advised, informed, complimented, assured, or aided but also by virtue of having created (or sustained) an understanding of the task, identities, and relationship involved. If we fail to consider how well enactments of support are adapted to these symbolic purposes, we miss critical features that make some enactments of support better than others. [emphasis added] (p. 151)

How a person frames their support-seeking messages may influence the types of support received as well as the audiences' evaluations of the support seeker (Caughlin et al., 2009). For example, if a person's HIV disclosure is limited to their HIV+ status, they are likely to receive informational support (e.g., advice) but not emotional support; however, if they expressly indicate that their reason for disclosure was to seek support, they were able to elicit emotional support and suppress unsolicited (and often unwanted) advice (Caughlin et al., 2009). Similarly, how a person responds to a sibling's disclosure of distress may influence whether his or her provision of social support is successful. In particular, a response that is sensitive to the support seeker's multiple goals (e.g., task, identity, and relational goals) is rated more favorably than those that are limited to the speakers' perspective or adopts normative statements (Caughlin et al., 2008). In short, social support is successful not simply because of the form it takes nor the amount offered, but is dependent on conversational partners' ability to collaborate and coordinate their tasks, identities, and relationships in a way that they find mutually agreeable, meaningful, and beneficial. Successful social support is a coordinated achievement between multiple parties (Goldsmith & Brashers, 2008).

An Integral Fusion approach highlights that one's understanding of others' perspectives and needs is essential to the success of support provision. For example, Crocker and Canevello (2008) found that support recipients' perception of support providers' intent (e.g., to get something for themselves versus genuine concern for the recipients' wellbeing) can influence the beneficial effects of social support. We argue that invisible support (i.e., when a support provider reported offering support, but the support recipient did not report receiving it) reflects an Integral Fusion approach of social support. By recognizing that support recipients may experience face threats or feel an additional burden, support providers actively disguise their supportive behaviors as routine interactions. For example, rather than offering a loan to help a friend to save his business, a person may suggest that she is looking for investment opportunities, and the friend's business, though not currently profitable, represents an important trend for future markets. Elderly Chinese grandparents may add Chinese herbal medicine in their cooking as they prepare meals for the family, hoping such food therapies can safeguard other family members' health (Kong & Hsieh, 2012). In the movie, *Farewell*, rather than informing grandma about her terminal illness, a Chinese family decided to hold a wedding – inviting all relatives from Japan and the United States for a "happy gathering" in grandma's hometown and allowing all to spend quality time with grandma (Wang, 2019). In these scenarios, support recipients enjoy the benefits of support without the burdens of identity threats, risks, or obligations.

Finally, an Integral Fusion approach suggests that the interactive process and complex relationships of providing and receiving social support can be fluid and multilayered. As Goldsmith (2004) explained, "One problem with the provider/recipient conceptualization is that in close relationships, it may not be entirely clear who is the provider and who is the recipient of support" (p. 117). For example, as discussed earlier, support providers may make extensive efforts and meticulous planning to offer *invisible* support. However, what if the support recipients were aware of such efforts and decided to pretend that they were unaware of such efforts? Many of us had pretended ignorance and acted shocked when we already knew about a surprise party or a Christmas present that was meant for us.

In a Chinese funeral attended by the first author, she overheard the deceased's adult children talking among themselves about whether their mother pretended not to be aware of her diagnosis of terminal cancer in support of their efforts to conceal the devastating news from her. In these scenarios, the intended support recipients became the support providers, allowing the initial support providers to enjoy their "invisible" support. Although the literature has traditionally treated support providers and support recipients as two distinctive entities through which support is offered in a unidirectional manner, these examples highlight the malleable and interactive dynamics of social support.

B. Challenges to In-Group Definitions and Negotiations

1. In-Group Memberships Essential to Social Support

Because in-group membership is essential to social support enacted through Magic Consciousness and Mythic Connection, how a community (or an in-group) is defined shapes the boundaries of support provision by these cultural perspectives. In contrast, because social relationships under Perspectival Thinking are transactional, the boundaries of communities have little influence over social support in interpersonal relationships. However, even in the most modern, perspectival societies, when communities are faced with a crisis, they often resort to cultural values and social norms to solidify community cohesion. For example, three days after the 9/11 Terrorist Attack, President Bush (2001a) proclaimed September 14, 2001, as a National Day of Prayer and Remembrance (see Figure 10.4). In his remarks at the National Cathedral, Bush (2001b) stated:

> God's signs are not always the ones we look for. We learn in tragedy that his purposes are not always our own. Yet the prayers of private suffering, whether in our homes or in this great cathedral, are known and heard, and understood.
>
> There are prayers that help us last through the day or endure the night. There are prayers of friends and strangers, that give us strength for the journey. And there are prayers that yield our will to a will greater than our own.
>
> This world He created is of moral design. Grief and tragedy and hatred are only for a time. Goodness, remembrance, and love have no end. And the Lord of life holds all who die, and all who mourn. (para. 10–12)

The appeal to sacred symbolism is mythic. And such symbols are strong binders of community. But as much as they bind in-group members, so too they distinguish one group and its mythological foundation from another. This is the bounded nature of in-group, out-group identities. This can form the basis of profound conflict because the more sacred and exclusive the symbolic community, the more the out-group is excluded and even defined as profane.

During such a crisis, when the physical world is endangered, humans tend to move to what Ernest Becker (1971/2010) called the "symbolic," a realm beyond the physical

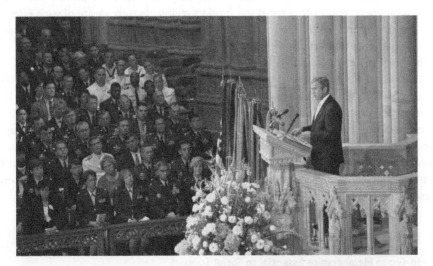

Figure 10.4 During the newly proclaimed National Day of Prayer and Remembrance, president George W. Bush addresses the congregation and the nation friday, September 14, 2001, at the national cathedral in Washington, D.C. *Source:* The U.S. National Archives.

space and time, which often entails Magic Consciousness and Mythic Connection. The shift to the symbolic gives us a sense of immortality. It also gives us a collective identity insofar as we believe we are part of something bigger than our limited physical existence. The sacredness of the symbolic structure also casts the Other as the opposite of the sacred: the profane. The Other is a profanity. Once this takes place, symbolic and/ or physical violence against the Other is no longer prohibited. One cannot be wrong in their pursuit of sacred peace and justice. This is the dangerous side of extreme group cohesion and community. Community posits a shared identity, which is a common source of strength for social relationships in adversities and against adversaries.

An Integral Fusion approach is responsive to the worldviews of the participants involved, reflecting a blending of different cultural perspectives. An Integral Fusion approach appreciates the primal emotions under Magic Consciousness, the value aspiration under Mythic Connection, and the analytic reflection under Perspectival Thinking. Although the boundaries of group membership are straightforward and unambiguous in communities with Magic Consciousness and Mythic Connection, the definitions of in-group memberships can be overlapping, conflicting, or contentious from an Integral Fusion approach.

For example, although infertility is a shared problem for couples, disclosure of infertility struggles for support-seeking may involve disclosing information related to the couples' personal, medical, or financial struggles. As a result, couples struggling with infertility concerns face challenges in terms of whom they can seek support from, and what (and to what extent) they feel comfortable disclosing. In an interesting study, Steuber and Solomon (2011) found that when husbands reported higher internalized stigma (see self-stigma in Chapter 8) and disclosure concerns, the couples, both husbands and wives, are less likely to share their infertility issues with their support network. In contrast, when wives reported internalized stigma, they were more likely to disclose their struggles with their support network. In other words, with male-factor infertility, the husband and wife acted as a unit in guarding their privacy and restraining from support-seeking from friends and family, and even offering vague or inaccurate reports of the cause of their infertility (Steuber & Solomon, 2011). However, when wives struggled with self-stigma of infertility, wives included their friends and family in the coping process (Steuber & Solomon, 2011). The differences may be caused by how infertility stigma functions differently for men and women – as women may disclose their infertility struggles to negate a potentially more damaging stigma – selfish, career-driven women who choose to be voluntarily childless (Bute & Vik, 2010). Women reported that they avoided disclosure to family members who were unhelpful in their coping process, often modifying their disclosure and shifting their privacy boundaries throughout their journey of infertility struggles (Bute, 2013; Bute & Vik, 2010). From this perspective, an Integral Fusion approach to social support highlights the dynamic and interactive nature of "community." In-group membership is dependent on the issues involved, risks entailed for individuals, and resources available.

2. Rethinking Communication Privacy Management Theory

Disclosing illness-related information is an essential part of individuals' managing of identity, relationship, and tasks in order to solicit the support needed for illness management (Fair & Albright, 2012; Peterson et al., 2012). **Communication Privacy Management Theory (CPM)**, proposed by Petronio (2002), aims to explain individuals' management of private information in social relationships. By noting that individuals believe that they own private information (i.e., **privacy ownership**) and have the right to that information, an "information owner" actively manages control of their **privacy boundaries** (i.e., people with whom the information owner share his or her private information). By recognizing the co-existence of different layers of privacy boundaries (e.g., husband-wife boundary, family boundary, and community boundary), CPM suggests that individuals rely on **privacy rules** (i.e., a set of rules that determine when, how, with whom, and in what way others might be granted or denied access to someone's private information) to determine with whom, and to what extent, they share private information (Petronio & Durham, 2008). As private information is shared, the trusted individuals become co-owners or shareholders of the information and, thus, enjoy a shared privacy boundary around that information (Petronio & Child, 2020). When co-owners of the private information disclose information to other parties, the information owner may experience **privacy boundary turbulence** (i.e., when the management of private information violates one's expectation; e.g., confidants breaking social norms/rules in disclosing the private information to others), resulting in a **recalibration** of the privacy boundaries of their private information (Petronio & Child, 2020). In other words, when an information owner becomes concerned about increased costs due to their lack of control of private information, they "recalibrate privacy rules or establish new rules to meet their risk-benefit threshold in a given situation or in terms of meeting an overall need" (Petronio, 2010, p. 180). CPM has been applied in various contexts, including family communication, health communication, and computer-mediated communication.

Although CPM may first appear as an Integral Fusion approach to social support as one actively coordinates with others in a dynamic process of management of information, CPM has a strong Perspectival Thinking undertone. For example, it is Perspectival Thinking to conceptualize information as being "privately own" by an individual who has a "right" to "control" access and dissemination of the information. The information owner's personal agenda determines a focused strategy to maximize one's benefits through the control of private information (e.g., obtaining social support through disclosure of illness). Violations to an information owner's expectations do not result in renegotiations of identities or relationships but center on the information owner's change of "privacy rules" (Petronio & Child, 2020) – a relatively information owner-centered, mechanical, and rule-based process that is indicative of a Perspectival Thinking worldview.

Although CPM emphasizes a dialectic perspective, which may suggest an Integral Fusion approach, the approaches to the management of private information centered on the information owner's perspective and control, relying on risk-benefit analysis for decisional balance (Petronio, 2010) – a Perspectival Thinking perspective. Information is conceptualized as an asset, a "thing" that can be owned, shared, parsed, and concealed by the owner in strategic ways. CPM does not directly address the components of Magic Consciousness (e.g., how one's identity is impacted by self-disclosure) or Mythic Connection (e.g., relationship building through shared narratives/storytelling), which are presumed and remain somewhat hidden. We argue that if CPM appears intuitive to our readers, it is a result of us living in a modern, perspectival society: We are accustomed to viewing information as a resource to be shared or withheld to achieve specific ends (i.e., maximizing individual benefits).

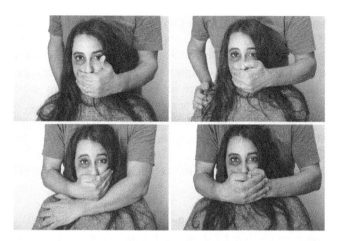

Figure 10.5 Family secrets. Because domestic abuse in a family is a common taboo topic where all family members safeguard the secret to avoid stigmatization from outsiders, interventions must address the Magic Consciousness that binds the family unit. *Source:* ahmetnaim/AGE Fotostock

However, we propose that recognizing CPM as a predominately Perspectival Thinking worldview can also provide opportunities to reconsider how CPM may operate in other cultural contexts and perspectives. CPM posits that cultural-specific norms and rules may guide individuals' management of private information (Bute et al., 2017; Petronio & Child, 2020). However, for people with Magic Consciousness, the concepts of privacy and ownership do not exist. All is shared – a collective One. There is very little "privacy." Thus, it would be unthinkable for a person with Magic Consciousness to consider that there are privacy boundaries or privacy rules. However, this does not mean that a person with Magic Consciousness does not have control over private information – rather, under Magic Consciousness, all information is free-flowing within the community but strong distinctions are made for people outside of the magic community. In her work on family secrets, Vangelisti (1994) found that taboo topics (i.e., activities that are often condemned and stigmatized by both family members and the larger society; e.g., incest, substance abuse, illegalities, and physical/psychological abuse) are often treated as a *whole* family secret: Although all members of the family were aware of the secret, it was not shared with non-family members (see Figure 10.5). Although the most stigmatizing topics are shared by the greatest number of family members (i.e., lack of privacy) and despite the negative consequences of withholding such information (e.g., emotional distress), the whole family acted together to guard against outsiders' evaluation and to defend the family name (Vangelisti, 1994; Vangelisti & Caughlin, 1997). We argue that due to the highly stigmatizing nature of taboo topics, the "self" of individual family members disappears; at the same time, the magic community of a blood-bound family unit is invoked. As a result, information is shared freely within the magic community yet outsiders are indiscriminately denied access to the information.

On the other hand, for people with Mythic Connection, sharing information may become a symbolic act to display cultural or community values (as opposed to maximizing individual gain) and to develop and maintain relationships. For example, rule violations (e.g., getting a tattoo or piercing) is often shared between individual family members, but not necessarily the whole family, to bond with one another (Vangelisti & Caughlin, 1997). Similarly, individuals may choose to disclose their vulnerability to solicit social support and to perform relational closeness (Goldsmith et al., 2007). Sharing information under Mythic Connection is not about individual gain per se, but about individuals' desire to conform to societal-level norms that speak to specific social values, such as honesty, privacy, or restraint (Bute, 2013; Bute et al., 2017). For example, some people may choose to disclose family secrets to a person they are not familiar with if there is an urgent need (e.g., helping a person in crisis; Vangelisti et al., 2001). From this perspective, individuals' management of private information is not driven by individual-level risk-benefit analysis but incorporates considerations for cultural values within their communities.

3. An Integral Fusion Approach to Social Relationships

An Integral Fusion approach to CPM means that the coordinated management of private information is not limited to information owners' cost-benefit analysis. Rather, we propose that individuals manage their privacy boundaries through their understanding of the in-group community. Individuals in the in-group community are viewed as co-owners of the "private" information. The boundaries of the community shapes (a) whether and how certain information may stay private or even be considered private at all, and (b) how the information should be managed. One may recognize that the husband-wife unit is a magic community and thus, they have no concerns about "privacy" per se; similarly, one may argue that a family clan serves as a magic community and thus, not differentiating the "ownership" of property, whether it's information or resources, between members. For example, it would have appeared that with male-factor infertility, couples treated the husband-wife unit as an in-group; in contrast, when wives struggle with infertility-related self-stigma, the wives treated their whole support networks as in-groups (Steuber & Solomon, 2011). As a result, the disclosure of private information varies due to how couples construe their in-group membership for support-seeking purposes.

The understanding of "ownership" is essential in distinguishing communities of Magic Consciousness from other cultural perspectives. Because there is no concept of self, individuals of magic communities would not consider themselves having a "right" to "private" information or properties. For example, Western biomedical traditions (i.e., a perspectival worldview) assume that an individual's health data and biospecimens are considered his or her individual "property" and thus, the individual can choose to give access to the private information via informed consent. However, indigenous participants emphasized the need to consult tribal elders before participating in biobank projects – noting that their biospecimen is not theirs to give since their biological materials also include group information (e.g., a cultural group's migration patterns or genetic history; Burgess & Tansey, 2009). Similarly, Chinese people often resisted organ donation because their cultural values (e.g., filial piety) emphasize that a person's body is not his or her own (e.g., a person's body is given by one's parents and ancestors) and thus, one has a duty, "to return his or her body to the ancestors in the same intact condition that he or she received it from his or her parents out of respect" (Lam & McCullough, 2000, p. 452). In other words, for some indigenous people and Chinese people, they do not even consider themselves having sole ownership of their bodies.

Recognizing that the inclusion and exclusion of members of a magic or mythic community can be dynamic *and* symbolic, an Integral Fusion approach to CPM suggests that individuals may make decisions against their own personal (individual) interests. For example, individuals may experience social and cultural pressures in how they determine the membership of their magic or mythic community. A mother may feel hurt when her daughter struggles with infertility or miscarriage without telling her. When a Chinese father allows his son to take over the responsibilities of information management and to be a proxy decision-maker (e.g., making decisions about treatments), he is demonstrating his commitment to his family and community (Ellerby et al., 2000). Although individuals may choose to disclose or withhold private information for self-interest purposes (e.g., obtaining social support), individuals were found to disclose *or* conceal private, distressing, negative information *against their personal preferences* due to their moral beliefs and ethical obligations (e.g., disclosing one's HIV+ status because their relational partner has a right to know) and relational considerations (e.g., disclosing/concealing one's cancer diagnosis would be devastating to a parent's psyche; Derlega et al., 1998; Derlega et al., 2000; Goldsmith et al., 2007). From this perspective, whether one chooses to conceal or reveal private information may be best understood from a multiple-goal approach (Caughlin & Vangelisti, 2009).

A **multiple-goal approach** is inherently integral because it is responsive and accommodating to the perspectives of multiple parties, including their diverging purposes, needs, and resource availability. Recognizing that there may be competing and even conflicting goals within a single person as well as between a person and his/her supportive others, an Integral Fusion approach recognizes that soliciting social support through communication may create dilemmas and challenges to identities, relationships, and tasks involved. As a result, a person may choose to disclose or withhold certain information (e.g., cancer-related concerns) for the needs of others – even when such a decision conflicts with her personal interests, preferences, or needs. The disclosure of information for support-seeking is not construed as a dualistic process (i.e., disclose or not) but complex coordination between parties involved. Greene et al. (2006) explained,

> [S]elf-disclosure (including "who" discloses, "what" is divulged, "how" the partners influence one another to disclose or not, and "when" and "where" disclosure occurs) is a process that unfolds over time – within a single conversation as well as across days, weeks, months, and even years of a personal relationship. ... Also, despite the conceptual distinction between "discloser" and "disclosure recipient," partners in a relationship are likely to exchange roles of discloser and recipient within a conversation and across time as they coordinate their needs and expectations about disclosing or listening. (p. 415)

In summary, an Integral Fusion approach to social support recognizes that social support is a complex with magic unity, mythic group, and perspectival individuated aspects. Like shifting a heavy burden from one muscle group to another in order to carry the load, integral support takes into account how a person can shift from one source to another as need dictates. An integral understanding and appreciation for support recognize the efforts of rational scientists working to find a cure for us, our church friends praying for and with us and reading scripture to us, and the comfort we take from even a strange dog, with its magic touch that calms us. An Integral Fusion approach is a fluid process coordinated between individuals. Individuals' supportive acts are constructed through communication, appraising, and negotiating the meanings and impacts of their support coordination. An Integral Fusion approach aims to reconcile differences in individuals' perspectives and to achieve mutually agreeable and beneficial outcomes. Support (and care) may seek no final outcome but rather to be here now comfortably (Dass, 1971/2010, 2011).

An Integral Fusion approach to social support blurs the lines of support giving and receiving support. A support provider may intentionally disguise her support to minimize the risks and burdens faced by the support recipient. Similarly, a support recipient may actively perform ignorance to the support provider's effort to show their appreciation *and* support to the support provider. In other words, support providers and recipients do not act as "individuals" but as a "team," a community. An Integral Fusion approach recognizes that individuals can learn to see meanings of supportive actions from another person's perspective and respond to others' perspectives in a way that is understanding, responsive, and accommodating. Rather than focusing on individual needs or perspectives, it calls for empathy and compassion. As a result, what can be perceived as "nagging" or "controlling" to an outsider is interpreted as "caring" or "reminding"(Goldsmith et al., 2006). Support was given *and* received even when the form it takes may not be perfect.

In the midst of COVID-19 pandemic, local businesses, community members, and even children worked to donate food supplies, medical supplies, homemade facemasks to local hospitals, homeless shelters, and food pantries. People reached out: not to seek support, but to offer it in endless forms. "I'm contributing some good to where it's going to be needed. [... It] gives me purpose," said a 70-year-old volunteer who has been sewing masks to be donated to local hospitals (Huber, 2020). As University of Dayton faculty members donated personal protection equipment (e.g., gloves and masks) to healthcare workers, a professor commented, "I think this effort shows how giving something, even if it's a small amount, can help, and it empowers people to feel they can do something to help. When people are feeling helpless and hopeless in a crisis like this, giving or doing just a little bit can make a big difference" (Spicker, 2020, para. 3). An Integral Fusion approach to social support is a non-zero-sum relationship. It energizes the support providers, inspires community members, and embraces support recipients. It recognizes we are all connected as one.

IV. Additional Resources

A. Key Terms and Theories

Forms of support
instrumental support = tangible support
informational support
emotional support ↔ esteem support
   appraisal support
   network support
buffering effects

stressful life events
matching model
perceived social support
received social support
support structure
direct effect model = main effect model
social integration
paying it forward (PIF)
invisible support
hysterical strength
clan culture
compassionate goals
self-image goals
moral capital
reciprocity
empathy
enacted support
Communication Privacy Management Theory
    privacy ownership
    privacy boundaries
    privacy rules
    privacy boundary turbulence
    recalibration
multiple-goal approach

B. Discussion Questions

1. Please give examples of the following types of support when you are preparing for an important exam for an undergraduate course. Please explain who are the likely support givers and whether they are likely to be useful or not?
   a. instrumental support
   b. informational support
   c. emotional support
   d. esteem support
   e. appraisal support
   f. network support
2. Do you think timing makes a difference on when you are likely to need the support you identified in Question 1? In what ways?
3. Please compare and contrast buffering effects and direct effects of social support.
   a. What are the functions and impacts of social support when you are facing adversities?
   b. What are the functions and impacts of social support in everyday life?
4. Do you agree that the support you need must match the support that was offered for social support to have positive effects? Why or why not?
   a. Why do you think Pay-It-Forward as a social movement can transform the whole community? Does the matching model explain this effect?

    b. Do you think social support offered would not be effective as long as it is not what the support recipient needs?

5. Why do you think perceived social support is a better predictor of health than received social support?

    a. If this is the case, why is it that invisible support (i.e., support received but not perceived) is so effective?

    b. Have you tried to offer invisible support? How did you do it?

    c. Based on the two the lines of research (i.e., (a) perceived support is a better predictor than received support for health outcomes, and (b) invisible support has some of the best outcomes), what are your suggestions for people who want to offer support to their loved ones?

6. Please answer the following questions by using each of the four cultural perspectives (i.e., Magic Consciousness, Mythic Connection, Perspectival Thinking, and Integral Fusion).

    a. Think about your experiences of offering social support. Give examples of the support you offered under each of the four cultural perspectives. Why do they belong to these cultural perspectives?

    b. Whether people would avoid support-seeking (even when they need the support) under Magic Consciousness? Why or why not? What are the possible reasons that they would do so? (How about other cultural perspectives?)

    c. When offering social support, what are the likely emotional impacts (e.g., empowered, fulfilled, drained, or exhausted) under different cultural perspectives? Why do you think people feel that way?

7. When you offer social support to others? Do you expect them to pay you back later? Why or why not?

    a. Are there people that you would always offer support even if they would not have paid you back (e.g., symbolically with praises and/or literally with other favors)? Why?

    b. Are there people you would not have offered support if they would not pay you back? Why?

    c. Are there strangers that you would still offer support even if they would not have paid you back? Why would you do that?

    d. Do you think you may have different decisions based on different types of support (e.g., instrumental versus emotional support)?

C. References

Bales, K., & Soodalter, R. (2010). *The slave next door: Human trafficking and slavery in America today.* University of California Press.

Banerjee, A. V., & Duflo, E. (2019). *Good economics for hard times.* PublicAffairs.

Baron-Cohen, S. (2012). *The science of evil: On empathy and the origins of cruelty.* Basic Books.

Becker, E. (2010). *Birth and death of meaning.* Free Press. (Original work published 1971)

Bolger, N., Zuckerman, A., & Kessler, R. C. (2000). Invisible support and adjustment to stress. *Journal of Personality and Social Psychology, 79*(6), 953–961.

Bowling, N. A., Beehr, T. A., Johnson, A. L., Semmer, N. K., Hendricks, E. A., & Webster, H. A. (2004). Explaining potential antecedents of workplace social support: Reciprocity or attractiveness? *Journal of Occupational Health Psychology*, *9*(4), 339–350.

Brashers, D. E., Hsieh, E., Neidig, J. L., & Reynolds, N. R. (2006). Managing uncertainty about illness: Health care providers as credible authorities. In R. M. Dailey & B. A. Le Poire (Eds.), *Applied interpersonal communication matters: Family, health, and community relations* (pp. 219–240). Peter Lang.

Braswell, H., & Kushner, H. I. (2012). Suicide, social integration, and masculinity in the U.S. military. *Social Science & Medicine*, *74*(4), 530–536.

Brissette, I., Cohen, S., & Seeman, T. E. (2000). Measuring social integration and social network. In S. Cohen, L. G. Underwood, & B. Gottlieb (Eds.), *Social support measurement and intervention: A guide for health and social scientists* (pp. 53–85). Oxford University Press.

Brown, B. (2010, June). *The power of vulnerability.* TED Talk. https://www.ted.com/talks/brene_brown_the_power_of_vulnerability

Burg, M. M., & Seeman, T. E. (1994). Families and health: The negative side of social ties. *Annals of Behavioral Medicine*, *16*(2), 109–115.

Burgess, M., & Tansey, J. (2009). Cultural authority of informed consent: Indigenous participation in biobanking and salmon genomics focus groups. In O. Corrigan, J. McMillan, K. Liddell, M. Richards, & C. Weijer (Eds.), *The limits of consent: A socio-ethical approach to human subject research in medicine* (pp. 199–211). Oxford University Press.

Burleson, B. R., & MacGeorge, E. L. (2002). Supportive communication. In M. L. Knapp & J. A. Daly (Eds.), *Handbook of interpersonal communication* (3rd ed., pp. 374–424). Sage.

Bush, G. W. (2001a, September 13). *National Day of Prayer and Remembrance for the victims of the terrorist attacks on September 11, 2001.* The White House. https://georgewbush-whitehouse.archives.gov/news/releases/2001/09/20010913-7.html

Bush, G. W. (2001b, September 14). *President's remarks at National Day of Prayer and Remembrance.* The White House. https://georgewbush-whitehouse.archives.gov/news/releases/2001/09/20010914-2.html

Bute, J. J. (2013). The discursive dynamics of disclosure and avoidance: Evidence from a study of infertility. *Western Journal of Communication*, *77*(2), 164–185.

Bute, J. J., Brann, M., & Hernandez, R. (2017). Exploring societal-level privacy rules for talking about miscarriage. *Journal of Social and Personal Relationships*, *36*(2), 379–399.

Bute, J. J., & Vik, T. A. (2010). Privacy management as unfinished business: Shifting boundaries in the context of infertility. *Communication Studies*, *61*(1), 1–20.

Buunk, B. P., Doosje, B. J., Jans, L. G. J. M., & Hopstaken, L. E. M. (1993). Perceived reciprocity, social support, and stress at work: The role of exchange and communal orientation. *Journal of Personality and Social Psychology*, *65*(4), 801–811.

Campbell, J. (with Moyers, B.). (2011). *The power of myth.* Knopf Doubleday. (Original work published 1988)

Caplan, R. D., Cobb, S., & French, J. R. (1975). Relationships of cessation of smoking with job stress, personality, and social support. *Journal of Applied Psychology*, *60*(2), 211–219.

Caughlin, J. P., Brashers, D. E., Ramey, M. E., Kosenko, K. A., Donovan-Kicken, E., & Bute, J. J. (2008). The message design logics of responses to HIV disclosures. *Human Communication Research*, *34*(4), 655–684.

Caughlin, J. P., Bute, J. J., Donovan-Kicken, E., Kosenko, K. A., Ramey, M. E., & Brashers, D. E. (2009). Do message features influence reactions to HIV disclosures? A multiple-goals perspective. *Health Communication, 24*(3), 270–283.

Caughlin, J. P., & Vangelisti, A. L. (2009). Why people conceal or reveal secrets: A multiple goals theory perspective. In T. D. Afifi (Ed.), *Uncertainty, information management, and disclosure decisions: Theories and applications* (pp. 279–299). Routledge.

Chang, Y.-P., Lin, Y.-C., & Chen, L. (2012). Pay it forward: Gratitude in social networks. *Journal of Happiness Studies, 13*(5), 761–781.

Chen, F., Liu, G., & Mair, C. A. (2011). Intergenerational ties in context: Grandparents caring for grandchildren in China. *Social Forces, 90*(2), 571–594.

Chen, X., & Silverstein, M. (2000). Intergenerational social support and the psychological well-being of older parents in China. *Research on Aging, 22*(1), 43–65.

Chen, Y., Hicks, A., & While, A. E. (2014). Loneliness and social support of older people in China: A systematic literature review. *Health & Social Care in the Community, 22*(2), 113–123.

Cheung, C.-K., & Kwan, A. Y.-H. (2009). The erosion of filial piety by modernisation in Chinese cities. *Ageing and Society, 29*(2), 179–198.

Chou, R. J.-A. (2011). Filial piety by contract? The emergence, implementation, and implications of the "family support agreement" in China. *The Gerontologist, 51*(1), 3–16.

Chu, C. (2020, March 17).「我OK, 你先領」口罩禮讓運動, 是無私大愛, 還是隱藏的優越感? Commonwealth Magazine. https://www.cw.com.tw/article/article.action?id=5099421

Cobb, M. (2015, February 11). *Volunteer to practice random acts of kindness.* United Way Blog. http://www.unitedway.org/blog/volunteer-to-practice-random-acts-of-kindness

Cohen, S. (2004). Social relationships and health. *American Psychologist, 59*(8), 676–684.

Cohen, S., Murphy, M. L. M., & Prather, A. A. (2019). Ten surprising facts about stressful life events and disease risk. *Annual Review of Psychology, 70*, 577–597.

Cohen, S., & Wills, T. A. (1985). Stress, social support, and the buffering hypothesis. *Psychological Bulletin, 98*(2), 310–357.

Cosley, B. J., McCoy, S. K., Saslow, L. R., & Epel, E. S. (2010). Is compassion for others stress buffering? Consequences of compassion and social support for physiological reactivity to stress. *Journal of Experimental Social Psychology, 46*(5), 816–823.

Crocker, J., & Canevello, A. (2008). Creating and undermining social support in communal relationships: The role of compassionate and self-image goals. *Journal of Personality and Social Psychology, 95*(3), 555–575.

Curtis, M. (Writer) & Holland, T. (Director). (1999, April 8). The one where Rachel smokes (Season 5, Episode 18) [TV series episode]. In Crane, D., Kauffman, M., Bright, K. S., Curtis, M., Chase, A., & Malins, G. (Executive Producers), *Friends.* Bright/Kauffman/Crane Productions; Warner Bros. Television.

Dass, R. (2010). *Be here now.* HarperOne. (Original work published 1971)

Dass, R. (2011). *Be love now: The path of the heart.* HarperOne.

Dass-Brailsford, P., Thomley, R., & de Mendoza, A. H. (2011). Paying it forward: The transformative aspects of volunteering after Hurricane Katrina. *Traumatology, 17*(1), 29–40.

Dean, A., & Lin, N. (1977). The stress-buffering role of social support. *Journal of Nervous and Mental Disease, 165*(6), 403–417.

Derlega, V. J., Lovejoy, D., & Winstead, B. A. (1998). Personal accounts on disclosing and concealing HIV-positive test results: Weighing the benefits and risks. In V. J. Derlega & A. P. Barbee (Eds.), *HIV and social interaction* (pp. 147–164). Sage.

Derlega, V. J., Winstead, B. A., & Folk-Barron, L. (2000). Reasons for and against disclosing HIV-seropositive test results to an intimate partner: A functional perspective. In S. Petronio (Ed.), *Balancing the secrets of private disclosures* (pp. 53–69). Erlbaum.

Ellerby, J. H., McKenzie, J., McKay, S., Gariepy, G. J., & Kaufert, J. M. (2000). Bioethics for clinicians: 18. Aboriginal cultures. *Canadian Medical Association Journal, 163*(7), 845–850.

Fair, C., & Albright, J. (2012). "Don't tell him you have HIV unless he's 'the One'": Romantic relationships among adolescents and young adults with perinatal HIV infection. *AIDS Patient Care and STDs, 26*(12), 746–754.

Feeney, B. C., & Collins, N. L. (2015). A new look at social support: A theoretical perspective on thriving through relationships. *Personality and Social Psychology Review, 19*(2), 113–147.

Flynn, M. (2020, March 16). *From Bourbon Street to Miami Beach, America's party people ignored pleas for social distancing.* The Washington Post. https://www.washingtonpost.com/nation/2020/03/16/coronavirus-bars-lockdowns-closures

Fowler, J. H., & Christakis, N. A. (2010). Cooperative behavior cascades in human social networks. *Proceedings of the National Academy of Sciences, 107*(12), 5334–5338.

Fulkerson, G. M., & Thompson, G. H. (2008). The evolution of a contested concept: A meta-analysis of social capital definitions and trends (1988–2006). *Sociological Inquiry, 78*(4), 536–557.

Goldsmith, D. J. (2004). *Communicating social support.* Cambridge University Press.

Goldsmith, D. J., & Brashers, D. E. (2008). Communication matters: Developing and testing social support interventions. *Communication Monographs, 75*(4), 320–329.

Goldsmith, D. J., Bute, J. J., & Lindholm, K. A. (2012). Patient and partner strategies for talking about lifestyle change following a cardiac event. *Journal of Applied Communication Research,* 40(1), 65–86.

Goldsmith, D. J., Lindholm, K. A., & Bute, J. J. (2006). Dilemmas of talking about lifestyle changes among couples coping with a cardiac event. *Social Science & Medicine,* 63(8), 2079–2090.

Goldsmith, D. J., & Miller, G. A. (2013). Conceptualizing how couples talk about cancer. *Health Communication, 29*(1), 51–63.

Goldsmith, D. J., Miller, L. E., & Caughlin, J. P. (2007). Openness and avoidance in couples communicating about cancer. *Annals of the International Communication Association, 31*(1), 62–115.

Greene, K., Derlega, V. J., & Mathews, A. (2006). Self-disclosure in personal relationships. In A. L. Vangelisti & D. Perlman (Eds.), *The Cambridge handbook of personal relationships* (pp. 409-427). Cambridge University Press.

Haber, M. G., Cohen, J. L., Lucas, T., & Baltes, B. B. (2007). The relationship between self-reported received and perceived social support: A meta-analytic review. *American Journal of Community Psychology, 39*(1-2), 133–144.

Hadhazy, A. (2016, May 1). *How it's possible for an ordinary person to lift a car.* BBC. https://www.bbc.com/future/article/20160501-how-its-possible-for-an-ordinary-person-to-lift-a-car

Hawkins, D. N., & Booth, A. (2005). Unhappily ever after: Effects of long-term, low-quality marriages on well-being. *Social Forces, 84*(1), 451–471.

Heaney, C. A., & Israel, B. A. (2008). Social networks and social support. In K. Glanz, B. K. Rimer, & K. Viswanath (Eds.), *Health behavior and health education: Theory, research, and practice* (4th ed., pp. 189–210). Jossey-Bass.

Horne, C. (2009). *The rewards of punishment: A relational theory of norm enforcement.* Stanford University Press.

Huber, M. (2020, April 1). *'It gives me purpose': Volunteers, businesses sew face masks during COVID-19 outbreak.* Argus Leader.

Johns Hopkins Coronavirus Resource Center. (2020). *Coronavirus COVID-19 global cases by the Center for Systems Science and Engineering (CSSE) at Johns Hopkins University (JHU).* Retrieved July 10, 2020, from https://coronavirus.jhu.edu/map.html

Johnston, K. L., & White, K. M. (2003). Binge-drinking: A test of the role of group norms in the theory of planned behaviour. *Psychology and Health, 18*(1), 63–77.

Jung, C. G., von Franz, M.-L., & Freeman, J. (Eds.). (2012). *Man and his symbols.* Random House.

Klein, S. (2014). *Survival of the nicest: How altruism made us human and why it pays to get along* (D. Dollenmayer, Trans.). Workman.

Kong, H., & Hsieh, E. (2012). The social meanings of traditional Chinese medicine: Elderly Chinese immigrants' health practice in the United States. *Journal of Immigrant and Minority Health, 14*(5), 841–849.

Krause, N. (2006). Church-based social support and mortality. *The Journals of Gerontology: Series B, 61*(3), S140-S146.

Kulczycki, A., & Windle, S. (2011). Honor killings in the Middle East and North Africa: A systematic review of the literature. *Violence Against Women, 17*(11), 1442–1464.

Lai, D. W. L. (2009). Filial Piety, caregiving appraisal, and caregiving burden. *Research on Aging, 32*(2), 200–223.

Lam, W. A., & McCullough, L. B. (2000). Influence of religious and spiritual values on the willingness of Chinese–Americans to donate organs for transplantation. *Clinical Transplantation, 14*(5), 449–456.

Lévy-Bruhl, L. (2018). *Revival: How natives think.* Routledge. (Original work published 1926)

Logan, J. R., & Bian, F. (2003). Parents' needs, family structure, and regular intergenerational financial exchange in Chinese cities. *Sociological Forum, 18*(1), 85–101.

Louis, W., Davies, S., Smith, J., & Terry, D. (2007). Pizza and pop and the student identity: The role of referent group norms in healthy and unhealthy eating. *The Journal of Social Psychology, 147*(1), 57–74.

Luhmann, N. (2012). *Theory of society* (R. Barrett, Trans.; Vol. 1). Stanford University Press. (Original work published 1997)

Maier, C., Laumer, S., Eckhardt, A., & Weitzel, T. (2015). Giving too much social support: Social overload on social networking sites. *European Journal of Information Systems, 24*(5), 447–464.

Maner, J. K., & Gailliot, M. T. (2007). Altruism and egoism: Prosocial motivations for helping depend on relationship context. *European Journal of Social Psychology, 37*(2), 347–358.

Manne, S. L., Ostroff, J. S., Norton, T. R., Fox, K., Goldstein, L., & Grana, G. (2006). Cancer-related relationship communication in couples coping with early stage breast cancer. *Psycho-Oncology, 15*(3), 234–247.

McGonigal, K. (2013, June). *How to make stress your friend.* TED Talk. https://www.ted.com/talks/kelly_mcgonigal_how_to_make_stress_your_friend?

Merleau-Ponty, M. (2002). *Phenomenology of perception* (C. Smith, Trans.). Routledge. (Original work published 1945)

Mounk, Y. (2020, March 19). *Four theories for why people are still out partying: Our moral instincts don't match this crisis.* The Atlantic. https://www.theatlantic.com/ideas/archive/2020/03/moral-instincts-coronavirus/608305

Park, H.-J. (2015). Legislating for filial piety: An indirect approach to promoting family support and responsibility for older people in Korea. *Journal of Aging & Social Policy*, *27*(3), 280–293.

Perrine, R. M. (1993). On being supportive: The emotional consequences of listening to another's distress. *Journal of Social and Personal Relationships*, *10*(3), 371–384.

Peterson, J. L., Rintamaki, L. S., Brashers, D. E., Goldsmith, D. J., & Neidig, J. L. (2012). The forms and functions of peer social support for people living with HIV. *Journal of the Association of Nurses in AIDS Care*, *23*(4), 294–305.

Petronio, S. (2002). *Boundaries of privacy: Dialectics of disclosure.* State University of New York Press.

Petronio, S. (2010). Communication privacy management theory: What do we know about family privacy regulation? *Journal of Family Theory & Review*, *2*(3), 175–196.

Petronio, S., & Child, J. T. (2020). Conceptualization and operationalization: Utility of communication privacy management theory. *Current Opinion in Psychology*, *31*, 76–82.

Petronio, S., & Durham, W. T. (2008). Communication privacy management theory: Significance for interpersonal communication. In L. A. Baxter & D. O. Braithwaite (Eds.), *Engaging theories in interpersonal communication: Multiple perspectives* (pp. 309–322). Sage.

Pressman, S. D., Kraft, T. L., & Cross, M. P. (2014). It's good to do good and receive good: The impact of a 'pay it forward' style kindness intervention on giver and receiver well-being. *The Journal of Positive Psychology*, *10*(4), 293–302.

Roy, R. (2011). *Social support, health, and illness: A complicated relationship.* University of Toronto Press.

Schuller, T., Baron, S., & Field, J. (2000). Social capital: A review and critique. In S. Baron, J. Field, & T. Schuller (Eds.), *Social capital: Critical perspectives* (pp. 1–38). Oxford University Press.

Silverstein, M., Conroy, S. J., & Gans, D. (2012). Beyond solidarity, reciprocity and altruism: Moral capital as a unifying concept in intergenerational support for older people. *Ageing and Society*, *32*(7), 1246–1262.

Silverstein, M., Gans, D., & Yang, F. M. (2006). Intergenerational support to aging parents: The role of norms and needs. *Journal of Family Issues*, *27*(8), 1068–1084.

Spicker, K. (2020, April 1). *Coronavirus: UD donates 500 face masks, other PPE to health care workers.* Dayton Daily News. https://www.daytondailynews.com/news/local/coronavirus-donates-500-face-masks-other-ppe-health-care-workers/RiWEVi2LuLYLbypqL2uymM/

Steuber, K. R., & Solomon, D. H. (2011). Factors that predict married partners' disclosures about infertility to social network members. *Journal of Applied Communication Research*, *39*(3), 250–270.

Taylor, S. E., Sherman, D. K., Kim, H. S., Jarcho, J., Takagi, K., & Dunagan, M. S. (2004). Culture and social support: Who seeks it and why? *Journal of Personality and Social Psychology*, *87*(3), 354–362.

Tedros, A. G. (2020, March 16). *WHO Director-General's opening remarks at the media briefing on COVID-19*. World Health Organization. https://www.who.int/dg/speeches/detail/who-director-general-s-opening-remarks-at-the-media-briefing-on-covid-19---16-march-2020

Thoits, P. A. (1982). Conceptual, methodological, and theoretical problems in studying social support as a buffer against life stress. *Journal of Health and Social Behavior, 23*(2), 145–159.

Tsvetkova, M., & Macy, M. W. (2014). The social contagion of generosity. *PLoS One, 9*(2), Article e87275. https://doi.org/10.1371/journal.pone.0087275

Uchino, B. N. (2006). Social support and health: A review of physiological processes potentially underlying links to disease outcomes. *Journal of Behavioral Medicine, 29*(4), 377–387.

van Doorn, G. S., & Taborsky, M. (2012). The evolution of generalized reciprocity on social interaction networks. *Evolution, 66*(3), 651–664.

Vangelisti, A. L. (1994). Family secrets: Forms, functions and correlates. *Journal of Social and Personal Relationships, 11*(1), 113–135.

Vangelisti, A. L., & Caughlin, J. P. (1997). Revealing family secrets: The influence of topic, function, and relationships. *Journal of Social and Personal Relationships, 14*(5), 679–705.

Vangelisti, A. L., Caughlin, J. P., & Timmerman, L. (2001). Criteria for revealing family secrets. *Communication Monographs, 68*(1), 1–27.

Wang, L. (Director). (2019). *The farewell*. [Film]. A24.

Westman, M., Eden, D., & Shirom, A. (1985). Job stress, cigarette smoking and cessation: The conditioning effects of peer support. *Social Science & Medicine, 20*(6), 637–644.

Whitehead, A. N. (2010). *Process and reality* (D. R. Griffin & D. W. Sherburne, Eds.; Corrected ed.). Free Press. (Original work published 1929)

Williams, A. (2020, March 19). *'Stay at home for us': Health care workers post pleas for social distancing amid COVID-19*. Fox10 Phoenix. https://www.fox10phoenix.com/news/stay-at-home-for-us-health-care-workers-post-pleas-for-social-distancing-amid-covid-19

World Health Organization. (2014, May). *Eliminating forced, coercive and otherwise involuntary sterilization*. https://www.who.int/reproductivehealth/publications/gender_rights/eliminating-forced-sterilization/en

Yuen-Tsang, A. W. K. (2018). *Towards a Chinese conception of social support: Study of the social support networks of Chinese working mothers in Beijing*. Routledge.

Zhang, C. (2019). Family support or social support? The role of clan culture. *Journal of Population Economics, 32*(2), 529–549.

11

Transformative Technologies

Cultural Approaches to Technologies in Health Contexts

Rather than seeing technology as a tool for health communication and health intervention, Chapter 11 asks how technology as a cultural phenomenon shapes our experiences and understanding of the body, health, and illness. This chapter begins with an examination of the relationships between science, technology, and ethics. By exploring the cultural approaches to technology, we will consider how technologies shape our understanding of realities. By using genetic technologies and big data technologies as examples, we will examine the interactive relationships between humans and technologies: How such technologies transformed our understanding of health and illness, our cultural consciousness, and even our humanity. The chapter concludes by proposing how an Integral Fusion worldview is necessary to ensure ethical creation, development, and application of emerging technologies.

I. Science, Technology, Ethics, and Medicine

Technology is ubiquitous in health communication and public health. As telemedicine becomes part of our everyday life, rather than talking about how prevalent and important technology is in shaping the landscape of healthcare services and transforming medical research (e.g., Kruse et al., 2018; World Health Organization, 2017), we will explore how technology challenges our fundamental understanding of health and illness – our understanding of our bodies and human consciousness.

A. Three Categories of Knowledge

Although we often think of science and technology interchangeably in today's world, technology has a much longer history than science. Aristotle (2019) divides knowledge into three categories: theoretical (*episteme*), productive (*techne*), and practical (*phronesis*; Haney, 1999). **Science** is the theoretical knowledge of the world, what Aristotle called *scientia* (*episteme*) – the knowledge about causes and reasons for the functioning of the world apart from personal (and often subjective) opinions (*doxa*), technology (*techne*), and the arts (*ars*; Weingart, 2010). Science is theory-oriented (Biswas, 2007). Science concerns itself with first principles and the attempt to identify universal laws that govern the behavior of all things. Only scientific knowledge can claim to be

Rethinking Culture in Health Communication: Social Interactions as Intercultural Encounters, First Edition. Elaine Hsieh and Eric M Kramer.
© 2021 John Wiley & Sons, Inc. Published 2021 by John Wiley & Sons, Inc.

universally valid. Science is a relatively recent cultural phenomenon, barely 200 years old in its present form (Weingart, 2010). In Chapter 4, we have detailed how the emergence of science shaped the development of modern medicine.

In contrast, **technology** is the systematic study of techniques for making and doing things. Works of art are a result of techne. The term technology is a composite of the Greek *techne*, meaning art and craft, and *logos*, meaning word or speech. Although at first, it meant the discussion of the applied arts, but over time, it began to denote these "arts" themselves (Biswas, 2007). In the past, techniques or practical arts rarely involved any clear scientific basis. Technology was not always science-based. In fact, historically, technological innovations often preceded the growth of science (Biswas, 2007). Science is much more abstract and, thus, very Perspectival. Technology is the practical application of *tools* humans create, allowing us to have better control in altering our realities.

Techne is the means to change things. *Techne* is an attitude or approach to achieving what one wants. The search for and operationalization of technical alterations of the world are themselves prompted by desires and judgments. It is applicable to material efforts to build machines that will accomplish what we, with our hands alone, cannot. Technology, as Archimedes explained, is the amplification of our abilities. Given a lever long enough, Archimedes says, "I can move the Earth." Technology is leverage, the most basic material form of amplifying the power and directing desire to achieve what we want.

With the first historical emergence of perspectival consciousness in Classical Greece, *techne* began to separate from **phronesis** (Greek for prudence), leading to a crisis and a felt need to overtly address the dangers of *techne* without moral guidance. *Phronesis* is the domain of ethics, a "state grasping the truth, involving reason, concerned with action about things that are good or bad for a human being" (Aristotle, 2019, p. 105). *Techne* aims to achieve a specific objective through the means created by a craftsman's technique; in contrast, *phronesis* is its own domain, a moral domain. *Phronesis* is concerned with whether an action is intrinsically good and thus done for its own sake. Ethics are inherent in one's actions and practices. Immoral things could not be beautiful or good. Without *phronesis*, there is no real ethical check on *techne*. *Phronesis* or prudence is what determines *if* we should do something. *Techne* is concerned with can we do it and how. Technical answers follow a yes or no form. Yes, we have technologies to clone animals. That we know. The ethical issue is *should* we (Savulescu, 1999). Unlike science that is limited to objective, universal knowledge or technique that is focused on a means to a specific end, prudence is concerned about actions (i.e., "pursuit of the best good that is achievable in action for a human being") specific to particulars (Aristotle, 2019, p. 108). In other words, ethical actions are situation- and context-specific. The separation of ethics from objective "disinterested" universal science and goal-oriented techniques remains a major issue that only increases in importance as science and technologies become more powerful and expansive (Husserl, 1970).

Aristotle repeatedly uses medicine as an example to explore the nuances between science, technology, and ethics. Traditional medicine involves *techne*, as healers identify and utilize different means to help patients to manage illness symptoms and achieve specific health outcomes (Irwin, 2019; Waring, 2000). As we discussed in Chapter 4, modern medicine could not have existed without the perspectival pursuit of science. In addition, patient-centered care is inherently situational and contextual – treating a patient is not about validating a specific medical theory or applying the most effective cure but about finding the one that is most *appropriate* for the particular patient in question (see also Chapter 6).

"The medical reasoning of a skilled and conscientious physician is analogous to *phronetic* reasoning" (Waring, 2000, p. 143). The clinical practice of medicine often involves a blending of science, technology, and ethics – though not always in equal portions. Nevertheless, the practice of medicine without sufficient care of ethics can lead to lasting consequences (and damages) to our social relationships and humanity (Reiser, 2009).

B. Is Technology Magic, Mythic, or Perspectival?

Technology is a means to change the world to meet our needs. Humans have always relied on means as extensions of human bodies and minds to achieve specific goals – to socialize, communicate, perform, and accomplish our identity, relationship, and task goals (Gibson & Ingold, 1993). The "tools" need not be concrete and visible, like a tree branch that allows us to reach higher fruits or a walking stick that helps us go further. Researchers have noted that human gestures and vocal languages are some of the most important tools created by early hominids during our evolutionary journeys (Gibson & Ingold, 1993). Because *Homo sapiens* have the biological capacity (i.e., the anatomical specialization of the speech apparatus and a very large brain) and a species tendency to live in groups where resources are shared, it is possible that they have the skills to produce lengthy vocal sequences, allowing them to "take advantage of extant cognitive capacities for representation and intentional communication," to "share resources and to cooperate," and "to coordinate interactions" (Savage-Rumbaugh & Rumbaugh, 1993, p. 86). Technology has been an essential element in all stages of human evolution.

As a means to an end, technology is not inherently magic, mythic, or perspectival. It is the attitudes that people hold toward technology that creates cultural meanings to the technology we use. For example, the magic wand is the most common and best example of technologies in Harry Potter's wizarding, magic world (Sheltrown, 2008). A wooden stick in the hands of Harry Potter is a magic wand, which is alive (i.e., it chooses its wizard) and becomes the wizard's extension in creating a focus of the wizard's power. However, a magic wand in the hands of a non-magic muggle is no more than a wooden stick. During the medieval period, the practice of magico-religious medicine is pervasive. Medieval physicians often relied on amulets, charms, incantations, and prayers as a means of treating patients (Olsan, 2003). For medieval physicians, those were the latest technologies of their times and thus, deserving of intense debates between theologians, physicians, and philosophers in distinguishing how such technologies can influence individuals' bodies and health (van der Lugt, 2013).

Technologies can take on mythic qualities as well. **Cargo cults**, first captured the public's fascination and imagination in the mid-1940s, was termed by colonizers but later popularized by anthropologists to describe attitudes toward modern technologies by indigenous natives in Melanesia (Lindstrom, 2019; see also Raffaele, 2006). According to an article from Los Angeles Times:

> Cargo cults develop when primitive societies are exposed to the overpowering material wealth of the outside industrialized world. Not knowing where the foreigner's plentiful supplies come from, the natives believe they were sent from the spirit world. They build makeshift piers and airstrips and perform magic rites to summon the well-stocked foreign ships and planes. (Lindstrom, 2019, p. 1)

Many scholars have later criticized the exploitations of cargo cults by colonizers in colonized communities (Lindstrom, 2019), which are beyond the scope of this book. Our interests lie in the mythic values that were attached to new technologies. As predominantly magic locals came to appreciate the foreign technologies, they did not simply view them as value-free tools for the betterment of their everyday lives. As hermeneutics would predict, they made sense of them the only way they could – in accordance with their worldviews. The technologies were incorporated into their belief systems, restructuring their understanding of their spiritual *and* material world – creating a new worldview that was different from what it had been prior to the arrival of the foreign technologies (see Figures 11.1 and 11.2). This is a form of cultural fusion.

It is important to note that attaching mythic qualities to technologies is not unique to "primitive" people. We can be (and often are) enchanted by our own technologies as well. In an analysis of over 55,000 user reviews of Amazon's digital assistant Alexa, researchers concluded that 30% of users humanized the technology-enabled speaker. Some "even developed a close relationship with Amazon Echo, such as a best friend, girlfriend, family, mistress, and wife" (Gao et al., 2018, p. 379). Researchers have raised concerns about how modern society is increasingly developing a cargo cult-like fascination with our own emerging technologies, such as artificial intelligence, robots, and even statistical software (Fernaeus et al., 2009; Stark & Saltelli, 2018). In his TED Talk, *A Doctor's Touch*, Dr. Verghese (2011) commented, "I joke, but I only half-joke, that if you come to one of our hospitals missing a limb, no one will believe you till they get a

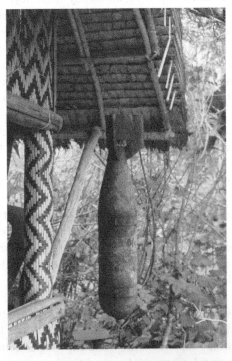

Figure 11.1 Cargo cult bomb. During World War II, when American troops, resources, and artifacts poured from the skies and seas into the islands in the South Pacific, local villagers developed "cargo cult" to make sense of the foreign technologies and cultures. Here, a World War II bomb is venerated and hangs outside a wooden house. *Source:* ©Eye Ubiquitous/AGE Fotostock

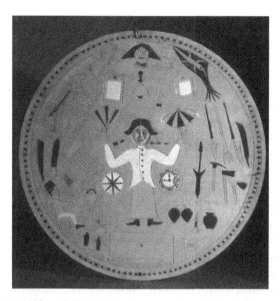

Figure 11.2   A *henta-koi* from Indian Nicobar Islands in Southeast Asia. A henta-koi is made at times of sickness at the direction of the Shaman and acts as a magical charm. If the patient recovers, the henta-koi is kept for future service; but if the patient dies, it is thrown away into the jungle (Temple, 1903). This particular henta-koi is painted with an image of a White man who appears to be dressed in the jacket of a sea captain. He is surrounded by the numerous magical symbols of European omnipotence: mirrors, clocks, umbrellas, knives etc. Date/Period: Late 19th/early 20th C. Material Size: Painted wood. *Source:* Werner Forman Archive/AGE Fotostock

CAT scan, MRI or orthopedic consult" (01:03). We have come to rely on our technologies to "see" our realities.

Many of us, including physicians and scientists, rely on results and outcomes provided through technologies (e.g., results provided by big data mining through AI and statistics; lab results performed and analyzed by sophisticated equipment) with little conscientious reflexivity about how and why the results are presented as such. Rather, we adopted almost ritualistic, faith-like affirmations about the accuracy and reliability of the results. For example, without a good understanding of the underlying assumptions of statistical analysis but equipped with powerful statistical software for data analysis, one can "demote statistics from a way of thinking about evidence and avoiding self-deception to a formal 'blessing' of claims" (Stark & Saltelli, 2018, p. 41). When we stop being reflective, critical, and cognizant over the assumptions, limitations, or interpretations of our technologies, we no longer view technologies from a Perspectival Thinking approach (e.g., an objective, clinical, and impersonal reflectivity of the technologies employed).

Under Perspectival Thinking, technology faces increasing specialization. The focus of advanced technological power is channeled through precision (fragmentation) and complexity. Expertise becomes deeper and narrower (perspectival). Simple technology such as a knife can be used to achieve many ends, from skinning to killing to spreading to prying to carving. A knife can be an heirloom and a work of art. The more complex a technology becomes, the more focused and limited (precise) its use. For instance, an air conditioner is basically only useful for cooling air, a Zamboni machine is only good for smoothing icy surfaces, and a microwave oven for heating things. In fact, certain technologies cannot emerge without Perspectival Thinking.

In a Perspectival Thinking world, what cannot be measured is not valued. Technologies in perceived through a Perspectival worldview can be dangerous, if not devastating, to our environment and even humanity. In Chapter 4, we have used eugenics to illustrate how the use of technology and science without ethics can have devastating consequences. The long history of environmental exploitation has led to extinctions of animal and plant species and even human cultures (Kramer et al., 2014). In April 2020, President Trump issued an executive order, which states that for resources in outer space (e.g., water and certain minerals), "Americans should have the *right* to engage in *commercial* exploration, recovery, and use of resources in *outer space*" [emphasis added] (White House, 2020).

In the modern Perspectival world, value exists when something is available for exploitation. The world as given, prior to exploitation, has only potential value. Value-addition is the application of technical manipulation, converting base resources into commodities. Once so transformed, value can be realized via exchange. But this process is still rooted in actual resources such as minerals, livestock, agricultural produce and such. As the Perspectival world becomes increasingly abstract, meaning and value are believed to be either nonexistent or not inherent in things. Value becomes a moment of exchange. It is not a thing but the difference between things. Value is nothing but difference. And so, it makes sense that in this world we would see the emergence of the most magical of technologies – machines that create metavalue. This is the rise of information technology, which is based on the conversion of anything and everything into digitized information and then manipulated at will. The most advanced technologies are reducing all things to information opening everything to manipulation. This is the great leap forward in the late-Perspectival world and its form of technology. AI and genetic engineering, which reduces all of life to codes, are extremely flexible and powerful because they can penetrate all aspects of life. A Zamboni machine lacks flexibility. But we can computerize almost any operation. The new forms of technology are revolutionizing medicine.

New technologies allow us to identify new resources – and thus, new "values." Because value itself is unreal (nonmaterial), and exists only as a consequence of technical manipulation, techne is separated from ethics and morality. When technologies are used with little reflection on their moral consequences and with a singular focus on prespecified objectives, the resulting outcome inevitably *discriminates* all that is not measured and valued.

In summary, technology can be magic, mythic, and/or perspectival. In fact, the same technology may hold very different meanings for different people. Although certain technologies cannot be developed without a Perspectival Thinking worldview, a person need not have Perspectival Thinking to wield a technology. For example, a person of Magic Consciousness can still benefit (or suffer) from antibiotics and anesthesia, two of the greatest medical advances since 1840 (Ferriman, 2007). Nevertheless, as individuals wield those technologies, they may develop new understandings of the technologies. The accrual of cultural dimensions is not linear (See also Accrual of Cultural Dimensions in Chapter 5). A person with Magic Consciousness cannot comprehend a Perspectival Thinking worldview, until and unless they become perspectival themselves. In contrast, a person with the Perspectival Thinking worldview can develop perspectives of Mythic Connection or Magic Consciousness with the technologies they wield because those modalities persist in the Perspectival world.

II. Transformative Technologies in Modern Medicine

Whereas realities in magic and mythic worlds are relatively stable, realities in perspectival worlds can change on a dime as a result of new scientific discoveries. Scientific advances can create revolutionary changes in how we understand realities. Lewis Mumford (1934/2010) proposed the term **technological complex**, noting human civilizations are marked by technologies that created revolutionary and paradigm-shifting changes to our realities:

> Each phase [of human history] has its origin in certain definite regions and tends to employ certain special resources and new materials. Each phase has its specific means of utilizing and generating energy, and its special forms of production. Finally, each phase brings into existence particular types of workers, trains them in particular ways, develop certain aptitudes and discourage others, and draws upon and further develop certain aspects of the social heritage. (pp. 109–110)

The technological changes marked by not only changes in raw materials (e.g., stone age, bronze age, and iron age) and new tools, but also how problems are identified, and solutions are developed. It favors certain ways of thinking and understanding of realities than others.

   The history of medicine is marked by changes in technologies (Reiser, 2009). Antoni van Leeuwenhoek's first simple microscope constructed in 1677 paved the way for the emergence of the **germ theory** (i.e., certain diseases are caused by an invasion of the body by microorganisms that are too small to be seen by the naked eye) in medicine in the 1800s (Gaynes, 2011). New instruments, such as the stethoscope and x-rays, did not just provide new ways of diagnosing illnesses but also shifted the power balance and social relationships between providers and patients – they allowed providers to discount patients' narratives, and increase and reinforce clinical authority (Reiser, 2009). By observing the changes in technologies in medicine, Reiser (2009) concluded, "It has become the norm in the battle for the succession of technologies in medicine to have winners and losers. Also, a significant factor in this story is a vision held for centuries by doctors: of medicine becoming a science and thus eliminating subjective elements when they seem to be replaceable with objective ones" (pp. 29–30).

   However, as we discussed in Chapter 4, the "objective realities" envisioned in Perspectival Thinking can be distorted and/or limited (and limiting). In recent years, changes in technology (and medicine) have been accelerating, creating rippling effects beyond medicine and transforming our understanding of health and illness in everyday life (i.e., a pan-evolution). In the following sections, we will focus on two major technological trends in medicine to illustrate the complexities and nuances of cultural approaches to health communication: genetic technologies and big data technologies.

A. Genetic Technologies in Medicine

1. Humans as Genetic Gold and Intellectual Properties

Under Perspectival Thinking, the development and testing of technology require ever-increasingly meticulous measurement to achieve "perfect" precision. One may be quick to believe that Perspectival Thinking is much more "concrete" and thus, "real," especially when contrasted with the world of Magic Consciousness where spirits, animals, and the dead are just as present, vital, and equal as the living humans. Such an understanding fails to appreciate that what is "real" under Perspectival Thinking is what is "measurable," which may or may not be concrete. Perspectival thinking tends to be more abstract than magic or myth, often presenting a world in terms of mathematical formulas and models.

The recent rise of genetic medicine and research provides a good example of how the pursuit of precision in Perspectival Thinking can also result in a significant disconnect between one's lived experiences and scientific modeling. An example that speaks to the importance of ethics in the face of emerging technologies is in how researchers conceptualize (and thus, measure) the "value" of human genes. In the backdrop of the concerns and tensions in conducting genetic research are indigenous groups' experiences of exploitation in the name of science. In the early days of genetic research, some researchers advocated that genetic populations untainted by modern medicine and lifestyles could provide useful materials for the research of affluence-related disease (Sleeboom-Faulkner, 2008). Many indigenous groups had remained geographically isolated, presented a high rate of inbreeding and were resistant to certain diseases. For example, the Hagahai from Papua New Guinea are resistant to leukemia: They carry a rare virus, a pathogen similar to ones that cause leukemia, in their white blood cells but remain unaffected (Salopek, 1997). Arhuaca Indians of Columbia have proven resilient to a type of virus that is associated with leukemia and HIV (Salopek, 1997). The genetic degree of Cherokee ancestry is positively correlated to one's resistance to Alzheimer's disease (Rosenberg et al., 1996). These indigenous groups provide a valuable treasure trove of unique genomes to advance biomedical research and improve healthcare delivery (Fox, 2017).

Many scholars raised concerns that people "will be mined for 'genetic gold' by scientists from industrialized countries and large corporations" (Ossorio, 2007, p. 428). Professor Stephen R. Munzer (2013) explained,

> In the United States, scientists since the nineteenth century and earlier have frequently treated Native Americans as a repository of specimens for measurement, experiment, and deeper understanding of human beings. To this end, scientists have exhumed the bodies of American Indians and studied them. Even today, some thousands of these bodies are kept in museums. A still more dramatic example is the case of Ishi, who, after he emerged from the wilderness, resided in a California museum as a living exhibit, and, in that capacity, served as an educational tool for those, mainly whites, who came to watch him. Thus, the American Indian experience with science reflects colonial domination. White scientists in the United States, at least from the perspective of Native Americans, often treated them as raw material to advance "science" and a way to get at the "truth" about them that would somehow satisfy non-Indians' curiosity about Indians. (pp. 17–18)

The indigenous peoples' genetic materials are "valuable" because these groups are often on the verge of extinction. For example, the **Human Genome Diversity Project**

(HGDP), a genetic research project that actively seeks out indigenous populations, is a 20-year effort funded at an estimated cost of twenty billion dollars by the U.S. National Institutes of Health and the Department of Energy (Amani & Coombe, 2005). In total, HGDP has identified 722 populations as "rapidly disappearing" and in danger of dying out or being assimilated (Lock, 1999). Although the HGDP aggressively pursued "genetic mining" of these populations to preserve the genetic record of human heritage, the survival or suffering of the *people* of these groups "were not considered relevant" to the project (Amani & Coombe, 2005, p. 155). Individuals' human existences are reduced to genetic materials, bits and pieces of unique DNA sequences. In the scientific world of Perspectival Thinking, indigenous peoples – their existence as living *people*, along with their unique cultures – are diminished. Only the unique *and* "valuable" (e.g., commercially profitable) elements of their DNA segments are retained and protected.

The fragmentation of human bodies does not end with the fragmentations of human bodies into DNA sequences. The courts in the United States have consistently ruled that individuals do not have ownership of their bodies in the context of medical research. In *Moore v. Regents of the University of California* (1990), the California Supreme Court ruled that Moore did not have an ownership interest in his spleen, which was removed during treatment for leukemia at UCLA. In addition, the Mo cell line, which was created from Moore's spleen cells, was patented by the researchers and has generated an estimated worth of $3 billion, was ruled to be the property of the researchers who had been granted a patent upon it (Amani & Coombe, 2005). The court reasoned that once the cells were removed from his body, Moore's ownership over them ceased because "research on human cells plays a critical role in medical research" – to grant the patient proprietary rights would threaten to "hinder research by restricting access to the necessary raw materials" *(Moore v. Regents of the University of California*, 1990, p. 144). In *Greenberg v. Miami Children's Hospital* (2003), the federal court not only concluded that (a) the patients did not have ownership over their bodily tissues and (b) the genes responsible for their illness were the property of the scientists who isolated it and the hospital that patented it – despite the fact that the gene is still in the patients' bodies. The *Greenberg* court reasoned that granting ownership rights to tissue donors "would bestow a continuing right for donors to possess the results of any research conducted by the hospital" and thus interfere with or de-incentivize medical research (p. 1076). In *Washington University v. Catalona* (2007), the Eighth Circuit Court of Appeals concluded that the ownership of *the intellectual property* in the body and the *tangible physical parts* of the body belongs to the University that operates the biobank, rather than the original owner of these biomaterials. These strong legal precedents suggest that the courts are unwilling to recognize tissue donors' property right for fear of stifling medical research. Nevertheless, as genetic technologies advance, bodies are no longer just "bodies." Instead, they are segmented into "tangible physical parts" of tissues as well as the invisible "intellectual property" that can now be "owned," "isolated," and even "patented" by a person or an entity that is not the owner of the "body."

In summary, the world of Perspectival Thinking is only "precise" and "real" to the objectives of its pursuit (i.e., what can be measured). With the help of genetic technologies, human beings are reduced to not just bodies or tissues, but genes – which cannot be experienced by any living person nor observed by any naked eyes. Even when a gene is identified and valued, the person with the gene can become invisible to the scientists looking for genetic gold. Genetic technologies changed our realities. As genes are further fragmented into tangible physical parts (e.g., genetic sequences that can be edited in genetic therapy) and the invisible, yet nevertheless *real*, "intellectual properties" (e.g., patents that can be traded commercially), the Perspectival Thinking world creates its own versions of invisible realities governing how "bodies" can be conceptualized and treated. The Perspectival worldview is also filled with abstractions, invisible realities that structure our understandings and experiences of the world.

2. Genetic Technologies in Preventive Care

In Chapter 8, we have detailed how a Perspectival Thinking approach to public health has led to the rise of eugenics movements in the United States in the first half of the 20th century, which, for some people, also involved cultural perspectives of Magic Consciousness and Mythic Connection tied to racism, social stigma, and structural discrimination. More recently, researchers have critiqued how the rise of biotechnologies can fuel a resurgence of eugenics, allowing people to adopt "scientific" screening to shield their behaviors from criticism. This enables stigmatization, discrimination, and marginalization of minority, marginalized, and underserved populations (Duster, 2003). Rather than elaborating on its potentials to reinforce social stigma (see also discussions about the "warrior gene" hypothesis for Māori Australians in Chapter 4), we will shift our attention to how genetic technologies can redefine the meanings of health and illness, resulting in tensions in our social relationships and "health" management.

Genetic technologies have redefined our understanding of health and illness. Unlike the prior models of illness that defined illness through observable changes in, invasions to, or anomalies of one's body (e.g., bacterial infections or a brain tumor), genetic screenings rely on probabilistic models. When Angelina Jolie found out in 2013 that she carries the "faulty" BRCA1 gene, a gene that is associated with 86% risk of developing breast cancer and 50% risk of developing ovarian cancer (although "the risk is different in the case of each woman"), she decided to undergo preventative bilateral mastectomy despite the fact that she was free of cancer (Jolie, 2013). She is "ill" because she is *at risk* of getting ill, not because she is not healthy. A patient is expected to make her individualized decision based on the scientific knowledge of generalized risks. As a result, individuals are likely to experience uncertainties in a wide range of topics (e.g., understanding genetic information, evaluating future cancer risks, managing known genetic information or mutation status, and assessing the utility of genetic information; Hong, 2020).

With an increase in scientific evidence of a significant reduction in the occurrence and mortality rate of cancer (Nelson et al., 2019), the public appears to have embraced relying on genetic tests as a tool for preventive care (Hann et al., 2017). When asked about her thoughts about learning of her gene mutation, a doctoral student who also carries the BRCA1 gene commented, "I'm lucky in that I have the chance now to take the preventative measures, and hopefully stay cancer-free" (Harris, 2020). In an analysis of websites that covered Jolie's announcement, Dean (2016) found that the majority of websites framed Jolie's decision positively, with only a few questioning her decision (e.g., whether her decision was too extreme or whether others have the same resources to make comparable decisions). The public learned to identify their health status and make health decisions, not based on how they feel or changes to their bodies, but based on statistical models of risks.

Trust (and reliance) in (genetic and statistical modeling) technologies is not without problems. According to a 2019 article in the *Wall Street Journal*, seven women in a family opted to have cancer-preventing surgeries to remove their breasts, ovaries, and/or fallopian tubes after learning about their BRCA genetic mutation (Marcus, 2019). However, these women questioned their decisions when the genetic screening company reclassified their risks from "harmful" to "unknown significance" four years later, based on new data and findings (Marcus, 2019). One may argue that this is a failure of "measurements" rather than technologies. However, when the interpretation of measurements is dependent on the scientific knowledge that is constantly evolving, one can never be certain about the accuracy or objectivity of the interpretation (see also Uncertainties in Medicine in Chapter 9). In addition, researchers have found that individuals' perceptions of risks can be influenced by how risks are presented (see also The Interactive Nature of Uncertainty Management in Chapter 9). For example, a person is likely to perceive a greater risk when a denominator of 10 or less is used (e.g., one in four) than equivalent percentages (e.g., 25%; Kessler et al., 1987). In short, although identifying the "faulty" gene may appear as an objective method in assessing one's health status, genetic technologies have motivated individuals to embrace aggressive treatments and alterations to their "healthy bodies" based on subjective tolerances of risks.

Some of the most intense debates over genetic technologies center on genetic selections and gene editing in reproductive care. Prenatal diagnosis of genetic disorders is not a new technology. Couples have relied on prenatal tests in their decision-making for a long time. For example, a review of seven population-based studies of prenatal Down syndrome diagnoses found a weighted termination rate of 67% (Natoli et al., 2012). With advances in fertility treatments, couples at risk of children with gene defects can use IVF along with preimplantation genetic testing to transfer only unaffected embryos (Handyside, 2018). Couples have used genetic screening to eliminate embryos carrying genetic diseases (e.g., Huntington's disease) and to have healthy children (Ledford, 2019). Genetic screening is touted as the future of preventive medicine (Sandler et al., 2018). However, researchers have raised concerns on how the breakthrough in genetic technologies can lead to **designer babies** (i.e., couples relying on technologies to choose character traits unrelated to health, such as sex selection, choice of eye/hair color, intelligence, and personality traits). One may argue that human beings have always selected mates with an eye to having children with preferred traits. Thus, relying on new technologies for the same purpose, may not be morally problematic (e.g., Segers et al., 2019). Same goal, different means.

Such an argument fails, however, to recognize how emerging genetic technologies have the potential to completely transform the meanings of "being human." **CRISPR** (pronounced "crisper") is a simple but powerful technology that allows scientists to edit genomes, allowing them to alter an organism's DNA sequences and modify its gene functions (National Human Genome Research Institute, n.d.). Scientists have used gene therapies (i.e., treatments involving genome editing) to prevent and treat disease in humans (National Human Genome Research Institute, n.d.). However, the world changed in 2018. With assistance from scientists from the United States, a Chinese scientist, He Jiankui, announced that he had created the worlds' first genetically edited babies – twin girls to be resistant to HIV by using CRISPR to modify DNA sequences in the embryos (Cyranoski, 2019; Wee, 2019; see Figure 11.3). The scientific community raised concerns about the lack of knowledge of the impacts and meanings of such technologies (e.g., the lack of knowledge on how modification of a DNA sequence may have unforeseen impacts and consequences on other genetic activities, health outcomes, and human behaviors; Ledford, 2019). The Chinese scientist was later sentenced by a court in China for three years in prison, which held that "in the pursuit of fame and profit, [He] deliberately violated the relevant national regulations on scientific and medical research and crossed the bottom line on scientific and medical ethics" (Wee, 2019, para. 5). Despite the outcry of the global scientific community, Jonathan Kimmelman, a bioethicist specializing in human trials of gene therapies noted that the event "would stimulate, not hinder, meaningful advance in this area" (Cyranoski, 2019, para. 6).

Although scientists have regularly used genetic technologies to treat genetic defects, at issue was whether it is appropriate to use the same technologies to *enhance* human traits. As we contemplate whether performance-enhancing drugs are fair or appropriate in sports or for academic performance (Dodge et al., 2012; Savulescu et al., 2004), genetic technologies have now opened up the possibility for human enhancement at the genetic level.

Transhumanism represents a movement to understand and evaluate technological opportunities for enhancing human conditions and the human organism (Bostrom, 2003). Among the multiple possibilities (e.g., human cyborgs or eternal life/consciousness in digital forms; see also Kramer et al., 2014), genetic engineering has promised

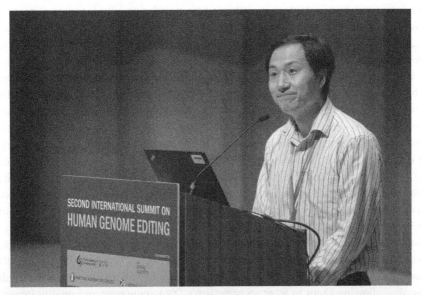

Figure 11.3 Chinese geneticist He Jiankui. He Jiankui, associate professor of the Southern University of Science and Technology in Shenzhen, China, presented his work during the Second International Summit on Human Genome Editing at the University of Hong Kong on November 28, 2018. Earlier, the Chinese geneticist claimed to have altered the genes of the embryo of a pair of twin girls before birth, prompting an outcry from scientists of the field. *Source:* ZUMA Press, Inc. / Alamy Stock Photo

great potential (e.g., alleviating unnecessary human suffering) and raised significant concerns (e.g., redefining the very meaning and nature of humanity). We know that individuals' height and physical attractiveness are correlated with reproductive and financial status (Frieze et al., 1991; Prokop & Fedor, 2011). Is it morally wrong for parents to use genetic engineering to ensure that their children are not only disease-free but also enjoy future success? What does it mean when technologies allow us to create "perfect" babies? What are the traits that will be preserved and what will be eliminated? Do children have rights to their genetic compositions? What are the kinds of powers that should be enhanced? Will such technologies truly "enhance" human traits or will it highlight our biggest flaws – our vanity, greed, and pursuits that have led to the extinction of not just many plants and animals, but also many cultures and peoples (Kramer et al., 2014)?

Faced with advances in technologies, researchers have warned against **ableism**, which refers to "a set of beliefs or practices that devalue and discriminate against people with physical, intellectual, or psychiatric disabilities and often rests on the assumption that disabled people need to be 'fixed' in one form or the other" (Smith, n.d.). For example, Deaf communities faced intense debates about whether cochlear implants pose challenges to the legitimacy of deafness as a disability (Tucker, 1998). Reflecting on the cultural impacts of transhumanism, Suter (2007) warned,

> On a societal scale, the more we use technology to select against lesser conditions and traits, the more perfectionist we may become as a culture, and the more demanding we may become with respect to what is acceptable, normal, or healthy. The distinction between disease and normalcy may evolve. If enhancement and trait selection are widely used, it is easy to imagine that what was once normal will start to seem abnormal and perhaps disease-like. If we begin to medicalize what we now consider normal traits, enhancement and trait-selection will become more "legitimate" because they will be understood as part of medical treatment, driving people toward using these technologies. (p. 936)

Most people would be quick to recognize the danger of people with Magic Consciousness or Mythic Connection wielding the power of nuclear weapons. When individuals' use of advanced technologies is driven by primal beliefs or symbolic values, the tools created through Perspectival Thinking come to exist in differing contexts where restraint through reflexivity may not exist. An Integral Fusion worldview also provides an ethical check on the power of *techne*. However, the history of science tells us that advances in technologies can lead to breakthroughs in scientific knowledge. In other words, at the time of wielding the technologies, we do not necessarily know the doors they will open.

Although CRISPR could not have been developed without scientific knowledge of genomes and we have developed sufficient technologies (e.g., stem cell technologies, nuclear transfer, epigenetic modulation, and gene-editing methods) to broadly manipulate human genome, Mukherjee (2016) cautioned,

> We have no knowledge of the fidelity or efficiency of these techniques in practice. Does making an intentional change in a gene run the risk of creating an unintended change in another part of the genome? Are some genes more easily "edited" than others – and what governs the pliability of a gene? Nor do we

know whether making a directed change in one gene might cause the entire genome to become dysregulated. [... Altering] one gene may cause far-reaching consequences for gene regulation – potentially unleashing a volley of downstream consequences, akin to the proverbial butterfly effect. (pp. 489–490)

Nevertheless, we possess the *techne* of genetic engineering. Are our uncertainties about genetic technologies limited to information and consequences of genetic testing or something more fundamental – about the definitions of "being human"? Is the desire to live disease-free driven by Magic Consciousness, Mythic Connection, or Perspectival Thinking? What is the cultural perspective driving the pursuit of ensuring the future success of offspring? What cultural approaches should drive the development of transhuman technologies? Are these cultural trends still under our control, or are we passive subjects at the mercy of the emerging technological complex (Gardner, 1995)? This question goes to the issue of technological determinism. Do the technologies developed by a few powerful interests determine the future for us all?

B. Big Data Technologies as Health Surveillance

Another technological trend that is transforming the landscape of public health and healthcare delivery is big data technologies. Nearly all aspects of modern life are in some ways being changed by big data and machine learning (i.e., artificial intelligence). Our daily movements and routines are now monitored by mobile and/or wearable technologies (e.g., GPS on cell phones and heartrates on Fitbit watches), cataloged by smart appliances (e.g., Wi-Fi-enabled scales that calculate your weight, body fat, BMI, and hydration levels), and tracked by mobile applications and social media (e.g., apps that track your blood sugar or blood pressure, and location-enabled notifications when you visit new locations or are close to new friends). Khoury and Ioannidis (2014) explained,

> The term "Big Data" refers to volumes of large, complex, linkable information. Beyond genomics and other "omic" fields, Big Data includes medical, environmental, financial, geographic, and social media information. Most of this digital information was unavailable a decade ago. This swell of data will continue to grow, stoked by sources that are currently unimaginable. Big Data stands to improve health by providing insights into the causes and outcomes of disease, better drug targets for precision medicine, and enhanced disease prediction and prevention. (p. 1054)

In this chapter, big data technologies include a wide range of surrounding technologies (e.g., mobile, wearable, and smart technologies) and applications (e.g., social media) that provide the information for big data analysis. We will begin the section by examining how such technologies have shaped and transformed our cultural consciousness and relationships with all these emerging technologies in our everyday lives.

1. Mobile Technologies and Social Media as Magic Consciousness

Magic Consciousness is essential to our existence as social beings. It is part of our primal instinct to connect with others (Kramer & Hsieh, 2019). Under Magic Consciousness, we were part of nature. Our ancestors lived in extended groups, mostly blood relatives. We knew each other from birth to death. This was the world we evolved in — as highly social beings who cared deeply about each other and our environment. As such, it is inevitable that many people's understanding and use of these highly personalized technologies can be shaped by Magic Consciousness.

Under Magic Consciousness, an individual experiences deep bonds with their environment so much so that they can experience anxiety and distress when the "oneness" is threatened. **Attachment Theory** refers to a profound and persistent bond that connects a person to another beyond the scope of time and space (Holmes, 2006). As a theory for human development, the theory was first developed to explore how a caregiver-infant bond is formed and the corresponding consequences when the bond is threatened. For example, an infant may experience **separation anxiety** (i.e., experiences of distress when the caregiver is not in proximity) when a caregiver leaves the room, resulting in the infant's **proximity-seeking behaviors** (i.e., attempts to be closer to the caregiver) when the caregiver returns (Holmes, 2006). **Nomophobia**, an abbreviation for no-mobile-phone phobia, is defined as the fear of being out of mobile phone contact, which can be caused by disruptions in network connection, power depletion, and lack of access. The literature has demonstrated that humans develop an attachment to cell phones (Yildirim & Correia, 2015). For example, they experience distress when they are separated from it (i.e., separation anxiety) and work to maintain proximity to the phone (i.e., proximity-seeking; Konok et al., 2016, 2017). During a 75-minute experiment, when college students were unable to use their mobile phones, their anxiety increased significantly over time – even when the phone was in their possession (Cheever et al., 2014).

The literature has suggested that a greater level of loneliness is associated with higher usage of mobile communication, including smartphones and social media use (Jin & Park, 2013; Kim, 2017). Some researchers argued that the correlation is a result of the social messaging functions (e.g., texting and post-sharing) of these technologies to foster connections with others (Bayer et al., 2020). In other words, lonely people are driven to use these technologies more in an effort to connect with others (Kim, 2017). Yildirim and Correia (2015) proposed that nomophobia manifests through four dimensions: (a) not being able to communicate, (b) losing connectedness, (c) not being able to access information, and (d) giving up convenience. These arguments adopt a perspectival understanding of individuals' use of mobile technologies and social media, which focuses on the functionalities of such technologies.

However, if we were to approach these phenomena from a Magic Consciousness perspective, it is possible that our attachment to these technologies is not limited to its functionality but also to our identities and relationships *with* and through the technologies. The literature provides some evidence for this argument. For example, mobile phone users' separation anxiety was not alleviated even when they had access to computers that provide alternative modes of communication (Nie et al., 2020). When discussing their use and relationships with their smartphones, users recognized that their smartphones and social media represent their character "to the world" (i.e., an externalized identity) and reported "a pathological lack of agency with smartphone use" (e.g., uncontrolled or compelled use of smartphones; Harkin & Kuss, 2020, pp. 5, 7; Nie et al., 2020). In other words, these technologies are not replaceable to the users, who develop blurred lines between their identities and the tools they wield. These are hallmarks of Magic Consciousness. These devices become fetishes, talismans of sorts. And people become very emotional about them.

Starting in the 1920s, and accelerating since the 1960s, numerous movies and TV shows have explored the increasingly blurred lines between humans, robots, and cyborgs (e.g., *Metropolis* [1927], *My Living Doll* [1964–65], *2001 A Space Odyssey* [1968], *West World* [1973, remake 2016–19], *The Stepford Wives* [1975, remake 2004], *Blade Runner* [1982], *Terminator* [1984–2008], *Weird Science* [1985], *Ghost in the Shell* [1995–2006, remake 2017], *The Iron Giant* [1999], *Bicentennial Man* [1999], *A.I. Artificial Intelligence* [2001]; *I, Robot* [2004], *Her* [2013], *Humans* [2015–18], *Blade Runner 2049* [2017], *Zoe* [2018], *Alita Battle Angel* [2019]). Living with human-like automata (robots) is part of modernity. In the 1600s, the famous mathematician/philosopher Rene Descartes built a clockwork – a talking, walking simulacrum "Francine," named after his daughter, who had died of scarlet fever at age five. For many years, Descartes carried her/it with him everywhere in a casket, until, during a voyage to Sweden, when some sailors, spooked by the robotic child sat up to greet them, threw it overboard (Brake, 2019).

In Chapter 3, we discussed how **anthropomorphism** (i.e., non-human spirits and objects that exhibit human characteristics) shaped the worlds of Magic Consciousness and Mythic Connection. In the modern, perspectival world, anthropomorphism has been a major approach to human-computer interactions, influencing the forms and interfaces of computer-enabled technologies to facilitate social behaviors between users and computers (Duffy, 2003; Wang, 2017). Developers of technologies have worked diligently to invoke Magic Consciousness to encourage users to identify with the technologies in their everyday lives. Digital voice assistants have been given human names (e.g., Siri and Alexa). Voice assistants read bedtime stories, sing lullabies to children, update the latest news, tell jokes, and even play games with adults. The manufactures of these devices actively work to personify these technologies, and the users also actively personalize their smart speakers and smartphones – learning to identify specific persons with their voice and adopt personalized commands. It is not a coincidence when people personalize their smartphones and voice assistants – treating them as an active partner in close social relationships (e.g., a friend or a wife; Gao et al., 2018; Wang, 2017). Smartphones channel users' sense of self (like a magic wand in a wizard's hand) and become an extension of the user (Harkin & Kuss, 2020). Rather than being mindful of computer-person distinctions, we mindlessly (i.e., non-consciously) apply social rules and attribute personal characteristics to computers (Kim & Sundar, 2012). We become enchanted by our own technologies (see Figure 11.4).

Marshall McLuhan argued that our technologies hold dialogic and interactive relationships with humans. As much as we shape our tools, we are also shaped by the tools we created (McLuhan & Fiore, 1996). The evolving nature of modern technologies poses unique challenges to our relationships with these technologies. When Google Flu Trends (GFT), which relied on individuals' search terms to identify flu clusters, was found to able to predict flu clusters *two weeks ahead* of CDC's data, the public was excited about the potential of its life-saving insights (Lazer & Kennedy, 2015). However, researchers later found that Google's algorithm was vulnerable to seasonal variations unrelated to the flu (e.g., high school football), changes in individuals' search behaviors over time, and Google's own suggested search features (Lazer & Kennedy, 2015; Lazer et al., 2014). As a result, in 2014, Google ended the program because its big data

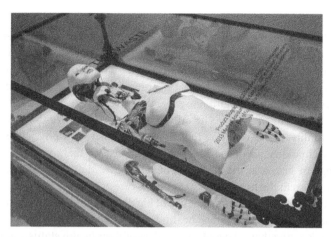

Figure 11.4   Robots. What defines humanity when AI and robots are increasingly "human-like"?
Source: Clément Philippe/AGE Fotostock

analysis was proven to be not only inaccurate but also "making it dangerous to rely on Google Flu Trends for any decision-making" (Lazer & Kennedy, 2015, para. 5). In other words, the big data technologies of GFT failed because it failed to accommodate humans' co-evolution (e.g., changing our search patterns as we become more familiar with the Google algorithm) along with its own evolving characteristics (e.g., new features of suggested search).

As our technologies learn to become more human-like, some have raised concerns about whether we may become more machine-like or how these technologies may change humanity. For example, as voice assistants penetrate all aspects of our everyday lives, people may adopt ways of speaking and thinking that are more responsive to AI and become less "appropriate" for human connection (McGarry, 2017). When digital voice assistants feature female voices and offering assistant-like services, researchers have questioned whether such technologies can reproduce indirect discrimination and gender stereotypes to be further entrenched in our cultural consciousness (Adams & Loideáin, 2019; UNESCO & EQALS Skills Coalition, 2019). "Obedient and obliging machines that pretend to be women are entering our homes, cars and offices," says Saniye Gülser Corat, Director of Gender Equality at UNESCO. "Their hardwired subservience influences how people speak to female voices and models how women respond to requests and express themselves. To change course, we need to pay much closer attention to how, when and whether AI technologies are gendered and, crucially, who is gendering them" (The United Nations, 2019, para. 6).

In summary, as we contemplate the role of big data technologies in health communication, we need to be vigilant against the Magic Consciousness that regularly emerges and often co-exists in our use of such technologies. Due to the prevalence and omnipresence of big data technologies, our worldviews and behaviors can be transformed by them with little knowledge or awareness of their influences. When Magic Consciousness and Mythic Connection creep into our relationships with technologies, we become faithful users with strong emotional attachment toward and identification with the technologies. Without reflexivity, we are at the mercy of algorithms that we do not understand but faithfully and dutifully follow (O'Neil, 2017).

2. Real-Time Surveillance of "Patients"

Big data technologies have transformed the meanings of "patients." Historically, a "patient" becomes visible when an individual experiences illness symptoms and seeks treatments at a point of service, usually a physician's clinic. Preventive care expanded the definition of "patients" by noting that healthy individuals may still be in need of health services and, thus, be legitimate patients. In response, many health interventions were designed to encourage "healthy" patients to recognize their illness symptoms, susceptibility, and severity so that they would visit their physicians to receive care (e.g., vaccinations, annual exams, colonoscopies, or mammograms). In short, before the age of big data, the first step of healthcare delivery was dependent on patients' initiatives in the help-seeking process.

However, the availability and prevalence of big data technologies have transformed the landscape of public health. Public health has always adopted an expansive view of "patients," recognizing that *all* people, regardless of their health status, are its domain and subject to its medical gaze. **Epidemiology** is an essential branch of public health. Epidemiology is a field of study that focuses on the causes and prevention of disease in populations (Pearce, 1996). Unlike clinical medicine, which has centered on disease pathology and individual treatments, epidemiology traditionally has centered on the prevention of disease and the health needs of the *population as a whole* (Pearce, 1996). As such, surveillance becomes an essential tool for public health interventions. **Public health surveillance** is "the systematic, ongoing collection, management, analysis, and interpretation of data followed by the dissemination of these data to public health programs to stimulate public health action" (Thacker et al., 2012, p. 3). Former Surgeon General David Satcher explained, "In public health, we can't do anything without surveillance. That's where public health begins" (Thacker et al., 2012, p. 3). In the United States, public health surveillance has focused historically on infectious diseases (e.g., required reporting of smallpox, yellow fever, and cholera; Thacker et al., 2012). In 1925, all states began participating in national morbidity reporting following several severe epidemics, including the 1918–1919 influenza outbreak (Thacker et al., 2012). By the 1950s, epidemiologists turned their attention to **risk factors** (i.e., specific factors, such as smoking, diet, obesity, or exposure to carcinogens that increase individuals' vulnerability against illness conditions) of specific groups (Pearce, 1996). The disease/risk-oriented and population-based approach to public health dominated the development of public health efforts until the 1980s.

Since then, the rise and advances of computer-based technologies have provided opportunities for public health interventions that were unimaginable before. Since the 2000s, many private companies have collected a wide range and large quantity of data that has significant implications for public health. For example, Google Flu Trends (2008–2014) was one of the first publicized efforts between a private company (i.e., Google) and a governmental agency (i.e., Centers for Disease Control and Prevention) in coordinating public health efforts. By relying on data from search engines and social media, big data technologies now have the capacity to predict epidemic diseases, such as dengue fever or influenza-like illnesses (Li et al., 2016; Strauss et al., 2017). Because smart thermometers and their corresponding software upload users' temperatures, collect attendant symptoms, and identify their geolocations, such technologies can provide insights to predict and avert epidemics by identifying spikes in users' usage in specific regions (Christakis, 2015). As individuals wondered if they were sick, checked their temperature, searched online information, or posted Instagram/Facebook comments, big data technologies had the capacity to see the clustering of information within a geographic area as well as the patterns of individual behaviors to see whether one is "sick" and thus, a patient needed medical attention. "Patients" no longer need to show up at a point of service to be identified.

Big data technologies make it possible to identify "patients" before they seek treatment, and even before they know they are sick. A physician is unlikely to be the first person to whom a patient discloses his or her troubles or concerns. Our first sign of trouble is often uttered privately or with friends. People engage in conversations to express suicidal thoughts through their social media (Carlyle et al., 2018). Researchers have investigated how digital voice assistants' responses to statements about mental health (e.g., "I want to commit suicide" or "I am depressed"), interpersonal violence (e.g., "my husband beats me"), or physical health (e.g., "my head hurts") can have important implications for the users' help-seeking behaviors (Miner et al., 2016). A study found that specific language-use on Facebook posts can predict depression approximately three months ahead of a clinical diagnosis (Eichstaedt et al., 2018). Using **machine learning**, Facebook developed suicide prevention tools to *forecast* and *classify* users' suicide risks based on word-choice, time of day of the post, content posted (photos, videos, plain text), and post reactions (Gomes de Andrade et al., 2018).

Although machine learning and AI are often used interchangeably, AI refers to the concepts of machines being able to carry out tasks that we would consider "smart;" in contrast, machine learning is an application of AI by giving machines access to data and letting them identify patterns and learn for themselves (Marr, 2016). Big data technologies provide possibilities of identifying at-risk individuals by enabling access to linked information from biobanks, electronic medical records, patient-reported outcome measures, automatic and semiautomatic electronic monitoring devices, and social media (Ehrenstein et al., 2017). By examining individuals' as well as populations' behavioral patterns along with other types of variables and data collected, big data technologies make it possible to identify people who are at risk *before* they themselves know that they are at risk.

Real-time health surveillance would not have been possible without mobile and wearable technologies. For example, smart thermometers are valuable real-time data to observe disease transmission dynamics and predict influenza (Ackley et al., 2020). Though such data is valuable, the data still requires individuals to take their temperature and input their symptoms. A person still needs to consider herself somewhat "sick" and take the initiative to assess the severity and urgency of their illness symptoms. **Wearable technologies** can be broadly defined as "any device that is worn by or attached to the body and is capable of providing the user with usable data" (Ackley et al., 2020; Kolodzey et al., 2017, p. 56). Wearable technologies, such as Fitbit and Apple watch, can now offer 24/7 real-time health surveillance by collecting individuals' **biometric data** (i.e., body measurements and calculations). For example, they monitor individuals' health status by collecting individuals' heart rate, hydration level, blood sugar, or exercise levels. Biometric data can also offer insights into individuals' mood, anxiety level, or behavioral patterns. Examples of biometric data also include a person's fingerprints, iris and retinal scans, voice recordings, walking gait, typing pattern of the fingers, and 3D facial scans. Biometric data are collected automatically, uploaded to the cloud, and analyzed (and even commercialized) by big data owners –

with minimal effort or continuous consent by the technology users (Pope, 2018). These data can also be used to compare to historical and/or aggregate data to identify individual-specific or season-specific variations. For example, by identifying weeks in which Fitbit users displayed elevated resting heart rate (which is often a result of infection, especially when accompanied by a fever) and increased sleep levels, researchers found Fitbit data significantly improved influenza-like illness predictions and had great potential to improve real-time and geographically refined influenza surveillance (Radin et al., 2020; see Figure 11.5).

Big data technologies make it possible to merge different areas and types of data for governmental actions to achieve *individual-level* public health interventions. As of July 2020, although Taiwan is only 110 miles off the coast of China and has a population of 23.8 million, it recorded less than 450 cases and 7 deaths during the COVID-19 pandemic. At the same time, confirmed cases had reached over 12 million cases and over half a million deaths globally (Johns Hopkins Coronavirus Resource Center, 2020). By merging national health insurance data with Customs and Immigration databases, physicians received patients' travel records and real-time alerts to help them identify vulnerable

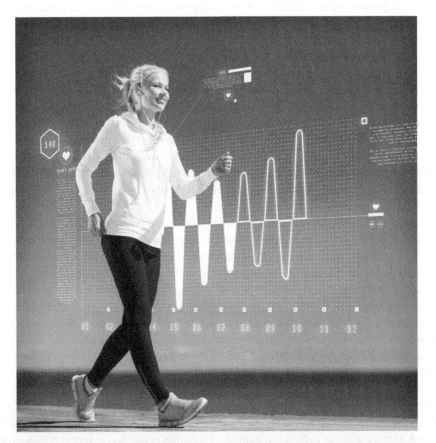

Figure 11.5   Real-time surveillance. In 2018, the Pentagon issued a policy banning service members from using certain fitness devices that track the distance and time they have exercised (Copp, 2018). Such devices can expose locations of bases and important facilities based on where the geo-tracking stops. *Source:* dolgachov/123RF

populations (Dewan et al., 2020). In addition, Taiwan also employed "digital fencing" for close to 55,000 people. This involved in-home quarantine, where alarms would sound if a quarantined person wandered too far from home (Dewan et al., 2020). Although public health has traditionally focused on aggregated, population-based data, big data technologies allow governments to enforce individual-level, real-time surveillance.

The use of real-time health surveillance has also been adopted outside of public health contexts. For example, a meta-analysis has found that text messaging to mobile phones can significantly increase individuals' treatment adherence (Thakkar et al., 2016). As a result, researchers have developed an AI-powered smart pillbox that monitors users' medication usage and sends reminders when the patient fails to take medication at appropriate times (Minaam & Abd-Elfattah, 2018). More recently, **ingestible technologies** (i.e., ingestible electronic sensors) are pushing the boundaries of health information collection. After the user co-ingest the sensor with medication, the sensors "can communicate with a wearable sensor capable of detecting and recording data such as time of medication intake or behavioral and physiological metrics" (Gerke et al., 2019, p. 329). Some researchers have raised ethical and legal concerns about the amount, complexity, and ownership of data collected through ingestible technologies (Gerke et al., 2019).

Finally, an important finding emerged in recent years is that despite the commercial popularization and public health implications for these emerging technologies, researchers have noted that individuals do *not* necessarily benefit from mobile or wearable technologies. A review of six studies found that mobile and wearable technologies have little impact on improving health outcomes for chronic disease management (e.g., improving cholesterol or blood pressure; Jo et al., 2019). The literature suggests that these technologies alone are only facilitators of behavioral change and are not sufficient to maintain long-term health benefits (Patel et al., 2015). However, combined uses of motivational strategies along with mobile and wearable technologies may have the ability to create sustainable changes that improve individuals' quality of life and health outcomes (Gell et al., 2020).

In short, the development of big data technologies has been so expansive and omnipresent that few can escape its medical gaze and surveillance. Without taking initiatives, submitting ourselves to healthcare systems, or knowing our risk levels, we are already being assessed and evaluated by AI algorithms. The benefits of real-time health surveillance and big data technologies are self-evident (Brownstein et al., 2009) – especially at a time when we face regular, global pandemics (e.g., swine flu 2009–2020; Ebola in 2014–2016; and COVID-19 in 2019-present). Tracking illness with global communication networks, big data can help trace outbreaks and slow or stop them.

However, surveillance is surveillance. With increased support for GPS tracking through individuals' cell phones in order to perform contact tracing and real-time surveillance amid the COVID-19 pandemic, many have raised concerns about how such ubiquitous surveillance systems by private companies and governmental agencies can intrude upon individual freedom (e.g., autonomy and privacy; Appleby &Knight, 2020; Owens & Cribb, 2019; see Figure 11.6). The collection of data allows the owners of big data technologies to track movements, behaviors, and variations both at an individual level and at a population-based level and to generate comparisons against historical records and real-time surveillance. Researchers have warned that problematic use of such technologies can result in "a tool for mass surveillance and population control" that further reinforces and exacerbates social inequalities and injustice (Rainie et al., 2019, p. 26). Humans' individual autonomy and agency will be compromised without transparency and understanding of algorithmic systems and their owners (Barnett & Torous, 2019; Rainie et al., 2019).

Reflecting on the future of technologies, Erik Brynjolfsson, director of the MIT Initiative on the Digital Economy wrote,

> I don't think the right framing is "will the outcome be good, or bad?" but rather it must be "how will we shape the outcome, which is currently indeterminate?" I'm hopeful that we will make the right choices, but only if we realize that the good outcomes are not at all inevitable. (Rainie et al., 2019, p. 5)

A major danger faced by our approach to big technologies is the "growing willingness to sacrifice the free will of humanity for the algorithms of machine" (Rainie et al., 2019, p. 36). In her TED Talk, *The Era of Blind Faith to Big Data Must End*, Cathy O'Neil (2017) explained,

> Algorithms are everywhere. They sort and separate the winners from the losers. The winners get the job or a good credit card offer. The losers don't even get an interview or they pay more for insurance. We're being scored with secret formulas that we don't understand, that often don't have systems of appeal. That begs the question: What if the algorithms are wrong? ... Algorithms are opinions embedded in code. It's really different from what you think- what most people think of algorithms. They think algorithms are objective and true and scientific. That's a marketing trick. It's also a marketing trick to intimidate you with algorithms, to make you trust and fear algorithms because you trust and fear mathematics. *A lot can go wrong when we put blind faith in big data.* [emphasis added] (00:09)

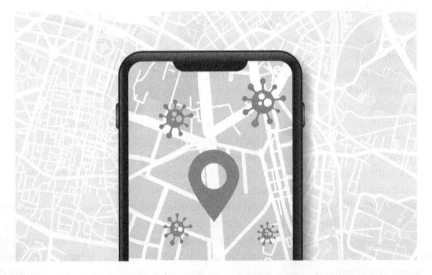

Figure 11.6 Surveillance through mobile phones. During the COVID-19 pandemic, program developers and policymakers have considered contemplated using mobile technologies for contact tracing and hotspot warning. *Source:* inkdrop / 123 RF

When we faithfully and uncritically rely on the results of big data, we no longer wield big data technologies as a tool of the Perspectival Thinking worldview. Blind faith is invoked and maintained through Mythic Connection – we just assume that the results are "true" and "accurate" (and thus virtuous). Perspectival Thinking encourages critical reflexivity. Advances in sciences are achieved by individuals' willingness to forego their presumptions and critically examine the underlying principles, procedures, and outcomes (see also Chapter 4).

3. Integral Fusion Worldviews Necessary to Address Inequality

One fascinating aspect of public health is that there is always an argument to be made for each perspective. During the COVID-19 pandemic, public health experts advocated for stay-at-home orders, noting that economic shutdown is a necessary price for the lives saved; others advocated that the mounting death toll is a necessary evil for society to survive as a whole. Who is right? Can we rely on big data analysis to help us figure this out? As O'Neil (2017) explained,

> To build an algorithm, you need two things: you need data – what happened in the past, and a definition of success – the thing you're looking for and often hoping for. You train an algorithm by looking, figuring out. The algorithm figures out what is associated with success. What situation leads to success? (00:36)

Once the meaning of success is defined, the Perspectival Thinking approach is singularly focused. This approach seeks to identify the measurements necessary to advance the agenda of defining and gauging that version of success. But it is just a version of success rooted in a perspective (i.e., what is measured).

Machine learning is not an objective tool. Rather, it reflects the bias and underlying tendencies of our societies as it learns to respond to and predict human behaviors. When Microsoft first launched its AI Twitter chatbot, Tay, on March 23, 2016, its aim was to "experiment with and conduct research on conversational understanding" (Hunt, 2016). According to Microsoft, "Tay is designed to engage and entertain people where they connect with each other online through casual and playful conversation. The more you chat with Tay, the smarter she gets" (Hunt, 2016). Within 16 hours of its release, Tay was taken offline. On March 25, Microsoft released an official apology, noting that it was "deeply sorry for the unintended offensive and hurtful tweets from Tay" who tweeted several racists, sexually-charged statements, as well as conspiracy theories related to 9/11 (Lee, 2016).

If we train our machines to learn from the patterns of the past to recommend and design a future for us, we are bound to repeat our own bias, discrimination, injustice, and inequalities of our societies (Husserl, 1970; Rainie et al., 2019). Algorithms are human artifacts, not naturally occurring things. As such, they manifestly reflect our limitations and prejudices. Self-learning technology expands our limitations but generally speaking, the trajectory is still traceable back to the inventor's capabilities, imagination, and desires. Algorithms are thus expressions of magic, mythic, and perspectival structures of awareness. As big data technologies learn that more Blacks have been arrested and convicted as criminals in the past and recommend sending more police to Black communities – they would be right: there will be more Blacks arrested as criminals. This is a self-fulfilling prophecy. O'Neil (2017) concluded that by choosing what data to collect and how success is defined, "We are the ones that are biased, and we are injecting those biases into the algorithms" (09:51).

Several studies have noted how AI programs often extend and exacerbate existing human biases and discriminations in our social worlds (Howard & Borenstein, 2018). For example, many states have adopted a popular computer program that has been used to predict which jail inmates are likely to commit future crimes. Researchers found that the program (a) "was particularly likely to falsely flag black defendants as future criminals, wrongly labeling them this way at almost twice the rate as white defendants;" and (b) "White defendants were mislabeled as low risk more often than black defendants" (Angwin et al., 2015). When Google delivers ads to job-seeking candidates, researchers found that Google showed male candidates more prestigious, high-paying positions than it did to female candidates, even though they shared the same credentials (Datta et al., 2015). Google delivered more images of men when searched for "doctors" but retrieved more images of women when searched for "nurses" (Kay et al., 2015). Reflecting on the society's increasing reliance on AI, Joanna Bryson, a researcher of machine learning, noted, "People expected AI to be unbiased; that's just wrong. If the underlying data reflects stereotypes, or if you train AI from human culture, you will find these things" (Buranyi, 2017). O'Neil (2017) noted, "We all are biased. We're all racist and bigoted in ways that *we wish we weren't*, in ways that *we don't even know*" [emphasis added] (09:20). As these technologies evolve, their evolutions are shaped by our cultural consciousness. As Eric Schmidt, CEO of Google from 2001 to 2011, noted, "We must remember that technology remains a tool of humanity" (Lazer & Kennedy, 2015, para. 8).

The strength of big data technologies is finding associations rather than the meanings of such associations (Khoury & Ioannidis, 2014). O'Neil (2017) noted that as we interpret the results of big data technologies, we "should not be the arbiters of truth. We should be translators of ethical discussions that happen in larger society" (12:25). The meanings of the tools we wield are not inherent but are socially constructed. Our cultural approaches shape not only how the tool is created, developed, or evolved but also how it will shape us – our cultural consciousness, how we understand and maintain fairness, justice, and humanity. As we subject ourselves to the surveillance of big technologies, it is important to remember that we still have choices: how we use these technologies and how we allow such technologies to define us (and humanity).

A world of pure Perspectival Thinking is ruthless in its pursuit of "success," a pursuit of efficiency. It has no care and does not care. More importantly, its reflexivity is often (though not always) limited to its measurements – rather than to the very definition of success. To interject reflexivity to the very meanings of success, we need ethics – prudence and care for the world. We need to interrogate the very definition of success – Is it right or appropriate to define success this way? For me, for others, and for all of us? For now *and* for past and future generations? We need an Integral Fusion worldview: We need the *care* to encompass ourselves, space, and time.

C. An Integral Fusion Worldview toward Technologies in Health Communication

The strength of an Integral Fusion worldview is not that it is always correct or the best. Often, we do not know the "correct" or "best" way to evolve as a society until we look back. The strength of an Integral Fusion worldview lies in its diversity, flexibility, and willingness to accommodate others, reconcile differences, and embrace change.

It does not deny nor fear the immense potentials of genetic and big data technologies. These technologies have demonstrated their capacities to eliminate and prevent unnecessary suffering, not just for humans but also for other animals/plants and our larger lived environment. It is vigilant against **instrumental reasoning** (i.e., believing that actions taken are just a means to a rational or better end) that often permeates a Perspectival Thinking world. More importantly, an Integral Fusion worldview is also capable of *seeing* and *seeing through* the injustice and danger embedded in the defined successes of a Perspectival Thinking world, the blind faith treasured in Mythic Connection, and the unquestioned, enchanted realities in Magic Consciousness. It recognizes the differences in these cultural approaches and does not presume that a correct answer is inherent or self-evident.

An Integral Fusion worldview acknowledges that "the" correct answer may be dependent on varying contexts and can be different for different groups of people. An Integral Fusion worldview demands exchanges of perspectives between parties. Randy Goebel, professor of computing science and developer of the University of Alberta's partnership with DeepMind, wrote,

> 'For the greater good' requires an ever-evolving notion and consensus about what the 'greater' is. Just like seat belt laws are motivated by a complex balance of public good (property and human costs), we will have to evolve a planet-wide consensus on what is appropriate for 'great' good. [emphasis added] (Rainie et al., 2019, p. 39)

Because consensus-building is essential in responding to the (co-)evolving environments, *transparency is a necessary condition* for an Integral Fusion worldview. One must be free to express herself for her perspectives to be heard (see also Chapter 14). Thus, an Integral Fusion worldview cannot emerge in an oppressive environment nor an authoritarian regime. In addition, because conversations to reconcile differences are contingent upon individuals' ability to engage in rational and informed dialogues, Integral Fusion worldviews cannot survive, let along thrive, when secrets abound. With both genetic and big data technologies, researchers have warned of a lack of transparency in the ownership, use, and application of the data and technologies, resulting in concerns about legal and ethical implications (Richards & King, 2013; Rodriguez & Galloway, 2017). Amy Webb, founder of the Future Today Institute and professor of strategic foresight at New York University, argued that we need to "rethink access to the internet, data ownership and algorithmic transparency, thus setting all of humanity on a better course for the future" (Rainie et al., 2019, pp. 40–41).

In summary, an Integral Fusion worldview is necessary because it is responsive to the ongoing and emerging challenges we encounter as we wield the tools to change our worlds. Its reflexivity is not limited to the measurements or the definitions of success. It continuously questions whether the world is truly better – for all of us and for all times. More importantly, it critically challenges us to ask: Are we, human beings, changing for the better? It recognizes that this is an evolving dialogue that we have to remain engaged in at the individual and societal levels, lest new technologies become normalized, routinized, and invisible. Social structures are invisible, but they can become impenetrable walls and unbreakable chains. It is through reflexivity and open conversations with all involved that an Integral Fusion worldview finds its strength to morally, ethically, and rationally respond to a world (with technologies) that are currently unimaginable and unpredictable to us today.

III. Additional Resources

A. Key Terms and Theories

science
technology
techne
phronesis
cargo cult
technological complex
germ theory
Human Genome Diversity Project
designer babies
CRISPR
transhumanism
ableism
attachment theory
separation anxiety
proximity-seeking behaviors
nomophobia
anthropomorphism
epidemiology
public health surveillance
risk factors
machine learning
real-time health surveillance
wearable technologies
biometric data
ingestible technologies
instrumental reasoning

B. Discussion Questions

1. Think about the different technologies that surround you in your everyday life. Please (a) identify a specific technology/*techne* and (b) explain which of the following cultural perspectives you hold with technology and why? Try to see if you can identify at least one technology for each cultural perspective.
    a. Magic Consciousness
    b. Mythic Connection
    c. Perspectival Thinking

2. Do you use voice assistants (e.g., Alexa, Siri, etc.)? Why or why not? Reflect on the following questions:
   a. Do you think you will feel differently about the voice assistant if they have a male voice? What do you think about having a voice assistant at home that sounds like a man?
   b. What do you think about their accent (or the lack of accent)? Do you think their (non-)accent can change how we feel about people who we interact with every day?
   c. What are the silliest or most private things you've asked/told your voice assistant?
   d. Why do you think people tell their voice assistant about their experiences with depression and domestic violence? Do you think people with different cultural perspectives have different reasons for such behaviors? Explain and delineate their reasoning.

3. The Human Genome Diversity Project is an ambitious research project that aimed to collect genetic variations of different populations, with a focus on indigenous and isolated populations. Reflect on the following questions.
   a. By reducing people to genetic components, the research project made it possible to "categorize" diversity among people. What do you think about this approach to understand human diversity?
   b. Is it appropriate to think of people as "genetic gold"? What are the possible pros and cons of such an approach?
   c. Do you think this approach can heighten the risk of racism or even genocide? How and why?

4. Do you think we should avoid developing certain technologies because they are too "dangerous," "immoral," or "unethical"?
   a. Looking back at history, what are the technologies that may have fitted such descriptions at one time?
   b. In your lifetime, what kinds of technologies are likely to fit such descriptions?
   c. Do you think people who hold different cultural perspectives may have different answers?
   d. How should people with different cultural perspectives work with one another if one insists on developing the technology and the other believes that it's absolute evil to do so?

5. Think about big data technology and the types and amount of information it can collect and analyze about you.
   a. What are the sources of information?
   b. Do you have control over how such information is used?
   c. How do you feel about other parties (e.g. private sectors) using, selling, and *profiting* from your data about your genes, movements, media viewing habits, purchase history, and other "private" information?
   d. Do you think people can control how such information would be "exchanged"? In other words, can people decide not to participate in the information economy that dominates the modern world? What are the likely consequences?

6. If we do not have a choice about the "world" we are born into, what are the different ways we can protect citizens from unfair/unjust exploitations of the infrastructure? (See also Chapter 14)

References

Ackley, S. F., Pilewski, S., Petrovic, V. S., Worden, L., Murray, E., & Porco, T. C. (2020). Assessing the utility of a smart thermometer and mobile application as a surveillance tool for influenza and influenza-like illness. *Health Informatics Journal, 26*(3), 2148–2158.

Adams, R., & Loideáin, N. N. (2019). Addressing indirect discrimination and gender stereotypes in AI virtual personal assistants: The role of international human rights law. *Cambridge International Law, Journal, 8*(2), 241–257.

Amani, B., & Coombe, R. J. (2005). The Human Genome Diversity Project: The politics of patents at the intersection of race, religion, and research ethics. *Law and Policy, 27*(1), 152–188.

Angwin, J., Larson, J., Mattu, S., & Kirchner, L. (2015, May 23). *Machine bias.* ProPublica. https://www.propublica.org/article/machine-bias-risk-assessments-in-criminal-sentencing

Appleby, J., & Knight, V. (2020, April 16). *Stopping COVID-19 will include monitoring and sharing personal data.* NBC News. https://www.nbcnews.com/health/health-news/stopping-covid-19-will-include-monitoring-sharing-personal-data-n1184716

Aristotle. (2019). *Aristotle: The Nicomachean ethics* (T. Irwin, Trans.; 3rd ed.). Hackett.

Barnett, I., & Torous, J. (2019). Ethics, transparency, and public health at the intersection of innovation and Facebook's suicide prevention efforts. *Annals of Internal Medicine, 170*(8), 565–566.

Bayer, J. B., Triệu, P., & Ellison, N. B. (2020). Social media elements, ecologies, and effects. *Annual Review of Psychology, 71*(1), 471–497.

Biswas, A. K. (2007). Technology in history with special reference to ancient and medieval India. In J. B. Das Gupta (Ed.), *Science, technology, imperialism, and war* (pp. 261–290). Pearson Longman.

Bostrom, N. (2003). Human genetic enhancements: A transhumanist perspective. *The Journal of Value Inquiry, 37*(4), 493–506.

Brake, M. (2019). *The science of the Big Bang Theory: What America's favorite sitcom can teach you about physics, flags, and the idiosyncrasies of scientists.* Skyhorse.

Brownstein, J. S., Freifeld, C. C., & Madoff, L. C. (2009). Digital disease detection — Harnessing the web for public health surveillance. *New England Journal of Medicine, 360*(21), 2153–2157.

Buranyi, S. (2017, August 8). *Rise of the racist robots – How AI is learning all our worst impulses.* The Guardian. https://www.theguardian.com/inequality/2017/aug/08/rise-of-the-racist-robots-how-ai-is-learning-all-our-worst-impulses

Carlyle, K. E., Guidry, J. P. D., Williams, K., Tabaac, A., & Perrin, P. B. (2018). Suicide conversations on Instagram: Contagion or caring? *Journal of Communication in Healthcare, 11*(1), 12–18.

Cheever, N. A., Rosen, L. D., Carrier, L. M., & Chavez, A. (2014). Out of sight is not out of mind: The impact of restricting wireless mobile device use on anxiety levels among low, moderate and high users. *Computers in Human Behavior, 37*, 290–297.

Christakis, D. A. (2015). Potential utility of a smart thermometer to predict and avert epidemics. *JAMA Pediatrics, 169*(11), 1067–1068.

Copp, T. (2018, August 6). *Fitbits and fitness-tracking devices banned for deployed troops.* MilitaryTimes.https://www.militarytimes.com/news/your-military/2018/08/06/devices-and-apps-that-rely-on-geolocation-restricted-for-deployed-troops

Cyranoski, D. (2019, March 11). *The CRISPR-baby scandal: What's next for human gene-editing.* Nature. https://www.nature.com/articles/d41586-019-00673-1

Datta, A., Tschantz, M. C., & Datta, A. (2015). Automated experiments on ad privacy settings: A tale of opacity, choice, and discrimination. *Proceedings on Privacy Enhancing Technologies, 2015*(1), 92–112.

Dean, M. (2016). Celebrity health announcements and online health information seeking: An analysis of Angelina Jolie's preventative health decision. *Health Communication, 31*(6), 752–761.

Dewan, A., Pettersson, H., & Croker, H. (2020, April 16). *As governments fumbled their coronavirus response, these four got it right. Here's how.* CNN. https://www.cnn.com/2020/04/16/world/coronavirus-response-lessons-learned-intl/index.html

Dodge, T., Williams, K. J., Marzell, M., & Turrisi, R. (2012). Judging cheaters: Is substance misuse viewed similarly in the athletic and academic domains? *Psychology of Addictive Behaviors, 26*(3), 678.

Duffy, B. R. (2003). Anthropomorphism and the social robot. *Robotics and Autonomous Systems, 42*(3), 177–190.

Duster, T. (2003). *Backdoor to eugenics* (2nd ed.). Routledge.

Ehrenstein, V., Nielsen, H., Pedersen, A. B., Johnsen, S. P., & Pedersen, L. (2017). Clinical epidemiology in the era of big data: New opportunities, familiar challenges. *Clinical Epidemiology, 9,* 245–250.

Eichstaedt, J. C., Smith, R. J., Merchant, R. M., Ungar, L. H., Crutchley, P., Preoţiuc-Pietro, D., Asch, D. A., & Schwartz, H. A. (2018). Facebook language predicts depression in medical records. *Proceedings of the National Academy of Sciences, 115*(44), 11203–11208.

Fernaeus, Y., Jacobsson, M., Ljungblad, S., & Holmquist, L. E. (2009). Are we living in a robot cargo cult? *Proceedings of the 4th ACM/IEEE international conference on Human robot interaction*, (p. 279–280). https://doi.org/10.1145/1514095.1514175

Ferriman, A. (2007). *BMJ* readers choose the "sanitary revolution" as greatest medical advance since 1840. *BMJ, 334*(7585), 111.

Fox, K. (2017, February 22). *The treasure trove of unique genomes hiding in plain sight.* TED. https://ideas.ted.com/the-treasure-trove-of-unique-genomes-hiding-in-plain-sight

Frieze, I. H., Olson, J. E., & Russell, J. (1991). Attractiveness and income for men and women in management. *Journal of Applied Social Psychology, 21*(13), 1039–1057.

Gao, Y., Pan, Z., Wang, H., & Chen, G. (2018, October 8–12). Alexa, my love: Analyzing reviews of Amazon Echo. *2018 IEEE smartworld, ubiquitous intelligence & computing, advanced & trusted computing, scalable computing & communications, cloud & big data computing, internet of people and smart city innovation* (pp. 372–380). https://ieeexplore.ieee.org/abstract/document/8560072

Gardner, W. (1995). Can human genetic enhancement be prohibited? *The Journal of Medicine and Philosophy: A Forum for Bioethics and Philosophy of Medicine, 20*(1), 65–84.

Gaynes, R. P. (2011). *Germ theory: Medical pioneers in infectious diseases.* Wiley.

Gell, N. M., Grover, K. W., Savard, L., & Dittus, K. (2020). Outcomes of a text message, Fitbit, and coaching intervention on physical activity maintenance among cancer survivors: A randomized control pilot trial. *Journal of Cancer Survivorship, 14*(1), 80–88.

Gerke, S., Minssen, T., Yu, H., & Cohen, I. G. (2019). Ethical and legal issues of ingestible electronic sensors. *Nature Electronics, 2*(8), 329–334.

Gibson, K. R., & Ingold, T. (Eds.). (1993). *Tools, language and cognition in human evolution.* Cambridge University Press.

Gomes de Andrade, N. N., Pawson, D., Muriello, D., Donahue, L., & Guadagno, J. (2018). Ethics and artificial intelligence: Suicide prevention on Facebook. *Philosophy & Technology, 31*(4), 669–684.

Greenberg v. Miami Children's Hospital Research Institute, 264 F. Supp. 2d 1064 (S.D. Fla. 2003). https://www.courtlistener.com/opinion/2507167/greenberg-v-miami-childrens-hospital-res-inst-inc

Handyside, A. H. (2018). 'Designer babies' almost thirty years on. *Reproduction, 156*(1), F75–F79.

Haney, D. P. (1999). Aesthetics and ethics in Gadamer, Lévinas, and romanticism: Problems of phronesis and techne. *PMLA: Publications of the Modern Language Association of America, 114*(1), 32–45.

Hann, K. E. J., Freeman, M., Fraser, L., Waller, J., Sanderson, S. C., Rahman, B., Side, L., Gessler, S., & Lanceley, A., & for the, P. s. t. (2017). Awareness, knowledge, perceptions, and attitudes towards genetic testing for cancer risk among ethnic minority groups: A systematic review. *BMC Public Health, 17*, Article 503. https://doi.org/10.1186/s12889-017-4375-8

Harkin, L. J., & Kuss, D. (2020). "My smartphone is an extension of myself": A holistic qualitative exploration of the impact of using a smartphone. *Psychology of Popular Media*. Advance online publication. https://doi.org/10.1037/ppm0000278

Harris, A. (2020, April 9). *BRCA1: 'I'm lucky that I have the chance to take preventative measures.'* The Irish Times. https://www.irishtimes.com/life-and-style/health-family/brca1-i-m-lucky-that-i-have-the-chance-to-take-preventative-measures-1.4217949

Holmes, J. (2006). *John Bowlby and attachment theory.* Routledge.

Hong, S. J. (2020). Uncertainty in the process of communicating cancer-related genetic risk information with patients: A scoping review. *Journal of Health Communication, 25*(3), 251–270.

Howard, A., & Borenstein, J. (2018). The ugly truth about ourselves and our robot creations: The problem of bias and social inequity. *Science and Engineering Ethics, 24*(5), 1521–1536.

Hunt, E. (2016, March 24). *Tay, Microsoft's AI chatbot, gets a crash course in racism from Twitter.* The Guardian. https://www.theguardian.com/technology/2016/mar/24/tay-microsofts-ai-chatbot-gets-a-crash-course-in-racism-from-twitter

Husserl, E. (1970). *The crisis of European sciences and transcendental phenomenology: An introduction to phenomenological philosophy* (D. Carr, Trans.). Northwestern University Press.

Irwin, T. (2019). Introduction. In *Aristotle: The Nicomachean ethics* (T. Irwin, Trans.; 3rd ed.). Hackett.

Jin, B., & Park, N. (2013). Mobile voice communication and loneliness: Cell phone use and the social skills deficit hypothesis. *New Media & Society, 15*(7), 1094–1111.

Jo, A., Coronel, B. D., Coakes, C. E., & Mainous, A. G., 3rd. (2019). Is there a benefit to patients using wearable devices such as Fitbit or health apps on mobiles? A systematic review. *The American Journal of Medicine, 132*(12), 1394–1400.e1.

Johns Hopkins Coronavirus Resource Center. (2020). *Coronavirus COVID-19 global cases by the Center for Systems Science and Engineering (CSSE) at Johns Hopkins University (JHU)*. Retrieved July 10, 2020, from https://coronavirus.jhu.edu/map.html

Jolie, A. (2013, May 14). My medical choice. The New York Times. https://nyti.ms/19l8bbY

Kay, M., Matuszek, C., & Munson, S. A. (2015). Unequal representation and gender stereotypes in image search results for occupations. *Proceedings of the 33rd annual ACM conference on human factors in computing systems* (pp. 3819–3828). https://doi.org/10.1145/2702123.2702520

Kessler, S., Levine, E. K., Opitz, J. M., & Reynolds, J. F. (1987). Psychological aspects of genetic counseling: IV. The subjective assessment of probability. *American Journal of Medical Genetics, 28*(2), 361–370.

Khoury, M. J., & Ioannidis, J. P. A. (2014). Big data meets public health. *Science, 346*(6213), 1054–1055.

Kim, J.-H. (2017). Smartphone-mediated communication vs. face-to-face interaction: Two routes to social support and problematic use of smartphone. *Computers in Human Behavior, 67*, 282–291.

Kim, Y., & Sundar, S. S. (2012). Anthropomorphism of computers: Is it mindful or mindless? *Computers in Human Behavior, 28*(1), 241–250.

Kolodzey, L., Grantcharov, P. D., Rivas, H., Schijven, M. P., & Grantcharov, T. P. (2017). Wearable technology in the operating room: A systematic review. *BMJ Innovations, 3*, 55–63.

Konok, V., Gigler, D., Bereczky, B. M., & Miklósi, Á. (2016). Humans' attachment to their mobile phones and its relationship with interpersonal attachment style. *Computers in Human Behavior, 61*, 537–547.

Konok, V., Pogány, Á., & Miklósi, Á. (2017). Mobile attachment: Separation from the mobile phone induces physiological and behavioural stress and attentional bias to separation-related stimuli. *Computers in Human Behavior, 71*, 228–239.

Kramer, E. M., Adkins, G., Kim, S. H., & Miller, G. (2014). *Environmental communication and the extinction vortex: Technology as denial of death.* Hampton.

Kramer, E. M., & Hsieh, E. (2019). Gaze as embodied ethics: Homelessness, the Other, and humanity. In M. J. Dutta & D. B. Zapata (Eds.), *Communicating for social change* (pp. 33–62). Palgrave Macmillan.

Kruse, C. S., Karem, P., Shifflett, K., Vegi, L., Ravi, K., & Brooks, M. (2018). Evaluating barriers to adopting telemedicine worldwide: A systematic review. *Journal of Telemedicine and Telecare, 24*(1), 4–12.

Lazer, D., & Kennedy, R. (2015, October 1). *What we can learn from the epic failure of Google Flu Trends.* Wired. https://www.wired.com/2015/10/can-learn-epic-failure-google-flu-trends

Lazer, D., Kennedy, R., King, G., & Vespignani, A. (2014). The parable of Google Flu: Traps in big data analysis. *Science, 343*(6176), 1203–1205.

Ledford, H. (2019, June 24). *CRISPR babies: When will the world be ready?* Nature. https://www.nature.com/articles/d41586-019-01906-z

Lee, P. (2016, March 25). *Learning from Tay's introduction.* Official Microsoft Blog. https://blogs.microsoft.com/blog/2016/03/25/learning-tays-introduction

Li, E. Y., Tung, C.-Y., & Chang, S.-H. (2016). The wisdom of crowds in action: Forecasting epidemic diseases with a web-based prediction market system. *International Journal of Medical Informatics, 92*, 35–43.

Lindstrom, L. (2019). *Cargo cult: Strange stories of desire from Melanesia and beyond.* University of Hawai'i Press.

Lock, M. (1999). Genetic diversity and the politics of difference. *Chicago-Kent Law Review, 75*(1), 83–111.

Marcus, A. D. (2019, December 21). *A genetic test led seven women in one family to have major surgery. Then the odds changed.* The Wall Street Journal. https://www.wsj.com/articles/seven-women-in-a-family-chose-surgery-after-a-genetic-test-then-the-results-changed-11576860210

Marr, B. (2016, December 16). *What is the difference between artificial intelligence and machine learning?* Forbes. https://www.forbes.com/sites/bernardmarr/2016/12/06/what-is-the-difference-between-artificial-intelligence-and-machine-learning/#44a18fea2742

McGarry, C. (2017, March 17). *Siri, Alexa, and robots could change how we talk.* Macworld. https://www.macworld.com/article/3181984/sxsw/siri-alexa-and-robots-could-change-how-we-talk.html

McLuhan, M., & Fiore, Q. (1996). *The medium is the massage: An inventory of effects.* HardWired.

Minaam, D. S. A., & Abd-Elfattah, M. (2018). Smart drugs: Improving healthcare using smart pill box for medicine reminder and monitoring system. *Future Computing and Informatics Journal, 3*(2), 443–456.

Miner, A. S., Milstein, A., Schueller, S., Hegde, R., Mangurian, C., & Linos, E. (2016). Smartphone-based conversational agents and responses to questions about mental health, interpersonal violence, and physical health. *JAMA Internal Medicine, 176*(5), 619–625.

Moore v. Regents of the University of California, 51 Cal. 3d 120 (Cal. 1990). https://law.justia.com/cases/california/supreme-court/3d/51/120.html

Mukherjee, S. (2016). *The gene: An intimate history.* Scribner.

Mumford, L. (2010). *Technics and civilization.* University of Chicago Press. (Original work published 1934)

Munzer, S. R. (2013). Research biobanks meet synthetic biology: Autonomy and ownership. In G. Pascuzzi, U. Izzo, & M. Macilotti (Eds.), *Comparative issues in the governance of research biobanks: Property, privacy, intellectual property, and the role of technology* (pp. 11–39). Springer.

National Human Genome Research Institute. (n.d.). *What is genome editing?* Retrieved October 10, 2020, from https://www.genome.gov/about-genomics/policy-issues/what-is-Genome-Editing

Natoli, J. L., Ackerman, D. L., McDermott, S., & Edwards, J. G. (2012). Prenatal diagnosis of down syndrome: A systematic review of termination rates (1995–2011). *Prenatal Diagnosis, 32*(2), 142–153.

Nelson, H. D., Pappas, M., Cantor, A., Haney, E., & Holmes, R. (2019). Risk assessment, genetic counseling, and genetic testing for BRCA-related cancer in women: Updated evidence report and systematic review for the US preventive services task force. *JAMA, 322*(7), 666–685.

Nie, J., Wang, P., & Lei, L. (2020). Why can't we be separated from our smartphones? The vital roles of smartphone activity in smartphone separation anxiety. *Computers in Human Behavior, 109*, Article 106351. https://doi.org/10.1016/j.chb.2020.106351

O'Neil, C. (2017, April). *The era of blind faith in big data must end.* TED Talk. https://www.ted.com/talks/cathy_o_neil_the_era_of_blind_faith_in_big_data_must_end

Olsan, L. T. (2003). Charms and prayers in medieval medical theory and practice. *Social History of Medicine, 16*(3), 343–366.

Ossorio, P. N. (2007). The human genome as common heritage: Common sense or legal nonsense? *The Journal of Law, Medicine & Ethics, 35*(3), 425–439.

Owens, J., & Cribb, A. (2019). 'My Fitbit thinks I can do better!' Do health promoting wearable technologies support personal autonomy? *Philosophy & Technology, 32*(1), 23–38.

Patel, M. S., Asch, D. A., & Volpp, K. G. (2015). Wearable devices as facilitators, not drivers, of health behavior change. *JAMA, 313*(5), 459–460.

Pearce, N. (1996). Traditional epidemiology, modern epidemiology, and public health. *American Journal of Public Health, 86*(5), 678–683.

Pope, C. (2018). Biometric data collection in an unprotected world: Exploring the need for federal legislation protecting biometric data. *Journal of Law and Policy, 26*(2), 769–803.

Prokop, P., & Fedor, P. (2011). Physical attractiveness influences reproductive success of modern men. *Journal of Ethology, 29*(3), 453–458.

Radin, J. M., Wineinger, N. E., Topol, E. J., & Steinhubl, S. R. (2020). Harnessing wearable device data to improve state-level real-time surveillance of influenza-like illness in the USA: A population-based study. *The Lancet Digital Health, 2*(2), e85–e93.

Raffaele, P. (2006, February). *In John they trust*. Smithsonian Magazine. https://www.smithsonianmag.com/history/in-john-they-trust-109294882/

Rainie, L., Stansberry, K., & Cohn, S. (2019, October 28). *Experts optimistic about the next 50 years of digital life*. Pew Research Center. https://www.pewresearch.org/internet/wp-content/uploads/sites/9/2019/10/PI_2019.10.28_The-Next-50-Years-of-Digital-Life_FINAL.pdf

Reiser, S. J. (2009). *Technological medicine: The changing world of doctors and patients*. Cambridge University Press.

Richards, N. M., & King, J. H. (2013). Three paradoxes of big data. *Stanford Law Review Online, 66*, 41–46.

Rodriguez, L. L., & Galloway, E. (2017). Bringing genomics to medicine: Ethical, policy, and social considerations. In G. S. Ginsburg & H. F. Willard (Eds.), *Genomic and precision medicine* (3rd ed., pp. 283–297). Academic Press.

Rosenberg, R. N., Richter, R. W., Risser, R. C., Taubman, K., Prado-Farmer, I., Ebalo, E., Posey, J., Kingfisher, D., Dean, D., Weiner, M. F., & Svetlik, D. (1996). Genetic factors for the development of Alzheimer disease in the Cherokee Indian. *Archives of Neurology, 53*(10), 997–1000.

Salopek, P. (1997, April 28). *Genes offer sampling of hope and fear*. Chicago Tribune. https://www.chicagotribune.com/news/ct-xpm-1997-04-28-9704280052-story.html

Sandler, S., Alfino, L., & Saleem, M. (2018). The importance of preventative medicine in conjunction with modern day genetic studies. *Genes & Diseases, 5*(2), 107–111.

Savage-Rumbaugh, E. S., & Rumbaugh, D. M. (1993). The emergence of language. In K. R. Gibson & T. Ingold (Eds.), *Tools, language and cognition in human evolution* (pp. 86–108). Cambridge University Press.

Savulescu, J. (1999). Should we clone human beings? Cloning as a source of tissue for transplantation. *Journal of Medical Ethics, 25*(2), 87–95.

Savulescu, J., Foddy, B., & Clayton, M. (2004). Why we should allow performance enhancing drugs in sport. *British Journal of Sports Medicine, 38*(6), 666–670.

Segers, S., Pennings, G., Dondorp, W., De Wert, G., & Mertes, H. (2019). In vitro gametogenesis and the creation of 'designer babies.' *Cambridge Quarterly of Healthcare Ethics, 28*(3), 499–508.

Sheltrown, N. (2008). Harry Potter's world as a morality tale of technology and media. In E. E. Heilman (Ed.), *Critical perspectives on Harry Potter* (pp. 47–64). Routledge.

Sleeboom-Faulkner, M. (2008). Human genetic biobanking in Asia: Issues of trust, wealth, and ambition. In M. Sleeboom-Faulkner & P. Garside (Eds.), *Human genetic biobanks in Asia: Politics of trust and scientific advancement* (pp. 3–24). Routledge.

Smith, L. (n.d.). *#Ableism*. Center for Disability Rights. Retrieved August 8, 2020, from http://cdrnys.org/blog/uncategorized/ableism

Stark, P. B., & Saltelli, A. (2018). Cargo-cult statistics and scientific crisis. *Significance*, *15*(4), 40–43.

Strauss, R. A., Castro, J. S., Reintjes, R., & Torres, J. R. (2017). Google dengue trends: An indicator of epidemic behavior. The Venezuelan case. *International Journal of Medical Informatics*, *104*, 26–30.

Suter, S. M. (2007). A brave new world of designer babies. *Berkeley Technology Law Journal*, *22*, 897–968.

Temple, R. C. (1903). *Census of India, 1901: The Andaman and Nicobar Islands* (Vol. 3). Office of the Superintendent of Government Printing. https://books.google.com/books?id=rixRAAAAYAAJ

Thacker, S. B., Qualters, J. R., & Lee, L. M. (2012). Public health surveillance in the United States: Evolution and challenges. *MMWR: Morbidity & Mortality Weekly Report Supplements*, *61*(3), 3–9.

Thakkar, J., Kurup, R., Laba, T.-L., Santo, K., Thiagalingam, A., Rodgers, A., Woodward, M., Redfern, J., & Chow, C. K. (2016). Mobile telephone text messaging for medication adherence in chronic disease: A meta-analysis. *JAMA Internal Medicine*, *176*(3), 340–349.

Tucker, B. P. (1998). Deaf culture, Cochlear implants, and elective disability. *Hastings Center Report*, *28*(4), 6–14.

UNESCO, & EQALS Skills Coalition. (2019). *I'd blush if I could: Closing gender divides in digital skills through education*. UNESCO. https://unesdoc.unesco.org/ark:/48223/pf0000367416

The United Nations. (2019, May 17). *Are robots sexist? UN report shows gender bias in talking digital tech*. UN News. https://news.un.org/en/story/2019/05/1038691

van der Lugt, M. (2013). The learned physician as a charismatic healer: Urso of Salerno (flourished end of twelfth century) on incantations in medicine, magic, and religion. *Bulletin of the History of Medicine*, *87*(3), 307–346.

Verghese, A. (2011, July). *A doctor's touch*. TED Talk. https://www.ted.com/talks/abraham_verghese_a_doctor_s_touch

Wang, W. (2017). Smartphones as social actors? Social dispositional factors in assessing anthropomorphism. *Computers in Human Behavior*, *68*, 334–344.

Waring, D. (2000). Why the practice of medicine is not a phronetic activity. *Theoretical Medicine and Bioethics*, *21*(2), 139–151.

Washington University v. Catalona, 490 F.3d 667 (8th Cir. 2007). https://www.courtlistener.com/opinion/798120/washington-university-v-william-j-catalona-md-washington-university

Wee, S.-L. (2019, December 30). *Chinese scientist who genetically edited babies gets 3 years in prison*. The New York Times. https://nyti.ms/356RaWR

Weingart, P. (2010). A short history of knowledge formation. In R. Frodeman, J. T. Klein, C. Mitcham, & J. B. Holbrook (Eds.), *The Oxford handbook of interdisciplinarity* (pp. 3–14). Oxford University Press.

White House. (2020, April 6). *Executive order on encouraging international support for the recovery and use of space resources.* https://www.whitehouse.gov/presidential-actions/executive-order-encouraging-international-support-recovery-use-space-resources

World Health Organization. (2017). *Global diffusion of eHealth: Making universal health coverage achievable: Report of the third global survey on eHealth.* https://www.who.int/goe/publications/global_diffusion/en/

Yildirim, C., & Correia, A.-P. (2015). Exploring the dimensions of nomophobia: Development and validation of a self-reported questionnaire. *Computers in Human Behavior, 49,* 130–137.

12

Health Disparities

Observations and Solutions Through Different Cultural Approaches

Chapter 12 provides a brief overview of minority health, identifying major themes and findings. Moving beyond the discussions of social stigma in Chapter 8, this chapter examines how different cultural approaches can provide insights into health disparities. We will first compare and contrast different ways researchers have identified and defined groups that face unique challenges in their experiences in all stages of care (i.e., access, process, and outcomes). We will then examine the health experiences of health disparity populations and explore potential solutions through different cultural approaches.

I. Introduction

In Chapter 8, we have offered an in-depth examination of social stigma, which, by definition, implies an in-group versus out-group distinction and is supported through sociocultural structures. Whereas in Chapter 8, our discussions centered on interpersonal and intergroup activities in response to social stigma, our goal for Chapter 12 is to adopt a bird's eye view to examine the larger sociocultural structures and mechanisms that maintain, support, and reinforce structural biases that result in health disparities among different populations.

Structural stigma is defined as "societal-level conditions, cultural norms, and institutional policies that constrain the opportunities, resources, and wellbeing of the stigmatized" (Hatzenbuehler & Link, 2014, p. 2). Another related concept is **structural discrimination**, which is defined as "institutional practices and policies that work to the disadvantage of the stigmatized group even in the absence of individual discrimination" (Angermeyer et al., 2014, p. 61). Structural discrimination can involve (a) *intended structural discrimination*, such as legislation and policies that intentionally discriminate against stigmatized groups and (b) *unintended structural discrimination*, such as policies and practices that do not intend to discriminate but result in discriminatory effects to certain groups of people (Angermeyer et al., 2014; Corrigan et al., 2004). In other words, specific groups may experience disparities in their health status and health services as a result of intentional practices or unintentional effects (also see Chapter 14 for discussions on structural barriers). Generally speaking, though structural stigma and structural discrimination are often used interchangeably, the two areas of research (i.e., stigma and discrimination) have emerged through different

Rethinking Culture in Health Communication: Social Interactions as Intercultural Encounters, First Edition. Elaine Hsieh and Eric M Kramer.
© 2021 John Wiley & Sons, Inc. Published 2021 by John Wiley & Sons, Inc.

traditions (Stuber et al., 2008). *Stigma* emerged from the literature in sociology and social sciences, examining the combined effects of prejudice and discriminatory behaviors against a minority group with "unusual" conditions (e.g., individuals with discrediting traits, such as HIV+ status or mental illness); in contrast, *discrimination* emerged through psychological studies on prejudice and is often used in legal and social policy analyses, focusing on the discriminatory *acts* and the corresponding impacts on everyday life (Goffman, 1963/2009; Stuber et al., 2008; Thornicroft et al., 2007).

The literature has provided conclusive evidence on how structural stigma and structural discrimination have damaging impacts on the health services for, and the health status of, a wide range of groups. As researchers develop systematic understanding and interventions for these groups, a crucial step is to identify the specific factors and manners that shape these groups' health experiences.

II. Defining Key Concepts and Populations

Healthy People is a national program to establish "a set of science-based objectives with measurable targets that provides a strategic framework to motivate, guide, and focus action on improving the nation's health and communicating a vision for achieving health equity" (McGowan et al., 2019, p. 63; see also Office of Disease Prevention and Health Promotion, 2020). Since 1990, Healthy People has set 10-year objectives for each decade for both the scientific community and the public to achieve better health in the United States (McGowan et al., 2019). Healthy People 2020 defines a **health disparity** as "a particular type of health difference that is closely linked with social, economic, and/or environmental disadvantage" (HealthyPeople.gov, n.d., para. 6). Elaborating on the underlying principles for the definition, Braveman et al. (2011) proposed that health disparities are "systematic, plausibly avoidable health differences adversely affecting socially disadvantaged groups; they may reflect social disadvantage, but causality need not be established" (p. S149). In other words, recognizing that not all causes and pathways of disparities in health status and health services are known, the investigations of health disparities maintain an *applied focus* and an emphasis on *social justice* by reducing *avoidable* health differences disproportionally affecting *socially disadvantaged* groups.

Historically, health disparities have been studied under the field of minority health. The National Institute on Minority Health and Health Disparities (NIMHD) defined **minority health** as "all aspects of health and disease in one or more racial/ethnic populations," including Blacks/African Americans, Hispanics/Latinos, Asians, American Indians/Alaska Natives, and Native Hawaiians/other Pacific Islanders (Alvidrez et al., 2019, p. S16). In recent years, however, health researchers have become wary of relying on racial/ethnic categories to conceptualize and investigate population-based health issues. Because racial/ethnic categories are sociopolitical (as opposed to biological) constructs which are often framed through political and commercial motivations, problematic use of racial/ethnic categorizations can lead to the conflation of race, ethnicity, and nationality with biological differences and/or discrimination of certain groups (Kahn, 2014; Lee, 2015; Paradies et al., 2007).

Whereas minority health has traditionally centered on racial/ethnic categories, what is considered a health disparity population has expanded significantly beyond racial/ethnic categorizations. A **health disparity population** is characterized by a *pattern* of poorer *access* to health services (e.g., lower socioeconomic status and lack of insurance coverage), *process* of healthcare delivery (e.g., social stigma and quality of provider-patient interactions), and *outcomes* of health status (e.g., the overall rate of disease incidence, prevalence, morbidity, mortality, or survival in the population as compared with the general population). Current NIMHD-designated health disparity populations include specific racial/ethnic minorities, socioeconomically disadvantaged populations, underserved rural populations, and sexual and gender minorities (Alvidrez et al., 2019).

To recognize the complexity of populations that face health disparities, governmental agencies and research communities have developed various terms to highlight specific characteristics and/or unique aspects of these groups. Some common groups identified include: underserved populations, vulnerable populations, at-risk populations, and marginalized populations. Although some of these terms are used interchangeably and individuals may qualify for multiple categories, the naming of these groups highlights different emphases of concerns (Centers for Medicare & Medicaid Services, n.d.; King & Wheeler, 2016). For example, **underserved populations** (which often are used in connection with **medically underserved areas**) refer to certain populations (and geographical locations) that face *limited access* to healthcare services (e.g., lack of health insurance or living in rural areas). In contrast, (medically) **vulnerable populations** highlight certain groups that may face *additional barriers* to healthcare services (e.g., complex treatment regimen, significant financial hardship, or communication/language/cultural barriers). A person may be vulnerable but not underserved (e.g., a Spanish-speaking child who lives in Chicago and has good insurance coverage).

At-risk populations reflect an epidemiological interest in identifying specific *risk factors* (e.g., obesity, smoking, food insecurity, and poverty) that can increase certain groups' illness susceptibility and severity. At-risk individuals are defined as "people with *access and functional needs* that may interfere with their ability to access or receive medical care" (U.S. Department of Health and Human Services, 2019, para. 1). **Access-based needs** can include individuals' ability to access a wide range of resources and services, including related social services, accommodations, information, transportation, medications to maintain health, among others. **Functional-based needs** refer to "restrictions or limitations an individual may have that requires assistance" (U.S. Department of Health and Human Services, 2019, para. 3). From this perspective, at-risk populations can overlap with underserved populations (who lack access to care) and vulnerable populations (who may face barriers to meet functional needs).

Marginalized populations refer to groups that are "*excluded* from mainstream social, economic, cultural, or political life," highlighting "*unequal power* between groups within society" [emphasis added] (Cook, 2008, p. 496). Individuals may be marginalized as a result of race/ethnicity, religion, political/cultural affiliation, age, gender, financial status, or education levels, among others. Because the marginalization is situated in relation to a groups' relationships with other, more dominant, groups, the process (e.g., formal v. informal; institutional v. individual; systematic v. incidental), pathways, extent, and impacts of marginalization are "context specific and reliant on the cultural organization of the social site in question" (Cook, 2008, p. 496). For example, LGBT+ group members may be considered as a single group marginalized by the larger society (Harper & Schneider, 2003); however, compared to other sexual minorities, transgender individuals, for example, tend to face additional inter-personal discrimination and structural barriers in the larger society *and* even within the LGBT+ community (Kcomt, 2019; Stone, 2009; Weiss, 2011). The exclusion can take place at all stages of care, including access, process, and outcomes of care.

The identification and naming of these populations are in themselves political acts. These labels categorize specific populations as unique groups. The process of categori-cal naming highlights their vulnerabilities and potential challenges, and implies inter-ventions that are available to these groups (Vallgårda, 2007). By naming these groups as such, however, one may unintentionally reinforce stigma to certain groups, an issue explored more in-depth later in this Chapter.

Finally, health disparities are closely tied to a concept we discussed in Chapter 7: **social determinants of health**, which was defined as "the conditions in which peo-ple are born, grow, live, work, and age" (World Health Organization, 2019, para. 1). Many of the social determinants of health also serve as critical factors in shaping the health of specific populations. Whereas social determinants of health focus on the spe-cific factors/conditions that shape individuals' health experiences, the population-based labels center on systematic, structural, and macro-level challenges faced by specific populations. For example, gender (equity) is a social determinant of health that result in women's health disparities; by contrast, women (and pregnant women in particular) are considered to be a vulnerable population due to their lack of represen-tation in medical research (Dresser, 1992; Lyerly et al., 2008).

In the following sections, we use *health disparity populations* (HDPs) as an umbrella term for all groups that face systematic, unique challenges and disparities in all stages of care (i.e., access, process, and outcomes). We also use *stigma* in the expanded sense to include attitudes (e.g., prejudice), behaviors (e.g., discrimination), and impacts (e.g., unequal power) against certain groups that are situated within situational, local, and cultural contexts (Phelan et al., 2008; Thornicroft et al., 2007). It is beyond the scope of the book to examine the specific disparities and unique challenges faced by each unique group. Rather, our goal is to provide a conceptual framework to facilitate the under-standing of health disparities faced by these groups and interventions that may apply.

III.   Cultural Approaches to Health Disparities

The literature on health disparities is extensive. Some researchers have urged that the literature should move beyond identifying the patterns of disparities and begin to identify the solutions (Srinivasan & Williams, 2014). To achieve meaningful solutions, Lo and Stacey (2008) argue that we must:

1. broaden our understanding of HDPs' culture (i.e., culture is not limited to individ-ual traits, beliefs, or values but also encompass cultural orientations);
2. conceptualize culture both systematically and flexibly (i.e., culture, social struc-tures, and their participants can exert influences on each other in response to his-torical forces as well as dynamic interactions); and
3. recognize how social actors can hold various cultural perspectives and "mix-and-match" various perspectives to meet situational demands (i.e., cultural perfor-mance is contingent and context-bound).

In the following section, our goals are to (a) situate the patterns of health disparities through different approaches to culture, (b) examine relevant concepts under different approaches, and (c) explore possible solutions for such disparities.

A. Culture as Group

There are extensive and comprehensive studies of health disparities among different racial groups (Williams & Mohammed, 2009). Minorities are disproportionately impacted by health disparities because they are often socially disadvantaged in other areas, which can compromise their health and healthcare services. For example, during the 2020 COVID-19 pandemic, racial/ethnic minorities were found to be dying at a higher rate than the general population (Devlin, 2020; Yancy, 2020). Researchers have argued that the prevalence of co-morbidity (e.g., other pre-existing conditions that compromise one's immune system, such as diabetes and hypertension), lower socioeconomic status (e.g., multigenerational family cohabitation), and other societal inequalities (e.g., lower-wage jobs at the service/hospitality industry, part-time jobs that do not provide health insurance, and incarceration disparities) all contribute to minorities' experiences of disparities in health *and* other areas in life (Perry et al., 2020).

Because racial/ethnic categories are often highly correlated with other social determinants of health, researchers have relied on racial/ethnic categories as a proxy for other variables. However, such an approach fails to recognize the real issues at stake and can create biases toward ethnic/racial and gender groups. Though it is impossible to identify all causes of disparities and biases, our goal is to inspire and challenge our readers to identify different pathways to health disparities.

1. Lack of Inclusion in Medical Research

Racial/ethnic minorities and various groups (e.g., women and children) experience health disparities as a result of the lack of inclusion and representation in medical research. Their absence in medical research was partially attributable to historical discrimination, sociocultural biases, and biopolitical paradigms (Epstein, 2007). **Biopolitical paradigms** are defined as "frameworks of ideas, standards, formal procedures, and unarticulated understandings that specify how concerns about health, medicine, and the body are made the simultaneous foci of biomedicine and state policy" (Epstein, 2007, p. 17). As the field of medicine and governmental policymakers contemplate the appropriate participants for medical research, their decisions reflect the intersections of "*knowledge formation* (how medical truths about human beings are uncovered), *the politics of institutional change* (how social movements and other political actors transform scientific, governmental, and corporate practices), and *the making of identity and difference* (how the human population is divided and what meaning is assigned to stratifying terms such as race and gender)" (Epstein, 2007, p. 18). In short, by excluding specific groups, members of those groups were made invisible in the sociopolitical structure of the larger society and their interests silenced in medicine.

Women and children traditionally have been absent in medical research. Until the mid-1980s, medical scientists often studied only White, middle-aged men, assuming that conclusions drawn from studying them can be generalized to the entire population (Epstein, 2007). Before then, children were often viewed as "miniature adults" (who require lower dosages – though the exact dose was approximated as it was not systematically nor rigorously studied). Similarly, women were considered inferior "specimens" due to their hormonal fluctuations that could create noise when interpreting findings (Dusenbery, 2018; Epstein, 2007). In fact, many researchers traditionally have worked only with male lab animals, fearing that the hormonal cycles of female animals would interfere with accurate findings (Rabin, 2014). Dr. Healy, former director of the National Institutes of Health, explained, "We tended to want to reduce the human to that 60 kilogram white male, 35 years of age, and make that the *normative standard* – and have everything extrapolated from that tidy, neat mean, 'the average American male'" [emphasis added] (Epstein, 2007, p. 1). This phenomenon is called "**androcentrism**" – where "the male health model is in the center of medical knowledge," marginalizing all others' perspectives (Recio-Barbero & Pérez-Fernandez, 2019, p. 868).

By constructing "(White) men" as a universal category that is inclusive of all people, researchers made little effort to distinguish children, women, or minorities, assuming that they would share the same mechanisms and responses to treatments the same way. Dusenbery (2018) explained,

> [W]omen had been left out of many of the largest, most important clinical studies conducted in the last couple of decades. The Baltimore Longitudinal Study of Aging, which began in 1958 and purported to explore "normal human aging," didn't enroll any women for the first twenty years it ran. The Physicians' Health Study, which had recently concluded that taking a daily aspirin may reduce the risk of heart disease? Conducted in 22,071 men and zero women. ...
>
> The default to studying men at times veered into absurdity: in the early sixties, observing that women tended to have lower rates of heart disease until their estrogen levels dropped after menopause, researchers conducted the first trial to look at whether supplementation with the hormone was an effective preventive treatment. The study enrolled 8,341 men and no women. ... An NIH-supported pilot study from Rockefeller University that looked at how obesity affected breast and uterine cancer didn't enroll a single woman. (p. 25)

Dr. Janine Austin Clayton, Associate Director for Research on Women's Health at the National Institutes of Health, concluded, "We literally know less about every aspect of female biology compared to male biology" (Rabin, 2014).

Concerns about the potential negative impacts on women, children, and minorities who are presumed to be more "vulnerable" than adult men often dominate the decisions to exclude these populations in medical research (Epstein, 2007). For example, the U.S. Food and Drug Administration (FDA) instituted a rule in 1977 to formally exclude women "of childbearing potential" from many drug trials, out of concern that an experimental drug might bring harm to a fetus if a woman became pregnant during the course of a clinical trial (Mastroianni et al., 1994). It was not until 1993, the NIH Revitalization Act was signed into law, requiring women and minorities to be included in NIH-funded studies beginning with the fiscal year 1995 (Epstein, 2007). Congress passed the Pediatric Research Equity Act (2003), allowing the FDA to compel drug companies to test products on children and provide pediatric labeling information (U.S. Food and Drug Administration, 2018). Alternatively, some argued that medical studies should not be required to recruit minorities because such institutional policies and regulations make minorities more likely to be exploited by researchers (Epstein, 2007).

Minorities' lack of representation in medical research is a complicated issue because there are historical and sociopolitical factors influencing the presence of minorities in medical research. First, minorities have been found to hold a deep distrust of health authorities who often hold alternative agendas that do not have their best interests in mind (see also Minority Groups' Historical Distrust of Healthcare Authorities in Chapter 7). A prominent case involved the acquisition of blood samples from the Havasupai Tribe by Arizona State University. The Havasupai Tribe (Havasupai: Havsuw' Baaja) is a Native American tribe that has lived in the Grand Canyon for over 1000 years (Charley et al., 2005). The Havasupai Tribe has 639 members, inhabiting a vast reservation at the bottom of the Grand Canyon, Arizona (Inter Tribal Council of Arizona, 2020). The Havasupai Tribe has the fourth highest prevalence of diabetes (46%) among any group in the world, affecting 45% of men and 50% of women in the tribe, a rate three times higher than other Native American Group (Van Assche et al., 2013). Interested in finding solutions to their high rates of diabetes among tribal members and determining whether they have a genetic predisposition for diabetes, over 200 Havasupai Indians offerred blood samples to researchers between 1990–1994 (Drabiak-Syed, 2010). The research team was unable to find a genetic link to diabetes, but the team then used the blood samples to conduct other studies to identify genetic causes of schizophrenia, the degree of inbreeding, and the geographical origins of the tribe (Drabiak-Syed, 2010). Researchers suggested that the high degree of inbreeding may have contributed to the increased risk of schizophrenia for Havasupai (Markow & Martin, 1993). Another study confirmed that Havasupai ancestors had crossed over the frozen Bering Sea into North America, which conflicted with traditional Havasupai stories that they had always lived in North America, specifically the Grand Canyon (Munzer, 2013). In total, 15 of the 23 academic publications that relied on Havasupai blood as the primary source material focused on schizophrenia, inbreeding, and migration (Rubin, 2004).

The Havasupai felt betrayed as they assumed that studies using their blood samples were limited to diabetes-related research. Studies on schizophrenia and inbreeding were considered offensive and discriminatory. Studies on their migration patterns, however, posed a risk to their tribal origin myth and even land rights (Harmon, 2010). A tribal member explained, "When people tell us, 'No, [the Grand Canyon] is not where you are from,' and your own blood says so – it is confusing to us. It hurts the elders who have been telling these stories to our grandchildren" (Harmon, 2010).

Minorities' bodies – their labor and their physical bodies, including genetic materials – are often the objects of (and subject to) exploitation by other groups they have trusted (see Chapter 11). As a result, minorities have become increasingly reluctant to participate in medical research for fear of further exploitation.

The lack of inclusion and representation in medical research, however, can reinforce healthcare disparities. In 2014, Attorney General of Hawaii filed a lawsuit for false, deceptive, and unfair marketing practices related to Plavix, a very popular antiplatelet drug (*Hawai'i ex rel. Louie v. Bristol-Myers Squibb Co.,* 2014). This is one of the first pharmacogenomics lawsuits focusing on differences in genotype according to ancestry (Bonham et al., 2016). It's been reported that "38–79% of Pacific Islanders and

40–50% of East Asians may respond poorly to Plavix due to a genetic predisposition to insufficiently metabolize the drug" (Abercrombie & Louie, 2014, p. 1). However, Bristol-Myers Squibb, the manufacturer of Plavix, continued to encourage prescriptions of the drug at a higher dose despite knowing that it has diminished or no effect on approximately 30% of the populations in Hawaii (Abercrombie & Louie, 2014). Without knowledge of their own genetic predisposition, 30% of the population in Hawaii would not have realized that Aspirin, which costs 1% of the price of Plavix, may be a more effective and cheaper medicine for their heart conditions. In this case, minority groups' knowledge of their genetic traits and gene-treatment interactions are essential in not only developing an effective treatment for the group but also critical in holding commercial enterprises accountable for exploitation of minority groups.

Similarly, despite the large number of women who take oral contraceptives or take pharmaceutical drugs during their pregnancy, there are few systematic efforts to investigate how newly approved drugs can create dangerous interactions that compromise women's health (Dusenbery, 2018; Recio-Barbero & Pérez-Fernandez, 2019). The lack of knowledge concerning treatments for chronic illness (e.g., diabetes and autoimmune disease) and mental illness (e.g., depression and bipolar disorder) during pregnancy and/or the corresponding impacts to fetuses have contributed to women's experiences of health disparities.

2. Exploitations by Group-Based Products and Policies

Minorities and women also are vulnerable to commercial exploitation in the healthcare marketplace. By marketing their products as race/gender-specific, manufactures may gain additional profits or advantages. One of the examples of such exploitation is the invention of race-specific medication, BiDil. In 2005, the U.S. Food and Drug Administration approved the first "ethnic drug," BiDil, to treat congestive heart failure in African Americans – only African Americans. NitroMed, the manufacturer of BiDil, sought a patent by combining two generic drugs that have been prescribed to patients (regardless of their race) for decades into a single pill. Because NitroMed was not able to establish BiDil's efficacy in the general population, it reinvented the drug as a race-specific medication and conducted clinical trials with only African Americans. Because the patent is race-specific, it also allows NitroMed to control the market longer – 13 years longer beyond the general methods (Sankar & Kahn, 2005). There is no scientific evidence to suggest that BiDil is designed to target specific genes or has demonstrated significant differences in health outcomes for different ethnic groups (Kahn, 2014; Roberts, 2011). Nevertheless, as pharmaceutical companies contemplate the commercial potential for "ethnic drugs" and the corresponding intellectual property rights advantages, the "biomedicalization" of race or ethnicity as a biological condition (as opposed to a social construct) can further increase the health disparities for marginalized populations who often face imbalance of information, power, finance, and medical research (Roberts, 2011). Sankar and Kahn (2005) concluded BiDil's success is "one not of personalized medicine but of exploiting race to gain commercial and regulatory advantage in the pharmaceutical marketplace" (p. 455) and that "[by] exploiting race in the service of product promotion, it distorts public understanding of health disparities and of efforts to address them" (p. 462).

Similarly, women are not unfamiliar with paying additional costs for gender-based policies, products, and services. **Pink tax** refers to pricing strategies and governmental policies that increase transactional costs for women (e.g., a higher price or higher tax; Yazıcıoğlu, 2018). Women in the United States make about 20% less than men (Blau & Kahn, 2017). Compared to earnings of White men, White and Black women make 18.5% and 34.7% less, respectively (Hegewisch & Hartmann, 2019). However, women pay higher interest rates despite having higher credit ratings than men (Goodman et al., 2016). In addition, women regularly pay a higher price for consumer goods and everyday products, including toys, shampoo, clothes, haircuts, dry cleaning, and even adult diapers (Dreher, 2019). It is worth noting that African American women are subject to additional costs to their already pink-taxed hair products and haircuts for their "textured," natural hair (Bryant, 2019; Evans, 2019). Compared to men, women's reduced earnings and added costs in their everyday lives can contribute to their experiences of health disparities.

Recently, **tampon tax**, a particular form of the pink tax, has been gaining attention in state legislatures in the United States and around the world (Crawford & Spivack, 2017; see Figure 12.1). Tampon tax refers to an umbrella term for the sales, value-added tax imposed on menstrual hygiene products (Crawford & Spivack, 2017). All U.S. states exempt non-luxury necessities like groceries and prescription medicine (Dreher, 2019). For example, Viagra, an erectile dysfunction medicine, is not taxed in any state except Illinois; similarly, Rogaine, a product for hair loss, is exempt from tax in 8 states as an over-the-counter treatment that does not require a prescription (Qiu, 2017). However, although menstrual cycles are unavoidable, making feminine hygiene products a necessity, 35 states charge sales tax on tampons and feminine pads (Zraick, 2019). Online campaigns such as "Don't Tax My Period" in Australia and the multinational "Bloody Disgrace" movement highlighted the gender inequities faced by women as they manage their everyday lives (Crawford & Spivack, 2017). It is estimated that a woman in her 60s will pay nearly $82,000 in fees that men do not have to pay – pink tax adds up (Dreher, 2019).

Women in the United States also face additional costs in managing their pregnancy. Currently, the United States is the only industrial country that does not mandate paid maternity leave, a striking policy compared to the 183 nations that guarantee paid leave for new mothers and the 79 nations that guarantee paid leave for new fathers (National Partnership for Women & Families, 2016). However, when women are able to take advantage of paid maternity leave, there is a lower risk of maternal and infant re-hospitalization and an increase in positive maternal health behavior, such as

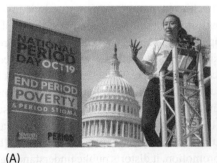
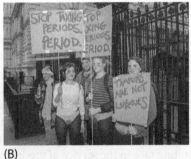

(A)   (B)

Figure 12.1 Protest against tampon tax. (A) Nadya Okamoto, founder of PERIOD, a non-profit organization working for menstrual equity, speaks at the Capitol during a National Period Day rally on Saturday, Oct.19, 2019, in Washington to raise awareness of period poverty and call for the elimination of the tampon tax. *Source:* AP photos (B) Campaigners at Downing Street to protest against the tampon tax. *Source:* Peter Maclaine/WENN.com/AGE Fotostock

exercise and stress management (Jou et al., 2018). In contrast, working mothers with limited options for paid leave may have to return to work immediately after childbirth, quit employment, or take unpaid leave, all of which can negatively impact not only the new mothers' health but also the overall wellbeing for other family members, including the infant and other children (Isaac et al., 2017). Recognizing that having children may pose risks to career trajectories, female college professors reported planning their delivery dates for their children to be born in the month of May (so that they can take advantage of the summer months) or to wait to have children after being tenured (Armenti, 2004a, 2004b). A study of 20 low- and middle-income countries found that each additional month of paid maternal leave was associated with approximately eight fewer infant deaths per 1,000 live births (Nandi et al., 2016). In short, without a national paid maternity leave mandate, women in the United States are left to shoulder the burden of childbearing and childrearing. This burden impacts not only their own and their children's health, but it also entails long-term negative impacts on their career trajectories and income.

B. Culture as Speech Community

1. Language and Cultural Barriers

When conceptualizing cultural differences as differences in speech communities, the literature has traditionally relied on patients with language barriers to illustrate the challenges to cross-cultural care. Patients with language barriers have been found to have low health literacy (McKee & Paasche-Orlow, 2012; Sentell & Braun, 2012). However, individuals' language-discordant status is a stronger predictor than their low health literacy status for poor health communication and problematic health outcomes (Sentell & Braun, 2012; Sudore et al., 2009). These findings suggest that the impacts of language barriers supersede the impacts of low health literacy for poor health outcomes. In an extensive review, Terui (2017) explained that patients with language barriers can experience health disparities through direct and indirect pathways that impact their *access* to care, *process* of provider-patient interactions, and *outcomes* of healthcare services. For example, patients with language barriers are likely to delay care (Karliner et al., 2012) and feel less satisfied with the quality of their care and interactions with providers (Harmsen et al., 2008; Ngo-Metzger et al., 2009). They are also more likely to experience problematic outcomes, such as having unplanned emergency department (ED) visits within 72 hours after discharging from the ED (Ngai et al., 2016).

Although many studies have noted that **language-concordant care** (i.e., providers and patients share the same language) result in higher ratings for patient satisfaction (Gany et al., 2007; Green et al., 2005), patient compliance (Manson, 1988), and perceived quality of care (Ngo-Metzger et al., 2007), such effects may be a function of rapport, rather than an indicator of quality care. Patients' illness experiences and concerns are socially and culturally situated in their everyday life. A short-term class on medical Spanish, though valuable, is unlikely to replace the need for professional interpreters. In fact, researchers found that ED physicians with medical Spanish training make minor errors in 50% of their consultations and major errors (e.g., misunderstanding of vocabulary or the duration of symptoms) in 14% of their consultations

(Prince & Nelson, 1995). Another study found that although short-term language courses allow providers to develop better inquiry skills and higher confidence during medical encounters, there is little change in their ability to provide emotional support (Farnill et al., 1997). In other words, medical Spanish may give providers false confidence that they are able to communicate directly with their patients, resulting in problematic assessments about the quality of care. Diamond and Jacobs (2010) concluded that "teaching 'Medical Spanish' or related courses may actually contribute to health care disparities if clinicians begin using these non-English language skills inappropriately with patients" (p. s189).

Interpreters have been traditionally viewed as the solution for language and cultural barriers in healthcare settings (Schouten et al., 2020). A comprehensive review by Diamond et al. (2019) found that when patients with limited English proficiency were provided with interpreters, including professional and untrained interpreters, they are likely to have better health outcomes in patient-reported measures (e.g., satisfaction and understanding of diagnosis) and objective measures (e.g., glycemic control and blood pressure). The literature is clear that there are positive impacts on the quality of care when professional interpreters are present (Greenbaum & Flores, 2004; Lee et al., 2006). There are also good reasons to recommend and rely on professional interpreters as part of ethical practices (Hadziabdic et al., 2010; Jacobs et al., 2010). In some studies, researchers found that that the quality of healthcare services and health outcomes of interpreted patients are equivalent to and, at times, *better* than that of English-speaking patients (Bernstein et al., 2002; Gany et al., 2007; Hampers & McNulty, 2002).

These findings are intriguing because language-concordant provider-patient interactions are often conceptualized as the gold standard for provider-patient interactions. However, low health literacy is a common problem in the United States, where 36% of the population has limited health literacy (National Network of Libraries of Medicine, 2013). An **interpreter-as-conduit** model is a traditional model that is incorporated many codes of ethics guiding interpreters' practices (Dysart-Gale, 2005; Loach, 2019). The model requires interpreters to adopt a passive, non-interfering role in medical encounters, faithfully transferring information from one language to another. In other words, interpreters are the voices of others and do not hold personal opinions or agendas (Hsieh, 2008). However, an interpreter-as-conduit model is likely to maintain patients' barriers to care by replicating patients' low health literacy in provider-patient interactions (Hsieh & Kramer, 2012; Watermeyer, 2011). Alternatively, interpreters, as communicative experts in bilingual, cross-cultural care, may be able to anticipate patients' communicative needs, convey providers' therapeutic goals, and facilitate provider-patient interactions in a way that enhances other speakers' abilities to seek, process, and utilize health information to make appropriate health decisions (Butow et al., 2012; Hsieh, 2013; Hsieh et al., 2013; Watermeyer, 2011). It is possible for interpreter-mediated medical encounters to be comparable and even better than language-concordant medical encounters (see Figure 12.2).

Interpreters are not passive conduits transferring information from one language to another. Rather, they are active agents in provider-patient interactions, mediating providers' and patients' communitive goals, including task, identity, and relationship goals (Guntzviller et al., 2017; Guntzviller & Wang, 2019; Hsieh, 2008, 2016; Hsieh & Nicodemus, 2015; Raymond, 2014). They have to exercise judgment in word choice, tone, and metalinguistic aspects even if that choice is to be as passive as a conduit. As

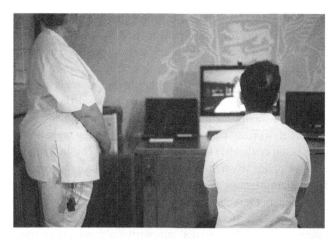

Figure 12.2   Remote interpreting. Many hospitals use remote interpreters to provide interpreting services to patients. LanguageLine solutions, one of the largest service agencies in the United States, has 11,000 professionally trained interpreters fluent in more than 240 languages, including American Sign Language. *Source:* Picture-Alliance/dpa/AGE Fotostock

Harold Lasswell (1948) noted, there are many implications to a message such as, who says what, to whom, in what channel, and we add, when, why, and how, and with what effect. For example, in American Sign Language (ASL), language production involves articulations of the hands, face, and body. Unfortunately, non-signing physicians have been reported misdiagnosing "an expressive Deaf person as having tics, inappropriate affection, and personality and mood disorder" (Barnett, 1999, p. 19), resulting in Deaf patients' negative experiences and avoidance behaviors (Steinberg et al., 2002). Miscommunication can arise when different cultures do not share the same understanding about the appropriateness and meanings of emotional displays and social norms (Jack et al., 2012; Koopmann-Holm & Matsumoto, 2011; Ozono et al., 2010). For example, although it may be appropriate for an oncologist to tease or joke with a patient with cancer in the United States to develop rapport, people from Japan or France would find it inappropriate or offensive to use humorous talk in such a context (Hsieh & Terui, 2015). As a result, interpreters play a critical role in mediating multiple participants' communicative goals to achieve quality care.

In the **Model of Bilingual Health Communication**, Hsieh (2016) proposed that interpreter-mediated medical encounters are goal-oriented communicative activities, requiring providers, patients, and interpreters to actively negotiate their task, identity, and relational goals to achieve quality and equality of care. Rather than prescribing a fixed role for interpreters (or providers), the model argues that both interpreters and providers need to be responsive and adaptive to the dynamic and emergent nature of provider-patient interactions and maintain clear boundaries for each participant's voice. In short, the model argues that successful interpreter-mediated medical encounters are not dependent on whether an interpreter faithfully or accurately transfers information from one language to another (i.e., silencing interpreters' presence, agenda, and voice). Rather, successful bilingual health communication requires providers, patients, and interpreters to accommodate, negotiate, and co-evolve with one another, allowing them to develop mutually agreeable and effective strategies to achieve their collaborative goal of optimal care.

For example, Guntzviller, Jensen, and Carreno (2017) found that when bilingual children serve as interpreters for their Spanish-speaking parents, they adopt a *team-effort model*, working together as a team to utilize both parties' strength, compensate for partner limitations, and achieve mutually desirable outcomes. Bilingual children worked to enhance their parents' self-efficacy while their parents assisted to improve the children's health literacy. When their children believed that interpreting was a shared task and responsibility for the parent-child dyad, Spanish-speaking mothers reported less frequent depressive symptoms even when they were ambivalent about such assessments (Kam et al., 2017). In contrast, bilingual children reported more frequent depressive symptoms when their mothers strongly disagree with their belief that interpreting for the family was a shared task and responsibility (Kam et al., 2017). In fact, Spanish-speaking mothers' support for their children's role as a family interpreter is a protective factor against these low-income, bilingual adolescents' depression – if the children were aware of the parents' supportive attitudes (Guntzviller & Wang, 2019). The parents and children thrived together when they coordinated and collaborated with one another to achieve mutually shared goals.

Finally, it is important to note that not all patients who face language barriers share similar experiences. Hsieh (2018) argued that (a) language discordance is a social phenomenon that may entail diverging meanings and experiences in different countries; (b) language-discordant patients may not share similar experiences even if they are in the same country; and (c) disparities in language concordance may be confounded with other disparities and cultural particulars that are unique to a host society. For example, in the United States, discordant language care generally means that the patient has limited English proficiency (rather than the provider using a second language); in contrast, in Japan, discordant language care may mean that both patients and their physicians communicate in their second language (e.g., English; Terui, 2017). In addition, depending on patients' ethnicity and/or country of origin, language discordant patients may experience preferential treatment (e.g., an English-speaking, White patient from France) or potential discrimination (e.g., a Bantu-speaking, Black patient from Zimbabwe) in a host society even though both would be considered to receive language-discordant care (i.e., providers and patients do not share the same language; Hsieh, 2018; Terui, 2017).

English-speaking patients' experiences of language barriers may be very different from those who do not speak English because English is the dominant language for medical education and healthcare settings in many countries around the world. For example, all healthcare providers in Taiwan are able to communicate in English through written, if not spoken English, because medical textbooks are often in English. Also, patients' medical records are kept in English, and prescriptions are typically written in English. A physician in Taiwan can comfortably rely on medical English to identify symptoms and write down diagnosis and treatment for an English-speaking patient to facilitate her understanding of the illness. In other words, when seeking healthcare services in Taiwan, a blue-collar patient from the Philippines, which adopts English as one of her two official languages, is more likely to have better communication than a blue-collar patient from Thailand. In fact, a Mandarin-only speaking physician in Taiwan even argued that it's harder to explain certain diagnoses to local patients who only speak Taiwanese, which does not have terms for the corresponding medical concepts, than to an English-speaking patient (Hsieh, 2018). In short, when conceptualizing health disparities as a result of language barriers and cultural differences, we need to consider patients' experiences in contexts.

2. Speech Community-based Normative Beliefs

Language barriers and cultural differences are some of the most observable challenges in cross-cultural care. However, health disparities due to differences in speech communities need not be about people who speak different languages. For example, gender stereotypes and gender role expectations about how men and women communicate differently (e.g., men are more stoic and women are more emotive) can lead to disparities in the diagnosis and treatment of illness that compromise women's quality of care. For example, historically, women's complaint of illness symptoms often is viewed as psychological distress or somatic symptoms. **Somatic symptoms** refer to physical experiences of illness that are caused by psychiatric conditions, such as depression, anxiety, or emotional distress. **Somatization** refers to "the propensity to experience and express psychiatric disorders and psychosocial distress as somatic distress and discomfort" (Wool & Barsky, 1994, p. 445). Because women are traditionally viewed as more emotionally expressive (or volatile), women's illness experiences are often attributed as psychiatric disorders, rather than a legitimate complaint of illness. Dusenbery (2018) explained,

> The terminology has morphed – from *hysteria* to *somatization* and *conversion disorders* to "*medically unexplained symptoms*" – but the idea has remained remarkably unchanged. And the idea that women are especially prone to such psychogenic symptoms has endured too. In other words, a stereotype that women's symptoms are likely to be "all in their heads" has been hard baked into medical knowledge itself. ... Women's symptoms are not taken seriously because medicine doesn't know as much about their bodies and health problems. And medicine doesn't know as much about their bodies and health problems because it doesn't take their symptoms seriously. [emphasis added] (p. 12)

These disparities are caused by differences in speech communities due to our normative beliefs of gender stereotypes and gender roles. For example, even though women are more likely than men to die from a heart attack, compared to male patients who also reported stressful life events, physicians are less likely to attribute symptoms to possible cardiac causes for female patients reporting stressful life events (Martin et al., 1998). In other words, when stress was reported, only female (but not male) patients' cardiac symptoms were misinterpreted or discounted, shifting from a diagnosis of coronary heart disease to a psychogenic disorder (Chiaramonte & Friend, 2006). Because women are perceived to be more emotive (and thus, their report is less "factual" or "reliable"), female patient's report of their pain is often discounted. As men's report of pain is situated in their gender stereotype (e.g., "stoic men" and "brave men"), men's report of their pain is taken seriously and more likely to refer to additional lab tests (Samulowitz et al., 2018). When men appear frustrated or angry about their pain management – they must be in serious pain; if they appear stoic, their complaint is equally real – because that's just the way they talk (Dusenbery, 2018). In contrast, women's reports of their pain are interpreted through gender stereotypes and social norms (e.g., "emotional" or "hysterical" women who are crybabies). As a result, if they appear emotional (e.g., crying or expressing anger/frustration), they are just being feminine and are not perceived to be experiencing a high level of pain; but if they calmly discuss their pain in an objective manner, they must not be experiencing that much pain after all (Dusenbery, 2018; Samulowitz et al., 2018). The gender bias is so pervasive and normative that adults are more likely to rate a child to be experiencing more pain when the child was described as a boy as opposed to a girl – despite identical behaviors and circumstances (Earp et al., 2019).

Because women's reports of their illness are more likely to be attributed to psychological problems and providers do not perceive their report of symptoms as reliable as men's, women also face disparities in diagnosis and treatment. For example, Lyratzopoulos et al. (2013) found that being a woman significantly *doubled* the likelihood of requiring or more pre-referral visits with their primary physicians before being diagnosed with bladder cancer by a specialist. For renal cancer, women's odds of requiring *three or more* pre-referral visits is nearly double that of men's as well. Compared to men, women experience delayed diagnosis (i.e., longer duration from the first presentation of symptoms to the official diagnosis) in a wide range of illnesses, resulting in prolonging unnecessary, avoidable suffering (Dusenbery, 2018).

Traditionally, research on health disparities and social determinants of health have often centered on the unique conditions of the HDPs. However, this line of research demonstrates that addressing health disparities is not limited to fixing what is "wrong" with the HDPs (e.g., low socioeconomic status or language barriers). Rather, our normative beliefs can result in bias and discrimination that contribute to HDPs' unnecessary and avoidable suffering. The solution to health disparities may require critical interrogation of our *natural attitudes* (see also Chapter 4), including our prejudice and biases.

C. Culture as Worldview

1. Minority Stress Rooted in Hostile Lived Environments

Worldviews are "what people in a community take as given realities, the maps they have of reality that they use for living" (Hiebert, 2008, p. 15). From this perspective, minorities and HDPs may hold very different worldviews than those of dominant groups. **Minority stress** is defined as "the excess stress to which individuals from stigmatized social categories are exposed as a result of their social, often a minority, position" (Meyer, 2003, p. 675). **Minority stress theory** proposes that minority groups experience health disparities because they are subject to constant, perpetual, and/or unique stressors in everyday life as a result of stigma, prejudice, and discrimination in the larger society due to their minority status (Meyer, 2003). Recognizing that they live in a hostile social environment, members of minorities regularly (a) experience external, objective stressful events and conditions (chronic and acute), (b) anticipate (and are vigilant against) reoccurrences of such events, and (c) internalize negative societal attitudes against themselves (Meyer, 2003). This state of affairs begins even before minorities are born. Minority mothers experiencing stress during pregnancy effects birth weight and mortality of babies. In fact, one study found that Black women with higher socioeconomic status and living in White neighborhoods had the worst outcomes (i.e., 14.5% infants have low birth weight); in contrast, Black women

with high socioeconomic status *and* living in Black neighborhoods had the best outcomes that are comparable to their White counterparts (i.e., 4% infants have low birth
weight; Kothari et al., 2016). In short, socioeconomic status alone is insufficient to
counteract race-based disparities (Kothari et al., 2016).

Similarly, concerns about "driving while Black," potential discrimination/harassment
at traffic stops, and corresponding criminal charges can effectively generate fear, anger,
and humiliation among Black people leading them to "voluntarily" limit their movement (Harris, 1999). Repeated exposure to and witnessing of aggressive policing that
results in fatal injuries of Black men and the injustice of the legal system (e.g., when a
grand jury failed to indict the police officer who killed Eric Garner, an unarmed Black
man who uttered "I can't breathe" during the arrest) can trigger traumatic reactions for
many Black people, with the cumulative, collective effects that can be passed across
generations (Aymer, 2016; Bryant-Davis et al., 2017). During the 2020 COVID-19 pandemic, many protesters flooded state congresses as the society contemplated whether to
reopen the economy. Dr. Samuel K. Roberts, director of Columbia University's Institute
for Research in African American Studies and an epidemiologist, commented,

> If you look at who these [protesters] are, I don't know many Black folks of any
> political stripe that would want to be in that crowd. ... These are the same people
> who called Obama all sorts of names, racist epithets, a lot of them overlap with
> the Tea Party, which was a very racially charged movement. Nothing about this
> movement is really black friendly. (Charles, 2020, para. 4)

Such experiences lead minorities to hold unique worldviews about their lived realities
that contribute to their health disparities.

Minority stress is a result of *objective* realities (i.e., objective stressors that do not
depend on individuals' interpretation, perception, or appraisals; e.g., public stigma,
chronic strains, and everyday microaggressions) and *subjective* experiences (e.g., self-
stigma, expectations of rejection and discrimination, and concealment of stigmatized
identity; see also Chapter 8). Minority stress has been extensively investigated in
LGBT+ populations, demonstrating that one's experiences with minority stress can
negatively impact one's overall well-being, including both physical and mental health
(Hatzenbuehler & Pachankis, 2016; Lick et al., 2013). Miller et al. (2007) explained,
"From early in childhood to late in adult hood, chronic stress is accompanied by worse
health, and the magnitude of this effect is substantial: In some cases, exposure to
chronic stress triples or quadruples the chances of an adverse medical outcome" (p.25).

2. Protective Effects of Ethnic Pride and Resilience

Although the literature has extensive evidence of minorities' health disparities,
researchers have noticed several intriguing phenomena. First, pride for one's minority
status has a protective effect against risk behaviors and is associated with greater well-
being, life satisfaction, and health status (also see **identity affirmation** in Chapter 8).
Unlike **ethnic differentiation**, which focuses on in-group versus out-group distinctions and a preference for in-group members, **ethnic pride** refers to one's attachment
to his or her ethnic group as a whole, feeling connected and belonging to the group and
expressing interests in the culture, history, and customs of the group (Valk & Karu,
2001). Because ethnic pride does not emphasize in-group/out-group distinctions but
highlights the role of community and solidarity, it promotes a sense of belonging

and minimizes feelings of isolation and marginalization by the larger society. Ethnic pride reduces smoking behaviors, alcohol use, and drug use for adolescents (Castro et al., 2009; Kong et al., 2012; Kulis et al., 2002). For African American and Latino adolescents, positive feelings about their racial/ethnic group identities are consistently associated with positive psychosocial adjustment and academic performance (Rivas-Drake et al., 2014). For African American and Latino young adults who are incarcerated, individuals who have high ethnic pride are (a) less likely to engage in illegal activities and be reincarcerated, and (b) more likely to hold positive attitudes toward avoiding violence in situations of conflict (Upadhyayula et al., 2017). Research also shows that attempts by those discriminated against and suffering undue stress to "fight back," to engage forces that cause stress and inequality improves mental and physical health. Resisting unfairness helps us feel engaged, not hopelessly depressed, and feel better (Fredriksen-Goldsen et al., 2017; Williams, 2018; Williams et al., 1997).

Researchers have argued that people have a "**psychological immune system**" that (a) is defensively protective and (b) promotes healing (Rachman, 2016). The psychological immune system can involve automatic, hidden processes that are triggered when one faces potential threats as well as purposeful, intentional interventions that proactively tackle potential stressors (Rachman, 2016). As a result, ethnic pride can function as a mechanism of the psychological immune system, helping minorities to maintain resilience against minority stress in a hostile social environment. **Resilience** is defined as "the capacity for adaptation to challenges that threaten the function or development of a dynamic system, manifested in pathways and patterns of positive adaptation during or following exposure to significant risk or adversity" (Motti-Stefanidi & Masten, 2017, pp. 20-21). In other words, resilience is an outcome of successful adaptation to adversity (Zautra et al., 2010). But adaptation does not mean simple conformity to a "mainstream" dominant culture especially if that means "deculturizing" and/or "unlearning" one's self. Rather adaptation in nature or in human behavior means taking on a new form or pattern that enhances survival (Kramer, 2019; Liu & Kramer, 2019).

Resilience can mitigate negative health effects and act as buffers against minority stress (Breslow et al., 2015), allowing individuals to develop self-acceptance, identity pride, self-esteem, and emotion-oriented coping (Grossman et al., 2011; Motti-Stefanidi & Masten, 2017). Meyer (2015) argued, "at its core, resilience is a process of stress buffering" – it's about how people respond when confronted with stressors/adversities (p. 210; see also buffering effects of social support in Chapter 10). Resilience has been associated with a wide range of variables, including personal agency, locus of control, hardiness, sense of coherence, hopefulness, and posttraumatic growth (Almedom, 2005; Meyer, 2015; O'Connor & Graham, 2019). From this perspective, (individual-level) resilience echoes with the concept of **self-mastery**, which is defined as "the sense that individuals feel that they can overcome obstacles and challenging circumstances based on their own effort" (Hobfoll et al., 2002, p. 856). Reflecting on veterans' responses to traumatic experiences, Waysman et al. (2001) concluded, "Those who view themselves as in charge of their fate (control), who are committed to meaningful goals and activities (commitment), and who view stress as a surmountable challenge are more likely in the long run to integrate the trauma into their lives and to enjoy a satisfactory level of adjustment" (p. 545). More importantly, resilience is situated in contexts and may take on different forms for different individuals. For example, for teens living in public housing and poverty, rebellions and resistance against social norms and identity expectations may be empowering, as they find a voice to call out the social injustice and inequalities in everyday life (Bottrell, 2009; Factor et al., 2011).

Although resilience has traditionally been studied as an individual trait, researchers have noted that such an approach may be a result of western bias, and even American ideology, which celebrates personal triumph over adversity (Meyer, 2015). A more collectivistic form of resilience has been recognized and studied. **Community resilience** can be essential in how the community, as a whole, develops coping strategies that empower minority members in the face of adversities. For example, **communal coping**, a major contributor to community resilience, refers to the process through which community members pool their resources, appraise the adversity as "our" (versus "my" or "your") problem, and coordinate their individual *and* collective actions to achieve optimal solutions (Lyons et al., 1998). Community resilience involves community efforts to empower its members to develop and sustain well-being and to collaborate with other communities (who share similar interests) in order to further their collective objectives (see Figure 12.3; see also discussions of LGBTQ as a Social Group in Chapter 8).

The **Theory of Resilience and Relational Load** proposes that when people validate their relational partners and family members on an ongoing basis (e.g., effective social support and affection), they accumulate emotional capital and social resources which can then function as a source of resilience during stressful times (Afifi et al., 2016). In a study of Latina/o early adolescents' coping strategies when serving as the

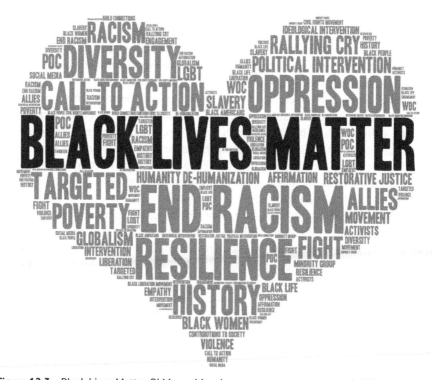

Figure 12.3 Black Lives Matter. BLM provides the necessary momentum to build a community that validates and strengthens positive personal qualities of ethnic pride. *Source*: arloo/123RF

family's interpreters, Kam et al. (2018) found communal copers reported greater efficacy even when they initially reported greater stress. Other family members' assistance and support during stressful events not only buffered their stress but also improved their efficacy when serving as interpreters for the family (Guntzviller et al., 2017; Guntzviller & Wang, 2019; Kam et al., 2018). Hobfoll et al. (2002) argued that such resilience is a result of **communal-mastery**, "the belief that being part of a closely knit social fabric in itself generates successful confrontation with life problems (i.e., 'I succeed because I am part of a social group that values me')" (p. 856). Community resilience can involve tangible resources (e.g., support group, role models, and affirmative policies) and intangible resources (e.g., ethnic pride and other cultural values, such as filial piety) that allow minority members to "tap into the community" and reap the benefits of group membership (Meyer, 2015). From this perspective, community resilience gains its strength through Magic Consciousness, a sense of blood tie, and/or Mythic Connection, and its sense of storied heritage and collective memory, energizing community members through their in-group membership. One can reinforce the other: as children become privy to the family stories and the bestowing of tales from older keepers of the collective biography makes them feel closer to their kin. The stories become their stories and they are initiated into them because they are already hereditary members of the family.

Community resilience, thus, sheds light into the second unique phenomenon of minority groups' experiences of health disparities: **Hispanic paradox** (also called Latino paradox, Hispanic/Latino health paradox, epidemiological paradox, or immigrant health paradox). Hispanic paradox refers to the tendency for Hispanic/Latino populations to have better health and lower mortality that are "paradoxically" comparable, or even better than those of their U.S. non-Hispanic, White counterparts – even though Latinos typically occupy lower socioeconomic status and lower formal educational attainment (Ruiz et al., 2018). There is strong evidence of Hispanic populations' advantage, including infant mortality, lower incidence of most major diseases, longer survival in the context of disease, lower all-cause mortality, and longer life expectancy (Patel et al., 2013; Ruiz et al., 2018). Ruiz et al. (2018) explained, "Hispanic cultural values for family (*familismo*), interpersonal harmony (*simpatía*), and the valuing of elder community members (*respeto*) facilitate greater social integration" (p. 25). This social integration proves to be essential in creating a sense of connectedness between members, and the accumulation of social capital/resources for communal coping (see Figure 12.4).

In other words, community resilience allows Hispanic populations to benefit from their social networks and cultural values, which act as essential buffers to mitigate stress and illness. The effects are particularly salient among individuals who hold strong affiliations with their communities (e.g., less acculturated, high ethnic pride, adopting, and maintaining traditional values). Recently, researchers have found a similar "paradox" in other minority populations (e.g., African Americans, Asian Americans, and immigrants to other countries), noting that their communities provide protective effects by building resilience in their members (John et al., 2012; Mulia et al., 2018; Urquia et al., 2012). At the same time, researchers also have cautioned that using terms like "paradox" oversimplifies the complex patterns, issue-specific nature, and between-(sub)group differences of minority health, masking other very real disparities these populations experience (John et al., 2012).

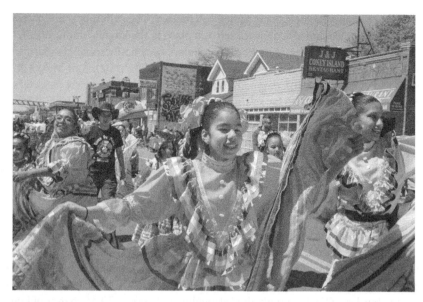

Figure 12.4   Community resilience. The Mexican-American neighborhood of southwest Detroit hosts the Cinco de Mayo parade every year. Such celebrations help the community to build a shared identity, allowing them to thrive as a whole. *Source:* Jim West / Alamy Stock Photo

Suicide is the ultimate failure of the psychological immune system (Rachman, 2016). In 2015, Case and Deaton (2015) warned that the increasing suicide rate among middle-aged White non-Hispanic Americans had resulted in a shorter average lifespan, which reversed decades of progress in mortality and presented a patterned not observed in any other industrial countries. In short, health and longevity appeared to be in decline in the United States among White non-Hispanics, particularly for those without college degrees (Case & Deaton, 2017). The **midlife mortality reversal** trend is *limited to* White non-Hispanics (but not other racial/ethnic groups) who live mostly outside of urban areas (Case & Deaton, 2015; Stein et al., 2017). Their causes of death are mostly suicide, accidental poisoning, and liver disease (Stein et al., 2017). Case and Deaton (2017) called these midlife premature deaths **"deaths of despair"** – which come from "a long-standing process of cumulative disadvantage for those with less than a college degree" (p. 398). Unlike Hispanics and Blacks who have developed individual- and community- resilience in the face of historical and current adversities pervasive in their everyday life, (middle-aged) White Americans appeared to have decreased in resilience as they confronted the perceived loss of the relative status of being members of the dominant group (Case & Deaton, 2017; Graham & Pinto, 2017; Siddiqi et al., 2019).

The social comparison aspect is vital. Under Magic Consciousness, individuals do not compete nor compare themselves with others. Jealousy or inferiority complex has no place for people with Magic Consciousness as they see the success of any members of the "clan" as the success for all (for more detailed discussion, see Social Support through Magic Consciousness: This is Who We Are in Chapter 10). However, experiences of dissociation under Perspectival Thinking can lead to experiences of alienation, a sociopsychological, not biological, malady. The suffering is not necessarily about material loss but also a loss of self and place in the larger community.

The social sciences were largely born as scholars became increasingly alarmed at what was unfolding across Europe. Max Weber (1905–1920/2002), Karl Marx (1935), Émile Durkheim (1953/2010), among others, all focused on the new set of social and psychological problems tied to increasing individualism/social isolation from extended agrarian kit and kin. Why were suicide rates rising in Europe, and more curiously, in a Europe that was rapidly industrializing and gaining in wealth? Why were suicide rates highest among the classes showing the most upward mobility? Why would they not be happier than their poorer country cousins who had no such opportunities? The answer was: when you have the opportunity to win, you also have the opportunity to lose. Winning and losing are social outcomes indicating relative success and failure, relative to others.

Perspectival Thinking worldview presumes agency, which entails individual responsibilities and self-control. The rise of capitalist society under Perspectival Thinking leads to two social phenomena: (a) the idea of progress, a chance for "betterment" within a new progressive ethos spread, and (b) the pursuit of betterment became largely the burden of the lone individual struggling to "make it." The chance of failure emerges (along with successful upward mobility), and the onus of success or failure is not shared but carried by the individual attempting to achieve a new social status and improve personal wealth. Money became not only the measure of relative success or failure but, at a magic level, a powerful indicator of identity for oneself and for others. Wealth could be exhibited. Often, life became a zero-sum game such that the more I can profit off of you, the more you lose. Life was neither stable nor "stagnant." Nor was the new industrial capitalism predisposed to win-win outcomes.

Being a "failure" not only became possible, but painfully so, obviously so. Social "climbing" became the new natural reality. Culture, values, beliefs, expectations, motivations were changing fundamentally. We are ultimately responsible for our own success and happiness. Braswell and Kushner (2012) argued that the masculinity culture of the military can even construe soldiers' suicide as failures to control their own emotions (as opposed to struggles with their suffering). In an analysis of 112 suicide notes of persons who succeeded in suicide in the Los Angeles, Jacobs (1967) found that the notes often included admissions of failure (e.g., "You did not fail, I did."; "I have failed at everything."). Jacobs (1967) concluded, "nearly all the others who attempt or succeed in suicide" have faced "the general condition of 'a progressive social isolation from meaningful relationships'" (p. 68). This is the source of many deaths of despair (see Figure 12.5). The promotion and expectation of self-determinism and hypertrophic individualism under Perspectival Thinking is not only deficient but also suicidal (Kramer et al., 2014).

In conclusion, different cultural groups can hold different cultural worldviews that impact their health behaviors and health status. This section highlights several complex and interesting phenomena of minority health. There is robust evidence of the impacts of minority stress on minorities' health disparities; nevertheless, minority groups also have developed mechanisms (e.g., identity affirmation, ethnic pride, and resilience) to cope with adversities at both individual and community levels. As a result, in some circumstances, minorities have been found to not only mitigate the negative impacts of stress and their social disadvantages but also do better than the general population (or the dominant groups). In contrast, the recent observations of

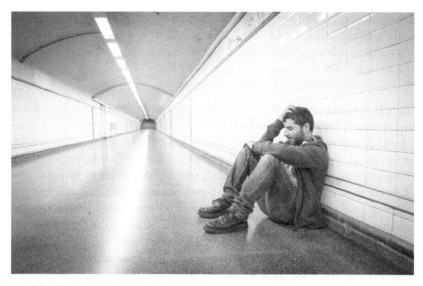

Figure 12.5 Death of despair. Under Magic Consciousness, when one experiences a loss of identity and relationships, the community actively reaches out to assure the person his/her identity and relationships can never be lost as long as s/he is a member of the group. In contrast, under Perspectival Thinking, one has no one but herself to blame if s/he cannot find a meaningful place for himself/herself. *Source:* ocusfocus/123RF

the epidemic of despair among middle-age White Americans highlight the devastating impacts of lack of resilience when ones' worldview (e.g., perceived relative status as a member of dominant groups) is threatened.

D. Culture as a Living Process: Situating Disparities in Pan-Evolution

Since the 1980s, there are consistent efforts to identify and recognize unique challenges and pathways that contribute to HDPs' experiences with health disparities (Alvidrez et al., 2019; Epstein, 2007; Terui, 2017). The identification of specific populations' experiences of health disparities can be powerful tools for health interventions. However, researchers also have raised concerns about how focusing on the unique traits (e.g., race and gender) or vulnerabilities (e.g., low socioeconomic status and language barriers) of these groups may have unintended consequences.

1. The Politics of Population Labels

First, focusing on specific traits/vulnerability creates a distorted view of the importance of these variables as predictors of disparities. Reflecting on the specific categories of populations that have been "labeled" and given protected status (e.g., gender, children, and ethnic minorities) in governmental policies, Epstein (2007) argued:

> [Categorical identities are recognized] when the identity is already socially salient, when the representative group is highly mobilized, when the group lays claim to a form of difference that is already authorized by state classifications, and when proponents are able to convincingly deploy frames that link justice arguments to biological difference claims. Conversely, the likelihood of recognition of a way of differing is reduced when the group is not well mobilized;

when it articulates demands in relation to a form of social difference that is not already institutionalized in state policies; and when its frames do not resonate with the public or policymakers, perhaps because of the difficulty of advancing a biological difference argument. (pp. 142-143)

For example, researchers have noted the importance of social class as a contributor to health disparities. **Social class** refers to "a social group defined relationally in social space by its possession and utilization of various capitals such as *economic, cultural, and social* capital" (Veenstra, 2007, p. 14). Although NIH has specific requirements for recruiting women, minorities, and children, there are no policies requiring the inclusion of people from different social classes. Nevertheless, people from different classes may adopt distinctive speech patterns, hold diverging worldviews, and occupy drastically different lived environments, including relational, social, and physical spaces. For example, individuals who are low in social class have reported poor relationships with neighbors and experiences of alienation/loneliness due to a lack of close and meaningful social relationships – which not only have implications to individuals' mental health but also to their ability to muster resources for coping in times of stress (Veenstra, 2007). Environmental health researchers have long recognized that communities of color are often disproportionately exposed to environmental pollutants and risk factors as their lived spaces are segregated in neighborhoods with high levels of poverty and material deprivation (Morello-Frosch & Lopez, 2006). Such fragmented and segregated residential spaces often overlap with food deserts (i.e., lack of access to affordable markets with fresh produce), low proximity to critical services and resources (e.g., health clinics, schools, parks, and libraries), and undesirable social and physical environments (e.g., higher crime rates and little open space; Morello-Frosch & Lopez, 2006). However, because (a) social class is much more fluid/mobile than racial categories, (b) community members may conceal, resist, or mislead their class labels, and (c) class-based social policies can be offensive to the public, social class (as opposed to racial categories) does not have a protected status in governmental policies.

When interventions are designed for specific population-based labels, we may overlook populations that are not named. For example, by focusing on racial disparities, we can inadvertently fuel racism and silence the suffering of the poor White Americans (Kawachi et al., 2005). As President Lyndon B. Johnson, the architect of the War on Poverty and various landmark civil rights legislation (e.g., the Civil Rights Acts of 1957 and 1960 and the Voting Rights Act of 1965), explained to an aide in 1960, "I'll tell you what's at the bottom of it. If you can convince the lowest white man that he's better than the best colored man, he won't notice you picking his pocket. Hell, give him somebody to look down on, and he'll empty his pockets for you" (Woods, 2007, p. 367). As Magic Consciousness and Mythic Connection seeps into poor White Americans' understanding of identities for self and others, they may not even recognize the sociocultural factors (e.g., poverty and racism) that shape their experiences of disparities (Bonilla-Silva, 2006; Siddiqi et al., 2019).

As we contemplate how we identify, categorize, and support different populations, it is important to remember the limits of Perspectival Thinking: Whatever is not measured becomes meaningless, invisible, and valueless. The labeling of HDPs is a political act. Some categories are named to facilitate social control yet others are not named due to difficulties in identifying boundaries of membership or pathologizing their differences. Although we do not advocate abandoning the labels for specific HDPs, we believe that when we tackle disparities faced by HDPs, sensitivity, and vigilant attendance to silenced suffering that results from labeling (and *not* labeling) is essential to developing a deeper understanding of the structural limitations people face.

2. The Interplays between Stigma, Structures, and Policies

Second, by highlighting specific characteristics, traits, or behaviors as risk factors, we may inadvertently pathologize these variables and overlook the underlying sociocultural issues that interact and even fuel the disparities. Several researchers have warned that by labeling race, gender, specific health behaviors, or even poverty as risk factors, we problematize and pathologize these variables – rather than recognizing the underlying issues that have contributed to these HDPs' experiences of disparities. For example, as we discussed earlier, by treating gender as a risk factor for disparities, we may overlook the impacts of gender bias from healthcare providers and the larger society as the cause of women's experiences of health disparities in pain management. When we focused on the vulnerabilities of HDPs, the consequent interventions inevitably highlight the "inadequacies" of those communities. In order to help, we must identify problems, which, in itself, can fuel prejudice.

Stigma is situated in communities and operates through dynamic, interactive social interactions. Stigma and public policies exert influences on each other bidirectionally (Hansen et al., 2014). For example, reflecting on how anti-smoking campaigns can become problematic, Bell et al. (2010) commented, "Historically, tobacco control policies have acted to entrench class-based health inequalities ... Indeed, they are likely to exacerbate them because they enable a political environment in which healthcare is increasingly seen as a privilege that smokers have negated the 'right' to access" (p. 798). By targeting current tobacco smokers as an at-risk group, anti-smoking legislation and campaigns create stigma toward smokers, motivating them to conceal smoking status to avoid scrutiny from insurance companies, organizational wellness programs, and healthcare providers.

By pathologizing social determinants of health (e.g., poverty) and medicalizing health disparities in specific groups, we can inadvertently reinforce existing stigma against the very people we aim to help (Hansen et al., 2014; Lantz et al., 2007). For example, researchers have raised concerns about the medicalization of the homeless. Although media coverage traditionally has provided sympathetic and positive views toward the homeless, it often centers on the deficits and deviant characteristics of homeless people (Buck et al., 2004). By constructing homelessness as a "disease" or deviancy to be avoided by self-awareness and responsible behaviors, shelter staff encourages the homeless to look into themselves to identify the causes of their homelessness, a practice that transforms the homeless to self-blaming and self-governing persons (Lyon-Callo, 2000). In other words, homeless people can only find redemption through submission to the regime of surveillance, discipline, and personal enhancement (Farrugia et al., 2016; Wasserman & Clair, 2012, 2013). For example, Luhrmann (2008) found homeless psychotic women refused to accept free housing provided by mental health services because the housing eligibility requires a psychiatric diagnosis. Accepting housing would imply that one agrees with the "mentally ill" identity assigned by the social system. As a result, these women talked about the need to be tough so that they can continue to face everyday violence in their street-life or to be "mentally strong" so that they can forgo their identities to accept the needed services. In short, policy efforts aiming to address health disparities also can become oppressive, stigmatizing the very people they aim to help.

Efforts to eliminate stigma (which often challenges the current social order) can also provoke resistance from the larger society. Hansen et al. (2014) noted, "Stigma and social structures, however, are dynamic, contextual, and evolve in interaction with one another; stigma can provoke neutralizing strategies among the stigmatized that, in turn, provoke counterstrategies among the stigmatizers" (p. 82). For example, when the social movement "Black Lives Matter," with the hashtag #BlackLivesMatter, emerged to highlight African Americans' disproportional suffering of structural racism, social injustice and police brutality, other social media users adopted hashtags such as #AllLivesMatter, #BlueLivesMatter, and #PoliceLivesMatter to engage in counter-protests. This amounted to hijacking content stemming from #BackLivesMatter advocates (e.g., adopting hashtags of a politically opposed group in order to inject their ideological beliefs; Gallagher et al., 2018). It also negated the effort to identify the Black experience in the United States as unique, erasing the difference and the point of the entire Black Lives movement. Similarly, Kosenko et al. (2019) observed that #ShoutYourAbortion, a hashtag originally intended to destigmatize abortion, was hijacked by anti-abortionists who linked it to hundreds of stigmatizing, anti-abortion messages, enforcing, and legitimizing public stigma for both women who receive and healthcare providers who perform abortion services. In short, as we contemplate solutions to address health disparities, we must recognize the dynamic interplays between stigma, structures, and policies.

3. An Integral Fusion Approach to Health Disparities

Although this Chapter begins with identifying specific HDPs and their corresponding disparities, such an organization of health disparities is largely an artifact of the literature and the field of minority health and health disparities. Since the 1980s, through collaborations between grassroots advocates, health professionals, medical researchers, and policymakers, there has been tremendous progress in addressing disparities by identifying and differentiating "unique" populations that are "vulnerable" to health disparities (Epstein, 2007). The approach highlights two principles: "the inclusion of members of diverse groups as research subjects and the measurement of outcome differences across medical subgroups" (Epstein, 2007, p. 278). The identification and segmentation of populations for measurements and targeting is a Perspectival Thinking approach to problem-solving. The Perspectival Thinking approach, however, is limited because the measurements center on the unique characteristics of the targeted populations. As the measurements become more precise, the more phenomena that are difficult or impossible to quantify are overlooked, becoming invisible. Populations that have yet to achieve recognizable, measurable labels or the complex, dynamic interplays between social/political actors, policy, and structure can become "noise" to those seeking to find solutions to health disparities.

To identify meaningful and effective strategies to address the challenges faced by HDPs, an Integral Fusion approach is essential. This is because HDPs' experiences of vulnerabilities and disparities are interconnected and multi-layered. For example, domestic violence (e.g., physical and sexual victimization and witnessing intimate partner violence) is one of the major contributors to homelessness (Martijn & Sharpe,

2006), especially in low socioeconomic populations who have limited housing options. Mallett et al. (2005) concluded that (a) family conflicts and family members' drug/ alcohol use often precede young people's homelessness and (b) homeless youth often use drugs as a coping mechanism for family conflicts prior to leaving home. In other words, addressing young people's drug use and/or homelessness should start *before* the youth become homeless and start with early-stage, strong support systems for the family and family members (as opposed to the young people) in addressing family conflicts and addiction problems.

Similarly, because housing insecurity poses major barriers to leaving domestic violence (Thurston et al., 2013), women with children and/or with limited resources can be particularly vulnerable when faced with domestic violence. Women who experience intimate partner violence in the last year are four times more likely to report housing instability than women who did not experience intimate partner violence (Pavao et al., 2007). A study found that 38% of women who experienced domestic violence reported homelessness immediately after separation and 25% reported having to leave their homes during the year after separation (Baker et al., 2003). From this perspective, addressing homeless women's suffering should not start at shelter housing but should begin with providing them sufficient resources (e.g., affordable public housing, family counseling services, meaningful employment placement, and livable wage to meet their basic needs) to mitigate housing insecurity and domestic violence in everyday life. An Integral Fusion approach provides opportunities to see beyond the "symptoms" of health disparities and to identify other causes that may offer "outside-the-box" solutions.

An Integral Fusion approach is empowering because it recognizes its participants' agency to identify problems and collaborate with one another to achieve mutually agreeable solutions. It encourages reflective thinking – awareness of and responsiveness to one's own bias and prejudice. An Integral Fusion approach embraces the perspectives of HDPs. Rather than conceptualizing HDPs as passive victims of health disparities that need to be "saved," an Integral Fusion approach engages and appreciates HDPs' agency and their capacity to thrive in the larger society and to co-develop solutions to challenges faced by their communities and the larger society (see also Culture-Centered Approach in Chapter 14). But an integral understanding is also aware that free will and choice are not the same things as access to resources. Indeed, not having access to resources is the opposite of free will and choice (see also Justice as Fairness in Chapter 14).

IV. Additional Resources

A. Key Terms and Theories

structural stigma
structural discrimination
    intended structural discrimination
    unintended structural discrimination
Healthy People
health disparity
health disparity population

medically underserved population
medically underserved areas
vulnerable populations
at-risk populations
    access-based needs
    functional-based needs
marginalized populations
social determinants of health (Chapter 7)
biopolitical paradigms
androcentrism
pink tax
tampon tax
language-concordant care
interpreter-as-conduit
Model of Bilingual Health Communication
somatic symptoms
somatization
minority stress
minority stress theory
identity affirmation (Chapter 8)
ethnic differentiation
ethnic pride
psychological immune system
resilience
self-mastery
community resilience
communal coping
Theory of Resilience and Relational Load
communal-mastery
Hispanic paradox
Midlife mortality reversal
death of despair
social class

B. Discussion Questions

1. Health disparity populations have been categorized in many different ways: underserved populations, vulnerable populations, at-risk populations, and marginalized populations.
   a. What are the different aspects highlighted by the label and naming of the populations?
   b. What are the pros and cons of each category?
   c. Would these labels create barriers to address health disparities? How?
   d. Are there populations that experience health disparities but are not labeled as a "group" to address their experiences of disparities? Why?
2. What are the groups of people who are likely not to be included in medical/pharmaceutical research? Why?

    a. What are the impacts when women are not included in medical/pharmaceutical research?

    b. What are the impacts when pregnant women are not included in medical/pharmaceutical research?

    c. What are the impacts when children are not included in medical/pharmaceutical research?

    d. What are the impacts when ethnic minorities are not included in medical/pharmaceutical research?

    e. Do you think the reasons to not include women, pregnant women, children, or minorities in medical/pharmaceutical research are appropriate? Is it ethical?

3. What are the different ways paying more for one's existence (e.g., pink tax for women or increased costs to obtain "ethnic" goods/services) can create economic and health disparities for the group?

4. The Chapter talked about how a society's normative belief about gender differences can create gender disparities for pain management. Researchers have also observed *racial* disparities for pain management. Racial/ethnic minorities consistently receive less adequate treatment for acute and chronic pain than non-Hispanic whites (Mossey, 2011). Black children are less likely to receive any pain medication for moderate pain and less likely to receive opioids for severe pain (Goyal et al., 2015). What are the likely normative beliefs and biases in our society that may have contributed such disparities?

5. Reflecting on your personal experience, do you think you being a member of a particular group subject you to "constant, perpetual, and/or unique stressors in everyday life as a result of stigma, prejudice, and discrimination in the larger society"?

    a. Do you think being a member of ethnic minorities gives a person more legitimacy to claim minority stress? Why? How?

    b. Do you think being a woman gives a person more legitimacy to claim minority stress? Why? How?

    c. What are the challenges for a poor, non-college-educated, non-Hispanic, White men to claim minority stress?

    d. How can we address the problems of the death of despair for non-college-educated Whites?

    e. Looking at the inclusive strategies for LGBT+ group membership (see LGBTQ as a Social Group in Chapter 8), what are the different ways to develop an inclusive group membership for minorities that also include non-college educated Whites?

6. What are the different ways people have worked to promote social causes and social justice social media?

    a. Why is "hashtag" important?

    b. Do you think people with different cultural perspectives (i.e., Magic Consciousness, Mythic Connection, and Perspectival Thinking) may view hashtags differently? How?

    c. Why do people try to "hijack" a hashtag?

    d. What to do when your hashtag is hijacked? Do you think people with different cultural perspectives (i.e., Magic Consciousness, Mythic Connection, and Perspectival Thinking) may feel differently?

C. References

Abercrombie, N., & Louie, D. M. (2014, March 19). *Attorney General files suit against manufacturers and distributors of the prescription drug Plavix.* Department of the Attorney General. https://ag.hawaii.gov/wp-content/uploads/2014/01/News-Release-2014-09.pdf

Afifi, T. D., Merrill, A. F., & Davis, S. (2016). The theory of resilience and relational load. *Personal Relationships, 23*(4), 663–683.

Almedom, A. M. (2005). Resilience, hardiness, sense of coherence, and posttraumatic growth: All paths leading to "light at the end of the tunnel"? *Journal of Loss and Trauma, 10*(3), 253–265.

Alvidrez, J., Castille, D., Laude-Sharp, M., Rosario, A., & Tabor, D. (2019). The national institute on minority health and health disparities research framework. *American Journal of Public Health, 109*(S1), S16-S20.

Angermeyer, M. C., Matschinger, H., Link, B. G., & Schomerus, G. (2014). Public attitudes regarding individual and structural discrimination: Two sides of the same coin? *Social Science & Medicine, 103*, 60–66.

Armenti, C. (2004a). May babies and posttenure babies: Maternal decisions of women professors. *The Review of Higher Education, 27*(2), 211–231.

Armenti, C. (2004b). Women faculty seeking tenure and parenthood: Lessons from previous generations. *Cambridge Journal of Education, 34*(1), 65–83.

Aymer, S. R. (2016). "I can't breathe": A case study – helping black men cope with race-related trauma stemming from police killing and brutality. *Journal of Human Behavior in the Social Environment, 26*(3-4), 367–376.

Baker, C. K., Cook, S. L., & Norris, F. H. (2003). Domestic violence and housing problems: A contextual analysis of women's help-seeking, received informal support, and formal system response. *Violence Against Women, 9*(7), 754–783.

Barnett, S. (1999). Clinical and cultural issues in caring for deaf people. *Family Medicine, 31*(1), 17–22.

Bell, K., Salmon, A., Bowers, M., Bell, J., & McCullough, L. (2010). Smoking, stigma and tobacco 'denormalization': Further reflections on the use of stigma as a public health tool. A commentary on *Social Science & Medicine's* Stigma, Prejudice, Discrimination and Health Special Issue (67: 3). *Social Science & Medicine, 70*(6), 795–799.

Bernstein, J., Bernstein, E., Dave, A., Hardt, E., James, T., Linden, J., Mitchell, P., Oishi, T., & Safi, C. (2002). Trained medical interpreters in the emergency department: Effects on services, subsequent charges, and follow-up. *Journal of Immigrant Health, 4*(4), 171–176.

Blau, F. D., & Kahn, L. M. (2017). The gender wage gap: Extent, trends, and explanations. *Journal of Economic Literature, 55*(3), 789–865.

Bonham, V. L., Callier, S. L., & Royal, C. D. (2016). Will precision medicine move us beyond race? *New England Journal of Medicine, 374*(21), 2003–2005.

Bonilla-Silva, E. (2006). *Racism without racists: Color-blind racism and the persistence of racial inequality in the United States.* Rowman & Littlefield.

Bottrell, D. (2009). Understanding 'marginal' perspectives: Towards a social theory of resilience. *Qualitative Social Work, 8*(3), 321–339.

Braswell, H., & Kushner, H. I. (2012). Suicide, social integration, and masculinity in the U.S. military. *Social Science & Medicine, 74*(4), 530–536.

Braveman, P. A., Kumanyika, S., Fielding, J., LaVeist, T., Borrell, L. N., Manderscheid, R., & Troutman, A. (2011). Health disparities and health equity: The issue is justice. *American Journal of Public Health*, *101*(S1), S149-S155.

Breslow, A. S., Brewster, M. E., Velez, B. L., Wong, S., Geiger, E., & Soderstrom, B. (2015). Resilience and collective action: Exploring buffers against minority stress for transgender individuals. *Psychology of Sexual Orientation and Gender Diversity*, *2*(3), 253–265.

Bryant, T. (2019, October 24). *Salons are charging extra fees for 'textured' hair. Black women have had enough.* Glamour. https://www.glamour.com/story/natural-hair-tax-salons

Bryant-Davis, T., Adams, T., Alejandre, A., & Gray, A. A. (2017). The trauma lens of police violence against racial and ethnic minorities. *Journal of Social Issues*, *73*(4), 852–871.

Buck, P. O., Toro, P. A., & Ramos, M. A. (2004). Media and professional interest in homelessness over 30 years (1974–2003). *Analyses of Social Issues and Public Policy*, *4*(1), 151–171.

Butow, P. N., Lobb, E., Jefford, M., Goldstein, D., Eisenbruch, M., Girgis, A., King, M., Sze, M., Aldridge, L., & Schofield, P. (2012). A bridge between cultures: Interpreters' perspectives of consultations with migrant oncology patients. *Supportive Care in Cancer*, *20*(2), 235–244.

Case, A., & Deaton, A. (2015). Rising morbidity and mortality in midlife among white non-hispanic americans in the 21st century. *Proceedings of the National Academy of Sciences*, *112*(49), 15078–15083.

Case, A., & Deaton, A. (2017). Mortality and morbidity in the 21st century. In *Brookings papers on economic activity* (pp. 397–476). Brookings Institute. https://www.brookings.edu/wp-content/uploads/2017/08/casetextsp17bpea.pdf

Castro, F. G., Stein, J. A., & Bentler, P. M. (2009). Ethnic pride, traditional family values, and acculturation in early cigarette and alcohol use among Latino adolescents. *The Journal of Primary Prevention*, *30*(3), 265–292.

Centers for Medicare & Medicaid Services. (n.d.). *Serving vulnerable and underserved populations.* Retrieved August 8, 2020, from https://marketplace.cms.gov/technical-assistance-resources/training-materials/vulnerable-and-underserved-populations.pdf

Charles, N. (2020, May 7). *For many cautious African Americans, the move to reopen America is not a 'black friendly' campaign.* NBC News. https://www.nbcnews.com/news/nbcblk/many-cautious-african-americans-move-reopen-america-not-black-friendly-n1200771

Charley, C., Slayton-Martin, R., Hallmark, S., & Vaidyanathan, C. (2005). *Havasupai.* Northern Arizona University. https://library.nau.edu/speccoll/exhibits/indigenous_voices/havasupai/overview.html

Chiaramonte, G. R., & Friend, R. (2006). Medical students' and residents' gender bias in the diagnosis, treatment, and interpretation of coronary heart disease symptoms. *Health Psychology*, *25*(3), 255–266.

Cook, K. (2008). Marginalized populations. In L. M. Given (Ed.), *The SAGE encyclopedia of qualitative research methods* (pp. 496). Sage.

Corrigan, P. W., Markowitz, F. E., & Watson, A. C. (2004). Structural levels of mental illness stigma and discrimination. *Schizophrenia Bulletin*, *30*(3), 481–491.

Crawford, B. J., & Spivack, C. (2017). Tampon taxes, discrimination, and human rights. *Wisconsin Law Review*, (3), 491–550.

Devlin, H. (2020, April 22). *Why are people from BAME groups dying disproportionately of Covid-19?* The Guardian. https://www.theguardian.com/world/2020/apr/22/why-are-people-from-bame-groups-dying-disproportionately-of-covid-19

Diamond, L., Izquierdo, K., Canfield, D., Matsoukas, K., & Gany, F. (2019). A systematic review of the impact of patient–physician non-English language concordance on quality of care and outcomes. *Journal of General Internal Medicine, 34*(8), 1591–1606.

Diamond, L. C., & Jacobs, E. A. (2010). Let's not contribute to disparities: The best methods for teaching clinicians how to overcome language barriers to health care. *Journal of General Internal Medicine, 25*(Suppl. 2), S189-S193.

Drabiak-Syed, K. (2010). Lessons from *Havasupai Tribe v. Arizona State University Board of Regents*: Recognizing group, cultural, and dignitary harms as legitimate risks warranting integration into research practice. *Journal of Health & Biomedical Law, 6*(2), 175–226.

Dreher, B. (2019, May 23). *What Is the pink tax? If you're a woman, it's costing you lots of money every year.* Good Housekeeping. https://www.goodhousekeeping.com/life/money/a27409442/what-is-pink-tax

Dresser, R. (1992). Wanted single, White male for medical research. *Hastings Center Report, 22*(1), 24–29.

Durkheim, E. (2010). *Sociology and philosophy.* Routledge. (Original work published 1953)

Dusenbery, M. (2018). *Doing harm: The truth about how bad medicine and lazy science leave women dismissed, misdiagnosed, and sick.* HarperOne.

Dysart-Gale, D. (2005). Communication models, professionalization, and the work of medical interpreters. *Health Communication, 17*(1), 91–103.

Earp, B. D., Monrad, J. T., LaFrance, M., Bargh, J. A., Cohen, L. L., & Richeson, J. A. (2019). Gender bias in pediatric pain assessment. *Journal of Pediatric Psychology, 44*(4), 403–414.

Epstein, S. (2007). *Inclusion: The politics of difference in medical research.* University of Chicago Press.

Evans, S. (2019, November 27). *Does it cost more to have natural hair?* Essence. https://www.essence.com/hair/the-cost-of-natural-hair

Factor, R., Kawachi, I., & Williams, D. R. (2011). Understanding high-risk behavior among non-dominant minorities: A social resistance framework. *Social Science & Medicine, 73*(9), 1292–1301.

Farnill, D., Todisco, J., Hayes, S. C., & Bartlett, D. (1997). Videotaped interviewing of non-English speakers: Training for medical students with volunteer clients. *Medical Education, 31*(2), 87–93.

Farrugia, D., Smyth, J., & Harrison, T. (2016). Moral distinctions and structural inequality: Homeless youth salvaging the self. *The Sociological Review, 64*(2), 238–255.

Fredriksen-Goldsen, K. I., Kim, H.-J., Bryan, A. E. B., Shiu, C., & Emlet, C. A. (2017). The cascading effects of marginalization and pathways of resilience in attaining good health among LGBT older adults. *The Gerontologist, 57*(Suppl. 1), S72-S83.

Gallagher, R. J., Reagan, A. J., Danforth, C. M., & Dodds, P. S. (2018). Divergent discourse between protests and counter-protests: #BlackLivesMatter and #AllLivesMatter. *PLoS One, 13*(4), Article e0195644. https://doi.org/10.1371/journal.pone.0195644

Gany, F., Leng, J., Shapiro, E., Abramson, D., Motola, I., Shield, D. C., & Changrani, J. (2007). Patient satisfaction with different interpreting methods: A randomized controlled trial. *Journal of General Internal Medicine, 22*(Suppl. 2), S312–S318.

Goffman, E. (2009). *Stigma: Notes on the management of spoiled identity.* Touchstone. (Original work published 1963)

Goodman, L., Zhu, J., & Bai, B. (2016, September 6). *Women are better than men at paying their mortgages.* Urban Institute. https://www.urban.org/research/publication/women-are-better-men-paying-their-mortgages/view/full_report

Goyal, M. K., Kuppermann, N., Cleary, S. D., Teach, S. J., & Chamberlain, J. M. (2015). Racial disparities in pain management of children with appendicitis in emergency departments. *JAMA Pediatrics, 169*(11), 996–1002.

Graham, C., & Pinto, S. (2017). Unhappiness in America: Desperation in White towns, resilience and diversity in the cities. In M. E. O'Hanlon (Ed.), *Brookings big ideas for America* (pp. 18–27). Brookings Institution Press.

Green, A. R., Ngo-Metzger, Q., Legedza, A. T. R., Massagli, M. P., Phillips, R. S., & Iezzoni, L. I. (2005). Interpreter services, language concordance, and health care quality: Experiences of Asian Americans with limited English proficiency. *Journal of General Internal Medicine, 20*(11), 1050–1056.

Greenbaum, M., & Flores, G. (2004). Lost in translation: Professional interpreters needed to help hospitals treat immigrant patients. *Modern Healthcare, 34*(18), 21.

Grossman, A. H., D'Augelli, A. R., & Frank, J. A. (2011). Aspects of psychological resilience among transgender youth. *Journal of LGBT Youth, 8*(2), 103–115.

Guntzviller, L. M., Jensen, J. D., & Carreno, L. M. (2017). Latino children's ability to interpret in health settings: A parent–child dyadic perspective on child health literacy. *Communication Monographs, 84*(2), 143–163.

Guntzviller, L. M., & Wang, N. (2019). Mother-adolescent communication in low-income, Latino families during language brokering: Examining the theory of resilience and relational load. *Journal of Family Communication, 19*(3), 228–242.

Hadziabdic, E., Albin, B., Heikkilä, K., & Hjelm, K. (2010). Healthcare staffs perceptions of using interpreters: A qualitative study. *Primary Health Care Research and Development, 11*(3), 260–270.

Hampers, L. C., & McNulty, J. E. (2002). Professional interpreters and bilingual physicians in a pediatric emergency department: Effect on resource utilization. *Archives of Pediatrics and Adolescent Medicine, 156*(11), 1108–1113.

Hansen, H., Bourgois, P., & Drucker, E. (2014). Pathologizing poverty: New forms of diagnosis, disability, and structural stigma under welfare reform. *Social Science & Medicine, 103,* 76–83.

Harmon, A. (2010, April 21). Indian tribe wins fight to limit research of its DNA. *The New York Times,* A1. https://www.nytimes.com/2010/04/22/us/22dna.html

Harmsen, J. A. M., Bernsen, R. M. D., Bruijnzeels, M. A., & Meeuwesen, L. (2008). Patients' evaluation of quality of care in general practice: What are the cultural and linguistic barriers? *Patient Education and Counseling, 72*(1), 155–162.

Harper, G. W., & Schneider, M. (2003). Oppression and discrimination among lesbian, gay, bisexual, and transgendered people and communities: A challenge for community psychology. *American Journal of Community Psychology, 31*(3), 243–252.

Harris, D. A. (1999). The stories, the statistics, and the law: Why driving while Black matters. *Minnesota Law Review, 84*(2), 265–326.

Hatzenbuehler, M. L., & Link, B. G. (2014). Introduction to the special issue on structural stigma and health. *Social Science & Medicine, 103*, 1–6.

Hatzenbuehler, M. L., & Pachankis, J. E. (2016). Stigma and minority stress as social determinants of health among lesbian, gay, bisexual, and transgender youth: Research evidence and clinical implications. *Pediatric Clinics, 63*(6), 985–997.

Hawai'i ex rel. Louie v. Bristol-Myers Squibb Co., Civ. No. 14-00180 HG-RLP (D. Haw. 2014). https://casetext.com/case/hawaii-ex-rel-louie-v-bristol-myers-squibb-co

HealthyPeople.gov. (n.d.). Disparities. Retrieved August 8, 2020, from https://www.healthypeople.gov/2020/about/foundation-health-measures/Disparities#6

Hegewisch, A., & Hartmann, H. (2019). *The gender wage gap: 2018 earnings differences by race and ethnicity*. Institute for Women's Policy Research. https://iwpr.org/iwpr-general/the-gender-wage-gap-2018-earnings-differences-by-race-and-ethnicity/

Hiebert, P. G. (2008). *Transforming worldviews: An anthropological understanding of how people change*. Baker Academic.

Hobfoll, S. E., Jackson, A., Hobfoll, I., Pierce, C. A., & Young, S. (2002). The impact of communal-mastery versus self-mastery on emotional outcomes during stressful conditions: A prospective study of Native American women. *American Journal of Community Psychology, 30*(6), 853–871.

Hsieh, E. (2008). "I am not a robot!" Interpreters' views of their roles in health care settings. *Qualitative Health Research, 18*(10), 1367–1383.

Hsieh, E. (2013). Health literacy and patient empowerment: The role of medical interpreters in bilingual health communication. In M. J. Dutta & G. L. Kreps (Eds.), *Reducing health disparities: Communication intervention* (pp. 41–66). Peter Lang.

Hsieh, E. (2016). *Bilingual health communication: Working with interpreters in cross-cultural care*. Routledge.

Hsieh, E. (2018). Reconceptualizing language discordance: Meanings and experiences of language barriers in the U.S. and Taiwan. *Journal of Immigrant and Minority Health, 20*(1), 1–4.

Hsieh, E., & Kramer, E. M. (2012). Medical interpreters as tools: Dangers and challenges in the utilitarian approach to interpreters' roles and functions. *Patient Education and Counseling, 89*(1), 158–162.

Hsieh, E., & Nicodemus, B. (2015). Conceptualizing emotion in healthcare interpreting: A normative approach to interpreters' emotion work. *Patient Education and Counseling, 98*(12), 1474–1481.

Hsieh, E., Pitaloka, D., & Johnson, A. J. (2013). Bilingual health communication: Distinctive needs of providers from five specialties. *Health Communication, 28*(6), 557–567.

Hsieh, E., & Terui, S. (2015). Inherent tensions and challenges of oncologist–patient communication: Implications for interpreter training in health-care settings. *Journal of Applied Communication Research, 43*(2), 141–162.

Inter Tribal Council of Arizona. (2020). *Havasupai tribe*. https://itcaonline.com/member-tribes/havasupai-tribe

Isaac, J., Healy, O., & Peters, H. E. (2017). *Paid family leave in the United States: Time for a new national policy*. Urban Institute. https://www.urban.org/sites/default/files/publication/90201/paid_family_leave_0.pdf

Jack, R. E., Garrod, O. G. B., Yu, H., Caldara, R., & Schyns, P. G. (2012). Facial expressions of emotion are not culturally universal. *Proceedings of the National Academy of Sciences, 109*(19), 7241–7244.

Jacobs, E. A., Diamond, L. C., & Stevak, L. (2010). The importance of teaching clinicians when and how to work with interpreters. *Patient Education and Counseling, 78*(2), 149–153.

Jacobs, J. (1967). A phenomenological study of suicide notes. *Social Problems, 15*(1), 60–72.

John, D. A., de Castro, A. B., Martin, D. P., Duran, B., & Takeuchi, D. T. (2012). Does an immigrant health paradox exist among Asian Americans? Associations of nativity and occupational class with self-rated health and mental disorders. *Social Science & Medicine, 75*(12), 2085–2098.

Jou, J., Kozhimannil, K. B., Abraham, J. M., Blewett, L. A., & McGovern, P. M. (2018). Paid maternity leave in the United States: Associations with maternal and infant health. *Maternal and Child Health Journal, 22*(2), 216–225.

Kahn, J. (2014). *Race in a bottle: The story of BiDil and racialized medicine in a post-genomic age.* Columbia University Press.

Kam, J. A., Basinger, E. D., & Guntzviller, L. M. (2017). Communal coping among Spanish-speaking mother–child dyads engaging in language brokering: A latent class analysis. *Communication Research, 44*(5), 743–769.

Kam, J. A., Pines, R., & Bernhold, Q. (2018). Using a theoretical model of communal coping to understand changes in language brokers' coping patterns: Implications for Latina/o early adolescents' brokering stress and efficacy. *Communication Monographs, 85*(2), 263–283.

Karliner, L. S., Ma, L., Hofmann, M., & Kerlikowske, K. (2012). Language barriers, location of care, and delays in follow-up of abnormal mammograms. *Medical Care, 50*(2), 171–178.

Kawachi, I., Daniels, N., & Robinson, D. E. (2005). Health disparities by race and class: Why both matter. *Health Affairs, 24*(2), 343–352.

Kcomt, L. (2019). Profound health-care discrimination experienced by transgender people: Rapid systematic review. *Social Work in Health Care, 58*(2), 201–219.

King, T. E., & Wheeler, M. B. (Eds.). (2016). *Medical management of vulnerable & underserved patients: Principles, practice, population* (2nd ed.). McGraw-Hill.

Kong, G., Camenga, D., Cavallo, D., Connell, C.M., Pflieger, J.C., & Krishnan-Sarin, S. (2012). The role of ethnic pride and parental disapproval of smoking on smoking behaviors among minority and White adolescents in a suburban high school. *The American Journal on Addictions, 21*(5), 424–434.

Koopmann-Holm, B., & Matsumoto, D. (2011). Values and display rules for specific emotions. *Journal of Cross-Cultural Psychology, 42*(3), 355–371.

Kosenko, K., Winderman, E., & Pugh, A. (2019). The hijacked hashtag: The constitutive features of abortion stigma in the #ShoutYourAbortion Twitter campaign. *International Journal of Communication, 13.* https://ijoc.org/index.php/ijoc/article/view/7849

Kothari, C. L., Paul, R., Dormitorio, B., Ospina, F., James, A., Lenz, D., Baker, K., Curtis, A., & Wiley, J. (2016). The interplay of race, socioeconomic status and neighborhood residence upon birth outcomes in a high Black infant mortality community. *SSM – Population Health, 2,* 859–867.

Kramer, E. M. (2019). Cultural fusion theory. In J. F. Nussbaum (Ed.), *Oxford research encyclopedia of communication.* Oxford University Press. https://doi.org/10.1093/acrefore/9780190228613.013.679

Kramer, E. M., Adkins, G., Kim, S. H., & Miller, G. (2014). *Environmental communication and the extinction vortex: Technology as denial of death*. Hampton Press.

Kulis, S., Napoli, M., & Marsiglia, F. F. (2002). Ethnic pride, biculturalism, and drug use norms of urban American Indian adolescents. *Social Work Research*, *26*(2), 101–112.

Lantz, P. M., Lichtenstein, R. L., & Pollack, H. (2007). Health policy approaches to population health: The limits of medicalization. *Health Affairs*, *26*(5), 1253–1257.

Lasswell, H. D. (1948). The structure and function of communication in society. In L. Bryson (Ed.), *The communication of ideas* (pp. 37–51). Harper and Row.

Lee, K. C., Winickoff, J. P., Kim, M. K., Campbell, E. G., Betancourt, J. R., Park, E. R., Maina, A. W., & Weissman, J. S. (2006). Resident physicians' use of professional and nonprofessional interpreters: A national survey. *JAMA*, *296*(9), 1050–1053.

Lee, S. S.-J. (2015). The biobank as political artifact: The struggle over race in categorizing genetic difference. *The ANNALS of the American Academy of Political and Social Science*, *661*(1), 143–159.

Lick, D. J., Durso, L. E., & Johnson, K. L. (2013). Minority stress and physical health among sexual minorities. *Perspectives on Psychological Science*, *8*(5), 521–548.

Liu, Y., & Kramer, E. (2019). Cultural value discrepancies, strategic positioning and integrated identity: American migrants' experiences of being the other in mainland China. *Journal of International and Intercultural Communication*. Advance online publication. https://doi.org/10.1080/17513057.2019.1679226

Lo, M.-C. M., & Stacey, C. L. (2008). Beyond cultural competency: Bourdieu, patients and clinical encounters. *Sociology of Health & Illness*, *30*(5), 741–755.

Loach, B. L. (2019). A time to speak and a time to keep silent: Professional ethics, conscience, and the medical interpreter. *Ethics, Medicine and Public Health*, *11*, 52–59.

Luhrmann, T. M. (2008). "The street will drive you crazy": Why homeless psychotic women in the institutional circuit in the United States often say no to offers of help. *American Journal of Psychiatry*, *165*(1), 15–20.

Lyerly, A. D., Little, M. O., & Faden, R. (2008). The second wave: Toward responsible inclusion of pregnant women in research. *IJFAB: International Journal of Feminist Approaches to Bioethics*, *1*(2), 5–22.

Lyon-Callo, V. (2000). Medicalizing homelessness: The production of self-blame and self-governing within homeless shelters. *Medical Anthropology Quarterly*, *14*(3), 328–345.

Lyons, R. F., Mickelson, K. D., Sullivan, M. J., & Coyne, J. C. (1998). Coping as a communal process. *Journal of Social and Personal Relationships*, *15*(5), 579–605.

Lyratzopoulos, G., Abel, G. A., McPhail, S., Neal, R. D., & Rubin, G. P. (2013). Gender inequalities in the promptness of diagnosis of bladder and renal cancer after symptomatic presentation: Evidence from secondary analysis of an English primary care audit survey. *BMJ Open*, *3*(6), Article e002861. http://dx.doi.org/10.1136/bmjopen-2013-002861

Mallett, S., Rosenthal, D., & Keys, D. (2005). Young people, drug use and family conflict: Pathways into homelessness. *Journal of Adolescence*, *28*(2), 185–199.

Manson, A. (1988). Language concordance as a determinant of patient compliance and emergency room use in patients with asthma. *Medical Care*, *26*(12), 1119–1128.

Markow, T. A., & Martin, J. F. (1993). Inbreeding and developmental stability in a small human population. *Annals of Human Biology*, *20*(4), 389–394.

Martijn, C., & Sharpe, L. (2006). Pathways to youth homelessness. *Social Science & Medicine, 62*(1), 1–12.

Martin, R., Gordon, E. E. I., & Lounsbury, P. (1998). Gender disparities in the attribution of cardiac-related symptoms: Contribution of common sense models of illness. *Health Psychology, 17*(4), 346–357.

Marx, K. (1935). *Wage-labour and capital: Value, price, and profit.* International Publishers.

Mastroianni, A. C., Faden, R. R., & Federman, D. D. (1994). *Women and health research: Ethical and legal issues of including women in clinical studies.* National Academy Press.

McGowan, A. K., Kramer, K. T., & Teitelbaum, J. B. (2019). Healthy People: The role of law and policy in the nation's public health agenda. *The Journal of Law, Medicine & Ethics, 47*(Suppl. 2), 63–67.

McKee, M. M., & Paasche-Orlow, M. K. (2012). Health literacy and the disenfranchised: The importance of collaboration between limited English proficiency and health literacy researchers. *Journal of Health Communication, 17*(Suppl. 3), 7–12.

Meyer, I. H. (2003). Prejudice, social stress, and mental health in lesbian, gay, and bisexual populations: Conceptual issues and research evidence. *Psychological Bulletin, 129*(5), 674–697.

Meyer, I. H. (2015). Resilience in the study of minority stress and health of sexual and gender minorities. *Psychology of Sexual Orientation and Gender Diversity, 2*(3), 209–213.

Miller, G. E., Chen, E., & Zhou, E. S. (2007). If it goes up, must it come down? Chronic stress and the hypothalamic-pituitary-adrenocortical axis in humans. *Psychological Bulletin, 133*(1), 25–45.

Morello-Frosch, R., & Lopez, R. (2006). The riskscape and the color line: Examining the role of segregation in environmental health disparities. *Environmental Research, 102*(2), 181–196.

Mossey, J. M. (2011). Defining racial and ethnic disparities in pain management. *Clinical Orthopaedics and Related Research, 469*(7), 1859–1870.

Motti-Stefanidi, F., & Masten, A. S. (2017). A resilience perspective on immigrant youth adaptation and development. In N. J. Cabrera & B. Leyendecker (Eds.), *Handbook on positive development of minority children and youth* (pp. 19–34). Springer.

Mulia, N., Ye, Y., Karriker-Jaffe, K. J., Zemore, S. E., & Jones-Webb, R. (2018). Protective factors as an explanation for the "paradox" of Black–White differences in heavy drinking. *Substance Use & Misuse, 53*(12), 2003–2016.

Munzer, S. R. (2013). Research biobanks meet synthetic biology: Autonomy and Ownership. In G. Pascuzzi, U. Izzo, & M. Macilotti (Eds.), *Comparative issues in the governance of research biobanks: Property, privacy, intellectual property, and the role of technology* (pp. 11–39). Springer.

Nandi, A., Hajizadeh, M., Harper, S., Koski, A., Strumpf, E. C., & Heymann, J. (2016). Increased duration of paid maternity leave lowers infant mortality in low- and middle-income countries: A quasi-experimental study. *PLoS Medicine, 13*(3), Article e1001985. https://doi.org/10.1371/journal.pmed.1001985

National Network of Libraries of Medicine. (2013). *Health literacy.* https://nnlm.gov/initiatives/topics/health-literacy

National Partnership for Women & Families. (2016). *Expecting better: A state-by-state analysis of laws that help expecting and new parents.* https://www.nationalpartnership.org/our-work/resources/economic-justice/expecting-better-2016.pdf

Ngai, K. M., Grudzen, C. R., Lee, R., Tong, V. Y., Richardson, L. D., & Fernandez, A. (2016). The association between limited English proficiency and unplanned emergency department revisit within 72 Hours. *Annals of Emergency Medicine, 68*(2), 213–221.

Ngo-Metzger, Q., Sorkin, D. H., & Phillips, R. S. (2009). Healthcare experiences of limited English-proficient Asian American patients: A cross-sectional mail survey. *The Patient: Patient-Centered Outcomes Research, 2*(2), 113–120.

Ngo-Metzger, Q., Sorkin, D. H., Phillips, R. S., Greenfield, S., Massagli, M. P., Clarridge, B., & Kaplan, S. H. (2007). Providing high-quality care for limited English proficient patients: The importance of language concordance and interpreter use. *Journal of General Internal Medicine, 22*(Suppl. 2), S324–S330.

O'Connor, K. J., & Graham, C. (2019). Longer, more optimistic, lives: Historic optimism and life expectancy in the United States. *Journal of Economic Behavior & Organization, 168*, 374–392.

Office of Disease Prevention and Health Promotion. (2020, August 18). *About Healthy People 2030*. https://health.gov/our-work/healthy-people-2030/about-healthy-people-2030

Ozono, H., Watabe, M., Yoshikawa, S., Nakashima, S., Rule, N. O., Ambady, N., & Adams, R. B. J. (2010). What's in a smile? Cultural differences in the effects of smiling on judgments of trustworthiness. *Letters on Evolutionary Behavioral Science, 1*(1), 15–18.

Paradies, Y. C., Montoya, M. J., & Fullerton, S. M. (2007). Racialized genetics and the study of complex diseases – the thrifty genotype revisited. *Perspectives in Biology and Medicine, 50*(2), 203–227.

Patel, M. I., Schupp, C. W., Gomez, S. L., Chang, E. T., & Wakelee, H. A. (2013). How do social factors explain outcomes in non–small-cell lung cancer among Hispanics in California? Explaining the Hispanic paradox. *Journal of Clinical Oncology, 31*(28), 3572–3578.

Pavao, J., Alvarez, J., Baumrind, N., Induni, M., & Kimerling, R. (2007). Intimate partner violence and housing instability. *American Journal of Preventive Medicine, 32*(2), 143–146.

Pediatric Research Equity Act of 2013. Pub. L. No. 108–115, 117 St. 1936 (2013). https://www.congress.gov/108/plaws/publ155/PLAW-108publ155.pdf

Perry, A. M., Harshbarger, D., & Romer, C. (2020, April 16). *Mapping racial inequity amid COVID-19 underscores policy discriminations against Black Americans*. Brookings. https://www.brookings.edu/blog/the-avenue/2020/04/16/mapping-racial-inequity-amid-the-spread-of-covid-19

Phelan, J. C., Link, B. G., & Dovidio, J. F. (2008). Stigma and prejudice: One animal or two? *Social Science & Medicine, 67*(3), 358–367.

Prince, D., & Nelson, M. (1995). Teaching Spanish to emergency medicine residents. *Academic Emergency Medicine, 2*(1), 32–37.

Qiu, L. (2017, January 22). *Are pads and tampons taxed but Viagra and Rogaine not?* Politifact. https://www.politifact.com/factchecks/2017/jan/22/ashley-judd/are-pads-and-tampons-taxed-viagra-and-rogaine-not

Rabin, R. C. (2014, September 23). *Health researchers will get $10.1 million to counter gender bias in studies*. The New York Times. https://www.nytimes.com/2014/09/23/health/23gender.html

Rachman, S. J. (2016). Invited essay: Cognitive influences on the psychological immune system. *Journal of Behavior Therapy and Experimental Psychiatry, 53*, 2–8.

Raymond, C. W. (2014). Epistemic brokering in the interpreter-mediated medical visit: Negotiating "patient's side" and "doctor's side" knowledge. *Research on Language and Social Interaction, 47*(4), 426–446.

Recio-Barbero, M., & Pérez-Fernandez, I. (2019). Gender bias in research: How does it affect mental health? In M. Sáenz-Herrero (Ed.), *Psychopathology in women: Incorporating gender perspective into descriptive psychopathology* (pp. 865–883). Springer.

Rivas-Drake, D., Seaton, E. K., Markstrom, C., Quintana, S., Syed, M., Lee, R. M., Schwartz, S. J., Umaña-Taylor, A. J., French, S., & Yip, T., & Ethnic and Racial Identity in the 21st Century Study Group. (2014). Ethnic and racial identity in adolescence: Implications for psychosocial, academic, and health outcomes. *Child Development, 85*(1), 40–57.

Roberts, D. E. (2011). What's wrong with race-based medicine? Genes, drugs, and health disparities. *Minnesota Journal of Law, Science & Technology, 12*(1), 1–21.

Rubin, P. (2004, May 27). *Indian givers*. The Phoenix New Times. http://www.phoenixnewtimes.com/news/indian-givers-6428347

Ruiz, J. M., Sbarra, D., & Steffen, P. R. (2018). Hispanic ethnicity, stress psychophysiology and paradoxical health outcomes: A review with conceptual considerations and a call for research. *International Journal of Psychophysiology, 131*, 24–29.

Samulowitz, A., Gremyr, I., Eriksson, E., & Hensing, G. (2018). "Brave men" and "emotional women": A theory-guided literature review on gender bias in health care and gendered norms towards patients with chronic pain. *Pain Research and Management, 2018*, Article 6358624. https://doi.org/10.1155/2018/6358624

Sankar, P., & Kahn, J. (2005). BiDil: Race medicine or race marketing? *Health Affairs, 24*(Suppl. 1), Article W5, 455–463. https://doi.org/10.1377/hlthaff.w5.455

Schouten, B. C., Cox, A., Duran, G., Kerremans, K., Banning, L. K., Lahdidioui, A., van den Muijsenbergh, M., Schinkel, S., Sungur, H., Suurmond, J., Zendedel, R., & Krystallidou, D. (2020). Mitigating language and cultural barriers in healthcare communication: Toward a holistic approach. *Patient Education and Counseling, 103*(12), 2604-2608.

Sentell, T., & Braun, K. L. (2012). Low health literacy, limited English proficiency, and health status in Asians, Latinos, and other racial/ethnic groups in California. *Journal of Health Communication, 17*(Suppl. 3), 82–99.

Siddiqi, A., Sod-Erdene, O., Hamilton, D., Cottom, T. M., & Darity, W. (2019). Growing sense of social status threat and concomitant deaths of despair among Whites. *SSM - Population Health, 9*, Article 100449. https://doi.org/10.1016/j.ssmph.2019.100449

Srinivasan, S., & Williams, S. D. (2014). Transitioning from health disparities to a health equity research agenda: The time is now. *Public Health Reports, 129*(1 Suppl. 2), 71–76.

Stein, E. M., Gennuso, K. P., Ugboaja, D. C., & Remington, P. L. (2017). The epidemic of despair among White Americans: Trends in the leading causes of premature death, 1999–2015. *American Journal of Public Health, 107*(10), 1541–1547.

Steinberg, A. G., Wiggins, E. A., Barmada, C. H., & Sullivan, V. J. (2002). Deaf women: Experiences and perceptions of healthcare system access. *Journal of Women's Health, 11*(8), 729–741.

Stone, A. L. (2009). More than adding a T: American lesbian and gay activists' attitudes towards transgender inclusion. *Sexualities, 12*(3), 334–354.

Stuber, J., Meyer, I., & Link, B. (2008). Stigma, prejudice, discrimination and health. *Social Science & Medicine*, *67*(3), 351–357.

Sudore, R. L., Landefeld, C. S., Pérez-Stable, E. J., Bibbins-Domingo, K., Williams, B. A., & Schillinger, D. (2009). Unraveling the relationship between literacy, language proficiency, and patient–physician communication. *Patient Education and Counseling*, *75*(3), 398–402.

Terui, S. (2017). Conceptualizing the pathways and processes between language barriers and health disparities: Review, synthesis, and extension. *Journal of Immigrant and Minority Health*, *19*(1), 215–224.

Thornicroft, G., Rose, D., Kassam, A., & Sartorius, N. (2007). Stigma: Ignorance, prejudice or discrimination? *The British Journal of Psychiatry*, *190*(3), 192–193.

Thurston, W. E., Roy, A., Clow, B., Este, D., Gordey, T., Haworth-Brockman, M., McCoy, L., Beck, R. R., Saulnier, C., & Carruthers, L. (2013). Pathways into and out of homelessness: Domestic violence and housing security for immigrant women. *Journal of Immigrant & Refugee Studies*, *11*(3), 278–298.

U.S. Department of Health and Human Services. (2019, March 28). *At-risk individuals*. https://www.phe.gov/Preparedness/planning/abc/Pages/atrisk.aspx

U.S. Food and Drug Administration. (2018). *Best Pharmaceuticals for Children Act and Pediatric Research Equity Act*. U.S. Food and Drug Administration. https://www.fda.gov/science-research/pediatrics/best-pharmaceuticals-children-act-and-pediatric-research-equity-act

Upadhyayula, S., Ramaswamy, M., Chalise, P., Daniels, J., & Freudenberg, N. (2017). The association of ethnic pride with health and social outcomes among young Black and Latino men after release from jail. *Youth & Society*, *49*(8), 1057–1076.

Urquia, M. L., O'Campo, P. J., & Heaman, M. I. (2012). Revisiting the immigrant paradox in reproductive health: The roles of duration of residence and ethnicity. *Social Science & Medicine*, *74*(10), 1610–1621.

Valk, A., & Karu, K. (2001). Ethnic attitudes in relation to ethnic pride and ethnic differentiation. *The Journal of Social Psychology*, *141*(5), 583–601.

Vallgårda, S. (2007). Health inequalities: Political problematizations in Denmark and Sweden. *Critical Public Health*, *17*(1), 45–56.

Van Assche, K., Gutwirth, S., & Sterckx, S. (2013). Protecting dignitary interests of biobank research participants: Lessons from *Havasupai Tribe v Arizona Board of Regents*. *Law, Innovation and Technology*, *5*(1), 54–84.

Veenstra, G. (2007). Social space, social class and Bourdieu: Health inequalities in British Columbia, Canada. *Health & Place*, *13*(1), 14–31.

Wasserman, J. A., & Clair, J. M. (2012). The medicalization of homelessness and the sociology of the self: A grounded fractal analysis. *Studies in Symbolic Interaction*, *37*, 29–62.

Wasserman, J. A., & Clair, J. M. (2013). The insufficiency of fairness: The logics of homeless service administration and resulting gaps in service. *Culture & Organization*, *19*(2), 162–183.

Watermeyer, J. (2011). "She will hear me": How a flexible interpreting style enables patients to manage the inclusion of interpreters in mediated pharmacy interactions. *Health Communication*, *26*(1), 71–81.

Waysman, M., Schwarzwald, J., & Solomon, Z. (2001). Hardiness: An examination of its relationship with positive and negative long term changes following trauma. *Journal of Traumatic Stress, 14*(3), 531–548.

Weber, M. (2002). *The Protestant ethic and the "spirit" of capitalism and other writings* (P. Baehr & G. C. Wells, Eds. & Trans.). Penguin. (Original work published 1905–1920)

Weiss, J. (2011). GL versus BT: The Archaeology of biphobia and transphobia within the U.S. gay and lesbian community. *Journal of Bisexuality, 11*(4), 498–502.

Williams, D. R. (2018, November 12). *Interview with David Williams, Professor, Harvard University*. WebsEdgeHealth. https://youtu.be/fum8vrDD15Y

Williams, D. R., & Mohammed, S. A. (2009). Discrimination and racial disparities in health: Evidence and needed research. *Journal of Behavioral Medicine, 32*(1), 20–47.

Williams, D. R., Yan, Y., Jackson, J. S., & Anderson, N. B. (1997). Racial differences in physical and mental health: Socio-economic status, stress and discrimination. *Journal of Health Psychology, 2*(3), 335–351.

Woods, R. B. (2007). *LBJ: Architect of American ambition*. Harvard University Press.

Wool, C. A., & Barsky, A. J. (1994). Do women somatize more than men? Gender differences in somatization. *Psychosomatics, 35*(5), 445–452.

World Health Organization. (2019). *Social determinants of health*. https://www.who.int/social_determinants/sdh_definition/en

Yancy, C. W. (2020). COVID-19 and African Americans. *JAMA, 323*(19), 1891–1892.

Yazıcıoğlu, A. E. (2018). *Pink tax and the law: Discriminating against women consumers*. Routledge.

Zautra, A. J., Hall, J. S., & Murray, K. E. (2010). Resilience: A new definition of health for people and communities. In J. W. Reich, A. J. Zautra, & J. S. Hall (Eds.), *Handbook of adult resilience* (pp. 3–29). Guilford.

Zraick, K. (2019, July 12). *22 states considered eliminating the 'tampon tax' this year. Here's what happened*. The New York Times. https://nyti.ms/2xJaZ8a

13

When Cultural Perspectives Collide
Community-Based Health Interventions in Marginalized Populations

Chapter 13 examines various health theories and cultural perspectives for community-oriented, field-based interventions in addressing health disparities in marginalized populations. The chapter explores how historical injustice and current disparities between marginalized communities and dominant groups in the United States and around the world create challenges to implementing health interventions. By exploring the different cultural approaches to community-based interventions, we will review different health theories and concepts that are critical to implementing community-based campaigns. We will conclude the chapter by comparing and contrasting different theoretical approaches to responding to the unique needs and cultural perspectives of marginalized communities.

I. Community-Based Interventions and Tensions in Cultural Perspectives

A. "Exploitations" When Cultural Perspectives Collide

1. Exploitation Exists Only in Perspectival Thinking
Exploitation is an act specific to Perspectival Thinking, though different cultural perspectives may have actions that appear exploitative. Under Magic Consciousness, people are complete as they are. They do not hold ulterior motives nor feel the need to have "more" for their own sake. Their culture is embodied through their existences and actions, flowing with the rhythm of nature and the community. Everyone and everything inside a community of Magic Consciousness is alive and fused as one. All are sacred and irreplaceable. However, out-group members (or "things"), the Other, are not "real" and thus, completely replaceable and disposable. There is no logic or persuasion needed. It is just the way things are. As a result, under Magic Consciousness, a person can justify the slave trade because of a sincere belief that Africans have no souls and, thus, can be traded like animals and commercial properties (Wilson, 1957).

Under Mythic Connection, people are driven by their cultural values and moral principles expounded in their sacred stories and texts (some of which are magic in the sense that the words are said to be literally those of a deity and if spoken have incantatory power). They act because they "have to" if they want to be good and moral.

Rethinking Culture in Health Communication: Social Interactions as Intercultural Encounters,
First Edition. Elaine Hsieh and Eric M Kramer.
© 2021 John Wiley & Sons, Inc. Published 2021 by John Wiley & Sons, Inc.

Because they are driven by a sense of right or wrong, they believe that they are doing the right thing. As they incorporate locals into their religion or community, even violent actions were done for the better good for all. Their ulterior motive, if any, is to pursue their cultural values and moral principles. Even though some of their actions may appear to be blatant and crass exploitation, a true mythic believer may well be convinced that he is doing a moral (not exploitative) act. For example, a Christian Prince, Henry of Portugal, known as Henry the Navigator, was the first White European to take slaves from the African coast as far as Sierra Leon in 1444 (Wilson, 1957). The Prince, who was also a scientist, had a motto: *Talent de Bien Faire*, which meant Desire to Do Good (Wilson, 1957). The Prince believed that by taking Africans as slaves to Europe, he could convert the natives to the true faith – it was "an unspeakable satisfaction to contemplate the salvation of those souls that but for him would have been forever lost" (Wilson, 1957, p. 408).

Under Perspectival Thinking, people engage in relentless pursuits to exploit our physical and social environments (Kramer et al., 2014). By relying on concepts such as **social Darwinism** (i.e., natural selection and survival of the fittest as applied to human society and our social world) and **the common good** (also known as the social good or the greater-good; i.e., what is shared and beneficial to all or the largest number of people; Hussain, 2018), Perspectival Thinking has promoted eugenics and genocide for "race betterment" (see also Chapter 8). However, unlike people with Magic Consciousness and/or Mythic Connection – who are sincere, true believers of the ingroup-outgroup divide, people with Perspectival Thinking can be cynical and exploitative. Because Perspectival Thinking involves dimensional accrual of magic and mythic dimensions, people with Perspectival Thinking can recognize and understand magic and mythic dimensions (Kramer, 2013). In fact, Perspectival Thinking can incorporate some aspects of magic and mythic dimensions, such as an identity-oriented subscription of Magic Consciousness (e.g., precision and efficiency defining who we are) and/or the value-orientated pursuit of Mythic Connection (e.g., the more precise and efficient we are, the better we are as sentient beings [and scientists, students, or parents, etc.]).

When any construct becomes hypertrophic, it becomes deficient – no longer promoting survival via successful replication but instead waning. What once sustained a people faulters. When Magic Consciousness fails, identity fragments; when Myth Connection fails, followers lose faith; when the Perspectival Thinking fails, the rational becomes dangerous (suicidal). As dissociation increases, identity shrinks: from the animistic whole of existence, to all the "people," down to the clan, down to the extended family, down to the nuclear family, down to the modern isolated and independent individual, and finally to identity crisis and nihilism – a worldview that denies the existence of anything that cannot be measured such as meaning. Correlating with this is the collapse of spirit from animism, to vague but identifiable titanic forces, to polytheism with multiple but specific gods, to an exclusive monotheism, to nothing. The universe empties, expands, and dies. Care too vanishes. The universe does not know humans exist, and it does not care. Time and space as empty fields exploded beyond human comprehension, and this occurred only in the last 150 years. We see the emergence of a philosophy of abject selfishness by writers such as Ayn Rand (1964).

Among the various forms of exploitation, the exploitation of people with other cultural perspectives includes some of the most egregious cases in human history. One of the prominent examples is the **nuclear testing at the Marshall Islands** (see Figure 13.1). From 1946 to 1958, the United States detonated 67 nuclear bombs at Bikini Atoll and Enewetak Atoll at the Marshall Islands in Micronesia, representing nearly 80% of all atmospheric tests ever conducted by the United State – the equivalent of *detonating 1.7 Hiroshima bombs every day for 12 years* (United States Congress House Committee on Resources, 2005). These tests caused devastating environmental damage and exposed the people of the Marshall Islands to horrendous health problems, including genetic abnormalities for generations (e.g., thyroid disease, leukemia, and cancers; Gilbert et al., 2002; Simon et al., 2006). Before 1946, people of the Marshall Islands had encountered various forms of colonization, including Spanish Christian missionaries, German economic exploitation, and Japanese wartime occupation. How was it possible that Americans were able to convince locals in Micronesia – who live in, by all accounts, a tropical paradise – to migrate to other islands and accept the catastrophic destruction to their homeland? Imagine giving up your entire city for a nuclear test by a foreign power.

Commodore Ben Wyatt, the military governor of the Marshall Islands, met with the locals on February 10, 1946, after their Sunday morning services (Keown, 2018; see Figure 13.2). By invoking the Christian values that had been well-established in Marshallese society, Wyatt asked if the locals would be willing to relocate so that the United States could begin testing atomic bombs for "the good of mankind and to end all world wars" (Weisgall, 1980, p. 77). He compared the locals to the "children of Israel whom the Lord saved from their enemy and led unto the Promised Land" (Keown, 2018; Weisgall, 1980, p. 77). By exploiting sacred cultural/religious values (i.e., God's will) and social norms (i.e., follow the chief's desire), Americans' arguments made it impossible for Marshallese to contemplate rejecting their sacred duty in the eyes of the Lord (Firth & Strokirch, 2004). In response, the local Chief Juda Kessibuki reported their decision after consulting with the locals:

> If the United States government and the scientists of the world want to use our island and atoll for furthering development, which with God's blessing will

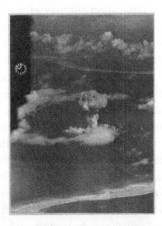

Figure 13.1 Nuclear testing at the Marshall Islands. Mushroom cloud with ships below during Operation Crossroads nuclear weapons test on Bikini Atoll. *Source:* Library of Congress Prints and Photographs Division[LC-DIG-ds-02946]

result in kindness and benefit to all mankind, my people will be pleased to go elsewhere. (Weisgall, 1980, p. 77)

Firth and Strokirch (2004) observed, "The Americans were happy to encourage their belief that forced migration were God's will and that nuclear tests would benefit all humankind" (p. 326). Weisgall (1980) noted some of the press coverage of the event:

> One U.S. military official, quoted in *Time* magazine, referred to the removal of the [locals] as "one hell of a good sales job." *The New York Times*, in an article entitled "The Strange People from Bikini," stated: "Primitive they are, but they love one another and the American visitors who took their home." (pp. 79–80)

Exploitation under Perspectival Thinking is not uncommon whenever a dominant group encounters indigenous or marginalized populations. Exploitation presumes that what you have is not mine; it is not universally shared. Thus, I must hatch a plan to get it for myself. By interpreting locals' actions of Magic Consciousness (i.e., they are one with "all mankind" – Marshallese and Americans belong to the same in-group) and/or Mythic Connection (e.g., following God's blessing will result in kindness and benefit to all mankind) through Perspectival Thinking, Americans were excited about their "sales job" in convincing the "primitive" locals that Americans who took their home had a fundamental kinship as part of their in-group. This is a prime example of deficient Perspectival Thinking, what Sloterdijk (1988) called **cynical reasoning** (i.e., being aware that one's beliefs and actions are based on some sort of lie but nevertheless continue to act as if everything is just fine). Even as they asked for their sacrifice for "all mankind," it is doubtful that Americans ever considered Marshallese as fellow American in-group kin, or as equals. In fact, the U.S. government shipped 130 tons of soil from its nuclear testing grounds in Nevada to the Marshall Islands in 1958 and even conducted a dozen biological weapons tests, including an aerosolized bacteria designed to kill enemy troops (Rust, 2019). These facts were not disclosed when the two countries signed a compact in 1986, which released the U.S. government from further liability (Rust, 2019). Under Perspectival Thinking, a lawyer would be quick to emphasize the voluntary nature of the forced migration, the ambiguity of promissory language during the "negotiation," and the contractual nature of the 1986 compact to mitigate the U.S. government's responsibilities.

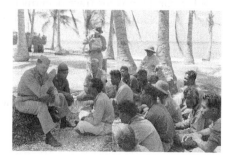

Figure 13.2 Commodore Ben H. Wyatt addressing the Bikini Island natives. On a Sunday afternoon a few months before the Army-Navy operation named Crossroads, Com. Ben Wyatt, the military governor of the Marshall Islands, traveled to Bikini. Commodore Wyatt can be seen sitting on the base of a palm tree, addressing the population moments before they were set to leave their home. (March 25, 1946) *Source:* Carl Mydans/ The LIFE Picture Collection/Getty Images

Alternatively, Marshallese may be startled and confused as to why the obvious would need to be stated and written at all. The Marshallese were basically a pre-literate culture that functioned based on Magic harmonics and implied trust. Firth and Strokirch (2004) explained,

> Marshallese accepted much of what was done to them without open complaint. Islanders, used to obeying chiefs, adapted to the Americans – the 'chiefs of the earth' – with apparent equanimity and a desire to please. ...
>
> Yet behind the politeness lay a determination to be compensated and a fierce attachment to the lands of their lineages. Chiefs, after all, were obligated to care for their people. (p. 326)

Marshallese took for granted their obligation (under Magic Consciousness), the natural equality of reciprocity and shared duty with their American brethren. They believed that one's word, that talk alone was sufficient to bind both parties (i.e., obligations are invoked as words are spoken, under Magic Consciousness; similarly, under the Mythic construct, the Americans were bound by the common covenant under a common God). They acted as their brother's keeper; in contrast, the American military did not see them that way.

The cultural differences are rooted in different realities and the corresponding assumptions and values. In the Magic world, good and evil do not exist as dualism does not exist. In the Mythic world, good and evil dissociate and become polarized but remain entangled. In the Perspectival world, what is legal and what is moral are completely severed via spatial dualistic thinking. The modern lawyer would stress that what was done was legal and ignore the morality of actions. Magic identity is not contingent but inherent and immutably permanent; in contrast, everything for the Perspectival person is contingent and mutable. Reality, value, meaning, and identity are all negotiable. Treaties and contracts can always be broken and/or renegotiated. Nothing is sacred. Everything is "for sale." Thus, reflecting on the meanings of treaties between the U.S. government and Indian nations, Prucha (1994) noted that it is "necessary to remember that formal written treaties were an Anglo-American, not an Indian, device" (p. XIV).

2. Exploitation through Strategic Communication

Sapir-Whorf hypothesis states that language and culture can influence one another through social interactions, resulting in worldviews that are unique and specific to the language (O'Neill, 2015). Language is an important resource to construct social realities. Through language (and social interactions), one can shift one's focus and understanding of an event (e.g., atmospheric nuclear testing is for "the good of mankind," and forced sterilization is for "race betterment," see also Chapter 8). We do not intend to suggest that Native Americans did not understand the meanings of treaties or that Marshallese did not agree to relocate. Rather, we argue that their cultural understanding regarding the functions of language, the meanings of their social interactions, and the corresponding implications to each parties' identities, relationships, and obligations are fundamentally different, resulting in misunderstanding, tensions, and conflicts.

People under Perspectival Thinking view language as mere tools, adopting signalic communication (see Chapter 4). Words are contingent. If this phrasing and this argument fail to win, change the phrasing and the argument. The more Perspectival a culture, the more meanings are parsed, and the complexity of legal literature grows enormously into giant libraries full of parsing. What a ruling means, precisely, becomes a focus of intense debate. In contract law, every comma and clause functions as semantic mechanics, carefully crafted for a precise fit. Language is just an instrument to achieve personal goals. It does not have inherent power other than its referential functions. Individuals may purposefully exploit the ambiguity and flout the linguistic rules to deceive others and to disguise intended objectives (Bavelas et al., 1990; Davis, 2007).

In contrast, under Mythic Connection, people use language to engage in symbolic communication (see Chapter 3). Languages are situated in social contexts, allowing community members to connect narratives to their cultural values and *perform* identities and relationships. Under Magic Consciousness, language has inherent power to create realities through idolic communication (see Chapter 2). In the Magic world, words are power. Words and deeds are who you are. As words are uttered, realities are invoked, defining who we are, what we do, and what is going on. Some language or linguistic devices are so sacred that no one (or only specific people) can say them. Indigenous people tend to hold Magic and/or Mythic worldviews. To them, a written, signed document encasing the specifics and limits of responsibilities and obligations of each party is no more "powerful" or "real" than the talk they engaged in during the social interactions. All are equally valid. Indigenous groups may consider mutual bonds and obligations cemented as they give each other their words in good faith (i.e., Mythic Connection) or at the moment the words are uttered (i.e., Magic Consciousness).

Moderns predominately hold a Perspectival worldview. From this perspective, the American governments may view formal, written treaties as the "official and final" referential tool to form the boundaries and limits of governmental obligations and intentionally rely on ambiguous, oral promises as strategic efforts to mitigate responsibilities during negotiations. In other words, although a perspectival person may say one thing but put something different in the contract, the final written contract is what "counts." They may also strategically exploit the ambiguity of written language to mitigate the binding "power" of a contract. This sort of purpose-driven construction of "wiggle room," this sort of strategic lying and prevarication such as lying by omission, evasion, and equivocation is unexpected by Magic people. When they are victims of such ploys, they are often confused, bewildered, and shocked.

Similar reactions occur when a Magic bond of identity is ruptured in the modern world: When a person is betrayed by another, whom they share a Magic bond (i.e., someone they had a complete commitment to and faith in). Such ruptures in "us" can only happen in a world of individuated egos. Otherwise, there is nothing for an individual to gain from deception because I am you and you are me. To betray you is to betray not myself, an individual ego, but *us collectively*. In the Mythic world, such treachery is regarded as evil. For a Magic person, it is not evil; it is unthinkable. It is as impossible as stealing from oneself.

Finally, although we adopted a somewhat dichotomous understanding to explore differences of cultural groups (e.g., Americans adopt Perspectival Thinking versus Marshallese or Native Americans adopt Magic Consciousness/Mythic Connection), it is important to note that not all members of a community share the same cultural perspective. For example, in the midst of congressional debates about whether the treaties with Indian nations were "legitimate" and "constitutional" since only nations with sovereignty can sign treaties, many politicians who fought to protect Native Americans' rights under the treaties were driven by "their deep Christian commitment to morality, to the honor and good faith of the nation" (Prucha, 1994, p. 165). For example, Senator Theodore Frelinghuysen of New Jersey, known as the "Christian statesman," asked,

> Do the obligations of justice change with the color of the skin? Is it one of the prerogatives of the white man, that he may disregard the dictates of moral princi-ples, when an Indian shall be concerned? ... The question has ceased to be – What are our duties? An inquiry much more embarrassing is forced upon us: How shall we most plausibly, and with the least possible violence, break our faith? (Prucha, 1994, p. 165)

Under Perspectival Thinking, it is perfectly "appropriate" and "justified" to discredit the legitimacy of the treaties by exploiting technicalities (e.g., whether an Indian tribe con-stitutes a "nation with sovereignty" that allowed them to create a legitimate treaty with its full legal force imposed upon both parties). It is perfectly "legal" and even "smart" to challenge the validity of a treaty based on whether all elements of legal language have been met. The parties' obligations were based on whether the legal language was precise enough to impose legal obligations (as opposed to an illusory promise that cannot be enforced by courts). However, challenging a good-faith agreement despite the imperfect legal language/conditions would be considered immoral for people who sub-scribe to Mythic Connection and unthinkable for people with Magic Consciousness. Frelinghuysen adopted a Mythic Connection perspective, arguing that we should not seek to relinquish our duties and break a good-faith agreement – even if the treaties may be flawed. In short, what distinguishes a person from one cultural perspective from someone from a different cultural perspective is not the "group" the person belongs to but how the person understands their social world through communication.

Researchers have proposed the concept **strategic racism**, which refers to "the manipulation of intentional racism, structural racism and unconscious biases for eco-nomic or political gain, regardless of whether the actor has express racist intent, although the very act of engaging in strategic racism is itself a form of racist behavior" (Hammer, 2019, p. 104). In public policies, politicians may adopt strategic racism through "dog whistle" politics by intentionally manipulating racialized beliefs in order to subvert support for welfare programs, promote a specific criminal justice agenda (e.g., war-on-crime), or to advance their own personal political objectives (López, 2015). Although these communication strategies aim to appeal to emotions of, and solicit support from, the public through Magic Consciousness and/or Mythic Connection, such strategies do *not* adopt an Integral Fusion approach. Alternatively, if the users of such strategies are genuine believers of their rhetoric, they have adopted the cultural perspectives of Magic Consciousness and/or Mythic Connection.

Indeed, the study of how to persuade people, of rhetoric itself, is a very perspectival pursuit. Magic and mythic peoples do not study rhetoric. They develop and deploy idolic ritual and mythic symbolic ceremony, not in order to persuade anyone of any-thing but rather to transform, divine, and commune. Race-baiting and ethnic agitation involve strategically designed and delivered messages that belie their Perspectival Thinking and directional targeting in the service of an implied agenda. The users of racist language as a strategic tool may claim not to be racist themselves, but only using racist tropes to achieve some other ends. But, to exploit racist tropes is itself to be racist. Perspectival thinkers who strategically exploit others' cultural perspectives for self-interested gains are pursuing narcissistic goals – they are disingenuous and cynical (Sloterdijk, 1988). Such exploitation within a society and between communities can fuel injustice over time, from one generation to the next.

We recognize that the events (e.g., eugenics, slave trade, nuclear testing, and American-Indian nations treaties) discussed in this section are rarely discussed in a typical health communication textbook. Nevertheless, these events continue to generate and perpetuate health disparities between marginalized and vulnerable populations and the better off within society. Our entry point to these events is not the outcome of health disparities but how the process of communication made such cases of exploitation and disparities possible. The encounters between dominant groups and marginalized communities provide ample opportunities for people of Perspectival Thinking to exploit the communicative process to maximize commercial benefits, maintain power hierarchy, and take strategic advantage of others' misunderstanding. It is true that magic and mythic people could not have appreciated the significant differences between a written contract and an oral promise in terms of their legal forces in protecting their rights. More importantly, perspectival people understood the differences and purposefully relied on magic and mythic people's lack of understanding (or misunderstanding) to achieve their objectives.

Health communication is more than communication that takes place in health settings or involves health contexts. How people engage in mundane, everyday talk can have profound implications for individual and population health. When people with different cultural perspectives engage in social interactions, there still can be significant misunderstanding or misalignment of perceived realities despite the appearance of "successful" interactions. Unjust exploitation happens when people of a cultural perspective intentionally and strategically rely on the ambiguity and gaps of understanding with people of other cultural perspectives for their own gain. Such an approach manipulates others' agency and fundamentally compromises any possibilities of developing an Integral Fusion worldview as others are not treated as equals in the communicative process.

B. Overview of Community-Based Health Interventions

1. Typology of Community-Based Health Interventions

Because experiences of health disparities often entail historical injustice and are situated in sociocultural and geopolitical contexts, researchers and public health experts have advocated for **community-based (health) interventions**. Historically, community-based interventions and developmental programs are rooted in the western values of self-reliance and self-determinism (Mansuri & Rao, 2004). The philosophy behind community-based interventions is an appreciation for community participation and ownership – which are essential to generate community support and efficacy (Merzel & D'Afflitti, 2003).

Despite the popularity of community-based health interventions, the term and the corresponding health campaigns have a wide range of meanings. Based on a survey of community-based interventions, McLeroy et al. (2003) proposed four ways through which "community" is framed: (a) community as setting, (b) community as target, (c) community as resource, and (d) community as agent. **Community as setting** refers to communities as the setting for intervention. It is the most common form of community-based interventions. As such, community is defined by its *geographic location* (as opposed to its membership) in which interventions are executed. Community inputs are sought through advisory committees or community coalitions to assist in tailoring interventions to meet the needs of target audiences. However, the focus of community input is to identify effective interventions, rather than to strengthen community capacity to address these issues themselves. These campaigns have primarily focused on changing individuals' behaviors as a way to reduce population risk – in other words, population change is defined as an aggregation of individual changes.

Community as target treats communities as a target of change. The goal is to create healthy community *environments* through systematic changes in public policy and institutional structures. In other words, a wide range of indicators can be used to track the health status and characteristics of the community (e.g., air quality, park availability, and percentage of residents living below the federal poverty level) over time to identify critical areas needed to improve community members' health.

Community as resource aims to marshal a community's institutions, internal resources or assets (e.g., informal social networks, schools, churches, among others) to strategically focus their attention on a selected set of health-related priorities, which may be predetermined by health authorities or selected by the community. Interventions adopting this model generally view community as a site of resources and often involve actors external to the community. Community-based health promotions often adopt this approach, believing that community *ownership* and *participation* are necessary to maintain long-term success in population-based health outcomes.

Community as agent, the least utilized form in public health interventions, emphasizes "respecting and reinforcing the natural adaptive, supportive, and developmental capacities of communities" (McLeroy et al., 2003, p. 530). Through combined utilization of resources *external* and *internal* to the community, these interventions incorporate the community's *"naturally occurring units of solution"* (e.g., family, church membership, teen peer groups, or other social units) to identify meaningful and effective entry points for interventions. In other words, the model is a bottom-up approach (i.e., "starting where people are") to develop solutions to address challenges faced by the community. The success of this approach is dependent on the campaigners' ability to understand, utilize, and leverage *community structures and processes* in ways as understood by community members.

These four forms of community-based interventions "reflect different conceptions of the nature of community, the role of public health in addressing community problems, and the relevance of different outcomes" (McLeroy et al., 2003, p. 530). The latter three forms (i.e., community as target, as resource, and as agent) consider not only changes in individual behaviors but also in *community capacity* to address health-related challenges as meaningful outcomes for their interventions (McLeroy et al., 2003). In addition, only the fourth form (i.e., community as agent) explicitly and actively integrates community members' understandings and cultural perspectives to identify problems and develop solutions. As such, the fourth form requires campaigners to see beyond their own perspectives and priorities, recognize the local community's perspectives and needs *in advance of* the actual campaign, and incorporate community members' agency at all stages of the campaign (e.g., planning, execution, and maintenance). In other words, community as agents requires campaigners to adopt an Integral Fusion approach to community-based health interventions.

More recently, researchers have used the term **community-driven interventions** (also called community-directed interventions) to highlight the paradigm shift in thinking about health priorities, power structures, and health service provisions in health campaigns (Amazigo et al., 2012). Community-driven interventions refer to community-based projects in which "communities have direct control over key decisions" (Mansuri & Rao, 2004, p. 2). Thus, an underlying principle in guiding community-driven interventions is a focus on building community capacity for problem-solving – building on "the strengths of a community to create change from within" (Lavery et al., 2005, p. 612). A review of community-driven health interventions (e.g., river blindness, human parasites, and malaria) in 16 countries concluded that such an approach is necessary to create sustained success in overcoming challenges of delivering services in very remote areas of poor countries with inadequate infrastructure (Amazigo et al., 2012).

2. Effectiveness of Community-Based Interventions

Despite the prevalence and popularity of community-based health interventions since the 1980s (Schensul, 2009), public health experts were confronted with puzzling findings. On the one hand, several studies noted that programs emphasizing community participation and collaboration have yet to demonstrate an impact on behavioral or health status outcomes (Ekman, 2004; Kreuter et al., 2000; Roussos & Fawcett, 2000). Often, community-based interventions have only weak or moderate effects in creating behavioral change (Black et al., 2002). A review of 32 community-based interventions, including several well-designed, large-scale, community-based interventions, concluded that most campaigns produced only limited effects in changing population risk behaviors (Merzel & D'Afflitti, 2003). A review of community-based interventions for elder abuse and neglect found that studies with high-quality evidence failed to demonstrate significant effects in reducing abusive behaviors (Fearing et al., 2017). A review of Signs of Suicide and Yellow Ribbon (i.e., two commonly applied school-based youth suicide prevention programs) and SafeTALK (i.e., the most widely adopted school-based and community-based suicide interventions in Canada) concluded that none of these community-based interventions demonstrated "sufficient evidence of effectiveness or of safety" (Kutcher et al., 2016, p. 383). The finding is also supported by other studies, noting the lack of evidence for the effectiveness of these school-based, community-based suicide prevention interventions despite many of these programs being framed as "evidence-based" programs (Bennett et al., 2015; Wei et al., 2015).

On the other hand, researchers have argued that community-based interventions are particularly valuable to engage minorities and marginalized populations and to develop effective interventions in their communities (De Las Nueces et al., 2012). A review of 67 community-based interventions concluded that community-based health workers can be "an effective intervention model that is also cost-effective for certain health conditions (e.g., high blood pressure, diabetes) or behaviors (e.g., mammogram and Pap test use) for low-income, underserved, and racial and ethnic minority communities" (Kim et al., 2016, p. e26). A study of 17 research projects by the Centers of Population Health and Health Disparities concluded that effective recruitment strategies for minority and underserved populations require using members of the target population in planning efforts, improving staff sensitivity, providing personal, culturally appropriate invitations to participate in studies, and providing either compensation or benefit to community members for their participation (Paskett et al., 2008).

In short, community-based interventions have become a widely accepted and commonly adopted model of health interventions despite a lack of evidence for its effectiveness. From this perspective, community-based interventions may be similar to patient-centered care, which has become a commonly embraced standard of care despite its mixed evidence in producing positive results (see Chapter 6). Similarly, despite the modest effects in most community-based interventions, one can argue that self-determinism and self-reliance through community ownership and participation are still worthy principles to maintain and protect.

Researchers have suggested that the limited effects may be a result of methodological issues (e.g., challenges in measuring community-level changes, incoherent outcome measures, lack of control groups, and varying levels of community participation), limitations of interventions (e.g., duration of intervention, insufficient tailoring, and low level of community participation/reach), and small effects of interventions in general (Ekman, 2004; Kreuter et al., 2000; Merzel & D'Afflitti, 2003; Roussos & Fawcett, 2000). These are useful, valid observations from the point-of-view of Perspectival Thinking.

The community-based interventions' lack of effectiveness can also be understood from a cultural approach by considering the way community is conceptualized, utilized, and incorporated in campaigns. Community-based interventions are particularly problematic when community and community resources are treated as sites and tools for interventions and/or when governmental authorities impose health priorities unilaterally. When community resources (i.e., organizational institutions and local governance) is conflated with community culture and equated as community-based interventions, the interventions are likely to adopt a top-down approach, privileging local authorities' perspectives and overlooking the diverse needs of community members (Asad & Kay, 2015). In addition, the historical injustice and widespread disparities faced by marginalized communities may make such interventions appear exploitative, hegemonic, and oppressive (Goddard & Myers, 2017). As a result, the beneficial effects of community-based interventions may be mitigated by **medical mistrust** (also called medical distrust; i.e., distrust of medical personnel and organizations; Guadagnolo et al., 2009). Medical mistrust is a known contributor to health disparities, resulting in reduced use of preventive care, poor treatment adherence, and lower patient satisfaction (Williamson & Bigman, 2018). Medical mistrust is particularly heightened in marginalized and vulnerable populations due to historical injustice and collective memories shared by members of these communities (Williamson & Bigman, 2018; see also Minority Groups' Historical Distrust of Healthcare Authorities in Chapter 7). Individuals' limited access to healthcare services (e.g., long wait time and high costs) also can significantly increase medical distrust (Nguyen et al., 2020).

Alternatively, community-based interventions that actively empower community members to engage in the decision-making processes can be particularly effective in marginalized populations. This is because the gaps in cultural perspectives are likely to be the greatest between marginalized populations and dominant groups, resulting in the strongest effects for culturally appropriate health interventions. For example, members of marginalized communities may engage in behaviors that appear risky or problematic by the standards and judgments of the dominant group, when, in fact, they are valuable resources for identity, relationship, and task goals. Without regular and continuous dialogue, the campaigners may simply attribute such behaviors as locals' ignorance or recklessness, instead of appreciating the essential functions served by these behaviors. Taking the locals' perspectives is essential to design, implement, and sustain a successful intervention.

For example, during the 2020 COVID-19 pandemic, hundreds of people defied stay-at-home orders to attend Church services, and hundreds of church leaders petitioned to open churches to the public (Presa et al., 2020). They did so despite the fact that epidemiologists warned that churches are high-risk clusters for COVID-19 because of the proxemics and the prolonged services and activities (e.g., singing and close social interactions), which can significantly increase individuals' exposure risks (Yong et al., 2020). A CDC report found that among the 92 attendees at a rural Arkansas church during March 6–11, 35 (38%) confirmed to contract COVID-19 and 3 died (James et al., 2020). An additional 26 cases in the community were linked to the church, including one death (James et al., 2020). It may appear that individuals who insist on attending church services and activities during a pandemic are irrational or ignorant. In response, health authorities may develop interventions to change these churchgoers' perceived susceptibility of risks or perceived severity of the illness.

Such an intervention can miss the fundamental meanings of attending church services for many of these churchgoers. Several studies have found that ethnic minorities, marginalized populations, and individuals with low socioeconomic status or low education level often actively incorporate **religious coping** in their illness management (Abraído-Lanza et al., 2004; Chatters et al., 2008; Harrison et al., 2001). Religious coping has been found to strengthen their sense of empowerment and resilience. Reflecting on the reasons for attending church events during the COVID-19 pandemic, a 24-year-old commented, "There is something great about praising the Lord when you're with other brothers and sisters. ... It's powerful, and it *strengthens your faith* and *encourages you*, especially during times like these" [emphasis added] (Presa et al., 2020). Such an attitude about attending church services indicates the performance of an in-group identity under Magic Consciousness and/or Mythic Connection.

Religious coping can entail both cognitive and behavioral strategies that are based on religious beliefs or practices (e.g., praying and seeking comfort/strength from God). Such forms of coping can be particularly valuable when one lacks other resources (e.g., marginalized populations). For example, low-income Latinos with chronic arthritis pain referred to their coping as putting oneself "en las manos de Dios" [in God's hands], which allowed them to accept what cannot be changed (Abraído-Lanza et al., 2004). Low-income Indonesian women viewed diabetes as an opportunity to demonstrate the cultural virtue of submission (e.g., opportunities to show patience, grace, and gratitude in the face of great difficulties, a testament to their humility) and to validate their faith (Pitaloka & Hsieh, 2015). For some, religious coping is not only an essential resource for coping with life difficulties but also represents indivisible facets of their identity and relationships (i.e., Magic Consciousness and/or Mythic Connection). Not attending church gatherings is unthinkable. Without understanding the social meanings of churches and the importance of attending church services, health authorities would not be able to develop meaningful interventions that address these marginalized communities' concerns (e.g., religious identities and community resilience).

Finally, the differences of cultural perspectives can exist not only between the dominant group and marginalized communities but also members of different subgroups within a community. Communities are *dynamic* and *multi-level* systems that "are internally connected via webs of relationships through which information, resources, and power flow and are exchanged" (Schensul, 2009, p. 246). Even within a marginalized community, there may still be significant differences and diversity of needs, perspectives, and agency between local partners (who tend to occupy more privileged positions, with higher education and better socioeconomic status) and targeted members (Asad & Kay, 2015). In addition, different marginalized communities may face unique struggles and challenges due to their sociohistorical relationships with the larger society. Schensul (2009) explained,

> For this reason, evidence based practices in prevention science which may have been tried and shown to be effective in one location under one set of historical and contextual conditions cannot be assumed to be effective in another. They must be weighed and judged to be suitable based on local criteria, with the anticipation that the endpoints or results may be somewhat or altogether different. (p. 243)

In other words, having mechanisms that incorporate community members' diverse perspectives at *all* stages of the campaign can be particularly valuable in creating *sustainable* success.

Schensul (2009) proposed that sustainability for a successful intervention is accomplished when a community has the capacity to engage in problem-solving that includes three components:

- *self-evaluation and monitoring* to assess whether the intervention continues to be well received and effective and when and how to modify it to continue that trajectory;
- *continued surveillance and review* of the environment to determine when the intervention needs to be changed to fit new conditions; and
- *responsive adaptation* to address the new conditions with a new approach.

This is because community-based interventions can trigger pan-evolutionary change not only within the targeted community but also in the larger society, making it necessary to take a holistic, ecological, and long-term approach to health interventions. This is an Integral Fusion approach to community-based health intervention because it adopts a temporal, adaptive, and multi-level approach, allowing the possibilities of multiple entry points to address health disparities.

C. Marginalized Populations and the Global South

Throughout this book, we have predominantly examined health disparities in the contexts of community/group-level struggles. We have explored various forms of disparities, noting that different understandings of culture can lead to different understandings and categorizations of marginalized groups (see also Chapter 12). For example, the **Black-nonblack divide** conceptualizes disparities through racial or ethnic categories (Shapiro et al., 2013; Yancey, 2003); the **urban-rural divide** centers on geographic location as the cause for economic and health disparities (Salinas et al., 2010); and the

digital divide recognizes that "the difference in the kinds of information and communication technologies to which people have access" can exacerbate existing inequalities, including health disparities, faced by communities (Howard et al., 2010, p. 110; Rains, 2008). How we conceptualize disparities and the corresponding causes frame our worldviews and shape our solutions.

One of the most important lessons learned from the COVID-19 pandemic is that health disparities in any vulnerable, marginalized populations are interconnected with all others in our communities, societies, and the rest of the world. As the United States is confronted with the disparities of death rates in African American communities (Pilkington, 2020; Yancy, 2020) – which are situated in the historical and sociocultural contexts of racial disparities, we should also recognize the disparities in our global communities. Marginalized populations can emerge through varying conditions and in different communities. Among nations, some countries may be marginalized within global "communities."

In the midst of the pandemic, President Trump announced that he planned to permanently end funding to the World Health Organization and pull out of the international body altogether because he "cannot allow American taxpayer dollars to continue to finance an organization that, in its present state, is *so clearly not serving America's interests*" [emphasis added] (Choi & Wheaton, 2020, para. 5). In contrast, reflecting on the devastating impacts of the COVID-19 pandemic, Dr. Anthony Fauci, Director of the U.S. National Institute of Allergy and Infectious Diseases and the leading medical expert in guiding the 2020 COVID-19 pandemic response in the United States noted:

> Right now, if you take southern Africa, sub-Saharan Africa, parts of Asia, South America and even parts of the Caribbean as areas that don't have the healthcare system to be able to respond the way one can respond in New York or LA or New Orleans or Chicago, we have really a *moral responsibility* for people throughout the world. (Powell et al., 2020, para. 6)

Whereas President Trump's comment highlights a focused self-interest through Perspectival Thinking, Dr. Fauci's call for moral responsibilities shifts America's pandemic response from a self-interest, Perspectival Thinking to the perspective of Mythic Connection and even Magic identification.

Do we really owe a moral responsibility to help other less developed countries? Should we help only if it is in the best interest of the United States to do so? Are we free to overlook other countries' suffering if such interventions do not serve "America's interests"? Before answering these questions, it may be helpful to understand how different "subgroups" (and thus in-groups and outgroups) can be conceptualized in the larger global community.

Researchers have noted that traditional categorization schemes that distinguish countries according to levels of developmental progress (e.g., "advanced" versus "primitive;" or "the First World," "the Second World," and "the Third World") can be insulting and confusing (Silver, 2015). For example, in the First World countries (e.g., the United States), there are still local communities that suffer from extreme poverty in rural and urban pockets. Instead of a ranked numbering system, many countries have welcomed the use of economic progress through the use of "developed," "developing," and "underdeveloped" countries, which can be more fluid and depicts their current economic reality. However, such an approach continues to imply a sense of progress and *hierarchy* between nations (Silver, 2015). In addition, when developed countries have depleted their natural resources and worked to exploit environmental and economic resources from underdeveloped countries for commercial benefits, is it truly appropriate to consider the industrialized countries more "developed" (Kramer et al., 2014)?

In response, the **Global South** becomes one of the latest terms researchers have used to conceptualize differences between nations in the global community. Dados and Connell (2012) explained,

> The phrase "Global South" refers broadly to the regions of Latin America, Asia, Africa, and Oceania. It is one of a family of terms, including "Third World" and "Periphery," that denote regions outside Europe and North America, mostly (though not all) low-income and often politically or culturally marginalized. The use of the phrase Global South marks a shift from a central focus on development or cultural difference toward an emphasis on *geopolitical relations of power.* [emphasis added] (p. 12)

The hierarchy of knowledge, what Michael Foucault (1966/2005) called "the order of things," is suddenly revealed to be highly Perspectival, very biased, and interested. What is ignored (e.g., what is not measured and why) is also critical. For instance, entire national economies have been brutalized by economic models deployed by the World Bank, leading to draconian policies. When a nation becomes a debtor, it becomes profoundly vulnerable within a global capitalist system. Everyone cheers for evermore "development," but it can be a money pit for poor countries. Once in debt, their creditors can keep making interest off them for decades. Poverty and bad credit ratings mean a country or even region, just like an individual, has a hard time gaining access to capital – money costs more for poor people and countries than for rich people and countries. It is expensive to be poor. Access to resources, including capital investment, is the basis of power. Who controls the access, who writes the rules and decides what counts and what does not matter, has power.

In recent years, the Global South is used in a way that goes beyond nation-state boundaries to capture the "a deterritorialized geography of capitalism's externalities and means to account for subjugated peoples within the borders of wealthier countries" (Mahler, 2017, para. 1). By looking beyond a territorial definition of nation-states, the Global South is used to refer to the shared *experiences* and shared *conditions* of marginalized populations – the subaltern groups across national, linguistic, racial, and ethnic lines – in the face of contemporary global capitalism (Mahler, 2017). From this perspective, the Global South "references an entire history of colonialism, neo-imperialism, and differential economic and social change through which large inequalities in living standards, life expectancy, and access to resources are maintained" (Dados & Connell, 2012, p. 13). In other words, the Global South is situated in the contexts of historical exploitation by the "Global North" and captured a network of resistance and social movements to demand justice and to empower resilience (see Figure 13.3).

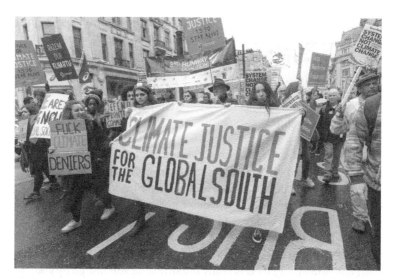

Figure 13.3 Justice for the Global South. By framing their funding as developmental aid to help the poor countries (as opposed to reparations), the Global North was able to disconnect the creation of their own wealth from their (colonial) exploitation of the Global South (Bogaert et al., 2019). *Source:* Peter Marshall / Alamy Stock Photo

From this perspective, the Global South adopts an Integral Fusion approach by situating identities as contingent and contextualizing their voice. Moving away from a hierarchical understanding of nation-states through developmental progress, the emerging meanings of the Global South have centered on the suffering of marginalized populations everywhere, encompassing African Americans in urban cities, indigenous people in Latin America and New Zealand, as well as rural communities in Africa, India, Pakistan, Bangladesh – everywhere. The Global South is not independent of or separated from the Global North. Rather, it recognizes the interconnectedness and the interdependence and globalization of capitalism in the current world order. It aims to identify solutions to address historical injustice, economic exploitation, and health disparities. In short, North and South are no longer used as geographical directions but as ways to identify the poor and systematically exploited populations everywhere. Solutions to disparities faced by the Global South entail pursuing social justice on a systemic scale – everywhere, from rural Alabama, which lacks healthcare infrastructure to Haiti, which also lacks healthcare infrastructure. The false assumption that rich countries, such as the United States, have no systemic inequality and no poor populations has been exposed. A 2017 report from the United Nations found that 40 million Americans (i.e., 12.7% of the population) live in poverty, among whom 18.5 million live in extreme poverty (i.e., family income below one-half of the poverty threshold; Alston, 2017a, 2017b). In fact, the United States has thrived on the exploitation of a massive underclass of underemployed and unemployed labor (for a documentary on unlivable wage, see Yamaguchi, 2020). This is an Integral Fusion way of seeing through ideologies deployed to mask inconvenient and unpleasant truths.

Now, let's return to our earlier questions. Do we owe a moral responsibility to help other less developed countries? If we believe that the United States is a country that is independent of and separate from the global communities, the answer is likely to be no. Under Magic Consciousness and/or Mythic Connection, we are obligated only to in-group members – moral obligations are for Americans only. Under Perspectival Thinking, morality does not come into play. The only calculation is: Does the United States *benefit* from such an action?

However, these are the moments that we are reminded of Dr. Fauci's (2014) reflection on the role of leadership:

> One of the things that I find with decision making is really important, and I tell everyone from my policy colleagues to the people in my laboratory, that when you're making a decision, whatever that might be, for your own career or for something that you want to do, you've got to do a combination of getting as much information as you possibly can, as well as listening to your gut.
>
> There's a certain something that when you build up your own training, your own moral values, your own principles, that your instinct and your gut about how something feels is really important. If you just go by your gut without any evidence, then you're just sort of a slave of your emotions. But if you go with evidence and never listen to how you really feel about it, I think you can make mistakes. (54:26)

Here, Dr. Fauci was talking about the value and importance of an Integral Fusion approach for decision-making. Despite his training as a medical expert and a scientist, he recognizes the limitations of Perspectival Thinking (i.e., you can make mistakes if you go with evidence and never listen to your gut instinct). On the other hand, he was also quick to note the dangers of Magic Consciousness and/or Mythic Connection (i.e., you are a "slave of your emotions" if you don't care about evidence). An Integral Fusion approach asks us to follow the evidence but never forget to do a gut-check.

In philosophy and in law, we recognize that there are **natural laws** and **natural rights** that are *morally valid, inherently just, self-evident,* and *universal* (Finnis, 2011). For example, the Declaration of Independence adopted a natural rights approach, arguing that *all* men are entitled to certain rights (e.g., life, liberty, and the pursuit of happiness) under natural law. The United Nations was founded on the principles of a Universal Declaration of Human Rights (1948). It represents another attempt to delineate natural rights for all humans. Natural rights are inherent in a person or a state and need no additional justification or jurisdiction to ensure their legitimacy or validity. Emmanuel Lévinas (1979/1987) noted that we all can recognize pain and fear in the Other despite linguistic and cultural barriers. We can even recognize it in other species such as horses and dogs. Such awareness is rooted in the shared reality at a Magic Consciousness level: We inherently know that no one likes pain, suffering, isolation, fear, and everyone wants to be respected and aided in times of crisis (Kramer & Hsieh, 2019). Cultural difference is not a good excuse for abandoning the Other (Kramer et al., 2014). This is the gut-check against positive law (i.e., laws instituted by humans). Now, do we owe a moral responsibility to help the Global South? What does the evidence say? What does your gut tell you?

II. Responding to the Cultural Perspectives of Marginalized Communities

A. Tailored Health Communication

Researchers have long recognized the importance of tailoring messages to target audiences to maximize the persuasive impacts of health interventions (Noar et al., 2007; Noar et al., 2009; Rimer & Kreuter, 2006). According to the **Elaboration Likelihood Model**, proposed by Petty and Cacioppo (1986), individuals are most likely to be persuaded by personally relevant messages because they are more likely to pay attention to the message and evaluate the message content more thoroughly. Traditionally, health interventions have relied on **message targeting**, which involves "defining a *subgroup* of a population-based on common characteristics and providing information in a manner consistent with those characteristics" (Schmid et al., 2008, p. 33). For example, to maximize the persuasive **impact** (i.e., defined as "population reach x efficacy;" Noar & Harrington, 2016, p. 251), an anti-drug abuse campaign that aims to stop young adults from engaging in the nonmedical use of prescription drugs (e.g., pain relievers, ADHD stimulants, and anti-anxiety drugs) would look very different from an anti-addiction campaign that is designed to help veterans who struggle with opioid addiction. The two campaigns may have very different message *content* and select *media* (e.g., venue/channel through which the message is delivered) that meets the preferences and needs of their target audience. Young adults who have high **sensation-seeking** needs (i.e., preference for thrill-seeking behaviors, including a strong tendency for experience-seeking, boredom susceptibility and adventure-seeking), a risk-taking personality, and an exaggerated sense of invulnerability are more likely to engage in risky health behaviors (Greene et al., 2000). Studies found that repeated exposures to high-sensation-seeking messages of televised health campaigns were effective in reducing high-sensation-seeking adolescents' risk-taking behaviors (Palmgreen et al., 2001; Zimmerman et al., 2007). In contrast, veterans' prescription opioid abuse is often connected to other health issues (e.g., chronic pain and mental health challenges, including depression and post-traumatic stress disorder; Bennett et al., 2019; Wilder et al., 2016). Their military identity also can discourage help-seeking behaviors (Braswell & Kushner, 2012; Cooper et al., 2018). As a result, successful campaigns must incorporate elements of clinical care that address mental health and pain management issues and respect veterans' desires to maintain independence and privacy (Vaughn et al., 2019).

  Audience segmentation is essential for message targeting as it is "the *necessary prerequisite* to creating messages that are responsive to the concerns, needs, and perspectives of specific populations" [emphasis added] (Slater, 1996, p. 267). Audience segmentation is a process through which a large, heterogeneous population is separated into more homogeneous subgroups based on the known or presumed shared characteristics of the group (Boslaugh et al., 2004). For example, in epidemiology, researchers use geographic variables (e.g., specific city or community), demographic variables (e.g., ethnicity, gender, age, education level, socioeconomic level, language proficiency, or nationality), and behavioral variables (e.g., people who are early versus late adopters of new technologies) to create subgroups. With the increasingly sophisticated technologies and techniques in collecting data, researchers and marketers also used

psychographics. Psychographics refers to the use of psychosocial variables (e.g., personality, lifestyles, attitudes, beliefs, values, opinions, and interests) for audience segmentation (Schmid et al., 2008). Although psychographic variables may not be as easily assessable as other variables, it can be a powerful tool in creating effective messages that directly target audiences who hold specific attitudes and behavioral intentions.

Whereas message targeting involves aiming a message at a subgroup of people, **message tailoring** fits a message to meet an *individual's* personal needs and characteristics, rather than a generalized targeting of group characteristics. Tailored communication has been defined as "any combination of strategies and information intended to reach one specific person, based on characteristics that are unique to that person, related to the outcome of interest, and derived from an individual assessment" (Kreuter et al., 1999, p. 277). Computer technologies have been essential in allowing health interventions to develop customized messages to their target audience (Noar & Harrington, 2016). In particular, **Web 2.0 technology** (i.e., web-based, multidirectional communication characterized by participation, collaboration, and openness [as opposed to read-only, unidirectional communication]), social media, and data mining artificial intelligence have made it possible to provide tailored health communication uniquely designed to target a particular person. Overall, a review of meta-analyses concluded that (a) tailored health interventions are often successful in encouraging behavioral change, and (b) messages that are more customized to an individual are more successful in influencing health behavior change (Noar & Harrington, 2016). In addition, although the tailoring of channel choice (e.g., print material, Internet, or in-person interventions) alone is not sufficient to make a difference, *how* tailoring is executed (e.g., choice of theoretical constructs and message designs) does appear to have a measurable impact on the effectiveness of an intervention (Noar & Harrington, 2016). Noar and Harrington (2016) concluded that researchers had shifted away from examining *whether* tailoring works to investigating the *specific conditions* that make tailored health communication effective.

For example, researchers may aim to match individuals' *information needs and interests* with tailored messages. Some of the common theories adopted for such interventions include the Health Belief Model (HBM), Theory of Reasoned Action/Theory of Planned Behavior (TRA/TPB), and Transtheoretical Model and Stages of Change (TTM; Noar & Harrington, 2016). The perceived susceptibility and perceived severity in HBM and the various beliefs (e.g., behavior, normative, and control beliefs) and the corresponding attitudes in TRA/TPB can be critical in addressing individuals' risky behaviors (see reviews of HBM and TRA/TPB in Chapter 6). During the COVID-19 pandemic, researchers found that counties that have a higher percentage of voters for President Trump in the 2016 election also have lower perceptions of risk, search less for information on the virus, and engage in less social distancing behavior (Barrios & Hochberg, 2020). Thus, meaningful interventions may require campaigners to rely on authorities that these voters identify with (e.g., conservative politicians and the White House) to provide information that specifically addresses their beliefs and attitudes (e.g., you can be susceptible because conservative politicians were tested positive and/or had to self-quarantine after exposure to COVID-19 at the annual CPAC meeting or at a White House event; White House agreed with the COVID-19 risks and have issued social distancing guidelines for the nation).

In contrast, the **Transtheoretical Model/Stages of Change** (TTM) is a theoretical model that adopts a *temporal* view of behavior change, noting that individuals may be at different stages of readiness for behavioral change (Prochaska et al., 2008). The stages of change include: **pre-contemplation** (i.e., no recognition of need for or interest in change), **contemplation** (i.e., thinking about changing), **preparation** (i.e., planning for change), **action** (i.e., adopting new habits), and **maintenance** (i.e., ongoing practice of new, healthier behavior; Glanz et al., 2015). Individuals do not always move through these stages in a linear manner as they often repeat and recycle certain stages (e.g., a person with addiction may relapse to an earlier stage or jump stages by quitting cold turkey). In addition, pre-contemplaters have very different needs than people who are in the maintenance stage. Whereas a pre-contemplater who is addicted to alcohol may need information to jolt her cognitive process (e.g., a friend killed in a DUI accident, education materials to change perceived susceptibility/ severity) to motivate behavioral change, a person in the action or maintenance stage would need resources and effective coping skills to maintain their self-efficacy (e.g., accessible AA meetings, the buddy system, and AA sponsors). Offering tools to increase self-efficacy for behavioral change would be useless to a person who is not even considering the need to adopt a target behavior; similarly, telling a person who has already adopted the target behavior about its corresponding benefits would be a waste of campaign resources. In short, under TTM, an effective, successful intervention must match the individual's stage-specific needs.

Finally, social marketing has become a popular model for health interventions. **Social marketing** is not a theory per se or a unique set of techniques; rather, it borrows from *commercial marketing* concepts and strategies to promote *socially beneficial* behaviors through voluntary behavioral change (Edgar et al., 2011; Grier & Bryant, 2005; see Figure 13.4). Because it is rooted in commercial marketing, the process of audience segmentation is essential to social marketing (Grier & Bryant, 2005). It adopts an interdisciplinary approach – drawing from fields of marketing research, advertising, psychology, communication, sociology, public health, among others – to create positive social change. Traditional health theories for behavioral change often incorporate elements of health education – believing that people should be informed decision-makers. In contrast, social marketing's primary focus is *voluntary behavioral change* – although improved knowledge or agency are desirable, they are not essential for a social marketing intervention (Storey et al., 2008). A social marketing campaign highlights a campaigner's Perspectival Thinking approach to health behavioral change in the sense that although it emphasizes *voluntary* behavioral change, it does not expect or require participants to exercise agency through informed, critical thinking for their health decisions. Rather, it focuses on appealing to consumers' self-interests and desire (i.e., the benefits most appealing to consumers) to induce changes in behaviors that are often predetermined by health authorities (Grier & Bryant, 2005). In other words, campaigners adopt strategies to *exploit* consumers' beliefs and attitudes for the benefit of accomplishing the *campaigner's* agenda. Until and unless the campaigners treat the participants as equal partners in all stages of the campaign (e.g., engaging target group's input in campaign design and decision making), social marketing campaigns cannot claim to have adopted an Integral Fusion approach even when it tailors its message to address the participants' beliefs and self-interests.

Researchers have raised ethical concerns about such goal-oriented, perspectival approaches to social marketing (Andreasen, 2001). For example, social marketers have relied on fear appeal (i.e., using messages to heighten a recipient's fear of impending

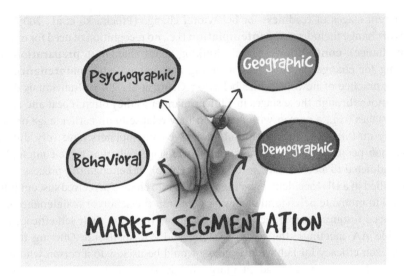

Figure 13.4 Audience segmentation. An essential component of social marketing campaigns is effective and meaningful market segmentations. *Source:* dizain/Shutterstock

danger or harm) to promote behavioral change. Although fear appeal can be an effective persuasion tactic, such strategies have been criticized for creating social stigma against the target population (Fairchild et al., 2018) and lead to maladaptive responses among those most vulnerable and thus, increase social inequity between those who respond to fear campaigns (e.g., people with higher education and income) and those who do not (e.g., marginalized populations; Hastings et al., 2004). Because what counts as "good" health behaviors are often predetermined by authorities in social marketing campaigns, marginalized populations' interests and perspectives may be overlooked or stigmatized. For example, although family planning can be a valuable health intervention, *how* (e.g., forced sterilization, instituting family caps for welfare, and offering available and accessible reproductive care) and *where* (e.g., ethnic minority communities, prisons, and low-income housings) such interventions are executed often reflect racial and social injustice, create coercive effects, and worsen health disparities in marginalized populations (Mengesha, 2017; Smith, 2006).

Finally, even if the underlying social issues are just and appropriate, it may still be problematic and unethical when the marketing strategies for those ideas are unethical and inappropriate (Lusch et al., 1980). Smith (2001) provided a real-life example: An African American ad agency in Southern California created a print ad that dramatized racism of White tobacco companies by targeting African American audiences. The ad featured two Ku Klux Kan hooded individuals – one carrying a flaming torch, with bold letters stating, "Nothing I like Better than Seeing a N---er Smoke." The "N" word was spelled out. Does it make a difference when the ad company is an African American agency? Would it be okay if the ad is produced by the National Institutes of Health, a federal agency? Does the ad stoke more racism, anger, and fear in African American communities? Is it ethical or appropriate to do so if it stops African Americans from smoking? Does the "greater" good or "social" good justify the use of racism as a social marketing tactic?

B. Cultural Sensitivity Approach

A **cultural sensitivity approach** aims to incorporate the cultural perspectives (e.g., characteristics, values, beliefs, experiences, and social norms) of the target population in the design, delivery, and evaluation of the health intervention (Resnicow et al., 1999). Resnicow et al. (1999) proposed that a cultural sensitivity approach can include interventions in two dimensions: surface structures and deep structures. Adaptations made to **surface structures** refer to matching intervention materials to observable, "superficial" characteristics of a target population (e.g., ethnicity, place, language, and food preferences), ensuring that the interventions fit within a specific culture. In contrast, adaptations made to the **deep structures** refer to recognizing the cultural, social, historical, environmental, and psychological forces that influence the target health behavior in the target population (e.g., African Americans' experiences of racial injustice and health disparities that shaped their low participation in preventive care), incorporating the target population's cultural perspectives and understanding as campaign features.

Resnicow et al. (2000) proposed that the tailoring of surface structure can increase receptivity and comprehension – making the intervention accessible and acceptable to the target audience; in contrast, tailoring of deep structure can increase self-efficacy and salience – increasing the impacts of the interventions. However, recent studies suggest the relationships between cultural adaptations and intervention outcomes may be more complicated and nuanced. For example, a meta-analysis found that although the effects of cultural adaptations in cancer communication are small, interventions that incorporated deep structure adaptations generate significantly stronger effects than those only incorporated surface structure adaptations (Huang & Shen, 2016). However, a study found that compared to those who received non-culturally adapted materials, Spanish-speaking participants had better recall of health information when they received pamphlets in *either* condition (i.e., deep structure adaptation and surface structure adaptation; Singelis et al., 2018). More importantly, the effects of these two adaptations are independent of one another and are additive, suggesting that they have different mechanisms in shaping intervention impact (Singelis et al., 2018). A review of five interventions of family-based interventions found that cultural adaptations can significantly improve ethnic minorities' participation and retention in health interventions, but only slightly improve their health outcomes (Kumpfer et al., 2002). In short, the literature suggests that different types of cultural adaptations are likely to have different impacts.

Tailored health communication can also include **cultural tailoring** that is responsive to target audiences' cultural perspectives (Barrera et al., 2013; Noar & Harrington, 2016). Despite the appreciation for "culturally tailored" interventions, health campaigns traditionally are limited to targeting ethnic minorities as cultural groups (e.g., Raj et al., 2001). Since the 2000s, researchers have proposed more sophisticated approaches to cultural tailoring and extend the understanding of culture beyond ethnic/racial groups. For example, Barrera et al. (2013) proposed that cultural adaptations in health interventions can be organized into five temporal stages: information gathering, preliminary design, preliminary testing, refinement, and final trial. Kreuter et al. (2003) proposed that common strategies for cultural tailoring include:

- **Peripheral strategies** that package the intervention in a way that appeals to a specific group. For example, by using certain colors, images, fonts, pictures of group members, or declarative titles (e.g., "A guide for African Americans"), a health pamphlet can explicitly convey relevance to the group.

- **Evidential strategies** that enhance perceived relevance to a specific group by presenting evidence of impacts on the group. For example, one can use epidemiological data for a specific group (e.g., the homeless) to increase the perceived relevance of information.
- **Linguistic strategies** that alter the language used in intervention materials to make them more accessible. For example, a campaign may avoid medical jargon for people with low health literacy and use the target audiences' native language to facilitate understanding.
- **Constituent-involving strategies** that utilize the cultural knowledge and experience of members of the subcultural group. For example, a health campaign may invite community insiders to identify health priorities and potential solutions when designing an intervention.
- **Sociocultural strategies** in which a subcultural group's "cultural values, beliefs, and behaviors are recognized, reinforced, and built upon" in campaign interventions (Kreuter et al., 2003, p. 136). For example, recognizing that Hmong people view epilepsy as a gift assigned by God for shamans, a health intervention may find ways to address the dangers of epilepsy in children and respect parents' concerns and appreciation for the child's divine destiny (Fadiman, 1997).

In addition, rather than conceptualizing marginalized populations as passive victims of health disparities who need to be "saved," we must engage and appreciate marginalized populations' agency and their capacity to thrive in adversities. Traditionally, health interventions of marginalized populations have often focused on improving their inadequacies (e.g., low health literacy, mental illness, or addictions) or training health care providers to develop **cultural competence** to accommodate marginalized populations' unique needs (Betancourt, 2004; Brach & Fraser, 2000; McCalman et al., 2017). Traditionally, cultural competence training in healthcare settings aims to improve providers' and health organizations' capacity to respond to racial/ethnic minorities' unique needs and perspectives, constructing the cultural groups' characteristics as fixed variables independent of any individual's life experiences and social contexts (Kirmayer, 2012). Such approaches, however, situate marginalized populations as passive recipients of disparities who are at the mercy of (healthcare) authorities.

Many medical schools now require training in cultural competence to ensure that providers have sufficient cultural and linguistic competence to assess patients' understanding of their illness and to elicit patients' use of folk medicine (Betancourt, 2004; Vela et al., 2015). With only ten weeks of medical Spanish, providers were found to reduce their use of interpreters but experienced an increase in patient satisfaction (Mazor et al., 2002). Such trainings, however, tend to adopt a biomedical perspective, emphasize physicians' informational needs, and focus on information gathering for clinical decision-making. A study found that when there is poor mutual understanding, language-discordant patients are likely to be silenced by providers' increased control over the content and process of communication (Meeuwesen et al., 2007). In fact, when compared to communicating with language-concordant patients, providers are likely to spend more time directly advising language-discordant patients and less time in engaging them in the decision-making process (Butow et al., 2011; Schouten et al., 2007). In short, providers may overestimate their linguistic skills or view communication as a means of gathering clinical information (as opposed to addressing patients' concerns; Diamond et al., 2009; Diamond et al., 2012). As a result, providers may feel satisfied because their informational needs have been met although they fail to address their patients' informational and emotional needs. The increase in patient satisfaction may be a result of rapport-building rather than patients' improved comprehension (Hsieh, 2016; see also language-concordant care in Chapter 12).

Increasingly, researchers have recognized that culture is neither a static nor fixed "thing" attached to a specific group of people. Rather, culture can entail varied meanings and perspectives. In addition, cultures and cultural perspectives are constantly being performed, negotiated, contested, and reconciled through the dynamic interactions and pan-evolutions between marginalized communities and the larger society. Kirmayer (2012) explained:

> An approach to cultural competence based on this more contemporary view of culture must consider how to meld recognition of, and respect for, the identity of individuals and communities with attention to the dynamic, contested, and often highly politicized nature of individuals' interactions with collectivities, both local and global. The cultural identity of an individual must be understood in terms of ongoing interactions within multiple networks or communities; similarly, the culture of an ethnic community can only be understood in terms of its interaction with the larger society. Each struggles to define, position, constrain and exploit the other. (p. 155)

More recently, some medical school curricula now seek to educate students about appreciating marginalized communities' experiences of social injustice and health disparities and develop awareness of their own potential biases when interacting with patients from different communities (Betancourt, 2004; Kirmayer, 2012; Vela et al., 2015). These approaches adopt a sociocultural, holistic approach by recognizing that both patients and providers are cultural participants who can work together to achieve the shared goals of equality and quality of care.

Since the 1970s, interventions for marginalized populations have embraced the incorporation of **community health workers** (CHWs; alternatively known as outreach workers, community health representatives, or patient navigator, many of whom also serve as language interpreters) to address health disparities in local communities around the world (Perry et al., 2014; see Figure 13.5). CHWs are defined as "a frontline public health worker who is a trusted member of and/or has an unusually close understanding of the community served" (American Public Health Association, 2020). Although they are not necessarily members of marginalized populations, they work with local communities to serve as advocates for patients and as bridges between different cultural perspectives (Natale-Pereira et al., 2011; Rosenthal et al., 2010; Terui et al., 2020). A review of 122 reviews concluded that CHW programs are highly context-specific and there are no standardized designs or interventions to ensure their success (Scott et al., 2018). Scott et al. (2018) summarized that CHWs generally offer six types of functions in healthcare settings:

1. deliver diagnostic, treatment, and other clinical services
2. assist with appropriate utilization of health services, make referrals
3. provide health education and behavioral change motivation to community members
4. collect and record data
5. improve relationships between health services and communities
6. provide psychosocial support

Themes of CHW interventions include four categories:

- *primary care interventions*: peer-support, phone calls, and home visits
- *reproductive, maternal, neonatal, and child health*: neonatal/child health (e.g., infant and childcare in resource-limited settings to reduce neonatal, infant, and child mortality and morbidity), immunization, contraception, maternal health, and breastfeeding
- *non-communicable diseases*: diabetes, cancer, mental health, asthma, and other chronic illness (e.g., hypertension)
- *infectious diseases*: HIV, malaria, hepatitis B, and tuberculosis

Factors that are likely to lead to positive outcomes include: community embeddedness (whereby community members have a sense of ownership of the program and positive relationships with the CHW), supportive supervision, continuous education, and adequate logistical support and supplies (Scott et al., 2018).

Finally, although cultural sensitivity approaches have demonstrated some success in addressing marginalized populations' health disparities, researchers also have cautioned against the efficacy and the limits of such approaches as they do not address (and can continue to perpetuate) the underlying *structural* inequalities and injustice that are at the roots of marginalized populations' experiences (Dutta, 2007; Swider, 2002). Incorporating marginalized communities' perspectives in tailored health communication or CHWs in health interventions does not guarantee equity or justice for

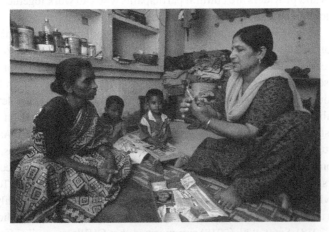

Figure 13.5 Community health workers. A community health worker explains how condoms should be used to avoid pregnancies as well as STDs in a slum in New Delhi, the capital of India. *Source:* Shehzad Noorani/AGE Fotostock

marginalized communities. Dutta (2007) explained a culturally sensitive campaign may still be problematic because "[the] expertise remains in the hands of the dominant external experts who determine the objectives, determine the relevant that cultural characteristics, configure the messages to fit these characteristics, and evaluate the messages based on externally defined criteria" (pp. 307–308).

Without an equitable distribution of *power* and an environment that supports and maintains marginalized communities' agency, these health interventions can continue to function as tools of the dominant group, enabling them to monitor, control, and coerce marginalized populations (Dutta, 2007; Mengesha, 2017). Smith et al. (2009) argued, "Conventional practice masks and supports status quo while it perpetuates the marginalization of the oppressed" (p. 159). As health interventions are developed to address poor diets, obesity, risky behaviors, and mental health problems in marginalized populations and ethnic minorities, we pathologize their existence without addressing the larger sociocultural structures and sociopolitical environments that make their suffering inevitable (Goddard & Myers, 2017; Smith et al., 2009; Viruell-Fuentes et al., 2012). A "culturally sensitive" intervention that targets the "at-risk" populations does not have answers for the structural barriers and challenges that constrain the target populations' everyday life.

In conclusion, a cultural sensitivity approach recognizes different types of cultural adaptations that are likely to have different effects. Cultural tailoring in health communication includes a wide range of strategies that address challenges faced by marginalized populations in both surface and deep structures. Traditionally, cultural competence training for healthcare providers has focused on improving providers' ability to seek information for clinical decision-making. In recent years, by recognizing culture involves dynamic and interactive processes between marginalized communities and the larger society, healthcare providers and health interventions have adopted a more holistic, contextualized approach to address marginalized populations' health disparities. CHWs are now a common element in community-based interventions in the United States and around the world. The literature suggests that (a) culturally sensitive interventions have a small but significant effect on improving campaign effectiveness, and (b) different cultural adaptations can have different intervention impacts. Researchers also have warned that without addressing the underlying structural injustices faced by marginalized populations, culturally sensitive/adapted interventions can serve as oppressive tools that perpetuate the inequalities and disparities between marginalized populations and dominant groups.

III. Additional Resources

A. Key Terms and Theories

> social Darwinism
> the common good
> nuclear testing at the Marshall Islands
> Sapir-Whorf hypothesis
> community-based health interventions
>> community as setting

community as target
community as resource
community as agent
community-driven interventions
medical mistrust
religious coping
Black-nonblack divide
urban-rural divide
digital divide
natural laws
natural rights
Elaboration Likelihood Model
message targeting
impact
sensation-seeking
audience segmentation
psychographics
message tailoring
Web 2.0 technology
Transtheoretical Model/Stages of Change (TTM)
    pre-contemplation
    contemplation
    preparation
    action
    maintenance
social marketing
cultural sensitivity approach
    surface structure
    deep structure
cultural tailoring
    peripheral strategies
    evidential strategies
    constituent-involving strategies
    sociocultural strategies
cultural competence (training)
community health workers (CHWs)

B. Discussion Questions

1. Do you agree that the nuclear testing at the Marshall Islands by the U.S. government are a result of "exploitations"?
   a. What constitutes exploitation? Do the exploited need to know that they are being exploited? Must the exploiter have the *intent* to exploit the Other?
   b. If a Magic/Mythic person cannot appreciate the intent and realities as perceived by a Perspectival person, are they always at the mercy of the Perspectival person then?

    c. If you were the negotiator on behalf of the U.S. government, would you do things differently? How?

    d. If you were to adopt an Integral Fusion approach when negotiating Magic/Mythic communities, what would you do? Can you use the nuclear testing at the Marshall Islands and/or treaties with Indian Nations as examples?

2. Compare and contrast the four different approaches to community-based campaigns: (a) community as setting, (b) community as target, (c) community as resource, and (d) community as agent.

    a. Which one is the easiest? Why?

    b. Which one is the most difficult? Why?

    c. Which one is likely to be expensive? Why?

    d. Which one is likely to be more successful? Why?

3. Do you agree that campaigns cannot be truly successful unless it ensures "community participation and ownership"?

    a. Can you think of any successful campaign that the participants were not involved in direct decision-making? (i.e., you do not have a choice of whether to do the health behavior or not.)

    b. Based on the Chapter, do you think we should always ensure "community participation and ownership" in community-based campaigns? Why or why not?

    c. If the target audiences adopt health behaviors and are becoming healthier, does it matter if they were not able to "choose" or that they were "coerced into" or "lied to" when adopting the health behaviors?

4. Do we owe a moral responsibility to help other less developed countries?

    a. Should we help only if it is in the best interest of the United States to do so?

    b. Are we free to overlook other countries' suffering if such interventions do not serve "America's interests"?

    c. Should we help other countries even if such actions may be at the expense of America's interests?

5. To maximize persuasive impacts for behavioral change, tailoring messages according to target audiences' unique characteristics is a common strategy for health campaigns. However, different cultural perspectives (i.e., Magic Consciousness, Mythic Connection, Perspectival Thinking, and Integral Fusion) may have different beliefs and attitudes about why and how to tailor messages. Try to answer the following questions:

    a. Which cultural perspective(s) are unlikely to tailor messages to increase their persuasive effects? Why?

    b. Which cultural perspective(s) are likely to tailor messages to adapt to target audiences' perspectives? Why?

    c. Which cultural perspective(s) are likely to tailor messages to maximize their persuasive effects even if they do not agree with the message? Would different cultural perspectives have different reasons to do so?

6. What are the pros and cons for physicians to have cultural competence training and/or second language training (e.g., medical Spanish)?

7. If you are a healthcare provider, how can you provide quality care to patients who do not share the same culture or language as you?

    a. Are there things you can do at an individual level?

b. What are the necessary support/resources at an organizational level?

c. How can community health workers facilitate healthcare delivery for minority, marginalized, or vulnerable populations?

C. References

Abraído-Lanza, A. F., Vasquez, E., & Echeverría, S. E. (2004). En las manos de Dios [in God's hands]: Religious and other forms of coping among Latinos with arthritis. *Journal of Consulting and Clinical Psychology, 72*(1), 91–102.

Alston, P. (2017a, December 15). *Extreme poverty in America: Read the UN special monitor's report.* The Guardian. https://www.theguardian.com/world/2017/dec/15/ extreme-poverty-america-un-special-monitor-report

Alston, P. (2017b, December 15). *Statement on visit to the USA, by Professor Philip Alston, United Nations Special Rapporteur on extreme poverty and human rights.* Office of the United Nations High Commissioner for Human Rights. https://www.ohchr.org/EN/ NewsEvents/Pages/DisplayNews.aspx?NewsID=225335

Amazigo, U. V., Leak, S. G. A., Zoure, H. G. M., Njepuome, N., & Lusamba-Dikassa, P.-S. (2012). Community-driven interventions can revolutionise control of neglected tropical diseases. *Trends in Parasitology, 28*(6), 231–238.

American Public Health Association. (2020). *Community health workers.* https://www. apha.org/apha-communities/member-sections/community-health-workers

Andreasen, A. R. (Ed.). (2001). *Ethics in social marketing.* Georgetown University Press.

Asad, A. L., & Kay, T. (2015). Toward a multidimensional understanding of culture for health interventions. *Social Science & Medicine, 144*, 79–87.

Barrera, M., Jr., Castro, F. G., Strycker, L. A., & Toobert, D. J. (2013). Cultural adaptations of behavioral health interventions: A progress report. *Journal of Consulting and Clinical Psychology, 81*(2), 196–205.

Barrios, J. M., & Hochberg, Y. (2020, April). *Risk perception through the lens of politics and the time of the covid-19 pandemic.* National Bureau of Economic Research. https:// www.nber.org/papers/w27008

Bavelas, J. B., Black, A., Chovil, N., & Mullett, J. (1990). *Equivocal communication.* Sage.

Bennett, A. S., Watford, J. A., Elliott, L., Wolfson-Stofko, B., & Guarino, H. (2019). Military veterans' overdose risk behavior: Demographic and biopsychosocial influences. *Addictive Behaviors, 99*, Article 106036. https://doi.org/10.1016/j.addbeh.2019.106036

Bennett, K., Rhodes, A. E., Duda, S., Cheung, A. H., Manassis, K., Links, P., Mushquash, C., Braunberger, P., Newton, A. S., Kutcher, S., Bridge, J. A., Santos, R. G., Manion, I. G., McLennan, J. D., Bagnell, A., Lipman, E., Rice, M., & Szatmari, P. (2015). A youth suicide prevention plan for Canada: A systematic review of reviews. *The Canadian Journal of Psychiatry, 60*(6), 245–257.

Betancourt, J. R. (2004). Cultural competence: Marginal or mainstream movement? *New England Journal of Medicine, 351*(10), 953–955.

Black, M. E., Yamada, J., & Mann, V. (2002). A systematic literature review of the effectiveness of community-based strategies to increase cervical cancer screening. *Canadian Journal of Public Health, 93*(5), 386–393.

Bogaert, K., Carlier, J., De Smet, B., Casier, M., Boer, D. V., & Mazin, B. (2019, October 5). *'Justice' not 'aid' for the Global South.* Governance in Conflict Network. https://www. gicnetwork.be/thinking-post-development-justice-not-aid-for-the-global-south

Boslaugh, S. E., Kreuter, M. W., Nicholson, R. A., & Naleid, K. (2004). Comparing demographic, health status and psychosocial strategies of audience segmentation to promote physical activity. *Health Education Research, 20*(4), 430–438.

Brach, C., & Fraser, I. (2000). Can cultural competency reduce racial and ethnic health disparities? A review and conceptual model. *Medical Care Research and Review, 57*(Suppl. 1), 181–217.

Braswell, H., & Kushner, H. I. (2012). Suicide, social integration, and masculinity in the U.S. military. *Social Science & Medicine, 74*(4), 530–536.

Butow, P. N., Bell, M., Goldstein, D., Sze, M., Aldridge, L., Abdo, S., Mikhail, M., Dong, S., Iedema, R., Ashgari, R., Hui, R., & Eisenbruch, M. (2011). Grappling with cultural differences; Communication between oncologists and immigrant cancer patients with and without interpreters. *Patient Education and Counseling, 84*(3), 398–405.

Chatters, L. M., Taylor, R. J., Jackson, J. S., & Lincoln, K. D. (2008). Religious coping among African Americans, Caribbean Blacks and non-Hispanic Whites. *Journal of Community Psychology, 36*(3), 371–386.

Choi, M., & Wheaton, S. (2020, May 19). *Trump: U.S. funding freeze to WHO could be permanent*. Politico. https://www.politico.com/news/2020/05/19/trump-world-health-organization-funding-267590

Cooper, L., Caddick, N., Godier, L., Cooper, A., & Fossey, M. (2018). Transition from the military into civilian life: An exploration of cultural competence. *Armed Forces & Society, 44*(1), 156–177.

Dados, N., & Connell, R. (2012). The global south. *Contexts, 11*(1), 12–13.

Davis, W. A. (2007). *Implicature: Intention, convention, and principle in the failure of Gricean theory*. Cambridge University Press.

De Las Nueces, D., Hacker, K., DiGirolamo, A., & Hicks, L. S. (2012). A systematic review of community-based participatory research to enhance clinical trials in racial and ethnic minority groups. *Health Services Research, 47*(3pt2), 1363–1386.

Diamond, L. C., Schenker, Y., Curry, L., Bradley, E. H., & Fernandez, A. (2009). Getting by: Underuse of interpreters by resident physicians. *Journal of General Internal Medicine, 24*(2), 256–262.

Diamond, L. C., Tuot, D., & Karliner, L. (2012). The use of Spanish language skills by physicians and nurses: Policy implications for teaching and testing. *Journal of General Internal Medicine, 27*(1), 117–123.

Dutta, M. J. (2007). Communicating about culture and health: Theorizing culture-centered and cultural sensitivity approaches. *Communication Theory, 17*(3), 304–328.

Edgar, T., Volkman, J. E., & Logan, A. M. B. (2011). Social marketing: Its meaning, use, and application for health communication. In T. L. Thompson, R. Parrott, & J. F. Nussbaum (Eds.), *The Routledge handbook of health communication* (2nd ed., pp. 235–251). Routledge.

Ekman, B. (2004). Community-based health insurance in low-income countries: A systematic review of the evidence. *Health Policy and Planning, 19*(5), 249–270.

Fadiman, A. (1997). *The spirit catches you and you fall down: A Hmong child, her American doctors, and the collision of two cultures*. Farrar, Straus and Giroux.

Fairchild, A. L., Bayer, R., Green, S. H., Colgrove, J., Kilgore, E., Sweeney, M., & Varma, J. K. (2018). The two faces of fear: A history of hard-hitting public health campaigns against tobacco and AIDS. *American Journal of Public Health, 108*(9), 1180–1186.

Fauci, A. (2014, May 6). *A leadership lesson: Turning the tide against AIDS.* Harvard University. https://www.hsph.harvard.edu/voices/events/fauci

Fearing, G., Sheppard, C. L., McDonald, L., Beaulieu, M., & Hitzig, S. L. (2017). A systematic review on community-based interventions for elder abuse and neglect. *Journal of Elder Abuse & Neglect, 29*(23), 102–133.

Finnis, J. (2011). *Natural law and natural rights.* Oxford University Press.

Firth, S., & Strokirch, K. V. (2004). A nuclear Pacific. In D. Denoon (Ed.), *The Cambridge history of the Pacific Islanders* (pp. 324–328). Cambridge University Press.

Foucault, M. (2005). *The order of things: An archaeology of the human sciences.* Routledge. (Original work published 1966)

Gilbert, E. S., Land, C. E., & Simon, S. L. (2002). Health effects from fallout. *Health Physics, 82*(5), 726–735.

Glanz, K., Rimer, B. K., & Viswanath, K. (Eds.). (2015). *Health behavior and health education: Theory, research, and practice* (5th ed.). Wiley.

Goddard, T., & Myers, R. R. (2017). Against evidence-based oppression: Marginalized youth and the politics of risk-based assessment and intervention. *Theoretical Criminology, 21*(2), 151–167.

Greene, K., Krcmar, M., Walters, L. H., Rubin, D. L., & Hale, L. (2000). Targeting adolescent risk-taking behaviors: The contributions of egocentrism and sensation-seeking. *Journal of Adolescence, 23*(4), 439–461.

Grier, S., & Bryant, C. A. (2005). Social marketing in public health. *Annual Review of Public Health, 26*(1), 319–339.

Guadagnolo, B. A., Cina, K., Helbig, P., Molloy, K., Reiner, M., Cook, E. F., & Petereit, D. G. (2009). Medical mistrust and less satisfaction with health care among Native Americans presenting for cancer treatment. *Journal of Health Care for the Poor and Underserved, 20*(1), 210–226.

Hammer, P. J. (2019). The Flint water crisis, the Karegnondi Water Authority and strategic–structural racism. *Critical Sociology, 45*(1), 103–119.

Harrison, M. O., Koenig, H. G., Hays, J. C., Eme-Akwari, A. G., & Pargament, K. I. (2001). The epidemiology of religious coping: A review of recent literature. *International Review of Psychiatry, 13*(2), 86–93.

Hastings, G., Stead, M., & Webb, J. (2004). Fear appeals in social marketing: Strategic and ethical reasons for concern. *Psychology & Marketing, 21*(11), 961–986.

Howard, P., Busch, L., & Sheets, P. (2010). Comparing digital divides: Internet access and social inequality in Canada and the United States. *Canadian Journal of Communication, 35*(1), 109–128.

Hsieh, E. (2016). *Bilingual health communication: Working with interpreters in cross-cultural care.* Routledge.

Huang, Y., & Shen, F. (2016). Effects of cultural tailoring on persuasion in cancer communication: A meta-analysis. *Journal of Communication, 66*(4), 694–715.

Hussain, W. (2018). The common good. In E. N. Zalta (Ed.), *Stanford encyclopedia of philosophy.* https://plato.stanford.edu/entries/common-good

James, A., Eagle, L., Phillips, C., Hedges, D. S., Bodenhamer, C., Brown, R., Wheeler, J. G., & Krirking, H. (2020, May 19). *High COVID-19 attack rate among attendees at events at a church — Arkansas, March 2020.* Centers for Disease Control and Prevention. https://www.cdc.gov/mmwr/volumes/69/wr/mm6920e2.htm

Keown, M. (2018). War and redemption: Militarism, religion, and anti-colonialism in Pacific Literature. In M. Keown, A. Taylor, & M. Treagus (Eds.), *Anglo-American imperialism and the Pacific: Discourses of encounter* (pp. 25–48). Routledge.

Kim, K., Choi, J. S., Choi, E., Nieman, C. L., Joo, J. H., Lin, F. R., Gitlin, L. N., & Han, H.-R. (2016). Effects of community-based health worker interventions to improve chronic disease management and care among vulnerable populations: A systematic review. *American Journal of Public Health, 106*(4), e3-e28.

Kirmayer, L. J. (2012). Rethinking cultural competence. *Transcultural Psychiatry, 49*(2), 149–164.

Kramer, E. M. (2013). Dimensional accrual and dissociation: An introduction. In J. Grace & E. M. Kramer (Eds.), *Communication, comparative cultures, and civilizations* (Vol. 3, pp. 123–184). Hampton.

Kramer, E. M., Adkins, G., Kim, S. H., & Miller, G. (2014). *Environmental communication and the extinction vortex: Technology as denial of death*. Hampton.

Kramer, E. M., & Hsieh, E. (2019). Gaze as embodied ethics: Homelessness, the other, and humanity. In M. J. Dutta & D. B. Zapata (Eds.), *Communicating for social change* (pp. 33–62). Palgrave Macmillan.

Kreuter, M. W., Lezin, N. A., & Young, L. A. (2000). Evaluating community-based collaborative mechanisms: Implications for practitioners. *Health Promotion Practice, 1*(1), 49–63.

Kreuter, M. W., Lukwago, S. N., Bucholtz, D. C., Clark, E. M., & Sanders-Thompson, V. (2003). Achieving cultural appropriateness in health promotion programs: Targeted and tailored approaches. *Health Education & Behavior, 30*(2), 133–146.

Kreuter, M. W., Strecher, V. J., & Glassman, B. (1999). One size does not fit all: The case for tailoring print materials. *Annals of Behavioral Medicine, 21*(4), 276–283.

Kumpfer, K. L., Alvarado, R., Smith, P., & Bellamy, N. (2002). Cultural sensitivity and adaptation in family-based prevention interventions. *Prevention Science, 3*(3), 241–246.

Kutcher, S., Wei, Y., & Behzadi, P. (2016). School- and community-based youth suicide prevention interventions: Hot idea, hot air, or sham? *The Canadian Journal of Psychiatry, 62*(6), 381–387.

Lavery, S. H., Smith, M. L., Esparza, A. A., Hrushow, A., Moore, M., & Reed, D. F. (2005). The community action model: A community-driven model designed to address disparities in health. *American Journal of Public Health, 95*(4), 611–616.

Lévinas, E. (1987). *Time and the other* (R. A. Cohen, Trans.). Duquesne University Press. (Original work published 1979)

López, I. H. (2015). *Dog whistle politics: How coded racial appeals have reinvented racism and wrecked the middle class*. Oxford University Press.

Lusch, R. F., Laczniak, G. R., & Murphy, P. E. (1980). The "ethics of social ideas" versus the "ethics of marketing social ideas." *Journal of Consumer Affairs, 14*(1), 156–164.

Mahler, A. G. (2017). Global South. In E. O'Brien (Ed.), *Oxford bibliographies in literary and critical theory*. https://www.oxfordbibliographies.com/view/document/obo-9780190221911/obo-9780190221911-0055.xml

Mansuri, G., & Rao, V. (2004). Community-based and -driven development: A critical review. *The World Bank Research Observer, 19*(1), 1–39.

Mazor, S. S., Hampers, L. C., Chande, V. T., & Krug, S. E. (2002). Teaching Spanish to pediatric emergency physicians: Effects on patient satisfaction. *Archives of Pediatrics & Adolescent Medicine, 156*(7), 693–695.

McCalman, J., Jongen, C., & Bainbridge, R. (2017). Organisational systems' approaches to improving cultural competence in healthcare: A systematic scoping review of the literature. *International Journal for Equity in Health, 16,* Article 78. https://equityhealthj.biomedcentral.com/articles/10.1186/s12939-017-0571-5

McLeroy, K. R., Norton, B. L., Kegler, M. C., Burdine, J. N., & Sumaya, C. V. (2003). Community-based interventions. *American Journal of Public Health, 93*(4), 529–533.

Meeuwesen, L., Tromp, F., Schouten, B. C., & Harmsen, J. A. M. (2007). Cultural differences in managing information during medical interaction: How does the physician get a clue? *Patient Education and Counseling, 67*(1–2), 183–190.

Mengesha, B. (2017). Racial injustice and family planning: An open letter to our community. *Contraception, 96*(4), 217–220.

Merzel, C., & D'Afflitti, J. (2003). Reconsidering community-based health promotion: Promise, performance, and potential. *American Journal of Public Health, 93*(4), 557–574.

Natale-Pereira, A., Enard, K. R., Nevarez, L., & Jones, L. A. (2011). The role of patient navigators in eliminating health disparities. *Cancer, 117*(15 Suppl), 3543–3552.

Nguyen, A. L., Schwei, R. J., Zhao, Y.-Q., Rathouz, P. J., & Jacobs, E. A. (2020). What matters when it comes to trust in one's physician: Race/ethnicity, sociodemographic factors, and/or access to and experiences with health care? *Health Equity, 4*(1), 280–289.

Noar, S. M., Benac, C. N., & Harris, M. S. (2007). Does tailoring matter? Meta-analytic review of tailored print health behavior change interventions. *Psychological Bulletin, 133*(4), 673–693.

Noar, S. M., & Harrington, N. G. (2016). Tailored communications for health-related decision-making and behavior change. In M. A. Diefenbach, S. Miller-Halegoua, & D. J. Bowen (Eds.), *Handbook of health decision science* (pp. 251–263). Springer.

Noar, S. M., Harrington, N. G., & Aldrich, R. S. (2009). The role of message tailoring in the development of persuasive health communication messages. *Annals of the International Communication Association, 33*(1), 73–133.

O'Neill, S. P. (2015). Sapir–Whorf hypothesis. In K. Tracy, T. L. Sandel, & C. Ilie (Eds.), *The international encyclopedia of language and social interaction* (pp. 1325–1334). Wiley.

Palmgreen, P., Donohew, L., Lorch, E. P., Hoyle, R. H., & Stephenson, M. T. (2001). Television campaigns and adolescent marijuana use: Tests of sensation seeking targeting. *American Journal of Public Health, 91*(2), 292.

Paskett, E. D., Reeves, K. W., McLaughlin, J. M., Katz, M. L., McAlearney, A. S., Ruffin, M. T., Halbert, C. H., Merete, C., Davis, F., & Gehlert, S. (2008). Recruitment of minority and underserved populations in the United States: The Centers for Population Health and Health Disparities experience. *Contemporary Clinical Trials, 29*(6), 847–861.

Perry, H. B., Zulliger, R., & Rogers, M. M. (2014). Community health workers in low-, middle-, and high-income countries: An overview of their history, recent evolution, and current effectiveness. *Annual Review of Public Health, 35*(1), 399–421.

Petty, R. E., & Cacioppo, J. T. (1986). *Communication and persuasion.* Springer.

Pilkington, E. (2020, May 20). *Black Americans dying of Covid-19 at three times the rate of white people.* The Guardian. https://www.theguardian.com/world/2020/may/20/black-americans-death-rate-covid-19-coronavirus

Pitaloka, D., & Hsieh, E. (2015). Health as submission and social responsibilities: Embodied experiences of Javanese women with type II diabetes. *Qualitative Health Research, 25*(8), 1155–1165.

Powell, A., Lewis, M., & Shumaker, L. (2020, May 20). *Julia Roberts, other stars hand over social-media spotlight to health experts.* Reuters. https://www.reuters.com/article/us-health-coronavirus-julia-roberts-fauc-idUSKBN22W2OS

Presa, L. R., O'Connell, P. M., & Villagomez, J. (2020, May 17). *Hundreds defy stay-at-home order to attend church while mayor's office warns that violators may be cited after review.* Chicago Tribune. https://www.chicagotribune.com/coronavirus/ct-coronavirus-illinois-churches-20200517-hawt4sd76jcmdorqquwytpqvx4-story.html

Prochaska, J. O., Redding, C. A., & Evers, K. E. (2008). The transtheoretical model and stages of change. In K. Glanz, B. K. Rimer, & K. Viswanath (Eds.), *Health behavior and health education: Theory, research, and practice* (4th ed., pp. 97–121). Jossey-Bass.

Prucha, F. P. (1994). *American Indian treaties: The history of a political anomaly.* University of California Press.

Rains, S. A. (2008). Health at high speed: Broadband internet access, health communication, and the digital divide. *Communication Research, 35*(3), 283–297.

Raj, A., Amaro, H., & Reed, E. (2001). Culturally tailoring HIV/AIDS prevention programs: Why, when, and how. In S. S. Kazarian & D. R. Evans (Eds.), *Handbook of cultural health psychology* (pp. 195–239). Academic Press.

Rand, A. (1964). *The virtue of selfishness.* Signet.

Resnicow, K., Baranowski, T., Ahluwalia, J. S., & Braithwaite, R. L. (1999). Cultural sensitivity in public health: Defined and demystified. *Ethnicity & Disease, 9*(1), 10–21.

Resnicow, K., Soler, R., Braithwaite, R. L., Ahluwalia, J. S., & Butler, J. (2000). Cultural sensitivity in substance use prevention. *Journal of Community Psychology, 28*(3), 271–290.

Rimer, B. K., & Kreuter, M. W. (2006). Advancing tailored health communication: A persuasion and message effects perspective. *Journal of Communication, 56(s1),* S184–S201.

Rosenthal, E. L., Brownstein, J. N., Rush, C. H., Hirsch, G. R., Willaert, A. M., Scott, J. R., Holderby, L. R., & Fox, D. J. (2010). Community health workers: Part of the solution. *Health Affairs, 29*(7), 1338–1342.

Roussos, S. T., & Fawcett, S. B. (2000). A review of collaborative partnerships as a strategy for improving community health. *Annual Review of Public Health, 21*(1), 369–402.

Rust, S. (2019, November 10). *How the U.S. betrayed the Marshall Islands, kindling the next nuclear disaster.* Los Angeles Times. https://www.latimes.com/projects/marshall-islands-nuclear-testing-sea-level-rise

Salinas, J. J., Al Snih, S., Markides, K., Ray, L. A., & Angel, R. J. (2010). The rural–urban divide: Health services utilization among older Mexicans in Mexico. *The Journal of Rural Health, 26*(4), 333–341.

Schensul, J. J. (2009). Community, culture and sustainability in multilevel dynamic systems intervention science. *American Journal of Community Psychology, 43*(3), 241–256.

Schmid, K. L., Rivers, S. E., Latimer, A. E., & Salovey, P. (2008). Targeting or tailoring? Maximizing resources to create effective health communications. *Marketing Health Services, 28*(1), 32–37.

Schouten, B. C., Meeuwesen, L., Tromp, F., & Harmsen, H. A. M. (2007). Cultural diversity in patient participation: The influence of patients' characteristics and doctors' communicative behaviour. *Patient Education and Counseling, 67*(1–2), 214–223.

Scott, K., Beckham, S. W., Gross, M., Pariyo, G., Rao, K. D., Cometto, G., & Perry, H. B. (2018). What do we know about community-based health worker programs? A systematic review of existing reviews on community health workers. *Human Resources for Health, 16*(1), Article 39. https://doi.org/10.1186/s12960-018-0304-x

Shapiro, T., Meschede, T., & Osoro, S. (2013, February). *The roots of the widening racial wealth gap: Explaining the Black-White economic divide* [Research and policy brief]. Institute on Assets and Social Policy, Brandeis University. https://heller.brandeis.edu/iasp/pdfs/racial-wealth-equity/racial-wealth-gap/roots-widening-racial-wealth-gap.pdf

Silver, M. (2015, January 4). *If you shouldn't call it the Third World, what should you call it?* NPR. https://www.npr.org/sections/goatsandsoda/2015/01/04/372684438/if-you-shouldnt-call-it-the-third-world-what-should-you-call-it

Simon, S. L., Bouville, A., & Land, C. E. (2006). Fallout from nuclear weapons tests and cancer risks: Exposures 50 years ago still have health implications today that will continue into the future. *American Scientist, 94*(1), 48–57.

Singelis, T. M., Garcia, R. I., Barker, J. C., & Davis, R. E. (2018). An experimental test of the two-dimensional theory of cultural sensitivity in health communication. *Journal of Health Communication, 23*(4), 321–328.

Slater, M. D. (1996). Theory and method in health audience segmentation. *Journal of Health Communication, 1*(3), 267–284.

Sloterdijk, P. (1988). *Critique of cynical reason* (M. Eldred, Trans.). University of Minnesota Press.

Smith, L., Chambers, D.-A., & Bratini, L. (2009). When oppression is the pathogen: The participatory development of socially just mental health practice. *American Journal of Orthopsychiatry, 79*(2), 159–168.

Smith, R. J. (2006). Family caps in welfare reform: Their coercive effects and damaging consequences. *Harvard Journal of Law & Gender, 29*(1), 151–200.

Smith, W. A. (2001). Ethics and the social marketer: A framework for practitioners. In A. R. Andreasen (Ed.), *Ethics in social marketing* (pp. 1–16). Georgetown University Press.

Storey, J. D., Satffitz, G. B., & Rimón, J. G. (2008). Social marketing. In K. Glanz, B. K. Rimer, & K. Viswanath (Eds.), *Health behavior and health education: Theory, research, and practice* (4th ed., pp. 435–464). Jossey-Bass.

Swider, S. M. (2002). Outcome effectiveness of community health workers: An integrative literature review. *Public Health Nursing, 19*(1), 11–20.

Terui, S., Goldsmith, J. V., Huang, J., & Williams, J. (2020). Health literacy and health communication training for underserved patients and informal family caregivers. *Journal of Health Care for the Poor and Underserved, 31*(2), 635–645.

The United Nations. (1948). *The Universal Declaration of Human Rights.* https://www.un.org/en/universal-declaration-human-rights/index.html

United States Congress House Committee on Resources. (2005). *The United States nuclear legacy in the Marshall Islands: Consideration of issues relating to the changed circumstances petition: Oversight hearing before the Committee on Resources, joint with the Committee on International Relations, U.S. House of Representatives, One Hundred Ninth Congress, first session, May 25, 2005.* U.S. Government Publishing Office.

Vaughn, I. A., Beyth, R., Ayers, M. L., Thornton, J. E., Tandon, R., Gingrich, T., & Mudra, S. A. (2019). Multispecialty opioid risk reduction program targeting chronic pain and addiction management in veterans. *Federal Practitioner: For the Health Care Professionals of the VA, DoD, and PHS, 36*(9), 406–411.

Vela, M., Fritz, C., & Jacobs, E. (2015). Establishing medical students' cultural and linguistic competence for the care of Spanish-speaking limited English proficient patients. *Journal of Racial and Ethnic Health Disparities, 3*(3), 484–488.

Viruell-Fuentes, E. A., Miranda, P. Y., & Abdulrahim, S. (2012). More than culture: Structural racism, intersectionality theory, and immigrant health. *Social Science & Medicine, 75*(12), 2099–2106.

Wei, Y., Kutcher, S., & LeBlanc, J. C. (2015). Hot idea or hot air: A systematic review of evidence for two widely marketed youth suicide prevention programs and recommendations for implementation. *Journal of the Canadian Academy of Child and Adolescent Psychiatry, 24*(1), 5–16.

Weisgall, J. M. (1980). The nuclear nomads of Bikini. *Foreign Policy, 39*, 74–98.

Wilder, C. M., Miller, S. C., Tiffany, E., Winhusen, T., Winstanley, E. L., & Stein, M. D. (2016). Risk factors for opioid overdose and awareness of overdose risk among veterans prescribed chronic opioids for addiction or pain. *Journal of Addictive Diseases, 35*(1), 42–51.

Williamson, L. D., & Bigman, C. A. (2018). A systematic review of medical mistrust measures. *Patient Education and Counseling, 101*(10), 1786–1794.

Wilson, R. D. (1957). Justifications of slavery, past and present. *The Phylon Quarterly, 18*(4), 407–412.

Yamaguchi, A. (Executive Producer). (2020). *Surviving an unlivable wage (Season 5, Episode 42)* [TV series episode]. In A. Yamaguchi, CBSN Originals. CBS News. https://www.cbsnews.com/video/surviving-an-unlivable-wage

Yancey, G. A. (2003). *Who is White?: Latinos, Asians, and the new Black/nonblack divide.* Lynne Rienner.

Yancy, C. W. (2020). COVID-19 and African Americans. *JAMA, 323*(19), 1891–1892.

Yong, S. E. F., Anderson, D. E., Wei, W. E., Pang, J., Chia, W. N., Tan, C. W., Teoh, Y. L., Rajendram, P., Toh, M. P. H. S., Poh, C., Koh, V. T. J., Lum, J., Suhaimi, N.-A. M., Chia, P. Y., Chen, M. I. C., Vasoo, S., Ong, B., Leo, Y. S., Wang, L., & Lee, V. J. M. (2020). Connecting clusters of COVID-19: An epidemiological and serological investigation. *The Lancet Infectious Diseases, 20*(7), 809-815.

Zimmerman, R. S., Palmgreen, P. M., Noar, S. M., Lustria, M. L. A., Lu, H.-Y., & Lee Horosewski, M. (2007). Effects of a televised two-city safer sex mass media campaign targeting high-sensation-seeking and impulsive-decision-making young adults. *Health Education & Behavior, 34*(5), 810–826.

14

Distributive Justice

Embedding Equity and Justice in Structural Barriers and
Health Policies

Chapter 14 examines the intersections of culture, ethics, and institutional policies. Shifting our focus away from individual- or group-based health interventions, we investigate how health policies and structural barriers shape the complex relationships between individuals' everyday lives and a society's management of resources. Using Medicaid work requirements and elements of the Patient Protection and Affordable Care Act (2010), we examine the meanings and functions of structural barriers. We then explore how distributive justice and other principles of justice can guide the development of health policies and the distribution of health resources. In the final section, we discuss the various theoretical approaches and methods that are valuable in helping policymakers and healthcare providers to address social barriers, ensure social justice, and achieve health equity.

I. Introduction to Structural Barriers

Researchers have noticed that compared to the general population (or the dominant groups), health disparity populations suffer disproportionally in their health management and maintenance due to structural barriers that encumber their *access* to health services, *process* of healthcare delivery, and *outcome* of health status (for detailed discussion, see Chapter 12). Addressing health disparities faced by marginalized and vulnerable populations has achieved some success by recognizing the unique characteristics and cultural perspectives of different patient populations (see Chapter 13). Such an approach, however, overlooks the everyday injustice and social inequalities that frame these populations' everyday life experiences and foreground their experiences of disparities (Viruell-Fuentes et al., 2012).

We define **structural barriers** as macro-level forces (e.g. governmental policies, institutional guidelines, and organizational cultures) that systematically impede marginalized and vulnerable populations' health management at all stages of care (see also Carrillo et al., 2011). From this perspective, social and economic policies are "equally or more important than health policies in maintaining and improving population health" (House et al., 2008, p. 5). Many of the social determinants of health involve nonmedical determinants, including various social, economic, and political issues (e.g. education, housing, food security, and political participation) in our society (see also Social Determinants of Health in Chapter 7; Boen et al., 2020; House et al.,

2008). How a society chooses to distribute our social and economic resources between different members of a society over time, from one generation to the next, can have profound implications as to whether we are able to maintain a just and fair system that maximizes benefits for all members and thrives in the face of adversities and unavoidable inequalities (Rawls, 2001).

Structural barriers are often historically rooted and culturally entrenched "through *mutually reinforcing inequitable systems* (in housing, education, employment, earnings, benefits, credit, media, health care, criminal justice, and so on) that in turn reinforce discriminatory beliefs, values, and distribution of resources, which together affect the risk for adverse health outcomes" [emphasis added] (Bailey et al., 2017, p. 1454; see also Viruell-Fuentes et al., 2012). Because structural barriers often are pervasive and integrated into institutional structures, policies, practices, and social norms, the corresponding stigmatization and discrimination can be normalized and even legitimized. As a result, community members, including members of marginalized populations, may not recognize the structural injustice at work in creating, maintaining, and reinforcing their experiences of disparities and suffering.

One topic of structural barriers that has received significant attention is structural racism. Structural racism is a major contributor to ethnic minorities' health disparities (Bailey et al., 2017; Williams et al., 2019). **Structural racism** refers to "the ideologies, practices, processes, and institutions that operate at the macro level to produce and reproduce differential access to power and to life opportunities along racial and ethnic lines" (Viruell-Fuentes et al., 2012, p. 2102). Structural racism involves interconnected institutions and refers to "the totality of ways in which societies foster racial discrimination" (Bailey et al., 2017, p. 1454). For example, the Social Security Act of 1935 is a valuable social safety net that offers employment-based old-age insurance and unemployment compensation. However, the Act excluded agricultural and domestic workers, a large percentage of whom were African Americans, from its coverage. Though researchers have debated whether such exclusions were racially-motivated, intentional discrimination (DeWitt, 2010), researchers have agreed that the effects (even if unintentional) have contributed to cross-generational injustice, as primarily White recipients were given resources to acquire wealth and pass it on to their children; in contrast, those excluded often became dependent on their children after retirement thus further curtailing the intergenerational accumulation of wealth (Bailey et al., 2017; Omi & Winant, 2014). *How Racism Makes Us Sick*, a TED talk by Dr. Williams (2016), and *Unnatural Causes: Is Inequality Making Us Sick*, a PBS series (Adelman & Smith, 2008) are great multimedia resources on this topic.

Structural racism in modern societies often manifests in disparate impacts between racial groups despite the lack of intentional discrimination through the "colorblind," neutral language in policies or legislation (Wiecek, 2011). Researchers have pointed out how our criminal justice system has failed as a fair system for marginalized and vulnerable populations. For example, federal law penalized crack cocaine offenses, which are almost exclusively charged against Black defendants, at a 100-to-1 sentencing ratio compared to powder cocaine, making crack the only drug that carried a five-year mandatory minimum federal sentence for first-time possession (Davis, 2010; Sklansky, 1995). The structural injustice embedded within legislation, laws, and policies have facilitated discriminatory arrests and incarceration of African Americans,

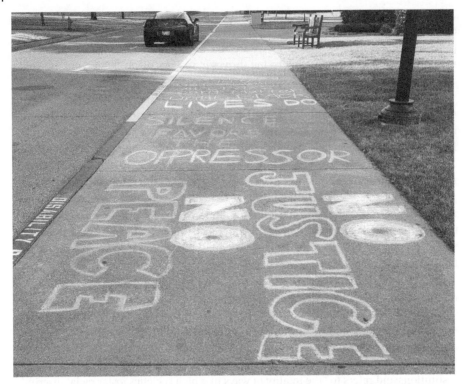

Figure 14.1 Sidewalk chalk signs at the University of Oklahoma: "No Justice, No Peace," "Silence Favors the Oppressor," and "All Lives Can't Matter Until Black Lives Do." *Source:* Elaine Hsieh

reinforced economic disparities in Black families, fueled unconscious bias in our society, heightened tensions against police brutality, and resulted in experiences of trauma across generations (Bailey et al., 2017; Bryant-Davis et al., 2017; Hart & Hart, 2019; see Figure 14.1). "I can't breathe," the last words uttered by Eric Garner in 2016, George Floyd in 2020, and many others during their arrests as they pleaded with the police, has now become a rallying cry against police brutality and everyday injustice faced by African Americans (Goyette, 2020; Passavant, 2015).

Racism exerts significant influences over the life course of African American lives and bodies, including higher risks for neonatal health (e.g., low birth weight and higher infant mortality), identity and physiological development in childhood, illness susceptibility due to exposure to everyday stress (e.g., increased risk for heart disease and depression), discrimination and limited life opportunities (e.g., unemployment and incarceration), and shared trauma as members of marginalized populations (Gee et al., 2012). In their analysis of life expectancies of Americans, Olshansky et al. (2012) concluded:

> Differences in longevity between subgroups of the US population are so pernicious and systemic that it is now reasonable to conclude that at least *two Americas* have formed... [Disparities] within racial and ethnic groups persist

even at the highest level of education. The same highly educated black men and women who live longer than less educated whites still live about 4.2 years less than comparably educated whites and 6.1 years less than comparably educated Hispanics. [emphasis added] (p. 1806)

Structural racism and racial inequality can *reinforce* and *normalize* one another. A 2020 CNN report found (Luhby, 2020):

- The median net worth of White households ($171,000) is about 10 times the median net worth of Black households ($17,600).
- The median income for Black households ($41, 000) is a little less than 60% of that of White households ($71,000).
- The unemployment rate for Black Americans (16.7%) exceeds that of Whites (14.2%) during the COVID-19 pandemic.
- The poverty rate for Black Americans (20.8%) is more than double that of Whites (8.1%).
- A larger share of Black Americans lacks health insurance (9.7%) compared to Whites (5.4%).
- Black people make up a larger share of U.S. Covid-19 deaths (23%) when they only account for 13% of the total population.

In the United States, these Black-White disparities can have significant implications for the Black-White divide in resources for childrearing (e.g., childcare and school facilities), neighborhood environment (e.g., open space availability and police surveillance), education, and economic opportunities. As we normalize inequalities, we often *moralize* disparities by attributing the cause to the inadequacy to character flaws or risk-taking behaviors of the marginalized populations rather than the structural injustice that is pervasive in limiting their everyday life. As a result, the System feels justified to adopt "tough" measures (e.g., work requirements for welfare recipients and three-strike law for criminals) to coerce "good" behaviors and submission from the marginalized.

In conclusion, as we consider the influences of culture on individuals' health management and on health disparities of specific communities, we must recognize that communication about health is not limited to clinical settings or health contexts. Our social and economic policies as well as political and legal systems have profound impacts on the health *and* prosperity of all members of a society. As such, these policies and systems provide a society with the necessary structures that collaboratively provide a fair and just system for all its members. Systematic injustice speaks volumes to the marginalized, informing them that their lives and bodies are dispensable, replaceable, and negligible. When these structures systematically and consistently fail to bring justice to certain populations within a society, these structural barriers can maintain and even ultimately result in social unrest and suffering that scars a society over time, from one generation to the next. The collective memories of marginalized populations and the trauma we experience together as a society will continue to demand truth and justice (Hom & Yamamoto, 2000; Nagata et al., 2019). Peace cannot be durable or sustainable without justice (Lederach, 1997).

II. Situating Structural Barriers in Contexts

Recent investigations of health disparities have highlighted several important issues in conceptualizing structural barriers. Rather than providing a blanket criticism against structural barriers, our goal is to explore the complex and nuanced interrelationship between structural barriers, social policies, and health disparities.

A. Work Requirements: Reinforcing Structural Barriers through Cultural Perspectives

Under cultural perspectives of Magic Consciousness and Mythic Connection, structural barriers are an extension of social stigma and, thus, are susceptible to manipulations through in-group versus out-group divide (see also Chapter 8). The recent impositions of work requirements for Medicaid recipients is a great example of intentional structural barriers under Mythic Connection. This is an issue that is heavily litigated in courts and debated among health scholars and policymakers. As of May 2020, four states' Medicaid work requirements have been approved but not yet implemented, four states' Medicaid work requirements have been blocked by courts, and ten states' Medicaid work requirements are currently under review by the Centers for Medicare & Medicaid Services (for the latest update, see The Commonwealth Fund, 2020).

Medicaid is an essential **social safety net** for many marginalized and vulnerable populations to access services that are critical to maintaining their health (Hahn, 2018). A social safety net can be broadly defined as structures and supports that have proven essential to a wide range of people (e.g., poor and vulnerable populations). They are established through government programs and policies, legislation, and structured benefits to which individuals are entitled (Loprest & Nightingale, 2018; The World Bank, 2019). A social safety net program can include: *cash* (e.g., unemployment benefits and workers' compensation), *in-kind transfers* of goods or services (e.g., food banks and free healthcare clinics), *social pensions* (e.g., social security), *public works* (e.g., short-term employment), and *school meal programs* (The World Bank, 2019).

Medicaid represents a public health insurance program that involves collaborations between the federal and state governments to provide "health coverage to millions of Americans, including eligible low-income adults, children, pregnant women, elderly adults and people with disability" (Centers for Medicare & Medicaid Services, n.d.-b, para. 1). As of June 2020, 67.9 million Americans were enrolled in Medicaid and nearly 6.7 million children were enrolled in the Children's Health Insurance Program (CHIP; Centers for Medicare & Medicaid Services, n.d.-a). In total, more than 36 million children are enrolled in CHIP or Medicaid, representing 50.1% of total Medicaid and CHIP enrollment (Centers for Medicare & Medicaid Services, n.d.-a). Medicaid covers 1 in 5 Americans and plays a critical role for certain populations, covering "nearly half of all births in the typical state; 83% of poor children; 48% of children with special health care needs and 45% of nonelderly adults with disabilities (such as physical disabilities, developmental disabilities such as autism, traumatic brain injury, serious mental illness, and Alzheimer's disease); and more than six in ten nursing home residents" (Rudowitz et al., 2019, p. 4). One of the primary objectives of Medicaid is to enable each State to furnish "medical assistance on behalf of families with dependent children and of aged, blind, or disabled individuals, whose income and costs are insufficient to meet the costs of medically necessary services." (Social Security Act, 2020). Medicaid represents the ideals of American federalism through which state and federal governments collaborate to provide health-services to states' poorest, elderly, and disabled citizens.

Requiring welfare recipients to work as an eligibility requirement to participate in welfare programs is not new. **Work requirements** generally include a wide range of activities; for example, a welfare recipient must be engaged in a job search, job training, or employment and community engagement activities (see Figure 14.2). As a result of the 1996 welfare reform law and debates in the 2000s, federal cash assistance (i.e., Temporary Assistance for Needy Families [TANF]), nutrition assistance (i.e., Supplemental Nutrition Assistance Program [SNAP], also known as food stamps), and some housing assistance agencies currently incorporate work requirements as a condition of program eligibility (Falk et al., 2014). In other words, if one does not satisfy work requirements, they will not receive welfare benefits.

Imposing a work requirement is consistent with the celebrated virtues of self-reliance and self-sufficiency (e.g., "God help those who help themselves") in western, capitalistic, individualistic societies (Greene, 2008). The famed "Protestant work ethic," a myth spread by social science as well as civic and religious leaders throughout the 20th century undergirds the ideology justifying work requirements: salvation comes from labor (Banerjee & Duflo, 2019; Hsieh & Kramer, 2019; Katz, 1996). This construct implies that Others (the poor) are lazy, stupid, and deceitful. This trope also expresses Social Darwinian notions that poverty and the poor are a burden to the larger community (Hsieh & Kramer, 2019).

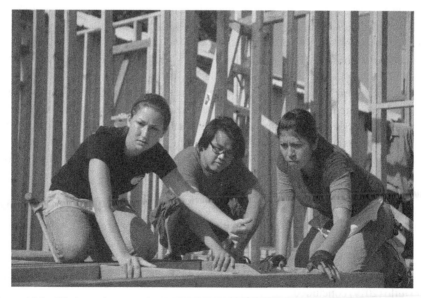

Figure 14.2 Work requirement. As an eligibility requirement, Habitat for Humanity (n.d.) expect an applicant to complete at least 400 hours of "sweat equity" towards the building of Habitat homes. *Source:* Hill Street Studios/Getty Images

According to a Congressional Research Services report, the rationale for imposing work requirements involve four primary goals: (a) offsetting work disincentives inherent in social assistance programs; (b) promoting a culture of work rather than one of *dependency*; (c) rationing scarce taxpayer dollars to the *truly* needy; (d) and combating poverty [emphasis added] (Falk et al., 2014). This rationale highlights a strong undertone of us versus "the Other" (Hsieh & Kramer, 2019). The in-group members, who are deserving of welfare support, embrace the "culture of work." Their tax contributions need to be rationed for those who really need them. By labeling those in need as "truly" needy, the public narrative *affirm* the government's historic commitment to helping those in need and echoes the Christian value of charity (Katz, 1996; Zarefsky et al., 1984). Yet, by conditioning support to those whose needs are "true," the narratives also imply that some others who are not "really" in need (Zarefsky et al., 1984).

The Other is from a culture of "dependency" and is not "truly" in need (i.e., the Other steals from those truly in need by frauds because they are lazy and cannot be self-sufficient). By receiving social assistance, the Other is disincentivized to work when their experiences of poverty can only be solved by forcing them to work (Hackworth, 2012). This is a call for social values and cultural norms – a call of pride for in-group to embrace work and to stigmatize the dependent, lazy, deceitful Other. "Two wedges are at work: one that separates hardworking good people from lazy thieves and one that separates the vulnerable from the robust. ... A moral imperative to help the weak while punishing the wicked is promoted" (Hsieh & Kramer, 2019, p. 143).

Questioning the poor's lack of motivation to work, which carries a strong, negative undertone about their moral character (e.g., laziness and dependency), is all too common in public policies (Banerjee & Duflo, 2019). For example, a **living wage** is the minimum hourly wage required to allow a worker to support her and her dependents, which should include the cost of food, housing, and basic needs. According to a report from the Massachusetts Institute of Technology, *the minimum wage does not provide a living wage for most American families*: The living wage in the United States in 2019 is $16.54 per hour (or $68,808 per year) before taxes for a family of four (for a living wage calculator for each state, please visit: https://livingwage.mit.edu; Nadeau, 2020). During the COVID-19 pandemic, as the federal and state governments worked to reopen sectors of the economy initially closed, many employers and government officials argued that employees are reluctant to return to work because their unemployment benefits are too high (Horsley, 2020; Luhby et al., 2020; Rainey & Mueller, 2020). It is true that two-third of laid-off workers received more money in unemployment benefits than they did from their jobs (Keshner, 2020). By challenging the moral character of the employees, the larger society was able to avoid discussions about the lack of living wages in our society (Luhby et al., 2020), the fact that 78% of American workers live paycheck to paycheck (Martin, 2019), or the fact that 27 million people are expected lose their health insurance following job loss during the pandemic (Garfield et al., 2020). These are structural problems that cannot be solved by forcing the poor to work harder.

Reflecting on a report on work requirements for non-cash welfare programs from The Council of Economic Advisers (2018), Nobel Prize winners in Economics Banerjee and Duflo (2019) concluded:

> The report argued that "the safety net – including government tax and [both cash and non-cash] transfer policies – has contributed to a dramatic reduction

in poverty [correctly measured] in the United States. However, the policies have been accompanied by a decline in self-sufficiency [in terms of receipt of welfare benefits] among non-disabled working-age adults. Expanding work requirements in these non-cash welfare programs would improve self-sufficiency, with little risk of substantially reversing progress in addressing material hardship." In other words, people had to be made to work for their supper, so they were not cheated of "the American work ethic, the motivation that drives Americans to work longer hours each week and more weeks each year than any of our economic peers [which] is a long-standing contributor to America's success." Sure, it might cause some pain, but it was worth it to prevent a large number of poor people from succumbing to sloth, one of the seven deadly sins. The Puritans would have applauded. (p. 287)

Work requirements in these welfare programs have been carefully investigated with irrefutable findings (see also Hahn et al., 2017): (a) Work requirements carry high administrative costs (Hahn et al., 2018), and (b) the complex administration yields high error rates that deny otherwise eligible individuals benefits, including individuals living with disabilities and chronic illnesses (USDA Office of Inspector General, 2016). In fact, various economic studies in different countries all consistently demonstrated that people are motivated to work – not just for money and survival but also for a sense of identity and accomplishment (Banerjee & Duflo, 2019). There is no evidence that recipients in welfare programs would work less as a result of governmental support (Banerjee & Duflo, 2019). Thus, it is particularly intriguing that state governments are willing to design and implement complex, costly reporting systems with high error rates.

An analysis from Kaiser Family Foundation found that in Kansas and Mississippi, due to their Medicaid income-eligibility requirement, "meeting Medicaid work requirements through 20 hours of work per week at minimum wage could lead to loss of Medicaid eligibility. In addition, these jobs are unlikely to have health benefits" (Musumeci et al., 2018, p. 2). In these states, individuals who are subject to work requirements are put in an impossible situation: "Damned if you do, damned if you don't" – If they do not meet the work requirements, they lose their Medicaid eligibility and access to health care; if they meet the minimum standard of work requirements, they lose Medicaid eligibility, have no health insurance, and are stuck with an income that barely supports the basic cost of living, let alone access to healthcare.

By imposing work requirements, the state Medicaid programs can expect that more participants will leave the program than the actual number of people who are targeted by the work requirements policy. For example, Kentucky anticipates "individuals with little to no claims activity choose to leave [Medicaid] rather than pay premiums" when they were not able to meet the work requirements. Kaiser Family Foundation explained, "Work requirements in Medicaid will *primarily affect people already working or exempt non-workers* by imposing new reporting requirements to document either their compliance or exemption with the rules regarding work" [emphasis added] (Garfield et al., 2018, p. 3). Because the majority of Medicaid adults are already working or exempt, they will constitute the majority of people who are disenrolled under the Medicaid work requirements "even if they may lose coverage at a lower rate than those who are not already working but subject to work requirements" (Garfield et al., 2018, p. 1). Depending on the different projected scenarios, Kaiser Family Foundation expected that between 1.4 to 4 million people may be disenrolled from Medicaid due to work requirements, among whom 77%-91% are expected to be people who remain eligible but lose coverage due to new administrative burdens (e.g., not reporting work activities or exemption; Garfield et al., 2018). By reducing the number of people covered by Medicaid, state governments can successfully control health expenditures.

In summary, we believe that structural barriers can be a result of magic, mythic, and perspectival worldviews. In addition, we argue that governments may invoke Magic Consciousness or Mythic Connection to corral public support. Similar to the eugenics movement that was driven by racism through Magic Consciousness and/or Mythic Connection (see Chapter 8), the U.S. federal and state governments have bound cultural values (and religious identities) to their policy decisions by connecting work ethics to self-sufficiency. By creating an in-group versus out-group divide, the suffering of the Other is not only negligible but also relished. On the other hand, like the scientific narratives that shaped the eugenics movement under Perspectival Thinking, policymakers also relied on narratives of economic efficiency (i.e., controlling health expenditures) to support their decision-making. The success of their policies is dependent on whether structural barriers can effectively curb certain groups' access to resources.

B. Rethinking Structural Barriers

Although structural barriers often have been viewed as a threat to public health and a contributor to health disparities in health disparity populations, structural barriers can serve strategic and functional purposes. In Chapter 8, we have provided an extensive discussion about the purposes and functions of social stigma. Although social stigma creates and silences suffering for the stigmatized groups, they are valuable (and may be effective) in maintaining the social order of the larger community (for a review, see Chapter 8). For example, Bayer (2008) has argued that stigma may be an effective *public health tool* – imposing normative sanctions that despite the short-term injustice may have long-term benefits to "the well-being of *the very people they burden* and on *those who might be dissuaded* from engaging in behaviors that have profound implications for health on a population level" (p. 470). Researchers have debated and investigated the effectiveness and appropriateness of using stigma as a public health tool to deter tobacco use, opioid addiction, and obesity (Corrigan & Nieweglowski, 2018; Puhl & Heuer, 2010). From this perspective, public health officials may decide to establish structural barriers to achieve common goods (i.e., what is shared and beneficial to all or the largest number of people; Hussain, 2018).

Imposing injustice onto a few for the common goods for all (e.g., "the greatest happiness for the greatest number") is a central principle of **utilitarian ethics** (Bentham, 1789/2007; see Figure 14.3). **Utilitarianism** is a moral theory according to which "an action is right if and only if it produces more utility (or welfare or well-being) for all people than any alternative" (Gandjour & Lauterbach, 2003, p. 230). By reducing ethical decisions to a *calculation* to achieve *one* intrinsic value (i.e., well-being for the greatest number), classical utilitarianism (e.g., hedonistic utilitarianism) envisions an *objective* and *rational* pursuit of happiness (Gandjour & Lauterbach, 2003). Utilitarianism avoids subjective interpretation and personal bias by focusing on an

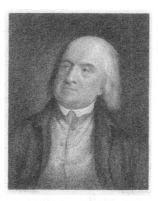

Figure 14.3 Jeremy Bentham. Jeremy Bentham was an English philosopher and was regarded as the founder of modern utilitarianism. *Source:* The Library of Congress

objective understanding of measurable outcomes (i.e., a means-end calculation): the most efficient means to achieve the end of maximal benefits for the largest number of people (rather than a specific person). In other words, individual interests are outweighed by obligations toward the community (Gandjour & Lauterbach, 2003). In the modern world where Perspectival Thinking predominates, a utilitarian approach is typically reduced to a *cost-benefit analysis* through which actions are evaluated through the maximization of efficiency, money, and outcome (Gandjour & Lauterbach, 2003). For example, cost-effectiveness analysis has played a long-standing and important role in the coverage of preventive services in Medicare, ensuring health gains are achieved at a reasonable cost (Chambers et al., 2015).

Though it may seem simple and objective, even when such a calculus is assumed, a cost-benefit analysis for structural barriers can be complicated, if not problematic. One of the examples is the efforts to reduce structural barriers through the Patient Protection and Affordable Care Act (2010), which as passed into law in 2010 and fully implemented in 2014 (ACA; Cogan, 2011; Gaffney & McCormick, 2017). The ACA requires (a) all individuals to have healthcare coverage and (b) mandates that patients have access to evidence-based preventive health services (e.g., vaccination) without **patient cost-sharing** mechanisms (i.e., the share of out-of-pocket costs not covered by insurance, which generally includes deductibles, coinsurance, and copayments; Cogan, 2011). These two strategies are critical to reducing barriers to health access because individuals now have insurance coverage to reduce the total cost of care. By eliminating cost-sharing, the ACA creates additional economic incentives for patients to seek preventive care. Cost-sharing is typically considered to be a cost-saving strategy by discouraging consumers from seeking health services as it creates economic disincentives and, thus, reduces overall healthcare costs. In other words, by eliminating cost-sharing requirements, patients are likely to utilize health services more frequently. The conventional wisdom assumes that preventive care is a worthwhile investment because the savings can exceed program costs (e.g., "An ounce of prevention is worth a pound of cure;" Warner, 1987).

However, reducing barriers may increase healthcare costs. Studies have found that when Oregon, Massachusetts, and Maryland increased individuals' Medicaid coverage, there was a significant to moderate increase, rather than a reduction, in individuals' use of emergency department utilization (Smulowitz et al., 2014; Taubman et al., 2014; Xu et al., 2018). When the cost of visiting emergency care is reduced, many used it more due to its convenience (Carroll, 2018). In fact, despite the common assumption that preventive care can save resources in the long run, analysis of over 599 research articles found that although "some preventive measures do save money, the vast majority reviewed in the health economics literature do not" (Cohen et al., 2008, pp. 662–663). An extensive review by Robert Wood Johnson Foundation found that only two preventive interventions (i.e., childhood immunizations and consulting adults to use low-dose aspirin) are truly **cost-saving** (i.e., decreases costs). Another 15 preventive services (e.g., screening for hypertension, cholesterol, diabetes, colorectal/breast/cervical cancer, HIV, among others) are **cost-effective** (i.e., benefits are sufficiently large compared to the costs, which was defined as cost less than $50,000–100,000 per quality-adjusted life-year gained [one QALY equates to one year of perfect health]; Cohen & Neumann, 2009). If the cost-benefit analysis is the basis to support ACA's mandates to reduce structural barriers, what should policymakers do when the cost-benefit analysis demonstrates that increased insurance coverage and access to preventive care are not necessarily cost-effective?

When confronted with cost-benefit analysis, important questions to ask are: *what* is considered cost or benefit, *who* bears the cost, and who enjoys the benefit? For example, economic analyses indicate that cessation of cigarette smoking will probably not lead to reduced health care expenditures in the *general population* because of increased health care utilization during those years of life saved as a result of cessation (Elixhauser, 1990). Nevertheless, for individual smokers, their regained health, extended productive years, reduction in pain and suffering, or quality time gained with family members may be too intangible to be included in the cost-benefit analysis (Scheffler & Paringer, 1980). Although a smoker may benefit from a workplace smoking cessation program by staying healthy and increasing productivity, the worker may also increase a company's retirement costs due to living longer (Warner, 1987). The danger of the cost-benefit analysis under Perspectival Thinking is: What is not measured is not valued. What is priceless becomes valueless. More importantly, the entities that determine the measurements of the costs and benefits determine the outcomes (see also Zarefsky et al., 1984).

We do not disagree that structural barriers can serve utilitarian functions. In fact, it is not uncommon for economists and health scholars to argue that certain discriminatory measures are necessary to ensure efficient use of health resources. For example, a review study found that workplace wellness programs cannot be cost-effective without being *discriminatory*, imposing **cost-shifting structures** (i.e., one party pays less than his/her share of the costs as the burden is shifted to others) such as making at-risk, unhealthy employees pay more to subsidize their healthier colleagues (Horwitz et al., 2013). When the Medicaid program increases copayments for nonurgent emergency department visits, patients are significantly less likely to visit emergency care for nonurgent reasons (Sabik & Gandhi, 2016).

The success of these utilitarian approaches is often dependent on the sacrifice of the most vulnerable. Individuals who are likely to be at-risk and unhealthy are also likely to be the ones who belong to minority, marginalized, vulnerable, or underserved populations. When workers' compensation programs adopt cost-shifting mechanisms, the costs are often shifted to the workers and their family members (Sears et al., 2020). As a result, vulnerable workers are more likely to underreport their occupational injuries/illness (Sears et al., 2020). Individuals with low socioeconomic status are more likely to be dissuaded by cost-sharing pressure. For example, in the midst of the COVID-19 pandemic, 1 in 7 U.S. adults reported that they would avoid seeking health-care for a fever and a dry cough for themselves or a family member due to concerns about their inability to pay for it (Witters, 2020).

Similarly, structural barriers that reduce individuals' access to insurance coverage (and thus, increases individual burden) can save costs for governments. For example, when the Supreme Court held that the federal government cannot coerce state govern-ments to accept Medicaid expansion by withholding existing Medicaid funding to the state (*National Federation of Independent Business v. Sebelius,* 2012), many states decided to not expand their Medicaid programs due to concerns about a significant increase in state spending after 2020, when the states were expected to contribute 10% of the cost of Medicaid coverage to more people (while the federal government funds the other 90%; Hays et al., 2019). As of October 2020, 12 states, mostly Southern states, have not yet expanded their Medicaid programs (for the latest update, see The Commonwealth Fund, 2020). Medicaid expansion can significantly reduce structural barriers faced by health disparity populations. For example, compared to their counterparts in non-expansion states, "low-income adults in ACA Medicaid expansion states experienced significant increases in coverage, improvements in access to care, and decreased finan-cial stress related to medical bills" (Miller & Wherry, 2019, p. 330). More importantly, the longer the states have adopted Medicaid expansion, the bigger the gap (Miller & Wherry, 2019). On the other hand, The Congressional Budget Office estimated that because states can reject federal funding to expand Medicaid, 3 million fewer people have insurance, which translates into $84 billion *savings* between 2012 and 2022 (Congressional Budget Office, 2012). In short, by *not* expanding Medicaid in some states, both federal and state governments benefit from reducing costs; in contrast, uninsured residents will individu-ally bear the costs of reduced healthcare access as well as increased healthcare costs.

It is from this perspective that utilitarian approaches to structural barriers become a glaring sore of a perspectival, modern society. We impose the costs and burden on the weakest few so that the majority can reap the greatest benefit. The classical utilitarian-ism principle is accomplished through overlooking and silencing individuals' rights and suffering (Gandjour & Lauterbach, 2003).

C. An Integral Fusion Approach to Structural Barriers

If structural barriers can be valuable tools in shaping the distribution of resources but utilitarian approaches to structural barriers can result in silencing individual suffer-ing, what are the possible solutions?

1. Incorporating Individual-Level Perspectives

First, it is important that we consider the costs and benefits not solely from aggregate (i.e., population-based) data but also from individuals' perspectives. Some researchers have proposed **preference utilitarianism** than a classical utilitarianism, which focuses on an objective cost-benefit analysis of utility. Preference utilitarianism argues that individuals' *subjective preferences* and their corresponding *intensity* should be considered in the cost-benefit analysis. In other words, "The goal of preference utilitarianism is to maximize the satisfaction of the preferences of all (i.e., the number and intensity of desires)" (Gandjour & Lauterbach, 2003, p. 242). For example, during the COVID-19 pandemic, President Trump issued an Executive Order, compelling meat processing plants to remain open to ensure "the continued functioning of the national meat and poultry supply chain" even though a large number of employees had become sick (White House, 2020, para. 4). Meat and poultry plant workers, however, have expressed concerns about risking their lives so that others can have meat at their dinner table (Colwell & McLean, 2020). A preference utilitarian approach would consider the amount and intensity of individuals' preferences (e.g., hundreds of thousands of meat plant workers' strong desire to remain healthy and stay alive versus 300+ million American people's moderate interests to avoid a meatless diet). By doing so, preference utilitarianism sidesteps the singular end of utility for the greatest number and accommodates minorities' interests and rights. Nevertheless, if the majority interests are high, the minorities' desires may still be silenced. For example, soldiers are expected to die for their countries. Meanwhile, deserters can be court-martialed even though their desire for life is extremely high.

Similarly, during the COVID-19 pandemic, some people have adopted Mythic Connection and even Magic Consciousness attitudes toward wearing facemasks as they fiercely and passionately rejected the use of masks, which has become a politicized issue (Syal, 2020). In response, Amy Arlund, a registered nurse who works at COVID unit, pleaded, "If I'm wrong, you wore a silly mask and you didn't like it. If I'm right and you don't wear a mask, you better pray that all the nurses aren't already out sick or dead because people chose not to wear a mask. Please tell me my life is worth a LITTLE of your discomfort?" (Almendrala, 2020, para. 16). The plead adopted a preference utilitarian approach by emphasizing the strong interests of a minority (i.e., healthcare providers) and the minimal costs to the general public.

The theory of preference utilitarianism, proposed by Singer (1972/2016), argues that "the more affluent should support the least privileged whenever this can be achieved without costing anything of comparable moral significance. Therefore, if we have the capacity to help others at minimal (relative) cost to ourselves, then it is our *moral duty to help*, regardless of their proximity to us" [emphasis added] (Stapleton et al., 2014, p. 3). Singer (1972/2016) explained,

> Moral attitudes are shaped by the needs of society, and no doubt society needs people who will observe the rules that make social existence tolerable. From the point of view of a particular society, it is essential to prevent violations of norms against killing, stealing, and so on. It is quite inessential, however, to help people outside one's own society.
>
> If this is an explanation of our common distinction between duty and supererogation, however, it is not a justification of it. The moral point of view requires us to *look beyond the interests of our own society*. ... From the moral point of view, *the prevention of the starvation of millions of people outside our society* must be considered at least as pressing as *the upholding of property norms within our society*. [emphasis added] (pp. 18–19)

From this perspective, preference utilitarianism takes on an Integral Fusion approach to structural barriers. Recognizing that institutional structures are necessary components in maintaining social order (e.g., upholding property rights to ensure individual safety and security; protecting food supply chain to the public) and the inherent incentives to protect "the interests of our own society" – preference utilitarianism embraces the consideration of the perspectives of the Other – "people outside of our society." When the suffering is significant and the cost for the in-group members to respond to their suffering is minimal (in comparison to their suffering), we have a moral obligation to act, to remedy the injustice of structural barriers. Singer (1972/2016) concluded, "Our obligation to the poor is not just one of providing assistance to strangers but one of compensation for harms that we have caused and are still causing them" (p. 66). By recognizing that impacts of structural barriers can connect past to present and to future times, preference utilitarianism contextualizes individual suffering and our moral obligations to one another. Preference utilitarianism is the most common utilitarianism in social and health policies in recent years (Gandjour & Lauterbach, 2003).

2. Situating Distributive Justice in Contexts

Second, we need to reconsider how we distribute benefits and burdens between different groups of people in our society. **Distributive justice** refers to the moral principles that guide the distribution of benefits and burdens in society. Distributive justice is grounded in the principles of social justice. In healthcare contexts, distributive justice offers "moral directives to a *just* allocation of resources, *fair* compensation to providers, and a *reasonable* range of services" (Dharamsi & MacEntee, 2002, p. 325). Distributive justice has become an underlying principle in health policies and healthcare reforms around the world. In Chapter 11, we explained that if we simply ask machine learning to provide suggestions from historical data, we are bound to repeat the injustice, bias, and discrimination of our history and our society. Similarly, recognizing the historical injustice and inherent disparities faced by health disparity populations, distributive justice emphasizes that justice can be achieved by modifying how a community distributes its resources/benefits and burdens/costs. However, distributive justice can be complicated in practice.

Three primary approaches to distributive justice are: libertarianism, egalitarianism, and contractarianism. A **libertarianism** approach believes that *freedom of choice* (e.g., freedom to choose preferred treatments without government interference) should be the guiding principle. For example, in Chapter 2, we discussed how the principles of freedom of religion had led 45 states and Washington D.C. to institute *religious exemptions* to mandatory vaccination requirements for children despite their potential to jeopardize the health of local communities (National Conference of State Legislatures, 2020). Should people be allowed to exercise their religion (i.e. benefits) at the expense of others' health status (i.e., burden)? Would eliminating the religious exemptions create a structural barrier that punishes the faithful? Similarly, does providing government-funded universal health care (e.g., Medicare for all), which reduces structural barriers, deny people their freedom of choice of private insurance (Hanson, 2007)? If they want to pay a commercial profit premium on top of healthcare costs and hamper universal healthcare by opting out, should they be allowed to?

An **egalitarianism** approach argues that every person should have an *equal* claim on all available resources (Dharamsi & MacEntee, 2002). In contrast, a **contractarianism** approach believes that because social inequalities are unavoidable and inherent in our social worlds, people hold a *social contract* with one another to creates a moral imperative to distribute basic needs to each other (the population) in a fair and unbiased manner that is responsive to such inequalities (i.e., the least advantaged should receive the greatest benefits; Rawls, 1971/2009). In other words, people make concessions to others' needs not because they must do so (e.g., as a moral imperative or to break an impasse) but because "they (ethically) should do so by virtue of living in a community with others" (Roemer, 1998, p. 93).

As Hochschild (1981) explained, "Aristotle's dictum 'treat equals equally' is useless until we specify who is equal to whom, what goods are subject to the dictum, and what equal treatment means in a particular case" (p. 51). Does distributive justice mean that every person has an equal claim on social resources, despite their differences (in race, sex, ancestry, talents, hard work, wealth, or luck), reflecting an egalitarianism approach (i.e., the **principle of equality**)? Or does it mean that their differences can create legitimate claims to different shares of social resources – reflecting a contractarianism approach (i.e., the **principle of differentiation**)?

Equality (i.e., every person is entitled to equal share) is easy to measure (e.g., whether one person's share is equal to another's). Equality principles are predominantly perspectival because its primary focus centers on a measurable quantity of distribution. In health contexts, equality generally translates into individuals having *equal opportunity* to access health resources (rather than having equal health status/outcomes). The resources needed to be healthy (i.e., the determinants of health, including living and working conditions necessary for health, as well as medical care) should be distributed *fairly* (as opposed to equally) regardless of the patients' age, race, gender, or social influence (Braveman et al., 2011). Rather than focusing on the equal amount of resource distribution, both adults and children appeared to be more sensitive about the *fairness* of resource distribution (Starmans et al., 2017). An Australian study found a strong egalitarian attitude among its participants (e.g. very little support to distribute lifesaving health sources for young people over the elderly; Nord et al., 1995). Equality is a common value embraced by Americans (Hochschild, 1981). It is also an essential value in guiding healthcare reforms in the United States (Braveman et al., 2011). During the debates of how to best distribute healthcare resources under the ACA, Sara Palin (2009), then-vice-presidential candidate and Alaska governor, called for egalitarianism and equality:

> Who will suffer the most when they ration care? The sick, the elderly, and the disabled, of course. The America I know and love is not one in which my parents or my baby with Down Syndrome will have to stand in front of Obama's "death panel" so his bureaucrats can decide, based on a subjective judgment of their "level of productivity in society," whether they are worthy of health care. Such a system is downright evil. (para. 2)

However, unlike Palin's rejection of government intervention in the distribution in health resources, a survey of 29 countries actually found that people who hold egalitarian attitudes are more likely to support government intervention for healthcare provision (Azar et al., 2018). This is because without governmental interventions and institutional policies, people who are wealthy or are powerful (having networks of strong influences among others) are likely to gain priority in the waiting list for organ transplants. Thus, government intervention may be necessary to ensure an egalitarian system. Palin was arguing for an egalitarian approach without any way to assure it actually occurring and instead, by default, assuring inequality. No change to policies means continued inequality.

On the other hand, social institutions may intentionally establish discriminatory policies and structural barriers to protect scarce resources. For example, most people would probably find it unfair (and offended) if a person who is actively addicted to alcohol receives a liver transplant – knowing that the liver, a scarce resource, is likely to be wasted (Albertsen, 2016). More recently, Medicaid and insurers have restricted coverage for expensive hepatitis C treatment (i.e. $1,000 per pill or $84,000 for a three-month course of treatment) that cures over 90% of the patients by requiring patients to demonstrate sobriety (e.g., no alcoholism or drug addiction) despite the fact that there is no evidence that sobriety improves the treatment success rate (Fox, 2018; Trooskin et al., 2015). Because concerns about personal responsibility as a contributor to one's illness condition may reduce the public's willingness to support an egalitarian approach, many vulnerable populations may be unfairly burdened (Schmidt & Hoffman, 2018). In short, equality (and in this case, the fairness of equal opportunity) is insufficient to make good social policies particularly when the resources are scarce.

Healthcare resources are often scarce, resulting in different groups of people competing for the same, limited resources. Following the principles of contractarianism, health equity aims to provide solutions and address existing inequalities. Healthy People 2020 defines **health equity** as the "attainment of the highest level of health for all people" (HealthyPeople.gov, n.d., para. 6). Achieving health equity requires "valuing everyone equally with focused and ongoing societal efforts to address avoidable inequalities, historical and contemporary injustices, and the elimination of health and health care disparities" (HealthyPeople.gov, n.d., para. 6). Health equity is "the value underlying a commitment to reduce and ultimately eliminate health disparities" (Braveman et al., 2011, p. S151). From this perspective, health equity follows contractarianism and echoes with preference utilitarianism – highlighting our moral duty to eliminate disparities faced by the Other (e.g., marginalized populations). This focus on eliminating health and healthcare disparities represents a Perspectival Thinking approach, a focused pursuit of measurable outcomes. Its commitment to "valuing everyone equally" represents cultural values under Mythic Connection. By integrating diverse cultural perspectives and appreciating the values of the Other, an Integral Fusion approach dominates the concept of health equity because it recognizes that solutions to suffering and disparities must consider and address historical and contemporary injustices faced by health disparity populations that may not be "my" group.

Integral Fusion does not claim to eliminate biases. An Integral Fusion mode of understanding, however, entails two important implications. First, by recognizing the Other as having a valid right to voice, my structure is exposed via difference. Second, this exposure frees me to be able to critically assess what had previously been invisible to me – my worldview. The Other enables me to see my own world, including its strengths and weaknesses (see Figure 14.4). Difference also liberates me. It enables me

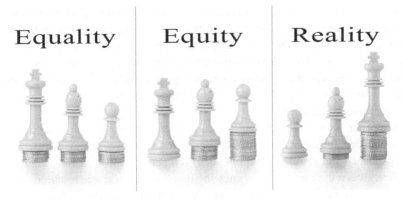

Figure 14.4 Equity-equality-reality. *Source:* Selu Gallego / Alamy Stock Photo.

to assess who I am, and how I might change, and how what I valued before is not so important after all, and how what I believed before, about myself and the Other (among other things), can be transformed.

In summary, structural barriers are not all bad. All structures discriminate. By embracing specific values, norms, guidelines, and even laws, structures aim to achieve what is considered just and fair for its participants. However, because inequalities are unavoidable and continuously evolve in our social worlds, we need to constantly monitor and assess how burdens and benefits are distributed as a result of social barriers.

III. Embedding Equity and Justice in Health Services and Policies

A. Justice as Fairness: Distribution of Health Services and Resources

Justice as fairness is a concept proposed by Rawls (2001) to explain how social institutions and basic structures of a well-ordered society can be formulated in a way that supports and maintains a fair, efficient, and productive system of social cooperation over time, from one generation to the next. A **well-ordered society** refers to a pluralistic society that is regulated by a *publicly recognized understanding of justice* that is shared by all community members. In other words, all members of a community can recognize that the basic structure of the community is just despite their differences in worldviews, perspectives, and interests. The shared understanding of justice does not presuppose any particular value but operates as *reasonable* values and principles that are acceptable and applicable to the social and political units within the cultural system. These values are subject to *public scrutiny and deliberation* – and the community is capable of *justifying* the substantive issues and procedures and *recognizing the diversities of worldviews in a democratic society*. This is a demand for truth and transparency – there can be no justice if community members do not have access to the truth (Lederach, 1997). There is no legitimacy to a society's principles of justice if it cannot be defended (i.e., not justifiable).

In addition, justice as fairness recognizes that in a democratic society in which pluralistic voices are embraced, justice cannot be achieved through hegemonic power but can only emerge through the dialogic space where different voices can be heard so that a *reasonable* solution can be agreed upon by different members of a society. From this perspective, justice as fairness takes on an Integral Fusion approach, recognizing that justice does not imply a singular or fixed answer but is contextually situated and inter-actively negotiated between a wide range of members and perspectives in a commu-nity. More importantly, justice is not accomplished in a moment in time but is measured "from one generation to the next."

Rawls (2001) noted that justice as fairness is only possible in a political structure of a democratic society where (a) all citizens are free and equal persons and (b) the soci-ety functions as a fair system of social cooperation over time, from one generation to the next. Justice as fairness presents two guiding principles of justice:

1. *First Principle*: Each person has the same indefeasible claim to a fully adequate scheme of equal basic liberties, which scheme is compatible with the same scheme of liberties for all (see also Figure 14.5);
2. *Second Principle*: Social and economic inequalities are to satisfy two conditions:
    a. They are to be attached to offices and positions open to all under conditions of fair equality of opportunity (principle of equality)
    b. They are to be to the greatest benefit of the least-advantaged members of society (principle of differentiation)

Justice as fairness represents Rawls' response to the different approaches to distribu-tive justice. The order of the principles is essential in establishing justice (Wenar, 2017). The first principle has priority over the second principle and the principle of equality is prior to the principle of differentiation.

The first principle governs political equality. It recognizes that all community mem-bers have the same basic rights and liberties: individuals' basic rights, including their choices (e.g., equal political liberties [e.g., freedom of speech and freedom of assembly]

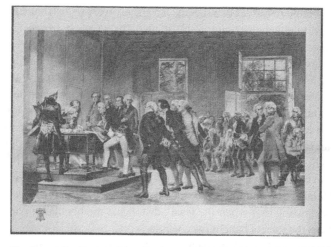

Figure 14.5 Signing at the Declaration of Independence. The Declaration of Independence states, "We hold these truths to be self-evident, that all men are created equal, that they are endowed by their Creator with certain unalienable Rights, that among these are Life, Liberty and the pursuit of Happiness." *Source:* The Library of Congress

and equal civil liberties [e.g., freedom of religion, freedom of association, and free choice of occupation]), are to be respected. This is a response to libertarianism and the most fundamental principle: "The basic rights and liberties must not be traded off against other social goods" (Wenar, 2017, "The Two Principles of Justice as Fairness" section). In other words, the shared justice must not require individuals to sacrifice their fundamental rights for the common good under normal circumstances. In health contexts, the first principle means that all people have a **right to health** (i.e., "the right of everyone to the enjoyment of the highest attainable standard of physical and mental health") and to a standard of living adequate for health (Braveman et al., 2011, p. S150). Only when the first principle is satisfied, can the second principle be triggered to address social and economic inequalities.

Echoing egalitarianism, the first condition of the second principle centers on the principle of equality, noting that all community members should have *equal opportunities* (i.e., a fair chance) in political participation. More importantly, equality is not just about having the same protection for all members of a community but also includes equality of having one's voice heard and be able to freely participate in decision-making. To ensure that equal opportunities are guaranteed for all across generations (i.e., powers cannot be concentrated to a few), Rawls (2001) emphasized that the sociopolitical and legal institutions of a society must ensure that all community members have equal opportunities for certain resources (e.g., education) as long as they are capable and willing. In health contexts, although the *right to health* does not mean the right to be healthy as there are many variables (e.g., natural disasters) that are beyond a society's control, the right to health entitles *all* citizens access to a system of health protection which provides equality of opportunity. This means being entitled (a) to enjoy the highest attainable level of physical and mental health (e.g., access to basic health services) and (b) to engage in public discourse and decision-making about how social, economic, and political resources are to be distributed so that everyone's right to health is equally protected (Braveman et al., 2011).

The second condition posits that because all citizens should have equal access to the social and economic resources of a society, if a society were to distribute the resources unequally, the unequal distribution must give the greatest benefit to the least-advantaged members of society. This is what holds a society together even when our lived realities are flawed. The second condition, the principle of differentiation, reflects an underlying assumption of justice as fairness – an ideal of social unity (Wenar, 2017). This shifts a perspectival focus of equality (e.g., does each member have the same share?) to an Integral Fusion understanding of equity (e.g., what is best for all of us as a whole?). "In justice as fairness," said Rawls (1971/2009), "men agree to share one another's fate" (p. 88). This is a contractarianism approach, recognizing that one is not truly free to choose any community or society one wants (e.g., we are born into our family with no choice of our race or sex) and that inequality is an unavoidable social condition. Members of a community, thus, have a moral duty to *cooperate* with one another – recognizing that when the least advantaged members of a community get more resources, the society benefits as a whole.

Rawls (2001) argued that a fair system of corporation implies **reciprocity**: "all who do their part, as the recognized rules require, are to benefit as specified by a public and agreed-upon standard" (p. 6). As a result, when all members of a community are free and *equal*, each member can reasonably and rationally recognize that it is to his/her own advantage to engage in cooperation, supporting the least-advantaged to receive more resources. In short, Rawls (2001) argued that when community members can believe that institutional structures and social practices are just and fair because the agreed-upon principles are established with their voices incorporated, they would be *ready and willing* to do their part to follow those arrangements if they can reasonably expect others do the same. The trust and confidence toward a fair system allows members of a community to accommodate differences of voices and interests even if it is temporarily at their expense: This is because shared cooperation is reciprocal and will be sustained over a long time. If they were ever in the Other's shoes (i.e., become the least advantaged), they can expect to benefit the most by receiving the most resources.

Essential to the success of justice as fairness, thus, is society's ability to include, appreciate, and honor different voices and perspectives as it delineates the principles of justice that make a system fair for all. In short, this is a polycentric, Integral Fusion mode of being that appreciates the validity of emotions, imagination, and rationality – of magic idolic, mythic symbolic, and perspectival signalic ways of understanding and communicating. Each contributes to our ability to survive. Each is valid in its way. Our emotions have served us well in our efforts to survive for millennia. Our imaginations have served us well over the millennia. And our analytic abilities have been valuable. Seeing the validity in all aspects is an Integral Fusion understanding. And it manifests ultimately as appreciation for all dimensions of human beings. Also, the ability to recognize the Other in us and us in the Other involves not merely reciprocity but the appreciation of differences. Diversifying understanding makes the social system more resilient, more interesting, more dynamic, more vital. The Integral Fusion mode of understanding also takes into account the changing fortunes of time. One day I may be able to help you, and tomorrow you can return the favor.

Rather than pursuing a pre-determined understanding of justice, community members engage in dialogue to achieve a reasonable overlapping consensus (Rawls, 2001). **Reasonable overlapping consensus** allows different members to endorse agreed-upon principles (e.g., institutional policies or practices) despite their varying reasons. This is not a pursuit of conformity or forced compliance. Rather, the dialogical community is never finished (Kramer, 1997). Justice is derived through dialogues that engage emotional, imaginative/rhetorical, and cognitive/analytic maturity. The rules of discourse must appreciate rationality to be sure but also the polycentricity of social existence, of the Others, including their emotional needs and their creative impulses. When we negotiate, debate, discuss policies and laws, we should listen for and appreciate all aspects of Other participants, including their Magic Consciousness, Mythic Connection, and Perspectival Thinking.

Because reasonable overlapping consensus is the most desirable form to maintain stability in a free society over time (as opposed to using brute power, such as military and hegemonic surveillance), it is essential that a society engage in continuous dialogue and create dialogic spaces for all members, particularly marginalized populations to voice their perspectives. When reflecting on and anticipating a forthcoming summer of riots like those that had consumed many Black inner cities in 1967, Martin Luther King Jr. (1968) explained,

> But it is not enough for me to stand before you tonight and condemn riots. It would be morally irresponsible for me to do that without, at the same time,

condemning the contingent, intolerable conditions that exist in our society. These conditions are the things that cause individuals to feel that they have no other alternative than to engage in violent rebellions to get attention. And I must say tonight that *a riot is the language of the unheard.* And what is it America has failed to hear? It has failed to hear that the plight of the negro poor has worsened over the last twelve or fifteen years. It has failed to hear that the promises of freedom and justice have not been met. And it has failed to hear that large segments of white society are more concerned about tranquility and the status quo than about justice and humanity. [emphasis added] (para. 6)

The goals of dialogue are more than "listening" to marginalized populations or "respecting" the rights "extended to them." Rather, the rules of engagement and the rights identified come from all. No one person or group presumes the power and privilege of bestowing rights.

In a polycentric Integral Fusion process, the validity of all is recognized. This does not mean mindless relativism. It means that the agenda and the processes themselves are developed through mutual engagement. The policy decisions that emerge will reflect the interests of all and should also manifest the best solutions available. In short, some proposals will be deemed better, meaning more desirable, than others. But initiatives to the process is the openness to hear, and be influenced by, the Other – to risk one's hermeneutic horizon so that we may evolve together – emotionally, rhetorically, and cognitively (Kramer, 2000).

Maturing is more than learning how to analyze things, it is also just as essential to mature emotionally and in our use of our imaginations. The fuel for imagination is **alterity** (i.e., differences and otherness), exposure to new things, ideas, places, people. Such is the raw material for fusional integration, innovation, and creation. As we engage in social interactions, our differences prompt the emergence of new forms of life and culture – transforming our ways of feeling, seeing, and thinking. This is fundamentally a communicative process (Kramer, 2019). An Integral Fusion approach to dialogic space means a commitment to suspend our judgment, recognize, and challenge our own bias/perspectives, and revise our worldviews. Rawls (2001) explained,

> Justice as fairness regards all our judgments ... as reasonable and rational, a certain intrinsic reasonableness. Yet since we are of divided mind and our judgments conflict with those of other people, some of these judgments must eventually be revised, suspended, or withdrawn, if the practical aim of reaching reasonable agreement on matters of political justice is to be achieved. (p. 30)

The better a society is in finding overlapping consensus by continuously incorporating all members' perspectives as its principles of justice that guide its functioning as a fair system, the more its citizens will have trust and confidence in the fairness of the system over time, from one generation to another – resulting in a stable, thriving society. Justice as fairness, thus, is not a set principle but a *fair process* that engages and evolves with all members of a community.

In conclusion, the meanings of justice and fairness are interactively negotiated and contextually situated in communities' historical tensions and sociopolitical relationships within a community and with the larger society. Principles of justice that guide a society's policies and practices cannot be a fixed or predetermined set of rules imposed by hegemonic powers or dominant groups. When we want to develop a social system that is stable, fair, and just over time, from one generation to the next, it is essential that its social structures provide a fair process that actively recognizes its citizens to be fair and equal, guarantees their basic rights to be free of governmental interference, and offers them equal opportunities and resources so that their voices and interests not only are protected but are also heard and incorporated into the structure. Because justice as fairness emerges through reasonable overlapping consensus among all members, each member can (a) have confidence that social goods are achieved (i.e., the community benefits as a whole) when community resources are distributed unequally to benefit the least-advantaged members and (b) trust that they can benefit from the system if their conditions satisfy the same rules. The trust and confidence in the fairness of the system allow community members to cooperate with one another even when we hold diverging perspectives and interests. Justice as fairness allows a pluralistic, democratic society to be fair and stable and yet flexible and evolving – conditions necessary for any society to thrive over time, from one generation to the next. It seeks free and equal expression as a principle. As a transcending principle, it seeks to protect diversity, including unpopular ideas.

B. Health Equity in A Pluralistic, Well-Ordered Society

1. Dialogic Spaces are Essential

> Pluralistic health care systems raise complex ethical and pragmatic issues and simply decrying the hegemony of biomedicine does not take us very far toward resolving the problems created by a naïve embrace of anything labelled "non-Western" or "traditional" as being inherently good and beyond critical appraisal. (Kirmayer, 2012, p. 156)

An Integral Fusion approach to social justice provides the best chance of developing the guiding principles to embed equity and justice in health policies and health services. This is because inherent to an Integral Fusion approach is a commitment to maintaining a dialogic space that protects, promotes, negotiates, and reconciles different ideas and perspectives. The pluralistic voices and perspectives in our communities cannot be maintained through a pre-determined set of rules but through each community member's willingness and capacity to engage in the dialogic process.

Due to limited space, we have decided to cover two methods that have helped healthcare providers, researchers, educators, activists, and marginalized and vulnerable populations to create and maintain dialogic spaces: Culture-Centered Approach and narrative medicine. Both methods place a great premium on the importance of listening as an entry point to interrogate one's own bias and presumptions (Charon, 2005; Dutta, 2014). Both methods also recognize the importance of embodiment, historical injustice, collective trauma, and community resilience in shaping one's lived experiences and understanding of realities (Charon et al., 2017; Dutta, 2011; Langellier, 2009). Researchers who adopted these methods have actively incorporated and welcomed a wide range of tools and expressive modes, such as embodied performances, storytelling, literary genres (e.g., poems and creative writing), and creative arts and performance, in dialogic spaces (Charon et al., 2017; Dutta & Zapata, 2019). Such an approach allows the cultural perspectives of Magic Connection or Mythic Connection to find their place in the dialogic space that has been long occupied by the analytical, biomedical narratives of Perspectival Thinking in medicine and institutional policies.

Mohan Dutta (2007, 2008) proposed **Culture-Centered Approach** (CCA) to address health disparities in marginalized populations (e.g., sex workers, migrant workers, and African Americans; Basu & Dutta, 2009; Dutta & Dutta, 2013; Dutta et al., 2017), which begins with listening to and including marginalized populations' voices and perspectives and, at the same time, critically and reflexively interrogate one's biases and presumptions. Culture-Centered Approach adopts an Integral Fusion approach to cultural perspectives as it invites members of marginalized communities, practitioners, the public, and the larger society to engage in dialogues that challenge existing social structure/order, address historically situated social injustice, and collaborate and co-create structures and knowledge that incorporates the perspectives of marginalized populations. In other words, CCA "seeks to build dialogic spaces in subaltern communities to interrogate, theorize, and formulate participatory communication in locally meaningful and contextually-situated ways, putting forth subaltern theories of health and wellbeing" (Dutta, 2018, p. 240). Because structural stigma and structural discrimination are foundational to marginalized populations' experiences of injustice and disparities, meaningful, and effective solutions can only emerge when marginalized populations' voices are not only heard but also integrated into the structures and cultural orientations of the larger society.

Whereas CCA is primarily concerned about fostering community-ownership, engaging community participation, and creating structural social change through community/field-based interventions, narrative medicine has centered on clinical care and social interactions in healthcare settings. **Narrative medicine** is a field of medicine that emerged in the 2000s. Narrative medicine is informed by interdisciplinary perspectives, including literature and medicine, narrative ethics, medical humanities, healthcare communication, and primary care medicine (Charon et al., 2017). Rita Charon (2008), who originated the field of narrative medicine, explained,

> Only when the doctor understands to some extent what his or her patient goes through can medical care proceed with humility, trustworthiness, and respect. I use the term narrative medicine to mean medicine practiced with these narrative skills of recognizing, absorbing, interpreting, and being moved by the stories of illness. (pp. 3–4)

By recognizing the power of language in shaping individuals' understanding of realities, clinicians learn to appreciate that the quality of care is dependent on their abilities and skills to engage the emotions and intricacies in patients' narratives that are interactively co-constructed in clinical interactions. In other words, their "narrative competence can widen the clinical gaze to include personal and social elements of patients' lives vital to the tasks of healing" (Charon et al., 2017, pp. 1–2). Narrative medicine shifts the medical gaze of biomedicine to collaborative coordination of patient-centered care. Three themes of narrative medicine have influenced the practice, research, and teaching of medicine (Charon, 2005):

- **Attention**: The state of heightened focus and commitment a listener can offer to a teller. The act of listening is not passive but a demanding action to capture and appreciate the teller's perspectives.
- **Representation**: A recreation of what is heard or perceived so that the emerging understanding is visible to both the listener and the teller for further dialogue. Through representation, the listener and teller co-create realities.
- **Affiliation**: Results from (a) deep, attentive listening and (b) the knowledge achieved through representation, which connects the participants as partners in achieving their shared goals.

There is no inherent hierarchy of power or knowledge in narrative medicine. Rather, the goals are for patients and clinicians to forge a partnership of patient-centered care. In particular, clinicians are encouraged to suspend and challenge their own cultural perspectives and biomedical presumptions, create dialogic spaces that engage the marginalized and silenced voices, and learn from Others through self-awareness and self-critique (Charon et al., 2017). Charon (2017) proposed that the principles of narrative medicine are: (a) action toward social justice, (b) disciplinary rigor, (c) inclusivity, (d) tolerance of ambiguity, (e) participatory and nonhierarchical methods, and (f) relational and intersubjective processes. From this perspective, narrative medicine is not just about contextualizing patients' narratives about health and illness, but also appreciating the historical, social, economic, and political forces that shape patients' lived experiences of marginalization and injustice.

2. Dialogic Spaces Under Different Cultural Worldviews

Different cultural consciousness structures can hold very different attitudes about whether and how to talk to the Other. People manifesting Magic Consciousness do not see the need to engage the Other. After all, under Magic Consciousness, people outside of the magic community (i.e., the out-group members) are not truly "human." Their perspectives and suffering are not "real." If the Other is not "real," then dialogues are not necessary. Whether a person holds the identity of an in-group member dictates whether the person will be heard or not by a person with predominantly Magic Consciousness.

A meta-analysis concluded that the stronger people project their in-groups to share similar interests and attitudes with them, the more they hold in-group favoritism attitudes, perceive the in-group to be homogeneous, and cooperate with in-group members (Robbins & Krueger, 2005). Whom we see through an in-group lens can be a result of early childhood socialization. When investigating children's socialization processes for ethnocentric bias between age 4–7, Aboud (2003) found that *in-group favoritism* did not appear until age five but reached significant levels; in contrast, out-group prejudice was weaker, but out-group members suffer due to high favoritism toward in-group members. Individuals often attribute cultural socialization (rather than their personal beliefs) to explain their unconscious biases against minorities (Uhlmann & Nosek, 2012). In short, it would appear that in-group identification and affiliation are essential to how we engage the Other.

How can we make a person who does not believe the Other is "real" or valid, to listen? Well, you can't. The only solution is to help them see that the Other as not an out-group being. How? In one of our studies about homelessness, undergraduate students were paired with a homeless person to hear about their life stories and perspectives. Hank, a participant of our study, explained this to our students:

> People have no idea. ... They think we're stupid and lazy. And they don't know what it's like until they've slept on this shit right here [pounds on concrete]. Until they do that, they have no idea what it's like. The people sleeping in their beds, they have no idea what it's like to wake up on the concrete [laughs] with a pair of shoes for a pillow, if you have that. (Kramer & Hsieh, 2019, p. 55)

Under Magic Consciousness, it is essential that we step outside of ourselves (i.e., the in-group self) if we are to create dialogic spaces with the Other. Though our personal experiences are directly experienced, others' experiences must be inferred – requiring additional effort and attention (Epley & Caruso, 2004). Although many educators and researchers have suggested role-play as a learning strategy to step into the Other's shoes (e.g., Stagner, 1977), such an effort can strengthen one's **egocentric biases** (i.e., a tendency to view things from one's personal perspectives and experiences) *unless* the perspective-taking is done *before* people adopt egocentric positions (Epley & Caruso, 2004; Vorauer & Sucharyna, 2013). Researchers have found that compared to monolingual individuals, people who grew up bilingual are less susceptible to egocentric biases because they have developed the sociolinguistic sensitivity of diverging worldviews embedded in different languages and have become attentive to interactional contexts to avoid inappropriate interference from a different language system (Rubio-Fernández & Glucksberg, 2012). Integral Fusion allows one to see through layered dimensions that make up our worldview and to be more vigilant against settling on a single bias.

We cannot disown our bodies or our eyes and most of us do not grow up as bilinguals. So then, how can we step outside of ourselves before taking the perspective of the Other? We argue that maybe the solution lies in non-goal-driven social interactions. When we see each other, we are beheld as an Other. Lévinas (1978) argues that we as human beings summon each other as moral beings and that this organic way of communicating with the Other *preempts* what may become competitive or instrumental communication. The event of encountering is a summons to respond – to reciprocate, to communicate. When we meet the Other without instrumental purposes, then we are free to connect, empathize, and identify with the Other – in that moment of mutual connection, a collective "we" is realized and a new magic bond is formed and the stronghold of Magic Consciousness of the original in-group is weakened. This is the power of compassionate goals – it is transformative (see Chapter 10). We all have Magic Consciousness in us. Maybe the way to connect with people with Magic Consciousness is not about "breaking down" their magic beliefs but to realize that we *can* connect because we understand that passion and loyalty for our magic groups as well. As we recognize our egocentric bias, it becomes available for reflection. It becomes the Other. And we are immediately able to empathize with the Other.

Bias cannot be totally avoided. But it can be challenged. The identity of each worldview is made possible (i.e., can be perceived) by comparing it to other worldviews. Identity is seen through differences. Comparison exposes each as different from the others. I am what you are not. And without you as different from me, I can have no identity. Seeing meaning and identity through difference is integral diaphaneity. I need the Other to have an identity. And the stronger the Otherness of the Other, the stronger my own identity. This is an essential issue in ethnocentrism, nationalism, racism, and other isms as ideological constructs. When a person or a group wants to accentuate their identity, they exaggerate the difference of the Other. In this sense, they need the Other to exist. When we see how this mechanism works, we can begin to understand our mutual dependence and see the positivity of difference.

On the other hand, dialogues with people under Mythic Connection may face the most difficulties. This is because mythic communities are driven by cultural values. At its extreme, people under Mythic Connection can be zealots of their beliefs – whoever does not share the same beliefs are not just different but "evil." Strong emotions and intense moral claims are attached to their beliefs, which are beyond reproach by analytical arguments under Perspectival Thinking. In addition, because people under Mythic Connection bond to one another through the shared cultural values of in-group membership, dialogue with the Other is unlikely to change their commitment to their cultural values.

As a result, dialogues with people under Mythic Connection must involve community insiders. In addition to building relationships directly with the community, *allies, interpreters, community health workers,* and bicultural community insiders are particularly valuable when maintaining dialogic spaces with mythic people (see Chapters 8 and 13). This is because mythic communities' shared identity and group membership are demarcated by shared values.

An outsider who does not share the same values may be regarded as not "real" or even evil (i.e., they do not have obligations toward the out-group members) and thus, their voices are resisted, if heard at all, in their communities. Thus, people who can serve as bridges and go-betweens in communities with different cultural perspectives are essential in engaging conversations with people under Mythic Connection – their in-group identity allows their voices to be heard and integrated into mythic communities. Over time, their integrated perspectives provide the necessary momentum to shape and change the cultural values and perspectives under Mythic Connection from within. Such an approach affords the communities the agency and efficacy to change in a manner of their choice.

It is from this perspective that the current cultural trends of online shaming through call-out culture and/or cancel culture can be particularly problematic and detrimental for dialogic spaces. **Call-out culture** refers to "the tendency among progressives, radicals, activists, and community organizers to publicly name instances or patterns of oppressive behavior and language used by others. People can be called out for statements and actions that are sexist, racist, ableist, and the list goes on" (Ahmad, 2015, para. 1). Similarly, **cancel culture** refers to having a person "canceled" by blocking their voice in public platforms and to "to effectively end their career or revoke their cultural cachet, whether through boycotts of their work or disciplinary action from an employer" (Romano, 2019, para. 2). Such strategies entrench the ingroup-outgroup divide by moralizing, blaming, and punishing a person's single statement or action, with little attention to the surrounding contexts (e.g., historical backgrounds and interactional dynamics) or the larger sociocultural environments (Dimitrakaki & Weeks, 2019).

Strategies of call-out/cancel cultures highlight differences and disagreements through public shaming of the Other. The more emotional the attack, the more identification through Magic Consciousness. Thus, what is canceled is not the act, but the actor. The action is occurring at the level of identity. In intensely emotional attacks, the actor is seen as evil, not just the actions. There is little to no dissociation between the two and this can become very violent, both symbolically and even physically. At this point, there is little chance to see anything of value in the Other and to attempt or care to try to communicate. As such, the Other is to be humiliated, made invisible, and silenced. Even apologies are rejected. Nothing is adequate and satisfying except for the elimination of the Other. There is little interest in understanding the Other as "people with complicated stories and histories" (Ahmad, 2015, para. 3). From this perspective, call-out/cancel cultures are transformed into performances of the Self. The actors of call-out/cancel cultures use these strategies to perform their identities, which are likely to be under Mythic Connection – moral claims about one's values and principles.

Unless we create and maintain dialogic spaces to foster a reasonable overlapping consensus of truth, peace, justice, and mercy, we can never have sustainable and durable reconciliation between groups (Lederach, 1997; Rawls, 2001). In short, online shaming through call-out or cancel cultures intensifies the Mythic Connection of the in-group members by publicly ousting, shaming, and denying out-group members a forum to voice their perspectives. As such, under Mythic Connection, these people and communities cut off bridges that connect with outsiders and, in the process, may eliminate the possibility of dialogue, which is the beginning of all efforts to form community and, in some cases, reconciliation.

It is important to note that we believe that people need to be held accountable for their actions. Acknowledging the truth, including wrongdoing and injustice, is a prerequisite for justice (Lederach, 1997). However, calling out for truth is only the first step. Dialogue is needed for *different parties* to engage and share their perspectives. When "truth" was called out by one party as the ultimate and only truth and the Other is silenced, it is a hegemony, not justice (Rawls, 2001).

Finally, it may appear that dialogue and dialogic spaces are readily embraced and accepted under Perspectival Thinking. It is true that open conversations and transparency are inherent values under Perspectival Thinking. But the imposition of a strict rationalist regime can also restrict interaction, especially between diverse populations. Perspectivism is, by definition, a narrowing. For example, science as a product of Perspectival Thinking always has welcomed public scrutiny and open challenges of its assumptions and findings (National Academies of Sciences, Engineering, and Medicine, 2019). But it can also become arrogant and dismissive of other ways of understanding the world, including illness. The danger of Perspectival calculation and lack of identification and care is the potential for exploiting the Other who holds a different worldview and disguising itself as an Integral Fusion approach (see Chapter 13).

An Integral Fusion approach requires individuals to accommodate and respond to the Other's cultural perspectives and unique needs. However, when one incorporates the Other's perspective for self-interest *and* without viewing the Other as "free and equal" (e.g., treating the Other's voice and perspectives as equally valid and legitimate as one's own and respecting the Other's agency for decision-making), then the person has engaged in exploitative, calculative Perspectival Thinking as an instrument of manipulation and compliance gaining. This is not an Integral Fusion approach for dialogues. For example, when interpreters are treated as tools to coerce submission from patients, to target audiences to enhance compliance, and to assist physicians in exerting their will and power over those patients, the provider has adopted a calculative Perspectival Thinking approach (Hsieh & Kramer, 2012). If the provider were to adopt an Integral Fusion approach, the interpreter and the patient would be treated as equal partners as they identify problems and challenges to achieve the desired process and outcomes of care (Hsieh, 2016).

IV.   Final Thoughts on Transformative Dialogues

> The world I live in is certainly first and foremost my world (and not the objec-
> tive" world of atoms and molecules), but to this very "mine-ness" also belongs
> otherness in the sense of the meaning of the world belonging to other people.
> The otherness of the world, however, is not only due to my sharing it with other
> people, but also to nature (as opposed to culture) as something resisting my
> understanding. (Svenaeus, 2013, p. 93)

Culture is more than a group, more than patterns of behaviors, or a speech community. The meanings of culture are constantly contested and negotiated as we engage in social interaction. The challenges posed by the Other is not only that they are different but also that we cannot understand them – their worldviews and realities. Throughout the book, we have relied on the **Theory of Dimensional Accrual and Dissociation** (Kramer, 2013; Kramer & Ikeda, 1998) and **cultural fusion theory** (Kramer, 2000, 2019) as the grounding framework for our exploration of cultural perspectives and approaches. To see from the Other's perspective, we do not believe that we should or can "unlearn" our own culture – at least, not in the sense of abandoning or forgetting who we are, what bonds us, or what makes realities real. Even in a modern, perspectival society, we often continue to hold Magic Consciousness with the "first" community worlds that we inhabit and that inhabit and define us (e.g., the magic bond we have with our children, the unquestioned patriotism for our homeland, or the taken-for-granted religious faith that defines us). Such bonds are difficult, if not impossible, to break or be forgotten. However, as we travel across different cultural perspectives and modalities, we can accumulate different layers of understanding and perspectives that enrich our worldview and provide solutions that were not visible or transparent to us before (Kramer, 2013, 2019; Liu & Kramer, 2019). An Integral Fusion worldview is the result of the dimensional accrual of cultures and is the best solution to cross-cultural communication (Gebser, 1949–1953/1985).

Dialogues or dialogic spaces may first appear to be a western-based concept and a western solution to resolving differences. The preference of *openness* in talk and the emphasis of individual voices reflect a western preference for "talk" as a solution to resolve conflicts (e.g., talking it out); in contrast, other cultures do not necessarily

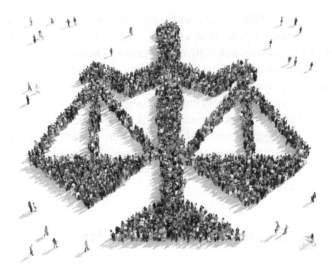

Figure 14.6 Justice means willingness to change. An Integral Fusion worldview of justice means that justice is not something external to be applied to us but something we embody, aspire, and contemplate continuously and reflexively. Justice and our communities co-evolve alongside with us, "We the People." *Source:* Arthimedes/Shutterstock

share the same preferences and may have preferred other strategies, such as avoidance, withdrawal, or other indirect communication strategies to resolve conflicts and differences (Glinow et al., 2004; Kim & Leung, 2000). However, we do not view dialogues and dialogic spaces merely as "talk." Just because two parties "talked" does not mean that there were dialogic spaces. One can walk away from a talk with a profound realization that s/he was silenced and truly unheard.

A dialogic space is where people with different perspectives and interests engage with one another – with *the goal to understand* the Other and a *willingness to change* (see Figure 14.6). Gadamer (1960/2005) characterized communication as a risk. Whenever we are exposed to something new (purposefully or accidentally), our horizon is affected. Freedom is how we respond to what happens to us and how we respond to changes with experience (van Inwagen, 1983). A dialogic space is created, not for the purpose of changing the Other, but for the commitment to be transformed together as a collective *We*. A transformative dialogue is successful not because the Other has changed but because *we*, together, are connected with one another and thus, are different because of it.

In practice, however, the cultural approaches to transformative dialogues may be easier said than done. First, we need to look beyond a group-based or risk-based approach to understand cultures. Although throughout this book, we have often relied on national, racial, or ethnic categories or western versus non-western dualism when discussing cultural differences, such distinctions are primarily an artifact of the existing literature. What distinguishes a person from a Magic Consciousness, Mythic Connection, Perspectival Thinking, or Integral Fusion worldview is *not* her group-, language-, or behavior-based affiliation; rather, it's one's understanding of one's self and potential realities – the meanings and functions of communities and communication

– that define our cultural approaches and perspectives. In addition, a person may hold different cultural consciousness on different issues. For example, a person may adopt Magic Consciousness when deciding to donate a kidney to her child but adopt Perspectival Thinking when deciding whether undocumented immigrants should have access to preventive care. As such, we must recognize that cultural approaches to dialogic spaces are highly contextualized and issue-specific. A group-based generalization or broad-brush categorization of cultural approaches can overlook the nuances individuals hold in their worldviews and miss the opportunities for meaningful dialogues

Second, we need to expand our understanding and appreciation of modes of communication. Although analytical arguments under Perspectival Thinking are essential to policymaking and clinical decision-making in modern societies, it is important to recognize that people with different cultural approaches do not communicate the same way. If we want to truly engage, listen, and understand the Other, it is essential that we appreciate the different modes and mediums of communication – to appreciate the validity of each other emotional needs and aspirations (imaginations). From this perspective, we echo with researchers of CCA and narrative medicine in embracing different modes of communication (e.g., embodied performance, storytelling, and creative arts, among others) in dialogic spaces. Our willingness to be flexible, adaptive, and responsive to the Other's worldviews and realities through the modes of communication is necessary to the success of transformative dialogues.

Finally, rather than assuming that dialogue can lead to the best or definitive solution that solves problems for all people, we believe that a dialogic space is a *process* through which members are engaged in creative problem-solving. In other words, rather than picking one perspective over another, a dialogic space creates the possibility of an Integral Fusion worldview that accommodates changing perspectives and pan-evolution within communities and in the larger society. Thus, a dialogue is never "finished." An open-dialogue and well-maintained dialogic spaces with the least advantaged members of our community provide a society immediate feedback and critique on the appropriateness and effectiveness of its principles of justice in maintaining a fair system – providing the best chance for the community as whole to respond to the injustice before its rippling effects compromise the sustainability and efficacy of our society.

Equity and Justice are public health issues. Without addressing structural injustice in our systems and institutions, we will continue to view marginalized populations as deviants and ills of our society – when the truth is, the suffering and disparities of vulnerable populations are the symptoms of an ill society that has failed to maintain a just and fair system for all its citizens.

V. Additional Resources

A. Key Terms and Theories

structural barriers
structural racism
work requirements

Medicaid
utilitarian ethics
utilitarianism
patient cost-sharing
cost-saving
cost-effective
cost-shifting structures
preference utilitarianism
distributive justice
libertarianism
egalitarianism
    principle of equality
contractarianism
    principle of differentiation
health equity
justice as fairness
    well-ordered society
    right to health
    reciprocity
    reasonable overlapping consensus
culture-centered approach
narrative medicine
    attention
    representation
    affiliation
egocentric bias
call-out culture
cancel culture
Theory of Dimensional Accrual and Dissociation
cultural fusion theory

B. Discussion Questions

1. Do you think social stigma should be used as a public health tool? Why or why not?
   a. Should social stigma be used as a public health tool against obesity?
   b. Should social stigma be used as a public health tool against HIV?
   c. If you have different answers to (a) and (b), why?
   d. Do you think social stigma may have different short-term versus long-term impacts? Does it matter?
2. Reflecting on your educational experiences, try to answer the following questions:
   a. What are the structural "barriers" you have to overcome to be where you are? Consider socioeconomic, sociocultural, and sociopolitical barriers as well.
   b. Do you think those barriers are necessary or "good"? Why or why not?
   c. What would happen if those barriers are eliminated? Would the world be better?

3. Do you agree that we have a moral obligation to people who are not "us"? What would people with different cultural perspectives respond to the answer?
   a. Do we have a moral obligation to help out our parents? How about our siblings? How about our children? Is there a limit to the "obligations"?
   b. Do we have a moral obligation to help out the homeless in our community? Is there a limit to the "obligations"?
   c. Do we have a moral obligation to stop a genocide in a different country? Is there a limit to the "obligations"?
   d. What are the upsides and downsides of helping out people who are not "us"?
4. Reflecting on your attitudes for distributive justice, which theory/approach (i.e., libertarianism, egalitarianism, and contractarianism) best explain your attitudes toward the distribution of the following resources. Do you hold different approaches to different issues?
   a. vaccination
   b. universal healthcare (i.e., all people and communities can access effective *and* affordable promotive, preventive, curative, rehabilitative, and palliative health services)
   c. receiving organ donation
   d. receiving expansive life-saving medications (e.g., $84,000 treatment for hepatitis C cure)
5. Two fundamental assumptions of justice as fairness is that (a) all citizens are free and equal persons, and (b) the society functions as a fair system of social cooperation over time, from one generation to the next.
   a. Can you identify countries/contexts when *not* all citizens are free or equal? What are they?
   b. When/How a society may stop being a fair system of social cooperation over time? What are the things we can do to ensure that the system continues to work?
6. Maintaining a dialogic space with people who hold completely different attitudes and beliefs than your own can be difficult. Are there certain beliefs, attitudes, or opinions that are absolutely unacceptable and even offensive to you?
   a. What are they? Why do you feel that way?
   b. Reflecting on your cultural perspectives, which cultural perspective do you hold?
   c. Do you think it is possible for people to change your mind about the issue? Why or why not? How?
   d. If the person who holds such beliefs or attitudes is your professor, your boss, or someone you know, what would you do? If you want to avoid strategies of call-out culture or cancel culture, what would you do?
   e. If you want to change what others feel/think about that issue, what would you do?
   f. How can you change the minds of people who do not want to talk to you or think that you are evil?
7. We suggested non-instrumental interactions (i.e., social interactions that are not goal-driven) as a way to engage people with Magic Consciousness.
   a. What are the kinds of environments and factors that may promote non-instrumental interactions?
   b. What are the kinds of environments and factors that may prohibit non-instrumental interactions?

8. Transformative dialogues are powerful because they can change us, our environments, and our cultural systems. What do you say to people who do not want to change?
   a. What do you say to people who hold Magic Consciousness and do not want to change?
   b. What do you say to people who hold Mythic Connection and do not want to change?
   c. What do you say to people who hold Perspectival Thinking and do not want to change?
   d. What do you say to people who hold Integral Fusion and do not want to change? (Ha, got you. People who hold the Integral Fusion worldview are not afraid of changes. They recognize that changes are a natural and necessary part of everyday life.)

C. References

Aboud, F. E. (2003). The formation of in-group favoritism and out-group prejudice in young children: Are they distinct attitudes? *Developmental Psychology*, *39*(1), 48–60.

Adelman, L., & Smith, L. M. (2008). *Unnatural causes: Is inequality making us sick?* [TV series]. California Newsreel. PBS. https://unnaturalcauses.org/about_the_series.php

Ahmad, A. (2015, March 2). *A note on call-out culture.* Briarpatch Magazine. https://briarpatchmagazine.com/articles/view/a-note-on-call-out-culture

Albertsen, A. (2016). Drinking in the last chance saloon: Luck egalitarianism, alcohol consumption, and the organ transplant waiting list. *Medicine, Health Care and Philosophy*, *19*(2), 325–338.

Almendrala, A. (2020, July 8). *A nurse's plea: 'Please tell me my life is worth a LITTLE of your discomfort?'.* Los Angeles Times. https://www.latimes.com/science/story/2020-07-08/nurses-beg-public-to-wear-masks

Azar, A., Maldonado, L., Castillo, J. C., & Atria, J. (2018). Income, egalitarianism and attitudes towards healthcare policy: A study on public attitudes in 29 countries. *Public Health*, *154*, 59–69.

Bailey, Z. D., Krieger, N., Agénor, M., Graves, J., Linos, N., & Bassett, M. T. (2017). Structural racism and health inequities in the USA: Evidence and interventions. *The Lancet*, *389*(10077), 1453–1463.

Banerjee, A. V., & Duflo, E. (2019). *Good economics for hard times.* PublicAffairs.

Basu, A., & Dutta, M. J. (2009). Sex workers and HIV/AIDS: Analyzing participatory culture-centered health communication strategies. *Human Communication Research*, *35*(1), 86–114.

Bayer, R. (2008). Stigma and the ethics of public health: Not can we but should we. *Social Science & Medicine*, *67*(3), 463–472.

Bentham, J. (2007). *An introduction to the principles of morals and legislation.* Clarendon Press. (Original work published 1789)

Boen, C., Keister, L., & Aronson, B. (2020). Beyond net worth: Racial differences in wealth portfolios and Black–White health inequality across the life course. *Journal of Health and Social Behavior*, *61*(2), 153–169.

Braveman, P. A., Kumanyika, S., Fielding, J., LaVeist, T., Borrell, L. N., Manderscheid, R., & Troutman, A. (2011). Health disparities and health equity: The issue is justice. *American Journal of Public Health, 101*(S1), S149-S155.

Bryant-Davis, T., Adams, T., Alejandre, A., & Gray, A. A. (2017). The trauma lens of police violence against racial and ethnic minorities. *Journal of Social Issues, 73*(4), 852–871.

Carrillo, J. E., Carrillo, V. A., Perez, H. R., Salas-Lopez, D., Natale-Pereira, A., & Byron, A. T. (2011). Defining and targeting health care access barriers. *Journal of Health Care for the Poor and Underserved, 22*(2), 562–575.

Carroll, A. E. (2018, Janurary 29). *Preventive care saves money? Sorry, it's too good to be true.* The New York Times. https://nyti.ms/2Fsh9vv

Centers for Medicare & Medicaid Services. (n.d.-a). *June 2020 Medicaid & CHIP enrollment data highlights.* Retrieved October 3, 2020, from https://www.medicaid.gov/medicaid/program-information/medicaid-and-chip-enrollment-data/report-highlights/index.html

Centers for Medicare & Medicaid Services. (n.d.-b). *Medicaid.* Retrieved October 3, 2020, from https://www.medicaid.gov/medicaid/index.html

Chambers, J. D., Cangelosi, M. J., & Neumann, P. J. (2015). Medicare's use of cost-effectiveness analysis for prevention (but not for treatment). *Health Policy, 119*(2), 156–163.

Charon, R. (2005). Narrative medicine: Attention, representation, affiliation. *Narrative, 13*(3), 261–270.

Charon, R. (2008). *Narrative medicine: Honoring the stories of illness.* Oxford University Press.

Charon, R. (2017). Close reading: The signature method of narrative medicine. In *The principles and practice of narrative medicine* (pp. 157–180). Oxford University Press.

Charon, R., DasGupta, S., Hermann, N., Irvine, C., Marchus, E.R., Colón, E.R., Spencer, D., & Spiegel, M. (2017). *The principles and practice of narrative medicine.* Oxford University Press.

Cogan, J. A., Jr. (2011). The Affordable Care Act's preventive services mandate: Breaking down the barriers to nationwide access to preventive services. *The Journal of Law, Medicine & Ethics, 39*(3), 355–365.

Cohen, J. T., & Neumann, P. J. (2009, September 1). *The cost savings and cost-effectiveness of clinical preventive care.* Robert Wood Johnson Foundation. https://www.rwjf.org/en/library/research/2009/09/cost-savings-and-cost-effectiveness-of-clinical-preventive-care.html

Cohen, J. T., Neumann, P. J., & Weinstein, M. C. (2008). Does preventive care save money? Health economics and the presidential candidates. *New England Journal of Medicine, 358*(7), 661–663.

Colwell, A., & McLean, R. (2020, April 29). *Meat plant workers to Trump: Employees aren't going to show up.* CNN. https://www.cnn.com/2020/04/29/business/meat-processing-plant-workers-reaction-executive-order/index.html

The Commonwealth Fund. (2020, May 28). *Status of Medicaid expansion and work requirement waivers.* https://www.commonwealthfund.org/publications/maps-and-interactives/2020/apr/status-medicaid-expansion-and-work-requirement-waivers

Congressional Budget Office. (2012, July). *Estimates for the insurance coverage provisions of the Affordable Care Act updated for the recent Supreme Court decision.* http://www.cbo.gov/sites/default/files/cbofiles/attachments/43472-07-24-2012-CoverageEstimates.pdf

Corrigan, P. W., & Nieweglowski, K. (2018). Stigma and the public health agenda for the opioid crisis in America. *International Journal of Drug Policy, 59*, 44–49.

The Council of Economic Advisers. (2018, July). *Expanding work requirements in non-cash welfare programs.* https://www.whitehouse.gov/wp-content/uploads/2018/07/Expanding-Work-Requirements-in-Non-Cash-Welfare-Programs.pdf

Davis, L. (2010). Rock, powder, sentencing-making disparate impact evidence relevant in crack cocaine sentencing. *Journal of Gender, Race & Justice, 14*(2), 375–404.

DeWitt, L. (2010). The decision to exclude agricultural and domestic workers from the 1935 Social Security Act. *Social Security Bulletin, 70*(4), 49–68.

Dharamsi, S., & MacEntee, M. I. (2002). Dentistry and distributive justice. *Social Science & Medicine, 55*(2), 323–329.

Dimitrakaki, A., & Weeks, H. (2019). Anti-fascism/art/theory. *Third Text, 33*(3), 271–292.

Dutta, M., Sastry, S., Dillard, S., Kumar, R., Anaele, A., Collins, W., Roberson, C., Dutta, U., Jones, C., Gillespie, T., & Spinetta, C. (2017). Narratives of stress in health meanings of African Americans in Lake County, Indiana. *Health Communication, 32*(10), 1241–1251.

Dutta, M. J. (2007). Communicating about culture and health: Theorizing culture-centered and cultural sensitivity approaches. *Communication Theory, 17*(3), 304–328.

Dutta, M. J. (2008). *Communicating health: A culture-centered approach.* Polity Press.

Dutta, M. J. (2011). *Communicating social change: Structure, culture, and agency.* Routledge.

Dutta, M. J. (2014). A culture-centered approach to listening: Voices of social change. *International Journal of Listening, 28*(2), 67–81.

Dutta, M. J. (2018). Culture-centered approach in addressing health disparities: Communication infrastructures for subaltern voices. *Communication Methods and Measures, 12*(4), 239–259.

Dutta, M. J., & Dutta, U. (2013). Voices of the poor from the margins of Bengal: Structural inequities and health. *Qualitative Health Research, 23*(1), 14–25.

Dutta, M. J., & Zapata, D. B. (Eds.). (2019). *Communicating for social change: Meaning, power, and resistance.* Palgrave Macmillan.

Elixhauser, A. (1990). The costs of smoking and the cost effectiveness of smoking-cessation programs. *Journal of Public Health Policy, 11*(2), 218–237.

Epley, N., & Caruso, E. M. (2004). Egocentric ethics. *Social Justice Research, 17*(2), 171–187.

Falk, G., McCarty, M., & Aussenberg, R. A. (2014). *Work requirements, time limits, and work incentives in TANF, SNAP, and housing assistance.* Congressional Research Service. https://greenbook-waysandmeans.house.gov/sites/greenbook.waysandmeans.house.gov/files/R43400_gb.pdf

Fox, M. (2018, May 6). *Hepatitis C cure eludes patients as states struggle with costs.* NBC News. https://www.nbcnews.com/health/health-news/hepatitis-c-cure-eludes-patients-states-struggle-costs-n870846

Gadamer, H.-G. (2005). *Truth and method* (J. Weinsheimer & D. G. Marshall, Trans.; 2nd rev ed.). Continuum. (Original work published 1960)

Gaffney, A., & McCormick, D. (2017). The Affordable Care Act: Implications for health-care equity. *The Lancet, 389*(10077), 1442–1452.

Gandjour, A., & Lauterbach, K. W. (2003). Utilitarian theories reconsidered: Common misconceptions, more recent developments, and health policy implications. *Health Care Analysis, 11*(3), 229–244.

Garfield, R., Claxton, G., Damico, A., & Levitt, L. (2020, May 13). *Eligibility for ACA health coverage following job loss.* Kaiser Family Foundation. https://www.kff.org/coronavirus-covid-19/issue-brief/eligibility-for-aca-health-coverage-following-job-loss

Garfield, R., Rudowitz, R., & Musumeci, M. (2018, June). *Implications of a Medicaid work requirement: National estimates of potential coverage loss* (Issue Brief). Kaiser Family Foundation. http://files.kff.org/attachment/Issue-Brief-Implications-of-a-Medicaid-Work-Requirement-National-Estimates-of-Potential-Coverage-Losses

Gebser, J. (1985) *The ever-present origin* (N. Barstad & A. Mickunas, Trans.). Ohio University Press. (Original work published 1949-1953)

Gee, G. C., Walsemann, K. M., & Brondolo, E. (2012). A life course perspective on how racism may be related to health inequities. *American Journal of Public Health, 102*(5), 967–974.

Glinow, M. A. V., Shapiro, D. L., & Brett, J. M. (2004). Can we talk, and should we? Managing emotional conflict in multicultural teams. *Academy of Management Review, 29*(4), 578–592.

Goyette, J. (2020, May 26). *Hundreds demand justice in Minneapolis after police killing of George Floyd.* The Guardian. https://www.theguardian.com/us-news/2020/may/26/george-floyd-killing-minneapolis-protest-police

Greene, T. W. (2008). Three ideologies of individualism: Toward assimilating a theory of individualisms and their consequences. *Critical Sociology, 34*(1), 117–137.

Habitat for Humanity. (n.d.). *Requirements for homeownership applicants.* Retrieved October 4, 2020, from https://habitatgnh.org/homeownership/requirements-for-homeownership-applicants

Hackworth, J. (2012). *Faith based: Religious neoliberalism and the politics of welfare in the United States.* University of Georgia Press.

Hahn, H. (2018). *Work requirements in safety net programs: Lessons for Medicaid from TANF and SNAP.* Urban Institute. https://www.urban.org/sites/default/files/publication/98086/work_requirements_in_safety_net_programs_0.pdf

Hahn, H., Kenny, G. M., Allen, E., Burton, R., & Waxman, E. (2018, Janurary 12). *Guidance on Medicaid work and community engagement requirements raises many important questions.* Urban Institute. https://www.urban.org/sites/default/files/publication/95846/2018.1.12.questions_final_for_pdf_v1_0.pdf

Hahn, H., Pratt, E., Allen, E. H., Kenny, G. M., Levy, D. K., & Waxman, E. (2017, December 22). *Work requirements in social safety net programs: A status report of work requirements in TANF, SNAP, Housing Assistance, and Medicaid.* Urban Institute. https://www.urban.org/research/publication/work-requirements-social-safety-net-programs-status-report-work-requirements-tanf-snap-housing-assistance-and-medicaid

Hanson, S. S. (2007). Libertarianism and universal health care: It's not what you think it is. *The Journal of Law, Medicine & Ethics, 35*(3), 486–489.

Hart, C. L., & Hart, M. Z. (2019). Opioid crisis: Another mechanism used to perpetuate American racism. *Cultural Diversity and Ethnic Minority Psychology, 25*(1), 6–11.

Hays, S. L., Coleman, A., Collins, S. R., & Nuzum, R. (2019, February 15). *The fiscal case for Medicaid expansion.* The Commonwealth Fund. https://www.commonwealthfund.org/blog/2019/fiscal-case-medicaid-expansion

HealthyPeople.gov. (n.d.). *Disparities.* Retrieved August 8, 2020, from https://www.healthypeople.gov/2020/about/foundation-health-measures/Disparities

Hochschild, J. L. (1981). *What's fair?: American beliefs about distributive justice.* Harvard University Press.

Hom, S. K., & Yamamoto, E. K. (2000). Collective memory, history, and social justice. *UCLA Law Review, 47*(6), 1747–1802.

Horsley, S. (2020). *For many, $600 jobless benefit makes it hard to return to work.* NPR. https://www.npr.org/2020/05/26/861906616/when-returning-to-your-job-means-a-cut-in-pay

Horwitz, J. R., Kelly, B. D., & DiNardo, J. E. (2013). Wellness incentives in the workplace: Cost savings through cost shifting to unhealthy workers. *Health Affairs, 32*(3), 468–476.

House, J. S., Schoeni, R. F., Kaplan, G. A., & Pollack, H. (2008). The health effects of social and economic policy: The promise and challenge for research and policy. In R. F. Schoeni, J. S. House, G. A. Kaplan, & H. Pollack (Eds.), *Making Americans healthier: Social and economic policy as health policy* (pp. 3–26). Russell Sage Foundation.

Hsieh, E. (2016). *Bilingual health communication: Working with interpreters in cross-cultural care.* Routledge.

Hsieh, E., & Kramer, E. (2019). Work as health: Tensions of imposing work requirements to Medicaid patients in the United States. In S. L. Arxer & J. W. Murphy (Eds.), Community-based health interventions in an institutional context (pp. 139–157). Springer.

Hsieh, E., & Kramer, E. M. (2012). Medical interpreters as tools: Dangers and challenges in the utilitarian approach to interpreters' roles and functions. *Patient Education and Counseling, 89*(1), 158–162.

Hussain, W. (2018). The common good. In E. N. Zalta (Ed.), *Stanford encyclopedia of philosophy.* https://plato.stanford.edu/entries/common-good

Katz, M. B. (1996). *In the shadow of the poorhouse: A social history of welfare in America* (10th Anniversary ed.). Basic Books.

Keshner, A. (2020, May 26). *Two-thirds of laid-off workers may temporarily be receiving more money in unemployment benefits than they did from their jobs.* MarketWatch. https://www.marketwatch.com/story/a-staggering-number-of-laid-off-workers-are-receiving-more-money-from-unemployment-benefits-than-when-they-were-employed-2020-05-26

Kim, M.-S., & Leung, T. (2000). A multicultural view of conflict management styles: Review and critical synthesis. *Annals of the International Communication Association, 23*(1), 227–270.

King, M. L., Jr. (1968, March 14). *The other America.* Crosse Pointe Historical Society. https://www.gphistorical.org/mlk/mlkspeech

Kirmayer, L. J. (2012). Rethinking cultural competence. *Transcultural Psychiatry, 49*(2), 149–164.

Kramer, E. M. (1997). *Modern/postmodern: Off the beaten path of antimodernism.* Praeger.

Kramer, E. M. (2000). Cultural fusion and the defense of difference. In M. K. Asante & J. E. Min (Eds.), *Socio-cultural conflict between African and Korean Americans* (pp. 182–223). University Press of America.

Kramer, E. M. (2013). Dimensional accrual and dissociation: An introduction. In J. Grace & E. M. Kramer (Eds.), *Communication, comparative cultures, and civilizations* (Vol. 3, pp. 123–184). Hampton.

Kramer, E. M. (2019). Cultural fusion theory. In J. F. Nussbaum (Ed.), *Oxford research encyclopedia of communication*. Oxford University Press. https://doi.org/10.1093/acrefore/9780190228613.013.679

Kramer, E. M., & Hsieh, E. (2019). Gaze as embodied ethics: Homelessness, the Other, and humanity. In M. J. Dutta & D. B. Zapata (Eds.), *Communicating for social change* (pp. 33–62). Palgrave Macmillan.

Kramer, E. M., & Ikeda, R. (1998). Understanding different worlds: The theory of dimensional accrual/dissociation. *Journal of Intercultural Communication*, *1*(2), 37–51.

Langellier, K. M. (2009). Performing narrative medicine. *Journal of Applied Communication Research*, *37*(2), 151–158.

Lederach, J. P. (1997). *Building peace: Sustainable reconciliation in divided societies*. United States Institute of Peace Press.

Lévinas, E. (1978) *Existence and existents* (A. Lingis, Trans.). Duquesne University Press.

Liu, Y., & Kramer, E. (2019). Cultural value discrepancies, strategic positioning and integrated identity: American migrants' experiences of being the Other in mainland China. *Journal of International and Intercultural Communication*. Advance online publication. https://doi.org/10.1080/17513057.2019.1679226

Loprest, P., & Nightingale, D. (2018, July). *The nature of work and the social safety net*. Urban Institute. https://www.urban.org/sites/default/files/publication/98812/the_nature_of_work_adn_the_social_safety_net.pdf

Luhby, T. (2020, June 3). *US Black-White inequality in 6 stark charts*. https://www.cnn.com/2020/06/03/politics/black-white-us-financial-inequality/index.html

Luhby, T., Yurkevich, V., & Hickey, C. (2020, April 30). *In some reopening states, unemployment can pay more than lost jobs*. CNN. https://www.cnn.com/2020/04/30/politics/unemployment-benefits-higher-than-work-wages

Martin, E. (2019, Janurary 10). *The government shutdown spotlights a bigger issue: 78% of US workers live paycheck to paycheck*. CNBC. https://www.cnbc.com/2019/01/09/shutdown-highlights-that-4-in-5-us-workers-live-paycheck-to-paycheck.html

Miller, S., & Wherry, L. R. (2019). Four years later: Insurance coverage and access to care continue to diverge between ACA Medicaid expansion and non-expansion states. *AEA Papers and Proceedings*, *109*, 327–333.

Musumeci, M., Garfield, R., & Rudowitz, R. (2018, Janurary). *Medicaid and work requirements: New Guidance, state waiver details, and key issues* (Issue Brief). Kaiser Family Foundation. http://files.kff.org/attachment/Issue-Brief-Medicaid-and-Work-Requirements-New-Guidance-State-Waiver-Details-and-Key-Issues

Nadeau, C. A. (2020, March 3). *New living wage data for now available on the tool*. Massachusetts Institute of Technology. https://livingwage.mit.edu/articles/61-new-living-wage-data-for-now-available-on-the-tool

Nagata, D. K., Kim, J. H. J., & Wu, K. (2019). The Japanese American wartime incarceration: Examining the scope of racial trauma. *American Psychologist*, *74*(1), 36–48.

National Academies of Sciences, Engineering, and Medicine. (2019). *Reproducibility and replicability in science*. National Academies Press.

National Conference of State Legislatures. (2020, Janurary 3). *State with religious and philosophical exemptions from school immunization requirements*. https://www.ncsl.org/research/health/school-immunization-exemption-state-laws.aspx

National Federation of Independent Business v. Sebelius, 567 U.S. 519 (2012). https://www.oyez.org/cases/2011/11-393

Nord, E., Richardson, J., Street, A., Kuhse, H., & Singer, P. (1995). Maximizing health benefits vs egalitarianism: An Australian survey of health issues. *Social Science & Medicine, 41*(10), 1429–1437.

Olshansky, S. J., Antonucci, T., Berkman, L., Binstock, R. H., Boersch-Supan, A., Cacioppo, J. T., Carnes, B. A., Carstensen, L. L., Fried, L. P., Goldman, D. P., Jackson, J., Kohli, M., Rother, J., Zheng, Y., & Rowe, J. (2012). Differences In life expectancy due to race and educational differences are widening, and many may not catch up. *Health Affairs, 31*(8), 1803–1813.

Omi, M., & Winant, H. (2014). *Racial formation in the United States* (3rd ed.). Routledge.

Palin, S. (2009, August 7). *Statement on the current health care debate*. Facebook. https://www.facebook.com/notes/sarah-palin/statement-on-the-current-health-care-debate/113851103434

Passavant, P. A. (2015). I can't breathe: Heeding the call of justice. *Law, Culture and the Humanities, 11*(3), 330–339.

Patient Protection and Affordable Care Act, Pub. L. No. 111-148, 124 Stat. 119 (2010). https://www.govinfo.gov/content/pkg/PLAW-111publ148/pdf/PLAW-111publ148.pdf

Puhl, R. M., & Heuer, C. A. (2010). Obesity stigma: Important considerations for public health. *American Journal of Public Health, 100*(6), 1019–1028.

Rainey, R., & Mueller, E. (2020, May 20). *Trump opposed to extending $600 unemployment boost*. Politico. https://www.politico.com/newsletters/morning-shift/2020/05/20/trump-opposed-to-extending-600-unemployment-boost-787765

Rawls, J. (2001). *Justice as fairness: A restatement* (E. Kelly, Ed.; 2nd ed.). Harvard University Press.

Rawls, J. (2009). *A theory of justice* (Rev. ed.). Harvard University Press. (Original work published 1971)

Robbins, J. M., & Krueger, J. I. (2005). Social projection to ingroups and outgroups: A review and meta-analysis. *Personality and Social Psychology Review, 9*(1), 32–47.

Roemer, J. E. (1998). *Theories of distributive justice*. Harvard University Press.

Romano, A. (2019, December 30). *Why we can't stop fighting about cancel culture*. Vox. https://www.vox.com/culture/2019/12/30/20879720/what-is-cancel-culture-explained-history-debate

Rubio-Fernández, P., & Glucksberg, S. (2012). Reasoning about other people's beliefs: Bilinguals have an advantage. *Journal of Experimental Psychology: Learning, Memory, and Cognition, 38*(1), 211–217.

Rudowitz, R., Garfield, R., & Hinton, E. (2019, March). *10 things to know about Medicaid: Setting the facts straight* (Issue Brief). Kaiser Family Foundation. http://files.kff.org/attachment/Issue-Brief-10-Things-to-Know-about-Medicaid-Setting-the-Facts-Straight

Sabik, L. M., & Gandhi, S. O. (2016). Copayments and emergency department use among adult Medicaid enrollees. *Health Economics, 25*(5), 529–542.

Scheffler, R. M., & Paringer, L. (1980). A review of the economic evidence on prevention. *Medical Care, 18*(5), 473–484.

Schmidt, H., & Hoffman, A. K. (2018). The ethics of Medicaid's work requirements and other personal responsibility policies. *JAMA, 319*(22), 2265–2266.

Sears, J. M., Edmonds, A. T., & Coe, N. B. (2020). Coverage gaps and cost-shifting for work-related injury and illness: Who bears the financial burden? *Medical Care Research and Review, 77*(3), 223–235.

Singer, P. (2016). *Famine, affluence, and morality*. Oxford University Press. (Original work published 1972)

Sklansky, D. A. (1995). Cocaine, race, and equal protection. *Stanford Law Review, 47*(6), 1283–1322.

Smulowitz, P. B., O'Malley, J., Yang, X., & Landon, B. E. (2014). Increased use of the emergency department after health care reform in Massachusetts. *Annals of Emergency Medicine, 64*(2), 107–115, 115.e101-103. https://doi.org/10.1016/j.annemergmed.2014.02.011

Social Security Act of 1935, 74 P.L. 271, 49 Stat. 620 (1935). https://www.ssa.gov/history/35actinx.html

Social Security Act, 42 U.S.C. § 1396-1 (2020). https://www.law.cornell.edu/uscode/text/42/1396-1

Stagner, R. (1977). Egocentrism, ethnocentrism, and altrocentrism: Factors in individual and intergroup violence. *International Journal of Intercultural Relations, 1*(3), 9–29.

Stapleton, G., Schröder-Bäck, P., Laaser, U., Meershoek, A., & Popa, D. (2014). Global health ethics: An introduction to prominent theories and relevant topics. *Global Health Action, 7*(1), Article 23569. https://doi.org/10.3402/gha.v7.23569

Starmans, C., Sheskin, M., & Bloom, P. (2017, May 4). *The science of inequality: Why people prefer unequal societies.* The Guardian. https://www.theguardian.com/inequality/2017/may/04/science-inequality-why-people-prefer-unequal-societies

Svenaeus, F. (2013). *The hermeneutics of medicine and the phenomenology of health: Steps towards a philosophy of medical practice.* Springer.

Syal, A. (2020, July 1). *Wearing a mask has become politicized. Science says it shouldn't be.* NBC News. https://www.nbcnews.com/health/health-news/wearing-mask-has-become-politicized-science-says-it-shouldn-t-n1232604

Taubman, S. L., Allen, H. L., Wright, B. J., Baicker, K., & Finkelstein, A. N. (2014). Medicaid increases emergency-department use: Evidence from Oregon's Health Insurance Experiment. *Science, 343*(6168), 263–268.

Trooskin, S. B., Reynolds, H., & Kostman, J. R. (2015). Access to costly new hepatitis C drugs: Medicine, money, and advocacy. *Clinical Infectious Diseases, 61*(12), 1825–1830.

Uhlmann, E. L., & Nosek, B. A. (2012). My culture made me do it. *Social Psychology, 43*(2), 108–113.

USDA Office of Inspector General. (2016, September). *FNS Controls over SNAP benefits for able-bodied adults without dependents.* https://www.usda.gov/oig/audit-reports/fns-controls-over-snap-benefits-able-bodied-adults-without-dependents

van Inwagen, P. (1983). *An essay on free will.* Oxford University Press.

Viruell-Fuentes, E. A., Miranda, P. Y., & Abdulrahim, S. (2012). More than culture: Structural racism, intersectionality theory, and immigrant health. *Social Science & Medicine, 75*(12), 2099–2106.

Vorauer, J. D., & Sucharyna, T. A. (2013). Potential negative effects of perspective-taking efforts in the context of close relationships: Increased bias and reduced satisfaction. *Journal of Personality and Social Psychology, 104*(1), 70–86.

Warner, K. E. (1987). Selling health promotion to corporate America: Uses and abuses of the economic argument. *Health Education Quarterly, 14*(1), 39–55.

Wenar, L. (2017). John Rawls. In E. N. Zalta (Ed.), *Stanford encyclopedia of philosophy.* https://plato.stanford.edu/archives/spr2017/entries/rawls

White House (2020, April 28). *Executive order on delegating authority under the DPA with respect to food supply chain resources during the national emergency caused by the outbreak of COVID-19.* https://www.whitehouse.gov/presidential-actions/

executive-order-delegating-authority-dpa-respect-food-supply-chain-resources-national-emergency-caused-outbreak-covid-19

Wiecek, W. M. (2011). Structural racism and the law in America today: An introduction. *Kentucky Law Journal, 100*(1), Article 2. https://uknowledge.uky.edu/klj/vol100/iss1/2/

Williams, D. R. (2016, November). *How racism makes us sick*. TED. https://www.ted.com/talks/david_r_williams_how_racism_makes_us_sick

Williams, D. R., Lawrence, J. A., & Davis, B. A. (2019). Racism and health: Evidence and needed research. *Annual Review of Public Health, 40*(1), 105–125.

Witters, D. (2020, April 28). *In U.S., 14% with likely COVID-19 to avoid care due to cost*. Gallup. https://news.gallup.com/poll/309224/avoid-care-likely-covid-due-cost.aspx

The World Bank. (2019, March 28). *Safety nets*. https://www.worldbank.org/en/topic/safetynets

Xu, T., Klein, E. Y., Zhou, M., Lowenthal, J., Sharfstein, J. M., & Peterson, S. M. (2018). Emergency department utilization among the uninsured during insurance expansion in Maryland. *Annals of Emergency Medicine, 72*(2), 156–165.

Zarefsky, D., Miller-Tutzauer, C., & Tutzauer, F. E. (1984). Reagan's safety net for the truly needy: The rhetorical uses of definition. *Central States Speech Journal, 35*(2), 113–119.

Index

Rethinking Culture in Health Communication: Social Interactions as Intercultural Encounters,
First Edition. Elaine Hsieh and Eric M Kramer.
© 2021 John Wiley & Sons, Ltd. Published 2021 by John Wiley & Sons, Ltd.

i

j

Printed and bound by CPI Group (UK) Ltd, Croydon, CR0 4YY

09/06/2025

14685921-0004